Pulmonary Rehabilitation
Guidelines to Success
Second Edition

Edited by

John E. Hodgkin, M.D.

Medical Director, Center for Health Promotion
Medical Director, Respiratory Care
  & Pulmonary Rehabilitation
St. Helena Hospital
Deer Park, California
Clinical Professor of Medicine
University of California, Davis

Gerilynn L. Connors, R.C.P., R.R.T., B.S.

Co-director, Pulmonary Rehabilitation
St. Helena Hospital
Deer Park, California

C. William Bell, Ph.D., M.B.A.

Administrative/Technical Director
Colorado Lung Center
Denver, Colorado

With 50 contributors

J.B. Lippincott Company   Philadelphia

Acquisitions Editor: Charles McCormick, Jr.
Sponsoring Editor: Wendy Greenberger
Project Editor: Mary Kinsella
Indexer: Victoria Boyle
Design Coordinator: Christopher Laird
Interior Designer: William Boehm
Cover Designer: Larry Pezzato
Production Manager: Helen Ewan
Production Coordinator: Maura C. Murphy
Compositor: Bi-Comp, Incorporated
Printer/Binder: RR Donnelly & Sons Company

Second Edition

6 5 4 3 2

Library of Congress Cataloging-in-Publication Data

Pulmonary rehabilitation: guidelines to success/edited by John E.
   Hodgkin, Gerilynn L. Connors, C. William Bell.—2nd ed.
        p.   cm.
   Includes bibliographical references and index.
   ISBN 0-397-51065-9
      1. Lungs—Diseases, Obstructive—Patients—Rehabilitation.
   2. Lungs—Diseases—Patients—Rehabilitation.   I. Hodgkin, John E.
   (John Elliott), 1939–   . II. Connors, Gerilynn Long.   III. Bell,
   C. William.
      [DNLM: 1. Lung Diseases, Obstructive—rehabilitation.   WF 600
   P9866]
   RC776.03P85   1993
   616.2'406—dc20
   DNLM/DLC
   for Library of Congress   92-15490
                                                                 CIP

The authors and publisher have exerted every effort to ensure that drug selection and dosage set forth
in this text are in accord with current recommendations and practice at the time of publication. However, in view of ongoing research, changes in government regulations, and the constant flow of information relating to drug therapy and drug reactions, the reader is urged to check the package insert for
each drug for any change in indications and dosage and for added warnings and precautions. This is
particularly important when the recommended agent is a new or infrequently employed drug.

We would like to dedicate this book to all those health care professionals who, by participating in pulmonary rehabilitation teams, have enhanced the quality of life for patients and their loved ones.

Contributors

Vito A. Angelillo, M.D.
Associate Professor of Medicine
    and Anesthesiology
Creighton University School of Medicine
Omaha, Nebraska
Associate Medical Director
St. Joseph Hospital
Omaha, Nebraska

C. William Bell, Ph.D., M.B.A.
Administrative/Technical Director
Colorado Lung Center
Denver, Colorado

Dale Robert Bergren, Ph.D.
Associate Professor of Physiology
Creighton University School of Medicine
Omaha, Nebraska

**Laura J. Reisman Beytas, B.S.P.H.,
R.R.T.**
Assistant Director, Pulmonary
    Rehabilitation Program
Duke University Medical Center
Durham, North Carolina

Mary Burns, R.N., B.S.
Assistant Clinical Professor
School of Nursing
University of California, Los Angeles
Supervisor, Pulmonary Rehabilitation
Little Company of Mary Hospital
Torrance, California

George G. Burton, M.D.
Medical Director, Respiratory Care
Kettering Medical Center
Kettering, Ohio
Clinical Professor of Medicine and
    Anesthesiology
Wright State University School of
    Medicine
Dayton, Ohio

Bartolome R. Celli, M.D.
Associate Professor of Medicine
Boston University School of Medicine
Boston, Massachusetts
Chief, Pulmonary Medicine and Critical
    Care
Department of Veterans Affairs
    Medical Center
Boston, Massachusetts

Catherine M. E. Certo, Sc.D., P.T.
Associate Professor and Chairman
Department of Physical Therapy
Sargent College of Allied Health
    Professions
Boston University
Boston, Massachusetts

**Gerilynn Long Connors, R.C.P.,
R.R.T., B.S.**
Co-director, Pulmonary Rehabilitation
    Program
St. Helena Hospital
Deer Park, California

Cele Darr, R.C.P., C.R.T.T.
Clinical and Marketing Liaison
Med-A-Rents
Healthcare Equipment and Supplies
Napa, California

David Daughton, M.S.
Behavioral Researcher
University of Nebraska Medical Center
Omaha, Nebraska

Patrick J. Dunne, M.Ed., R.R.T.
Managing General Partner
Southwest Medical Homecare Ltd.
Fullerton, California

Charles F. Emery, Ph.D.
Assistant Professor of Medical Psychology
Department of Psychiatry
Associate Director, Behavioral Medicine
    Program
Center for Living
Duke University Medical Center
Durham, North Carolina

A. James Fix, Ph.D.
Clinical Psychologist
Omaha, Nebraska

Mary E. Gilmartin, B.S.N., R.R.T.
Pulmonary Clinical Nurse Specialist
National Jewish Center for Immunology
    and Respiratory Medicine
Denver, Colorado

Lee W. Greenspon, M.D.
Clinical Associate Professor
The Medical College of Pennsylvania
Director of Critical Care
The Lankenau Hospital
Wynnewood, Pennsylvania

Sharon Grindal, R.R.T.
Pulmonary Rehabilitation Coordinator
Schumpert Medical Center
Shreveport, Louisiana

Karen L. Hill, Ph.D.
Assistant Professor
Department of Exercise and Sport Science
Pennsylvania State University
Delaware County Campus
Media, Pennsylvania

Lana R. Hilling, C.R.T.T., R.C.P.
Pulmonary Rehabilitation Coordinator
Mt. Diablo Medical Center
Concord, California

John E. Hodgkin, M.D.
Medical Director
Center for Health Promotion
Medical Director
Respiratory Care and Pulmonary
    Rehabilitation
St. Helena Hospital
Deer Park, California
Clinical Professor of Medicine
University of California, Davis, School of
    Medicine
Davis, California

Joyce W. Hopp, Ph.D., M.P.H.
Dean, School of Allied Health Professions
Loma Linda University
Loma Linda, California

Deborah Horne, P.T., M.B.A.
Director, Rehabilitation Services
National Jewish Center for Immunology
    and Respiratory Medicine
Denver, Colorado

John W. Jenne, M.D.
Professor of Medicine
Loyola University of Chicago
    Stritch School of Medicine
Maywood, Illinois
Medical Director, Respiratory Therapy
Edward Hines Jr. Veterans Administration
    Hospital
Maywood, Illinois

Robert M. Kacmarek, Ph.D., R.R.T.
Assistant Professor
Department of Anesthesiology
Harvard Medical School
Boston, Massachusetts
Director, Respiratory Care Services
Massachusetts General Hospital
Boston, Massachusetts

Richard E. Kanner, M.D.
Professor of Medicine
University of Utah College of Medicine
Salt Lake City, Utah
Medical Director
Pulmonary Function Laboratory
University Hospital
Salt Lake City, Utah

Robert M. Kaplan, Ph.D.
Professor, Community and Family
    Medicine
Chief, Division of Health Care Sciences
University of California, San Diego, School
    of Medicine
La Jolla, California

Lucy L. Kishbaugh, C.T.R.S., B.S.
Senior Pulmonary Outpatient Recreation
    Therapist
National Jewish Center for Immunology
    and Respiratory Medicine
Denver, Colorado

Howard M. Kravetz, M.D.
Medical Director, Respiratory Care
    Department
Yavapai Regional Medical Center
Prescott, Arizona

Donald A. Mahler, M.D.
Associate Professor of Medicine
Dartmouth Medical School
Hanover, New Hampshire
Chief, Section of Pulmonary and Critical
    Care Medicine
Dartmouth-Hitchcock Medical Center
Lebanon, New Hampshire

Barry J. Make, M.D.
Associate Professor of Medicine
Pulmonary Section
University of Colorado School of
    Medicine
Director, Pulmonary Rehabilitation
National Jewish Center for Immunology
    and Respiratory Medicine
Denver, Colorado

Susan L. McInturff, R.C.P., R.R.T.
Clinical Director
Bay Area Home Health Care
Novato, California

William F. Miller, M.D.
Professor of Internal Medicine
Pulmonary Division
University of Texas Southwestern Medical
    Center
Dallas, Texas

Kathleen V. Morris, R.N., M.S., R.R.T.
Co-director, Pulmonary Rehabilitation
   Program
St. Helena Hospital
Deer Park, California

Christine M. Neish, Ph.D., M.P.H.
Chairman, Department of Health
   Promotion and Education
School of Public Health
Loma Linda University
Loma Linda, California

Walter J. O'Donohue, Jr., M.D.
Professor and Chairman of Medicine
Creighton University School of Medicine
Omaha, Nebraska
Chairman, Department of Medicine
Creighton University Medical Center
Omaha, Nebraska

David M. Orenstein, M.D.
Associate Professor of Pediatrics
   and of Instruction and Learning
Exercise Physiology
University of Pittsburgh Schools of
   Medicine and Education
Pittsburgh, Pennsylvania
Director, Cystic Fibrosis/Pulmonology
   Department
Children's Hospital of Pittsburgh
Pittsburgh, Pennsylvania

James A. Peters, M.D., Dr.P.H., R.R.T., R.D.
Associate Professor, School of Public
   Health, School of Medicine, School of
   Allied Health
Department of Preventive Medicine
Loma Linda University
Loma Linda, California

Thomas L. Petty, M.D.
Professor of Medicine, University of
   Colorado Health Sciences Center
Denver, Colorado
Director, Academic and Research Affairs
Presbyterian-St Luke's Center
   for Health Sciences Education
Denver, Colorado

Nan Pheatt, M.T., M.P.H.
Elverta, California

Judith L. Radovich, B.A.
Pulmonary Rehabilitation Coordinator
Sutter General Hospital
Sacramento, California

Andrew L. Ries, M.D., M.P.H.
Associate Professor of Medicine
University of California, San Diego, School
   of Medicine
La Jolla, California
Director, Pulmonary Rehabilitation
   Program
University of California Medical Center
San Diego, California

Kevin P. Ryan, R.R.T., C.P.F.T.
Coordinator, Pulmonary Rehabilitation
Lower Bucks Hospital
Bristol, Pennsylvania

Miriam Scanlan, O.T.R., B.S.
Senior Occupational Therapist
National Jewish Center for Immunology
   and Respiratory Medicine
Denver, Colorado

Sharon Shnell-Hobbs, R.N., M.S.N.
Service Unit Manager, Internal Medicine
Kaiser Permanente
Santa Rosa, California

William A. Syvertsen, M.S., R.R.T.
Instructor, Business Division
Fresno City College
Fresno, California

Brian L. Tiep, M.D.
Director, Pulmonary Rehabilitation
Casa Colina Hospital for Rehabilitative
   Medicine
Pomona, California

Carlos A. VazFragoso, M.D.
Director, Pulmonary Function Laboratory
Pulmonary Medicine Division
Danbury Hospital
Danbury, Connecticut

Philip C. Weiser, Ph.D.
Research Associate Professor of Medicine
The Medical College of Pennsylvania
Philadelphia, Pennsylvania
Health Science Specialist, Pulmonary and
   Critical Care Section, Medical Service
Veterans Affairs Medical Center
Philadelphia, Pennsylvania

William K. Wilkison, B.A., R.R.T.
Executive Director, Mechanicsburg Rehab
   System
Mechanicsburg, Pennsylvania

**Patty Wooten, R.N., B.S.N.,
C.C.R.N.**
Director, Jest for the Health of It
Davis, California

Alan Russell Yee, M.D.
Director, Pulmonary Rehabilitation
Sutter General Hospital
Sacramento, California

Preface

The approach to caring for patients with chronic lung disease has evolved through the years from an attempt to improve their level of comfort with simple medications to the science of pulmonary rehabilitation. In 1942 the Council on Rehabilitation defined rehabilitation as "the restoration of the individual to the fullest medical, mental, emotional, social, and vocational potential of which he or she is capable." The principles of rehabilitation have been used widely for decades for individuals with neurologic and musculoskeletal disorders. Recently some patients with cardiovascular or pulmonary impairment have been offered the advantages of rehabilitation.

In 1984 the first edition of this book was published by Butterworths. In that edition the importance of using a team of health care professionals to improve the quality of care of patients with lung disease was emphasized. Support has continued to grow for the concepts presented in the first edition of this book. It is time to update our knowledge of this process for enhancing the ability to function of individuals with chronic lung disease.

In 1989 11.6 million people in the United States reported that they had asthma, 12 million reported that they had chronic bronchitis, and 2 million reported that they had emphysema. While individuals with a variety of pulmonary disorders can benefit from pulmonary rehabilitation, most patients participating in these programs have chronic obstructive pulmonary disease (COPD). The term COPD is best reserved for those individuals with chronic bronchitis or emphysema who have obstruction to airflow on a spirogram. Patients with COPD may also have a component of bronchial asthma.

COPD is a major source of morbidity and is the fifth leading cause of death in the United States. Between 1969 and 1989 there was a 54% increase in the age-adjusted death rate for COPD, compared to a 49% decrease for coronary artery disease.

The cost of health care in 1991 in the US was estimated to be approximately 740 billion dollars. In 1988 the estimated expenditure for COPD, including direct expenses and costs related to morbidity and mortality, was 13.2 billion dollars. This does not take into account the cost in terms of human suffering. Pulmonary rehabilitation can not only result in many benefits to patients and their families, but also can provide significant economic benefits (e.g., reducing the need for hospitalization).

This second edition of *Pulmonary Rehabilitation: Guidelines to Success* presents information which is crucial to those delivering pulmonary rehabilitation, including new knowledge which has become available since the first edition was published: the latest concepts regarding smoking cessation, pharmacologic therapy, aerosol therapy, oxygen therapy, nutrition support, and exercise training; the newest technology for providing out-of-hospital ventilator assistance; current concepts about marketing the program; and important advice regarding reimbursement. All the chapters from the first edition have been revised, and new chapters have been added, dealing with the history of pulmonary rehabilitation, biofeedback, respiratory muscle training, laughter as therapy, respiratory physiology, rehabilitation of the pediatric patient, and dyspnea.

One of the great challenges of the future is to acquaint primary care providers and third-party payors with the benefits of pulmonary rehabilitation, so more individuals with pulmonary impairment and their families can take advantage of these programs. All patients with COPD should be considered as candidates for pulmonary rehabilitation.

We would like to thank all of those individuals who shared their knowledge with us by contributing chapters. We also want to express our gratitude to Carol Lewis and Debra Duckett who assisted with the clerical challenges of multiple drafts of chapters, and to Wendy Greenberger of J.B. Lippincott Company who assisted with the production of this book.

John E. Hodgkin, M.D.
Gerilynn L. Connors, R.C.P., R.R.T., B.S
C. William Bell, Ph.D.

From the Preface
to the First Edition

One of the handicaps of patients with chronic disease is the fact that many health care professionals prefer to take care of patients who get well quickly. The field of rehabilitation developed as an attempt to deal with those individuals who have disorders resulting in long-term impairment or disability. Rehabilitation specialists first focused on patients with musculoskeletal or neurologic ailments, with the goal being to restore them to the highest level of functioning possible. Subsequently, those with cardiac or pulmonary disorders were also considered as candidates for the rehabilitation process.

There is no better area than pulmonary rehabilitation to demonstrate the value of team care. Patients with respiratory disorders can benefit from the talents of many health care disciplines in both the assessment of the individual and the development of a treatment plan.

It was this recognition of the importance of multiple disciplines in evaluating and caring for patients with pulmonary disease that led us to develop this book. The chapters in this book deal with the many disciplines that constitute good comprehensive respiratory care, i.e., pulmonary rehabilitation for patients with lung disorders. We recognize that every hospital or outpatient rehabilitation facility may not have a health professional trained to deal with pulmonary patients from each of the disciplines covered in this book. This problem, however, can often be alleviated by one health professional providing the services from more than one discipline.

The major goal of this book is to help physicians and allied health professionals as they attempt to outline a care program for patients with chronic lung disease. We feel that the material presented throughout the book can help health professionals develop pulmonary rehabilitation teams that will result in improved care for their patients. If the quality of care for these patients is enhanced by the efforts of the many authors in this book, we will be gratified that the long hours spent in compiling the book will have been well worthwhile.

We would like to acknowledge the inspiration that Thomas L. Petty has been to us, as well as to countless others who have taken care of patients with respiratory disorders. We feel honored that Dr. Petty was willing to write the Foreword for this book.

The many authors who contributed their time and expertise to the content of the book deserve a special note of thanks. We also want to express our gratitude to Carol Lewis and Donna Littlefield who assisted with the clerical challenges of typing multiple drafts of chapters, and to Kathleen Benn and Julie Stillman of Butterworths who assisted with the copyediting and structuring of the book. Without their contributions, there would be no book.

Contents

Pulmonary Rehabilitation

JOHN E. HODGKIN

Pulmonary Rehabilitation: Definition and Essential Components

Although rehabilitation has been practiced for several decades, its application to patients with pulmonary disorders is relatively recent. In 1942, the Council on Rehabilitation defined *rehabilitation* as the restoration of the individual to the fullest medical, mental, emotional, social, and vocational potential of which he or she is capable.

This process has found widespread acceptance throughout the medical profession for patients with musculoskeletal and neuromuscular disorders. Even rehabilitation programs for cardiac patients have become common. In spite of initial reports[1-7] suggesting that pulmonary rehabilitation programs result in benefits for patients with chronic obstructive pulmonary disease (COPD), it is only within the last decade that such programs have become common.

In the mid-1970s, a study by the Human Interaction Research Institute (HIRI) in Los Angeles, California, showed that many physicians in the United States were either not aware of or were not using various facets of care for patients with pulmonary disease that had been shown previously to be useful.[8] As part of this HIRI project, which was funded by the National Science Foundation, a state-of-the-art paper on the diagnosis and treatment of COPD was developed and published in the *Journal of the American Medical Association* in 1975.[9] Hundreds of physicians and allied health personnel around the country were invited to critique this paper, following which the article was modified, expanded, and published in 1979 as a book by the American College of Chest Physicians.[10] It was the goal of those involved in this project to disseminate widely to physicians and allied health professionals those principles of care that had been demonstrated to produce both subjective and objective benefits in respiratory patients. Although this goal, in large part, has been realized, there are still many primary care physicians who seem unaware of the benefits of pulmonary rehabilitation.

The term *chronic obstructive pulmonary disease* (COPD) is best reserved for those individuals with chronic bronchitis or emphysema who have indicated obstruction to airflow on a spirogram. Bronchial asthma should be considered as a separate

1

disorder, rather than being included under the term COPD; however, it should be recognized that those with COPD may also have a component of asthma. In 1989 in the United States, 11.6 million persons reported that they had asthma, 12 million reported chronic bronchitis, and 2 million reported emphysema.[11] An individual might have reported having more than one of these conditions. In comparison, 18.5 million persons reported the presence of heart disease. Since 1980, age-adjusted prevalence rates for COPD among men have been stable, with what recently appears to be a downward trend. However, in women the prevalence of COPD between 1979 and 1985 increased by 35%.[12] The prevalence of asthma is also increasing.[11]

TABLE 1-1.   Estimated Deaths, Death Rates, and Percentage of Total Deaths for the 15 Leading Causes of Death: United States, 1990*

Rank	Cause of death (Ninth Revision, International Classification of Diseases, 1975)	Number	Death rate	Total deaths (%)
	All causes	2,162,000	861.9	100.0
1	Diseases of heart	725,010	289.0	33.5
2	Malignant neoplasms, including neoplasms of lymphatic and hematopoietic tissues	506,000	201.7	23.4
3	Cerebrovascular diseases	145,340	57.9	6.7
4	Accidents and adverse effects	93,550	37.3	4.3
	Motor vehicle accidents	47,880	19.1	2.2
	All other accidents and adverse effects	45,680	18.2	2.1
5	Chronic obstructive pulmonary diseases and allied conditions	88,980	35.5	4.1
6	Pneumonia and influenza	78,640	31.3	3.6
7	Diabetes mellitus	48,840	19.5	2.3
8	Suicide	30,780	12.3	1.4
9	Homicide and legal intervention	25,700	10.2	1.2
10	Chronic liver disease and cirrhosis	25,600	10.2	1.2
11	Human immunodeficiency virus infection	24,120	9.6	1.1
12	Nephritis, nephrotic syndrome, and nephrosis	20,860	8.3	1.0
13	Septicemia	19,750	7.9	0.9
14	Certain conditions originating in the perinatal period	17,520	7.0	0.8
15	Atherosclerosis	16,490	6.6	0.8
	All other causes	295,100	117.6	13.6

* Data are provisional, estimated from a 10% sample of deaths. Rates per 100,000 population. Figures may differ from those previously published. Due to rounding, figures may not add to totals.
(Centers for Disease Control. Monthly vital statistics report, National Center for Health Statistics. Bethesda, MD: USDHHS, Public Health Service, Aug 28, 1991, with permission)

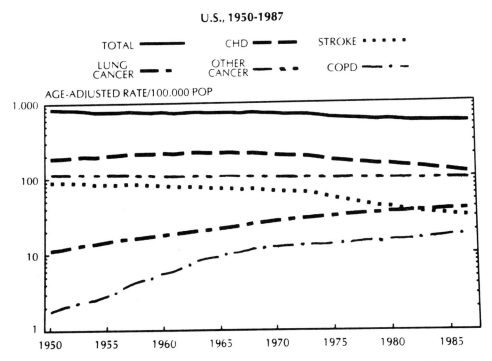

FIGURE 1-1 Death rates for selected causes. (National Heart, Lung, and Blood Institute. Morbidity and mortality chartbook on cardiovascular, lung, and blood diseases, 1990. Bethesda, MD: USDHHS, Public Health Services, National Institutes of Health, Feb 1991, with permission)

Chronic obstructive pulmonary disease and allied conditions have been the fifth leading cause of death in the United States since the late 1970s[13] (Table 1–1). Among the major causes of death from 1950 to 1987, only lung cancer and COPD mortality increased (Fig. 1–1).[14] Between 1969 and 1989, there was a 54% increase in the age-adjusted death rate for COPD in the United States, compared with a 49% decrease for coronary artery disease.[15] The death rate for asthma in the United States had been decreasing, but began increasing again in the late 1970s.[14] In 1985, COPD was considered to be the direct cause of death in 3.6% of all deaths in the United States and was a contributing factor in an additional 4.3% of deaths, with the sum of the two adding up to 164,650 deaths that year.[12] In 1987, COPD and allied conditions were considered to be the direct cause of death for 78,000 individuals in the United States, with the breakdown as follows: 70.2% due "to chronic airways disease," 18.5% to emphysema, 5.6% to asthma, 4.6% to chronic bronchitis, and 1.2% to bronchiectasis and extrinsic allergic alveolitis.[13] In 1989, COPD was estimated to be the direct cause of death for 79,000 people, with other airway diseases (including asthma) being listed as the direct cause of death for an additional 6000 individuals.[15] This compares with an estimated 498,000 deaths from coronary heart disease in 1989.[15] In 1990, COPD and allied conditions were considered to be the direct cause of death for 88,980 persons in the United States.[13] From 1979 to 1985, death from COPD increased by 16% in men (from 169 to 196 deaths per 100,000 population) and increased by 73% in women (from 47 to 81 per 100,000 population).[12] Mortality data for COPD in other countries worldwide show trends similar to those in the United States. The proportional mortality for COPD varies from less than 1% to 10% of all deaths in countries in the world.[16]

Morbidity related to COPD and asthma is considerable. In 1985, COPD was mentioned as the reason for 11,271,000 office visits to physicians in the United States (over 5% of the total), and asthma was listed as the reason for 6,503,000 office visits.[14] In 1985 in the United States, COPD was mentioned as a reason (not necessarily the first discharge diagnosis) for 1,939,906 hospitalizations (over 13% of the total).[12] In 1987, COPD was listed as the first discharge diagnosis for 357,000 hospitalizations, and asthma was listed as the first discharge diagnosis for 454,000 hospitalizations.[14] The estimated number of office visits to physicians in 1989 was 6,822,000 for asthma and 16,110,000 for COPD; asthma was the first-listed diagnosis for 475,000 hospitalizations, and COPD was the first-listed diagnosis for 229,000 hospitalizations in 1989 (The National Heart, Lung, and Blood Institute, unpublished data, 1991). From 1970 to the early 1980s, there was an upward trend in hospitalization for COPD, after which a steep decline began. However, hospitalization for asthma is still increasing.[14] Although age-adjusted rates of hospital discharges for COPD have been decreasing for men since 1981 and for women since 1983, and the duration of hospital stay for COPD has been declining in recent years, office visits for this disorder, for both men and women, have continued to increase.[12]

Between 1986 and 1988, of chronic conditions reported to cause a limitation of activity, heart disease was responsible in 4.8 million individuals, asthma in 1.9 million individuals, and emphysema in 0.9 million individuals. In the United States, COPD is second only to coronary heart disease in the number of patients receiving social security disability payments for their disease process. The patients with COPD, when compared with the general population, are more likely to rate their health as poor, to report limitations of usual activities, to visit physicians, to stay in hospitals, and to report bed disability days.[12]

The cost for health care in the United States is enormous. In 1990, Americans spent 666.2 billion dollars on health care, which was 10.5% more than in 1989 and more than twice the 5.1% growth rate of the gross national product. The cost of health care in 1991 was estimated to be about 740 billion dollars, representing 13.1% of the gross national product. By the year 2000, it has been estimated that spending for health care in the United States will reach 1.5 trillion dollars, an increase of 550% from 1980. The United States spends 40% more on health care than Canada, 90% more than the former West German republic, and more than twice as much as Japan.

The economic impact of obstructive airway disorders is substantial. In 1972, for asthma patients, the direct cost for physicians' services, hospital care, and medications was estimated to be 850 million dollars; costs associated with morbidity, 440 million dollars; and the cost of mortality in terms of lost productivity was estimated at 120 million dollars.[17] The cost for the care of patients with COPD (chronic bronchitis and emphysema) in 1977 in the United States was estimated at 1.0 billion dollars for direct costs, 3.8 billion dollars for morbidity, and 900 million dollars for costs from mortality.[17] By 1988, the estimated costs for asthma were 4.6 billion dollars for direct costs of treatment; 1.6 billion dollars for costs from morbidity; and

0.7 billion dollars for costs from mortality; totaling 6.9 billion dollars (The National Heart, Lung, and Blood Institute, unpublished data, 1991). In 1988, the estimated expenditure for COPD for the direct costs of treatment was 5.8 billion dollars; for costs from morbidity, 3.8 billion dollars; and for costs from mortality, 3.6 billion dollars; totaling 13.2 billion dollars (The National Heart, Lung, and Blood Institute, unpublished data, 1991). These estimates do not take into account the costs in terms of human suffering. As will be described in Chapter 31, pulmonary rehabilitation can result not only in direct benefit to patients and their families, but can provide significant economic benefits (e.g., reducing the need for hospitalization).

Most patients with COPD developed the problem as a direct result of smoking cigarettes. Although progress has been made in reducing the number of persons who smoke in the United States, efforts to help individuals avoid or cease smoking must be intensified. In the United States in 1988, tobacco companies spent 3.3 billion dollars on the advertising and promotion of cigarettes.[18] In 1965, 40% of adults in the United States smoked cigarettes. By 1987, only 29% were smoking. The decline began in the late 1960s for men and a decade later for women, whose rate of decrease has been much more gradual.[19] The percentage of men who smoked cigarettes decreased from 50.2 in 1965 to 31.7 in 1987. In women, smoking decreased from 31.9% in 1965 to 26.8% in 1987.[19] In spite of this decline in smoking in this country, it is estimated that more than 400,000 Americans died in 1988 as a result of smoking cigarettes.[20] Although only about 15% of smokers develop disabling airflow obstruction,[21] the impact for those who do, in terms of morbidity, mortality, and cost, is enormous.

The different trends in prevalence and death rates between men and women for COPD are thought to be consistent with changes in cigarette smoking among these groups. The increase in mortality from COPD for women lags behind that in men by about 15 years, as a result of the later acceptance and onset of cigarette smoking among women. Also, men are stopping smoking more rapidly than women. It is reasonable to assume that if the significant decrease in the number of people smoking persists, the increase in mortality from COPD will cease and, in fact, decline sometime during the next 25 years.

Since there are many facets of care, crossing disciplinary lines, that can be applied to pulmonary patients,[22] attempts have been made to clarify which aspects of care are useful and to define *pulmonary rehabilitation*. In 1974, a committee of the American College of Chest Physicians developed the following definition:[23]

> Pulmonary rehabilitation may be defined as an art of medical practice wherein an individually tailored, multidisciplinary program is formulated which through accurate diagnosis, therapy, emotional support, and education, stabilizes or reverses both the physio- and psychopathology of pulmonary diseases and attempts to return the patient to the highest possible functional capacity allowed by his pulmonary handicap and overall life situation.

In the late 1970s, pulmonary rehabilitation programs began to spring up around the country. Even though this seemed like progress, many pulmonary physicians became concerned that some of these so-called pulmonary rehabilitation programs were not providing good care for patients, but instead were business ventures intent on making money by selling and servicing respiratory therapy equipment. Because of this concern, as well as a growing recognition that the term *pulmonary rehabilitation* was defined differently by many pulmonary specialists, in 1979 an ad hoc committee of the Scientific Assembly on Clinical Problems of the American Thoracic Society was delegated the responsibility of defining pulmonary rehabilitation. This committee developed a statement that not only defined pulmonary rehabilitation but also listed the essential components of such a program. If a group is going to offer a "pulmonary rehabilitation program," it should be able to provide all the services described in this statement, which was published in 1981 as an official position statement of the American Thoracic Society.[24] Since this statement is still appropriate today, we are reprinting it by permission of the American Thoracic Society.

(*Text continues on p. 11*)

AMERICAN THORACIC SOCIETY POSITION STATEMENT ON PULMONARY REHABILITATION

Introduction

The purpose of this statement is to define pulmonary rehabilitation and to describe the essential elements of a pulmonary rehabilitation program. In order to provide comprehensive pulmonary rehabilitation services, a program should be able to carry out the described components of pulmonary rehabilitation and to provide the essential services required, as defined in this statement.

Definition of Pulmonary Rehabilitation

Rehabilitation was defined by the Council of Rehabilitation in 1942 as the restoration of the individual to the fullest medical, mental, emotional, social, and vocational potential of which he/she is capable. Instead of addressing solely the physical and mental aspects, rehabilitation should be tailored to maximize one's improvement and minimize the impact of an illness, or a state of progressive deterioration from optimal health, not only on the person, but also his/her family and community.

The American College of Chest Physicians' Committee on Pulmonary Rehabilitation adopted, at its annual meeting in 1974, the following definition:

> Pulmonary rehabilitation may be defined as an art of medical practice wherein an individually tailored, multidisciplinary program is formulated which through accurate diagnosis, therapy, emotional support, and education, stabilizes or reverses both the physio- and psychopathology of pulmonary diseases and attempts to return the patient to the highest possible functional capacity allowed by his pulmonary handicap and overall life situation.

The two principal objectives of pulmonary rehabilitation are to: (1) control and alleviate as much as possible the symptoms and pathophysiologic complications of respiratory impairment, and (2) teach the patient how to achieve optimal capability for carrying out his/her activities of daily living. Depending on the needs of the specific patient, comprehensive care may include the delivery of a structured, defined "rehabilitation program" as an element of the patient's care. However, in the broadest sense, pulmonary rehabilitation means providing good, comprehensive respiratory care for patients with pulmonary disease. A facility caring for such individuals should be capable of either providing or having access to a regional medical center that is able to offer such a comprehensive care program. The components of pulmonary rehabilitation described in this statement are most useful for patients with chronic obstructive pulmonary disease (COPD), e.g., emphysema, chronic bronchitis, and asthma. However, certain aspects may be selected for patients with other pulmonary disorders.

Sequence of Pulmonary Rehabilitation

A certain sequence should be followed when outlining an appropriate treatment plan. This process involves careful evaluation of the patient, developing a treatment program that best meets the patient's needs, proper assessment of the patient's progress, and a plan for patient follow-up. A logical sequence would proceed as follows:

A. Patient Selection

Any patient with symptomatic COPD should be considered for pulmonary rehabilitation. Those patients with either very mild or very severe disease will not generally be placed on as intensive and comprehensive a rehabilitation program as those with moderate to moderately-severe disease.

Multiple factors affect the ultimate success of rehabilitation for any individual. These include, in addition to severity of the disease, the presence of other disabling diseases such as cancer or arthritis, age, intelligence, level of education, occupation, family support, and personal motivation.

B. Evaluation

A careful assessment of the patient should be performed initially. This evaluation would include:

1. *Diagnostic Workup*

Proper identification of the patient's specific respiratory ailment is important because the treatment regimen prescribed should be geared to the patient's disease process. Essential diagnostic information would include: appropriate pulmonary function studies, a chest radiograph, an electrocardiogram, and, when indicated, arterial blood gas measurements at rest and during exercise, sputum analysis, and blood theophylline measurements.

2. *Behavioral Considerations*

The best rehabilitation results require personal commitment from the patient, determination, and persistence. Additionally, significant psychiatric symptoms of any sort profoundly disrupt compliance. For these reasons, the patient should receive emotional screening assessments and treatment or counseling when required.

Thorough understanding of the disease and its treatment is one of the more important factors in patient motivation, cooperation, and anxiety reduction. This is particularly true in pulmonary rehabilitation during which the patient must master a large amount of knowledge. Yet learning abilities among these patients are often subtly impaired. This can be remedied in two ways: (a) estimating the patient's learning skills and adjusting the program to the patient's ability, and (b) requiring the patient to demonstrate new knowledge and skills before progressing further.

The patient must be viewed in terms of the personal and environmental assets at his/her disposal. These include family and social support, potential employment skills, employment opportunities, and community resources. These all need to be evaluated and mobilized for practical help to the patient and to bolster his/her motivation.

(*Continues on p. 8*)

C. Determine Goals

It is crucial that short- and long-term goals be developed for each individual following the evaluation. The patient and his/her family need to help determine and fully understand these goals, so that they realistically approach the treatment phase.

D. Components of Pulmonary Rehabilitation

1. *Physical Therapy*

   Good bronchial hygiene, e.g., effective coughing, clapping, and bronchial drainage is particularly important to those patients who produce excess mucus within the airways. Pursed-lip breathing may help to slow the respiratory rate and lessen small airway collapse during periods of increased dyspnea. Relaxation techniques can be useful in anxious patients.

2. *Exercise Conditioning*

   A physical conditioning (exercise) program should be considered in any patient with exercise limitations. Selection of appropriate, safe exercise routines is enhanced by measuring workloads, gas exchange behavior, heart rate, and electrocardiogram. However, in selected patients, assessment of the functional work capacity may be possible with such techniques as determining the number of steps the individual can climb or the distance the patient can walk at a certain speed.

3. *Respiratory Therapy*

   Supplemental oxygen and aerosolization of medications such as bronchodilators and corticosteroids are useful for certain patients. In an attempt to limit the inappropriate and excess use of oxygen and respiratory therapy equipment in the home, the American Thoracic Society has developed statements regarding these treatment modalities.

4. *Education*

   If patient compliance is to be optimized, both the patient and his/her family need to understand the underlying pulmonary disorder. Those individuals outlining the treatment plan should instruct the patient and family about the purpose for medications, as well as their side effects. Proper nutrition, the use and cleaning of respiratory therapy equipment, techniques of physical therapy modalities, and details of an exercise conditioning program must all be carefully explained.

5. *General*

   The importance of smoking cessation must be emphasized. Attention should be paid to such environmental factors as temperature, humidity, inhaled irritants, and altitude. Although there is little objective data that adequate hydration liquefies airways secretions, it is agreed that dehydration should be prevented. Immunization with the influenza and pneumococcal vaccines is recommended. An appropriate use of such pharmacologic agents as β_2-agonists, methylxanthines, antimicrobials, and corticosteroids is important, and their indications must be understood by the primary care physician.

E. Assessment of Patient's Progress

While the treatment plan is being developed, the patient's progress should be monitored. This will help both the patient and the health care team objectively evaluate the plan outlined, so that any needed changes can be initiated.

F. Long-Term Follow-up

Ongoing care will generally be the responsibility of the primary care physician. Periodic reassessment can be beneficial to the patient, as a way of objectively evaluating progress and allowing for educational reinforcement.

Services Required for Pulmonary Rehabilitation

A variety of services are provided through a pulmonary rehabilitation program. Many patients with COPD will not need these services; however, they should be available for those patients with special needs or more severe disease.

A. Essential Services

1. *Initial Medical Evaluation and Care Plan*

   Perform a complete history and physical examination. Obtain appropriate laboratory tests. Make the correct diagnosis. Outline a proper therapy regimen for ongoing care.

2. *Patient Education, Evaluation, and Program Coordination*

   Educate patient regarding lung anatomy and physiology, disease process, useful therapeutic modalities, and other relevant matters. Coordinate allied health personnel involved in the patient's care. Make home visits, as necessary.

3. *Respiratory Therapy Techniques*

   Educate patient concerning proper use and cleaning of respiratory therapy equipment. Administer therapy as prescribed by attending physician. Make home visits as needed to ensure compliance.

4. *Physical Therapy Techniques, Including Exercise Conditioning*

   Educate patient regarding relaxation techniques, proper breathing, clapping, and bronchial drainage. Measure functional work capacity and develop an exercise conditioning program. Record physiologic changes resulting from exercise training.

5. *Daily Performance Evaluation*

   Evaluate activities of daily living. Teach energy conservation (work simplification) and self-care techniques.

6. *Social Service Evaluation*

   Obtain social history and determine patient's psychosocial assets and needs. Evaluate potential for compliance as well as actual compliance. Mobilize family or other interested individuals as part of extended support system to be used following discharge from the hospital. Evaluate third-party payer problems and help in resolving such problems. Assist in making arrangements for needed community resources, including financial aid, homemaker services, and extended care facilities.

7. *Nutritional Evaluation*

   Evaluate the patient's nutritional status. Outline dietary prescription based on the patient's specific nutritional needs.

B. Additional Services

1. *Psychological Evaluation*

   Administer psychometric battery that includes tests designed to measure organic brain dysfunction, IQ, personality profile, psychosocial assets, impact of illness on

(*Continues on p. 10*)

person, his/her family, etc. Help patient and family develop coping mechanisms to control not only chronic anxiety or depression but also acute exacerbations.

2. *Psychiatric Evaluation*

Categorize personality pattern. Make psychiatric diagnosis if one exists. Provide specific psychiatric support and/or therapy when needed. If necessary, make specific recommendations regarding optimal psychopharmacologic agents.

3. *Vocational Evaluation*

Assess vocational rehabilitation potential for those patients with significant impairment. Includes vocational tests, interviews, on-the-job observation, as well as determining whether the subject has the work capacity to meet the oxygen requirements of his/her job. Work output can generally be sustained for an eight-hour period if one does not exceed 30–40% of his/her attained maximum oxygen consumption.

A physician knowledgeable about respiratory diseases should perform the initial complete examination and assist in outlining a proper regimen of treatment.

The specific provider for the other services may vary from program to program. A multidisciplinary team that might include a professional nurse, respiratory therapist, physical therapist, occupational therapist, dietitian, social worker, and pulmonary or cardiopulmonary technologist is appropriate for those settings where large numbers of patients are referred and for teaching or research purposes. However, in other settings, it may be possible to provide similar services with fewer individuals if they are highly-qualified and specially-trained in evaluation and management of the patient with COPD. In selected patients, the evaluation and delivery of a comprehensive care program can be accomplished in an outpatient setting. Thus, the techniques of rehabilitation should be within the reach of all physicians, applying the principles expressed in this document.

Benefits and Limitations of Pulmonary Rehabilitation
A. Benefits

A comprehensive respiratory care program can result in definite benefits to the patient. There is overwhelming evidence that a comprehensive respiratory care program can result in an improved quality of life and a significantly improved capability for carrying out his/her daily activities.

Participation in a comprehensive pulmonary rehabilitation program has repeatedly been shown to decrease the hospital days required per patient per year. Some patients may be able to return to useful employment, thus making a contribution to the work force. Patients can achieve a significant reduction in anxiety, depression, and somatic concern, with an associated improvement in their own ego strength. Numerous studies have shown that the physical conditioning of patients with COPD can be substantially improved with a regular exercise training program.

Cessation of smoking can result in improved pulmonary function, reduction of cough, decreased sputum production, and lessened dyspnea. The course of COPD may be altered if the airway abnormality is detected early.

B. Limitations

Even though all of the above benefits have been documented, an extention of lifespan and slowing of pulmonary function deterioration have not been shown in the majority of published studies. Through the use of routine office spirometry, COPD can be detected at a much earlier stage when institution of a comprehensive respiratory care program may more effectively achieve an alteration in the patient's course.

A significant problem relates to the fact that only approximately 20–35% of the participants in smoking cessation programs quit permanently. More effort needs to be applied to the prevention of respiratory disease, rather than concentrating on treatment after significant disability has occurred.

Another major factor interfering with delivery of good care is the unevenness in our capacity to deliver community-based services. A visiting nurse association (or its equivalent) does not exist in every community, nor do socially-oriented service programs, such as Meals on Wheels, Homemakers, etc.

Which tests are required to appropriately determine impairment/disability needs to be more clearly determined. Ideally, patients should be adequately evaluated and treated comprehensively prior to a final disability determination.

Conclusion

In the 17th century, Jeremy Taylor said, "To preserve a man alive in the midst of so many diseases and hostilities, is as great a miracle as to create him." In the past, rehabilitation has been applied rather loosely to vaguely describe various approaches to long-term management of the chronically ill patient. The time has come for us to not only define what we mean by pulmonary rehabilitation, but to describe what we mean by services required. This comprehensive approach to patient evaluation will result in improved care for respiratory patients so that they may be restored to their most optimal potential.

This statement was prepared by an ad hoc committee of the Scientific Assembly on Clinical Problems. The committee members are as follows:

John E. Hodgkin, Chairman	Irving Kass
Michael J. Farrell	Lawrence M. Lampton
Suzanne R. Gibson	Margaret Nield
Richard E. Kanner	Thomas L. Petty

In 1987, the American Thoracic Society published a statement dealing with standards for the diagnosis and care of patients with COPD and asthma.[25] Many of the components of care used in pulmonary rehabilitation programs were discussed in this statement. Recent review articles have described the various components and benefits of pulmonary rehabilitation programs.[26]

Characteristics of pulmonary rehabilitation programs determined by a national survey in the United States were reported in 1988.[27] In 1987, the American Association for Respiratory Care and the American Association of Cardiovascular and Pulmonary Rehabilitation jointly conducted a survey to gain information regarding existing pulmonary rehabilitation programs. Responses were received from 150 programs in 37 states. The responses were divided equally across the United States (i.e., 47 from the western, 50 from the middle, and 53 from the eastern United States). There was a marked variation in the structure of the pulmonary rehabilitation programs responding to this survey. Programs met for anywhere between 1 and 8 hours per day, on 1 to 7 days per week, with the length of the program varying from 1 to 52 weeks. The average program enrolled six patients for approximately 2 hours/

day, 3 days/week, for 8 weeks, with the average program lasting approximately 48 hours. Most of the programs (97%) had outpatient rehabilitation programs, although 49% worked with inpatients as well. Only 3% of the programs worked with only inpatients. Directors of 52% of the programs held a respiratory therapy credential; 31% had a director with a nursing degree; and 8% had a director with both respiratory therapy and nursing credentials. The remaining program directors included exercise physiologists, physical therapists, occupational therapists, and cardiopulmonary technicians. The content of some of the programs was predominantly education provided in a group setting (e.g., getting a group together for a 1- or 2-hour lecture one evening a week for 6 weeks). Such a program (i.e., predominantly lectures in a group setting) may be of value to patients with pulmonary impairment and their families, but it does not meet the criteria for being a pulmonary rehabilitation program as described in the ATS Position Statement on Pulmonary Rehabilitation.[24]

SUMMARY

As the ATS Statement on Pulmonary Rehabilitation points out,[24] pulmonary rehabilitation programs may vary in size and configuration. All allied health professions may not be represented on every team in every hospital; however, all the services listed in the ATS statement must be available and provided by someone. Although every patient with COPD does not need all these services, many patients need them all.

Even though most of the patients participating in pulmonary rehabilitation programs have obstructive airway disease (COPD or asthma), these programs may also be very helpful for patients with other types of pulmonary dysfunction.[28,29] The definition and essential components of pulmonary rehabilitation are much more widely agreed upon and accepted now than in 1984, when the first edition of this book was published.[30] The remainder of this book is devoted to describing the components of pulmonary rehabilitation and providing guidelines that can lead to the successful rehabilitation of patients with pulmonary dysfunction.

REFERENCES

1. Barach AL. The treatment of pulmonary emphysema in the elderly. J Am Geriatr Soc 1956;4:884.

2. Miller WF. Rehabilitation of patients with chronic obstructive lung disease. Med Clin North Am 1967;51:349.

3. Balchum OJ. Rehabilitation in chronic obstructive pulmonary disease. Arch Environ Health 1968;16:614.

4. Haas A, Cardon H. Rehabilitation in chronic obstructive pulmonary disease: a five-year study of 252 male patients. Med Clin North Am 1969;53:593.

5. Cherniack RM, Handford RG, Svanhill E. Home care of chronic respiratory disease. JAMA 1969;208:821.

6. Petty TL. Ambulatory care for emphysema and chronic bronchitis. Chest 1970;58:441.

7. Kimbel P, Kaplan AS, Alkalay I, Lester D. An in-hospital program for rehabilitation of patients with chronic obstructive pulmonary disease. Chest 1971;60(suppl):6s.

8. Glaser EM. Strategies for facilitating knowledge utilization in the biomedical field. Final report to National Science Foundation, Grant No. DAR 73-07767 A06. Washington, DC: National Science Foundation, 1975.

9. Hodgkin JE, Balchum OJ, Kass I, et al. Chronic obstructive airway disease: current concepts in diagnosis and comprehensive care. JAMA 1975;232:1243.

10. Hodgkin JE, ed. Chronic obstructive pulmonary disease: current concepts in diagnosis and comprehensive care. Park Ridge, IL: American College of Chest Physicians, 1979.

11. Current estimates from the National Health Interview Survey, 1989. Hyattsville, MD: National Center for Health Statistics, U.S. Govt. Printing Office, 1990; DHHS publication no. (PHS) 90-1504. (Vital and health statistics: series 10, no. 176).

12. Feinleib M, Rosenberg HM, Collins JG, Delozier JE, Pokras R, Chevarley FM. Trends in COPD morbidity and mortality in the United States. Am Rev Respir Dis 1989;140:S9.

13. Centers for Disease Control. Monthly vital statistics report, National Center for Health Statistics. Bethesda, MD: U.S. Dept. of Health and Human Services, Public Health Service, Aug 28, 1991.

14. National Heart, Lung and Blood Institute. Morbidity and mortality chartbook on cardiovascular, lung and blood diseases/1990. Bethesda, MD: U.S. Dept. of Health and Human Services, Public Health Service, National Institutes of Health, Feb 1990.

15. National Heart, Lung, and Blood Institute fact book. Fiscal year 1990. U.S. Dept. of Health and Human Services. Public Health Service. National Institutes of Health, Feb. 1991.

16. Thom TJ. International comparisons in COPD mortality. Am Rev Respir Dis 1989;140:S27.

17. Respiratory Diseases Task Force report on prevention, control, education. DHEW publication no. (NIH) 77:1248. Bethesda, MD: National Heart, Lung, and Blood Institute, 1977.

18. Centers for Disease Control. Cigarette advertising—United States, 1988. MMWR 1990;39:261.

19. Dept. of Health and Human Services: Reducing the health consequences of smoking: 25 years of progress: a report of the Surgeon General. DHHS Publication No. (CDC) 89-8411. Rockville, MD: U.S. Dept. of Health and Human Services, Public Health Service, Center for Chronic Disease Prevention and Health Promotion, Office of Smoking and Health, 1989.

20. Centers for Disease Control. Smoking—attributable mortality and years of potential life lost—United States, 1988. MMWR 1991;40:62.

21. U.S. Dept. of Health and Human Services. Chronic obstructive lung disease. The health consequences of smoking. A report of the Surgeon General. Rockville, MD: U.S. Govt. Printing Office, 1984. Public Health Service Publication No. 84-50205.

22. Connors GL, Hodgkin JE. Pulmonary rehabilitation. In: Burton GG, Hodgkin JE, Ward JA, eds. Respiratory care: a guide to clinical practice, 3rd ed. Philadelphia: JB Lippincott, 1991.

23. Petty TL. Pulmonary rehabilitation. Basics of RD. New York: American Thoracic Society, 1975.

24. American Thoracic Society. Position statement on pulmonary rehabilitation. Am Rev Respir Dis 1981; 124:663.

25. American Thoracic Society. Standards for the diagnosis and care of patients with chronic obstructive pulmonary disease (COPD) and asthma. Am Rev Respir Dis 1987;136:225.

26. Ries AL. Position paper of the American Association of Cardiovascular and Pulmonary Rehabilitation: scientific basis of pulmonary rehabilitation. J Cardiopulm Rehabil 1990;10:418.

27. Bickford LS, Hodgkin JE. National pulmonary rehabilitation survey. In: Hodgkin JE, guest ed. Pulmonary rehabilitation symposium. J Cardiopulm Rehabil 1988;8:473.

28. Goldstein RS, McCullough C, Contreras MA. Approaches in rehabilitation of patients with ventilatory insufficiency. Eur Respir J 1989;2(suppl 7):655S.

29. Foster S, Thomas HM. Pulmonary rehabilitation in lung disease other than chronic obstructive pulmonary disease. Am Rev Respir Dis 1990;141:601.

30. Hodgkin JE, Zorn EG, Connors GL, eds. Pulmonary rehabilitation: guidelines to success. Boston: Butterworths, 1984.

WILLIAM F. MILLER

2

Historical Perspective of Pulmonary Rehabilitation

The concept of rehabilitation, involving organized holistic efforts to restore patients with debilitating and disabling disease to an optimally functioning state, is not new. However, application to patients with chronic pulmonary disease is a relatively recent practice. Before 1950, our understanding of pulmonary physiology and the nature of functional impairment was limited. Thus, it would have been difficult to formulate a physiologic approach to treatment. This chapter will review briefly the beginnings of pulmonary rehabilitation before 1970, at which time recognition of and interest in impairment and disability from chronic pulmonary disease intensified.

PHILOSOPHIC CONCEPT OF REHABILITATION

Charles G. Eustace presented a pertinent and concise philosophic review of general rehabilitation in 1966.[1] He emphasized the importance of a historical perspective to the understanding of where we are today and where we hope to be in the future. Eustace defined rehabilitation as a process that demonstrates the impulse of people of goodwill to make other people whole. Many different types of people are involved with rehabilitation activities, and each group thinks their contribution is the most important. Thus, interdisciplinary rivalries often result in a shift of care away from the physicians. Eustace found this to be a deplorable situation based on ethical and practical considerations. However, the nonmedical components of rehabilitation are not primarily the responsibility of the physician.

Eustace emphasized that all handicapped persons do not have the same potential or motivation for rehabilitation. He states, "We cannot escape the fact that the quality of the finished product will depend on the quality of the raw material that went into it." Eustace cites Dr. Howard Sprague of Boston, who noted that *the greatest resource for help* to the patient pursuing rehabilitation *is self-help*. An appropriate goal of rehabilitation effort is to return the patient to a state of self-help. Eustace refers to another medical giant from the past, Sir William Osler. He reminds us that some patients never have been, and never will be, able to stand entirely on their own feet. Therefore, when careful evaluation of the patient indicates a lack of potential for rehabilitation, the inappropriate use of valuable personnel time and talent as well as money and facilities, ". . . merely indicates an absence of clinical intelligence and personal courage," according to Osler. On the other hand, when patients are properly selected there is no doubt that pulmonary rehabilitation is economically both practical and valuable.

The background of a definition of pulmonary disability and pulmonary rehabilitation is presented in Chapter 1. I will discuss early developments on the processes of treatment.

PATIENT AND FAMILY EDUCATION

In the early days, patient and family education were given considerable attention because the physician had limited therapeutic options aside from counsel and reassurance. Ironically, with the advent of improved technology, emphasis on patient and family education waned. Moreover, an attitude of negativism emerged when it became apparent that therapeutic products might help symptoms, whereas the disease process seemed inexorably progressive. New and better agents, such as selective β-agonist bronchodilators, anticholinergic bronchodilators, and anti-inflammatory drugs, brought new interest and hope.

From 1945 through 1970, education of the patient and significant others as an essential part of treatment of all chronic diseases progressively gained attention. Many reviews and monographs appeared. Notable among these were Barach's books entitled *Physiologic Therapy in Respiratory Diseases*, 1948[2] and *Pulmonary Emphysema*, 1956;[3] Miller's reviews in 1954,[4] 1958,[5] and 1967[6] as well as Petty and Nett's monograph, *For Those Who Live and Breathe With Emphysema*, 1967.[7]

SMOKING CESSATION

Today, smoking cessation is accepted universally for management of these patients. However, since Dr. Barach was a cigarette smoker, as were many physicians in the 1940s and 1950s, there was seldom mention of smoking cessation in discussions of therapy. Moreover, Barach and others were critical of the antismoking programs for patients with chronic obstructive pulmonary disease (COPD). It is significant, however, that Dr. Barach did not inhale the cigarette smoke.

Animal studies dating back to the 1850s by Van Praeg and also Claude Bernard, as well as studies on humans in the early 1900s, demonstrated the toxic consequences of tobacco use. However, it was not until after the Surgeon General's first report on the health effects of tobacco smoke in 1964[8] that arguments[9,10] against cigarette smoking generally were accepted.

Since that time a large body of literature on the adverse health effects of tobacco use, as well as studies on smoking cessation techniques, has accumulated. Regular reports from the Surgeon General's office have sustained the initiatives to eliminate smoking. A coalition of the major voluntary health organizations brought together by the Surgeon General in 1964 was named the Interagency Council on Smoking and Health. In 1969, Diehl reviewed the early objectives and accomplishments of this group.[11]

Dr. Norman Hepper and colleagues at the Mayo Clinic were pioneers in the antismoking endeavor.[12,13] The state of Minnesota has been the world leader in developing programs to eliminate smoking in the general population. Since 1970 many people and agencies have been engaged actively in education of the public concerning the adverse effects of tobacco use. They are also aggressively promoting smoking cessation programs. J. L. Swartz has been a dominant figure in this activity.[14]

PSYCHOSOCIAL CONSIDERATIONS

Psychosocial aspects of chronic disabling lung disease are discussed usually as an afterthought in presentations on rehabilitation. Experience has taught us to consider these matters at the outset if other therapy is to be effective.

In 1950, Hurst noted that early workers—Binger Christie, Alexander, and Faulkner—recognized the influence of psychological factors on breathing.[15] The first systematic studies were published by Dudley, a psychiatrist and Martin, a pulmonary physiologist in 1969.[16] About the same time DeCencio and the Leshners defined the personality characteristics of the COPD patients.[17] The greatest danger that the candidate for pulmonary rehabilitation faces is a feeling of helplessness and a lack of self-worth that can, and often does, lead to depression, hopelessness, and suicide.[18] Prompt help to restore the patient's courage and dignity is crucial to successful rehabilitation. The most comprehensive summary of psychosocial considerations was presented by Dudley.[19] He stated: "The best thing to do with these patients is to treat their depression or anxiety or anger in a *subtle* way—that is with medication. At the same time give them emotional support and be the good listener they need." In addition he stated, ". . . emphysema patients generally can't tolerate insight-oriented group therapy; they feel more comfortable as *loners*." He also emphasizes honesty in dealing with disabled patients. Certain personality traits important in therapists and physicians are confidence, humility, courage, tolerance, compassion, and an optimistic casual sense of humor. It is essential to convince the patient that, even though the road to success is not always smooth or predictable, experience has taught us that often great things come out of adversity.

MEDICAL TREATMENT

The unquestioned pioneer of physiologic treatment of chronic pulmonary disease was Alvan L. Barach (Fig. 2–1). He began his career, after graduating in 1919 from the College of Physicians and Surgeons in New York, at Massachusetts General Hospital in Boston under the sponsorship of Dr. James H. Means, studying oxygen therapy and pulmonary physiology. He published his first reports with Dr. Margaret N. Woodwell, a series of three papers on oxygen therapy in the *Archives of Internal Medicine*, 1921; 28:367, 394, and 421. He returned to New York to stay in 1922, where he started working at Presbyterian Hospital under the sponsorship of Dr. Walter W. Palmer and Dr. Robert F. Loeb. The same year he published his first solo report on the therapeutic use of oxygen in the *Journal of the American Medical Association*. He wrote his first review article in 1938[20] and a monograph entitled

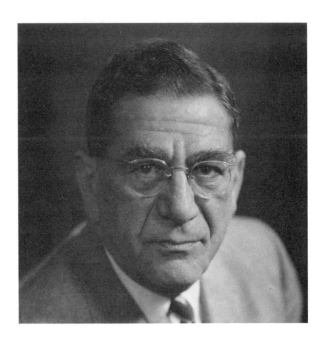

FIGURE 2-1 Alvan L. Barach, M.D., "Father" of modern day physiological therapy of chronic obstructive pulmonary disease

Principles and Practice of Inhalation Therapy in 1944.[21] In 1948 he revised and renamed the monograph *Physiological Therapy in Respiratory Diseases*.

Bronchodilator Therapy

Bronchodilator therapy was variably effective in early days because little was known about the pharmacodynamics of the limited agents available. Ephedrine and aminophylline have been used orally since the early 1930s. In most instances ephedrine was only a fair bronchodilator and caused side effects, especially in elderly men, who would develop urinary retention as well as nervousness and tachyarrythmia. Aminophylline, because of its propensity for causing gastrointestinal distress as well as nervousness and increased cardiac irritability, usually was given in doses inadequate to achieve therapeutic blood levels. Epinephrine by subcutaneous injection was effective, but, like ephedrine, frequently caused side effects.

Aerosol Sympathomimetics

In 1935 Graeser and Rowe[22] introduced to the United States the aerosol inhalation of 1 : 100 epinephrine for relief of bronchospasm and bronchial congestion.[22] This had been introduced in Germany in 1919 by Heubner.[23] Barach promptly adopted this great advance and, subsequently, promoted its use.[24] He also aerosolized 1% phenylephrine (Neo-Synephrine) a sympathetic agonist decongestant used for nasal congestion as spray or drops. This was not as effective a bronchodilator as epinephrine.

Lucien Dautrebande, a French physiologist, first published studies on aerosols in 1941.[25] He became the world authority on microaerosols. The results of his years of work, which include more than 100 papers, are summarized in his monograph

Microaerosols published in 1962.[26] With systematic, carefully conducted studies he produced what became the best bronchodilator solution. This consisted of 0.25% isoproterenol, a β-agonist; 0.5% cyclopentamine, a superior α-sympathetic agonist decongestant; and 0.1% atropine, an anticholinergic agent. Cyclopentamine was considered superior to both phenylephrine and ephedrine because of fewer side effects and longer duration of action. It is intriguing that this agent was never used subsequently as a mucous membrane decongestant. It was not until oxymetazoline appeared that a long-acting decongestant was available. To my knowledge long-acting decongestants have not been evaluated as adjuncts to bronchodilators in selected patients with bronchial inflammatory disease since Dautrebande did his studies. Later, atropine was removed from this combination because of rare serious cardiogenic side effects and because incidental deposition of aerosol in the eyes caused profound dilation and fixation of pupils. This was most often unilateral and led to clinical confusion, suggesting the presence of central nervous system problems. Today atropine is added, on a selective basis, or the cogener ipratropium bromide (Atrovent) is used. For a long time, isoproterenol was the standard aerosol bronchodilator. It is a potent bronchodilator, but often its very brief duration of action was not appreciated; hence when patients routinely were dosed two to four times daily, they were often undertreated.

In 1958, Lands[27] introduced the concept of β_2-bronchoselective adrenergic agonists as opposed to β_1-cardioselective agents for bronchodilator therapy. Isoetherine, a somewhat more selective bronchodilator, was a product of this early work. Its principal disadvantage, similar to isoproterenol, was a short duration of action. Only a few workers in the field recognized this shortcoming and adjusted the dosage and frequency to provide adequate bronchodilator action for patients with chronic recurring airways' obstruction.

Ariens in 1964 demonstrated that it was the deposition of large droplets in the mouth that was responsible for the side effects,[28] so microaerosol nebulizers and tube extenders were used to control this problem. In the late 1970s and early 1980s we learned that extenders and reservoirs also enhanced the deposition of fine particle aerosol.

In the United States there were only two nebulizers available in the 1940s, the Vaponephrin and DeVilbiss hand-held glass units. Wilson and LaMer indicated that the Vaponephrin device was more efficient because of more consistent small particle size (median 5.2 μm).[29] Most European workers, as reflected best by Dautrebande's work, found that pulmonary deposition required a preponderance of particles in the 1 μm or smaller range. Small-particle nebulizers did not become standard until the 1980s, following which there was a progressive development of more bronchoselective sympathomimetic agents. These had not only fewer side effects, but also had a longer duration of effectiveness. Thus, they could be given in larger doses. As a result, control of airways' obstruction moved into a new age.

Methylxanthines

Theophylline was introduced as a bronchodilator in the 1930s with varying success, because it was not until 1972 that Jenne clarified the clinical pharmacology of this substance.[30] Then the introduction of sustained-release agents, which allowed once- or twice-daily treatment with sustained blood levels of drug, revolutionized treatment with this substance. There was a period before 1975 when theophylline preparations were administered rectally as suppositories or solutions. This was a very effective method of administration for some patients, but often resulted in both local and systemic undesirable side effects. This method is no longer recommended.

Theophylline preparations were occasionally used by aerosol by some physicians. It is irritating and, in some cases, probably promoted bronchial evacuation of secretions; it was not a very effective agent.

Alternative preparations of theophylline, such as oxytriphylline, glyphylline, diphylline, dynophylline, and aminophylline, were generally unsatisfactory and more unpredictable than theophylline. Of these, aminophylline was the most widely used. It is a short-acting, rapidly absorbed agent that for oral use was replaced by the sustained-release theophylline preparations. However, it is still used as a standard parenteral preparation, and, per milligram, it is approximately equivalent to 0.8 mg anhydrous theophylline.

Anticholinergics

Atropine, stramonium, and belladonna were introduced to the Western World in the early 1900s in the form of medicated cigarettes. The first real attempt at investigation was by Herxheimer in 1959.[30] He used specially prepared cigarettes, from which the usual irritants were removed. Atropine was added at two dose levels: 0.5 and 1.45 mg. It was estimated that 80% was delivered to the patient. He found this method very effective in patients with COPD, without significant side effects. He commented that other investigators had not found larger doses of atropine aerosol to be effective. Moreover, they were plagued by a high incidence of side effects, such as dryness of the mucous membranes, tachycardia, urinary retention, and mental confusion. He felt that this was a result of the much larger droplets by the standard nebulizer method, compared with the cigarette. We confirmed these observations and suggestions by giving 1% atropine solutions administered in doses of 0.05 to 0.1 mg/kg body weight in 2 to 4 mL of water by an ultramicronebulizer designed by Dautrebande. Lowell also demonstrated that the side effects were due to the large droplets delivered by the standard nebulizers, leading to significant systemic absorption.[31] However, neither the special atropine cigarettes nor the special nebulizers were available in this country for clinical use, and it was not until the late 1970s that similar nebulizers were available. A safer anticholinergic, an atropine cogener, ipratropium bromide, was first described in 1975[32,33] as Sch 1000, but was not available until the mid-1980s for clinical use as the metered-dose inhaler, Atrovent.

Anti-Inflammatory Agents

Hench and colleagues first introduced corticotropin (ACTH) and corticosteroid therapy for treatment of the inflammatory component of arthritis. Bordley et al. and Randolph and Rollins in 1949 reported use of these agents in the treatment of inflammatory bronchial disease, especially allergic asthma.[34,35] The first definitive study was by Carryer et al., in 1950.[36] Rose provided the first authoritative review in 1954,[37] and Barach and associates reviewed their experience in 1955.[38] It is important to appreciate that most of what is known about the pharmacology of corticosteroids was described by Thorn and his associates, 1953 to 1955.[39] Nevertheless, therapy with these agents, to this day, is largely empirical. George Thorn and his colleagues are responsible for most major developments in the use of corticosteroids. These include the recommendation of a single daily early-morning dose, rather than multiple doses throughout the day, and the use of alternate-day doses[40] to reduce side effects of systemic therapy. Many workers have verified these observations, but these principles often are still ignored in current clinical practice.

Cromolyn Sodium

Roger Altounyan discovered cromolyn sodium in the mid-1960s. The first report of a controlled evaluation in patients with asthma was by Howell and Altounyan 1967.[41] Cromolyn sodium for many years was considered to be of value only in young asthmatics. As the true nature of this agent became better understood, it was apparent that prolonged use in patients with chronic nonspecific bronchial inflammatory disease decreased the reactivity of the airways. The result was improved control of obstructive disease and decreased dependence on corticosteroid therapy.

Bronchopulmonary Clearance

The effects of viscid bronchial secretions and exudates in causing aggravated breathing difficulties and fatiguing cough have been recognized since antiquity. Inhalations have been used, especially hot vapors of salt water, often with a variety of volatile substances added such as eucalyptus, menthol, creosote, ammonium chloride, and calcium salts, with varying results. None were ever evaluated in controlled studies, but the one consistent component was hot water vapor, which has withstood the test of time. Today we use the steam vaporizor. In the 1940s and 1950s a variety of agents, such as hyaluronidase, trypsin, pancreatic dornase, and acetyl-cystiene, were used in aerosols. Segal and his associates were active in this area. They were also enthusiastic promoters of (intermittent) inspiratory positive-pressure breathing (IPPB) as an adjunct to aerosols to promote bronchial evacuation. Much of their interesting work is reviewed in the book by Segal and Dulfano.[42]

Formerly, chronic productive bronchitis was a common manifestation of the patient with chronic airflow limitation; hence, good methods of bronchial clearance was a major concern. The advent of improved antibiotics, corticosteroids, and other agents to improve airways function and control inflammation has drastically reduced the frequency of this problem. Mucous plugging still occurs and often goes unrecognized.

The pattern of breathing during aerosol administration was first emphasized by Stalport[43] and later reaffirmed by Dautrebande.[44] They found that slow, deep breathing with an inspiratory pause was optimal for deposition of microaerosols in the airways. Simple relaxed normal-pattern breathing results in less than 40% deposition, whereas a slow exhalation, followed by slow inhalation to near total lung capacity, followed by an inspiratory pause of 5 seconds, could result in up to 85% deposition of aerosol.

In 1954, the first paper I published was to describe a clinical evaluation of these principles of aerosol administration.[45] With use of the OEM mask, I demonstrated the superiority of an expiratory–inspiratory–pause (E-I-P) method, compared with conventional methods of breathing aerosols. Surprisingly, it was not until current workers repeated the deposition studies with radioactive-labeled aerosols and metered-dose inhalers that these important considerations were universally adopted.

Mist Therapy

Those patients who demonstrate gas exchange impairment and volume limitation proportionate to the flow impairment should be suspected of having a bronchial-plugging problem and should receive aggressive bronchial hygiene therapy. In 1955 to cope with this problem, we adopted an idea that we had learned from Jack Emerson, who had heated the water reservoir of gas humidifiers to improve their efficiency. I was aware of the claims in the writings from the early and mid-1800s for heated inhalations, so we started by using a small laboratory heater to heat water in a stainless steel bucket into which we placed the nebulizer reservoir jar. This system was reported in *Anesthesiology* in 1957,[46] and was later revised to be heated by an immersion-type first made by Mist O-2 Gen Corp. and later adopted by Puritan-Bennett and others.

As soon as we began using the reservoir nebulizers (1953 to 1954), we began finding an increased frequency of pulmonary infections caused by gram-negative rods. I was convinced this was related to contamination of the nebulizer systems, but I could not convince the hospital administration that added personnel was necessary to maintain and change the equipment every 12 to 24 hours, especially since many infectious disease investigators at that time did not consider these common environmental contaminants as serious pathogens, even though they may be resistant to most antibiotics. However, when some of these patients began to demonstrate fatal gram-negative pneumonias, I was able to convince my colleagues Alan K. Pierce and Jay P. Sanford to study this problem. The results of those studies were published by Reinarz and colleagues in 1965.[47] We found high-density mist therapy very effective in achieving good bronchial clearance, even in patients with severe ventilatory insufficiency, if we provided ventilatory assistance.[48] Subsequent reports have confirmed that in patients who have adequate function, clearance can be affected with aerosols, voluntary augmented breathing, and chest physiotherapy.[49] Unfortunately, there was a reactionary rejection of this mode of treatment for many years. It now seems to be returning to use as an aid to bronchial clearance on a more selective and rational basis, with appropriate precautions to prevent nosocomial infection.[50]

Much research needs to be done in the area of bronchial clearance to determine the role of evacuant aerosols and pharmacologic expectorants in the treatment of chronic bronchitic syndromes.

Pressure-Breathing Methods

Welsh, in 1878, reported the use of inspiratory positive-pressure breathing (IPPB) to successfully treat acute pulmonary edema.[51] Norton reported use of IPPB to treat acute toxic pulmonary edema in 1896,[52] and Emerson in 1909,[53] again treated pulmonary edema with IPPB. It was not until 1936 that the next report by Poulton appeared.[54] From that point on Barach focused a great deal of attention on various modes of pressure breathing. In 1935, he introduced continuous positive-pressure breathing (CPPB), which he defined as 4 to 20 centimeters of water during both inspiration and expiration.[55] This was used at first with helium and oxygen to treat obstructive dyspnea and later, in 1937, with high oxygen mixtures to treat acute pulmonary edema of various causes.[56] These observations were verified by Segal and Aisner in 1943[57] and 1944,[58] by Ansbro in 1945,[59] and by Barach and associates in 1947.[60] This modality was often combined with increased inspiratory pressure and mechanical ventilation (IPPV). Thus, when Ashbaugh and Petty, in 1969,[61] added positive expiratory pressure (PEP) with inspiratory positive-pressure ventilators (IPPV) to treat adult respiratory distress syndrome (ARDS), they called it CPPB.[61] In a subsequent article,[62] they corrected the terminology and introduced the terms IPPV with positive end-expiratory pressure (PEEP).

Gregory and coworkers, apparently unaware of the previous publications on CPPB, described a method similar to Barach's and used it to treat infant inspiratory distress syndrome (IRDS).[63] They called it continuous positive airway pressure (CPAP). This term has been accepted and popularized. As a result few people realize that Barach first described the method.

In the interim IPPV became known as intermittent positive-pressure breathing (IPPB) when administered by a portable device on a short-term basis. This method was first used in clinical medicine as recommended by physiologists to ventilate patients with early ventilatory failure and carbon dioxide retention.[64,65] The approach lost popularity as aggressive endotracheal intubulation and mechanical volume ventilation gained interest. Motley popularized IPPB as a method of administering bronchodilator aerosols.[66] The unwarranted overuse of this method was created by a combination of several factors: a general lack of knowledge about pulmonary physiology, as it relates to therapy among clinicians; the liberal policies of the third-party payers including Medicare in payment for these devices, in spite of a lack of evidence to support a wide use without established criteria; and vigorous promotion by multiple manufacturers, especially to respiratory therapy technologists and general physicians and surgeons who were unable to critically assess the message.

There have been three studies that state the essence of the physiologic role of intermittent inspiratory breathing assistance.[67–69] These studies have a double message. The first, and most frequently cited, message is that in patients, especially those with emphysema, there is no advantage to using ventilatory assistance to administer bronchodilator aerosols. The second message is that in patients with ventilatory failure and cough with abundant tenacious secretions, often a better short-term response to aerosol bronchodilator was observed with ventilatory assistance. To my knowledge, there has never been a long-term study wherein patients were selected on the basis of clinical and physiologic indicators for ventilatory assistance. Such patients were specifically excluded in other short-[70] and long-term studies,[71,72] including the elaborate multicenter clinical trial reported in 1985.[73]

PHYSICAL REHABILITATION

The principal components of physical rehabilitation for patients with clinical pulmonary disease include stress control, breathing control training, and physical conditioning. Optimal medical control of the inflammatory components of the process, proper nutritional adjustments, and supplemental oxygen where indicated is addressed first. Certain therapy procedures such as pneumoperitoneum, emphysema belts, thoracoabdominal compressors, and exsufflation with negative pressure are of only historical interest.

Relaxation, Stress Control, and Biofeedback

From 1935 to 1948 there appeared many dissertations of a descriptive nature, concerning psychological factors in relation to breathing. Jacobson described classic relaxation techniques in 1938.[74] Some of these were modified by Fink, who first wrote his book *Release from Nervous Tension* in 1943.[75] This became a paperback in its third expanded edition 1962. Both authors used examples of patients with asthma and breathing difficulty. It was not until 1976, when Vachon did his formal studies on visceral learning in asthma,[76] that methods of objective assessment were applied to this area. The term biofeedback was not in use until the 1970s, even though the concepts of self-awareness, mind–body interrelations, and physiologic self-regulation existed long before. The term autogenic training was first used as early as 1959 by Schultz and Luthe.[77] The recognition of the role of both conscious and subconscious feedback to the process led to the term autogenic feedback training. It was later contracted to biofeedback. The development of this field is best and most colorfully reviewed by Elmer and Alyce Green.[78] They believe the concepts go back to ancient times and were aggressively pursued by the yogis.

Pursed-lips breathing is a form of biofeedback that helps the patient with emphysema to moderate expiratory effort, thereby reducing the tendency for the airways to close, exaggerating flow obstruction. In an effort to standardize the feedback, we used mouthpieces with selected small orifices that created a back pressure, which the patient sensed, causing them to control their expiratory effort. Biofeedback means the subjects are receiving immediate ongoing physiologic information about their own biologic processes, with the intent of using that information to control or change function in a desirable way. We also used a visual form of feedback to help patients control breathing and reduce dyspnea.[4,5] The patients monitored their breathing tracing and could see how increasing the frequency of breathing caused air trapping, with an increase in the functional residual capacity. They also saw how forced exhalation caused a slowing of the emptying rate, owing to airway closure. They learned that more relaxed exhalation actually led to increased flow. Others used the visual image of the flow–volume tracing on a video screen or plotter. Patients are taught to reproduce an ideal frequency or flow pattern.

Yet another approach was to use a simulated audible breathing signal. The specific characteristics of the signal were selected to optimize the patients breathing, with the least effort. These and even more sophisticated approaches to control of breathing frequency, pattern, and effort as adjuncts to breathing retraining have never been fully investigated.

There is a vast literature on biofeedback, with well-controlled studies in many areas, but very little has been published on its use in treatment of pulmonary problems. Relaxation techniques appear to be quite helpful in teaching breathing and dyspnea control.

Breathing Control Training

The principal aim of breath control techniques is to help the patient learn to breathe with the least expenditure of effort compatible with adequate alveolar ventilation for any given level of physical activity.[6] The physiologic basis for breathing control training was elucidated in part by many, including Hofbauer, 1951.[81] Methods were first described by Schutz[82] and Livingston.[83] Barach modified and popularized, "breathing exercises" in 1944[20] and 1948.[21] I preferred the designation *breathing control training* because the goal is to teach a slow, relaxed form of breathing. The term *exercise* implies a vigorously aggressive form of breathing. Barach did not believe that patients could be taught slow, relaxed breathing.

Our data on the physiologic assessment of the training was published in 1954.[4] The small group of patients showed the desired reduction in ventilation and breathing frequency with an increase in tidal volume. They also showed some improvement in ventilatory and gas exchange functions at rest and exercise. The magnitudes of the changes were quite small, but were consistently found, so statistical significance was achieved. The essence of our favorable effects was confirmed by Bolton and associates in 1955[84] and by Dayman in 1956.[85] Howard Dayman was one of my contemporaries from whom I learned much. He stated most succinctly in 1956, "In this disease expiration is fixed by the check valve mechanism and inspiration by the hyperinflated condition of the thorax. The purpose of therapy is to enhance the efficiency of breathing within these fixed limits."

Immediately following our study, a number of reports appeared that did not find measured improvement with breathing training. The key point here is that our goal was to train the patients to use a slow, deep pattern of breathing. This, in fact, was achieved as demonstrated by the data. In the other studies there was no evidence that training had been accomplished. An additional consideration is that our patients were quite active and showed signs of increased strength as reflected by the increased maximum expiratory pressure (MEP) and FCV. This suggests that the patients achieved an element of physical conditioning. This is an effect not specifically attributable to training in breathing control. It is also possible that our patients achieved some clinical improvement in their bronchitis. This also is an effect not specifically a consequence of the breathing control training, but coincidental to the regular bronchodilator and bronchial hygiene therapy. Even in retrospect, these are factors difficult to control in a variable disease condition. Even more impressive were some brief observatons reported 13 years later.[6] In those studies we studied persons with stable pulmonary emphysema of a very severe degree; all 1-second forced expiratory volume (FEV_1) values were less than 1 L/second. None of these persons had ever had any previous instruction in breathing control, and none had discovered pursed-lips breathing. They were asked to walk on a motor-driven treadmill at 2.5 miles/hour as long as they could. None of these patients was able to walk more than 2 minutes. Breathing frequencies ranged from 38 to 45 breaths per minute and most of the patients showed exercise-induced exaggerated hypoxemia and carbon dioxide retention. After the first walk, the patients were allowed 30 to 45 minutes of rest. During that time they were advised to note that they were comfortable breathing slowly. They observed the spirometer tracing of their breathing during the exercise. This demonstrated a progressive decrease in tidal volume and progressive air trapping associated with the rapid breathing. They were asked to try to keep their breathing rate as slow as they could when the exercise was repeated. The breathing frequencies varied from 24 to 30/minute and, in every instance, the duration of walking increased two-fold or more. This sequence was repeated two more times the same day, and each time the duration of walking increased strikingly. We used taped signals from a breathing simulator[86] to facilitate breathing control. The magnitude of the increase was proportional to the slowing of the breathing frequency. In several patients the arterial oxygen saturation and $PaCO_2$ improved strikingly, even though the patients were working at increased levels. The maximum duration of walking increased by five times or more above the initial duration. We also have noted patients who demonstrate exaggerated hypoxemia and carbon dioxide retention as a result of hyperpnea and air trapping, precipitated by a variety of reasons other than by exericse. This could be corrected with control of breathing frequency alone. These observations have been confirmed by others.[86–89] It is important that achieving slow controllable deep breathing, by whatever method available, is essential to optimal gas exchange and activity tolerance. Thorman and coauthors[89] and Meuller and associates[90] have confirmed the immediate effects of pursed-lips breathing. These include a decrease of required minute ventilation, a slowing of breathing frequency, and increasing tidal volume. This maneuver prevents premature airway collapse. Other adjuncts to breathing control training were described. Barach[91] emphasized use of a 20° to 30° head-down position with added weights (up to 15 lb) on the abdomen in conjunction with expiratory pursed-lips breathing. This has the same inspiratory muscle training effect as inspiratory resistors. Emphysema belts[91,92] and therapeutic pneumoperitoneum[93–95] are now only of historic interest. Muscle-strengthening exercises are a much more cost-effective approach and have fewer potential side effects. There probably are occasional patients, with very relaxed abdominal walls, who would benefit from an abdominal support if muscle strengthening is not feasible.

Exercise Reconditioning

The concept of therapeutic exercise is not new. Cristobal Mendez in 1553 published a monograph entitled *Book of Bodily Exercise*.[96] The modern era of therapeutic exercise for pulmonary disease was initiated by Barach.[2,3] On many occasions Barach was known to state, "I am of the opinion that a program generally dedicated to physical and mental rest is fraught with hazard!" He also stated,

> Measures which have as their purpose an expansion of the life of the patient as much as may be feasible is to my mind a proper objective. We should encourage these stimulating activities not simply because our patients deserve to live fully as human beings but also because constricting their activities for the sake of conserving their energies leads to psychosomatic disturbances that impair respiratory function itself. The heart of the matter is the physicians attitude.

Our first studies were reported in 1962[97] and 1963[98] followed by more extensive observations by Pierce and others in our laboratory in 1964.[99] The details of our techniques, summarized in 1967,[6] were independently developed, but embody many of the principles of Donaldson and colleagues in Australia.[100,101] Oxygen-supported exercise was first described by Barach in 1938.[20] The first physiologic evaluation was undertaken by Cotes in 1956.[102] Pierce and coworkers demonstrated the same training effects with oxygen-supported exercise as with exercise at ambient oxygen levels.[103] Paez and associates in 1967 demonstrated that in short-term exercise training the major element accounting for the improvement was a specific learning effect for the particular activity used for training.[104] There was no transference of training effect from the treadmill to the bicycle. The learning effect was predominantly a lengthening of stride and improved posture on the treadmill, so that the patient performed more efficiently. I suspect that if the patients had trained for a longer period, to a stable optimum degree of conditioning on the treadmill, there would be more evidence of training effect transference.

Finally, Pierce, in 1968 found that patients with moderate to severe chronic airway obstruction were able to achieve significantly greater flow during both inspiration and expiration on exercise, than they achieved during forced spirometry maneuvers.[105] This effect was accomplished as a result of modulation of the respiratory effort during exhalation to minimize the airways' closure, which is demonstrated on maximal force exhalation in the patients.

Once we were able to demonstrate to patients that they could exercise or work in a regimented program, it was possible, after reassurance, for patients to apply the same approach of progressive intensity to other activities of interest. These ranged from work functions to pleasurable pursuits, such as dancing or sexual intercourse. In our opinion, the secret of success is an interested and enthusiastic physician coupled with a motivated patient who has achieved effective breathing control. We always saw our primary objective as improvement in quality of life.

The year 1970 marked the beginning of the modern era for rehabilitation of patients with chronic obstructive pulmonary disease. Since that time, the numbers of publications have increased immensely. The other chapters in this text deal with these advances in our knowledge.

REFERENCES

1. Eustace CG. Rehabilitation: an evolving concept. JAMA 1966;195:1129.

2. Barach AL. Physiologic therapy in respiratory diseases. Philadelphia: JB Lippincott, 1948.

3. Barach AL, Bickerman HA. Pulmonary emphysema. Baltimore: Williams & Wilkins, 1956.

4. Miller WF. A physiologic evaluation of the effects of diaphragmatic breathing training in patients with chronic pulmonary emphysema. Am J Med 1954;17:471.

5. Miller WF. Physical therapeutic measures in the treatment of chronic bronchopulmonary disorders. Methods for breathing training. Am J Med 1958;24:929.

6. Miller WF. Rehabilitation of patients with chronic obstructive lung disease. Med Clin North Am 1967;51:349.

7. Petty TL, Nett LM. For those who live and breathe. A manual for patients with emphysema and chronic bronchitis. Springfield, IL: Charles C Thomas, 1967, 2nd ed., 1972.

8. Smoking and health: a report of the advisory committee to the surgeon general. Public Health Service, US Dept of Health, Education and Welfare, PHS publication 1103, 1964.

9. Anderson DO, Ferris BG Jr. Role of tobacco smoking in the causation of chronic respiratory disease. N Engl J Med 1962;267:787.

10. Thurlbeck WM. The incidence of pulmonary emphysema, with observations on the relative incidence and spatial distribution of various types of emphysema. Am Rev Respir Dis 1963;87:206.

11. Diehl HS. Tobacco and your health: the controversy. New York: McGraw-Hill, 1969.

12. Hepper NGG. Cigarette smoking and chronic respiratory disease. Minn Med 1969;52:1373.

13. Hepper NGG, Carr DT, Andersen HA, et al. Antismoking clinic: report of an experience and comparison with published results. Mayo Clin Proc 1970;45:189.

14. Swartz JL. A critical review and evaluation of smoking control methods. Public Health Rep 1969;84:483.

15. Hurst A, Henkin R, Lustig GL. Some psychosomatic aspects of respiratory disease. Am Practitioner 1950;1:486.

16. Dudley DL, Martin CJ, Masuda M, Ripley HS, Holmes TH. The psychophysiology of respiration in health and disease. New York: Appleton Century Crofts, 1969.

17. Decencio DV, Leshner M, Leshner B. Personality characteristics of patients with chronic obstructive pulmonary emphysema. Arch Phys Med 1968;49:471.

18. Agle DP, Baum GL, Chester EH, Wendt M. Multidiscipline treatment of chronic pulmonary insufficiency. I Psychological aspects of rehabilitation. Psychosom Med 1973;35:41.

19. Dudley DL, Glaser EM, Jorgenson MSW, Logan DL. Psychosocial concomitants to rehabilitation in chronic obstructive pulmonary disease. Part I Psychosocial and psychological considerations. Chest 1980;77:413. Part II Psychosocial treatment. Chest 1980;77:544. Part III Dealing with psychiatric disease. Chest 1980;77:667.

20. Barach AL. Physiological methods in diagnosis and treatment of asthma and emphysema. Ann Intern Med 1938;12:454.

21. Barach AL. Principles and practice of inhalation therapy. Philadelphia: JB Lippincott, 1944.

22. Graeser JB, Rowe AH. Inhalation of epinephrine. J Allergy 6:415, 1935.

23. Heubner W. Uber inhalation zerstaubter flussigkeiten. Z Gesamte Exp Med 1919;10:269.

24. Barach AL. Physiological methods in the diagnosis and treatment of asthma and emphysema. Ann Intern Med 1938;12:454.

25. Dautrebande L. Aerosols medicamenteux. III Possibites de traitment des etats asthmatiformes par aerosols de substances dites bronchodilatatrices. Arch Intern Pharmacodyn 1941;66:379.

26. Dautrebande L. Microaerosols. New York: Academic Press, 1962.

27. Lands AM, Luduena FP, Hoppe JO, Oyen IH. The pharmacologic actions of the bronchodilator drug isoetherine. J Am Pharm Assoc 1958;47:744.

28. Ariens EJ. Pharmacology of bronchodilating and bronchoconstricting drugs. In: Orie NGM, Sluiter HJ, eds. Bronchitis II. The Netherlands: Assen, Royal Van Gorcum, 1964:209.

29. Wilson IB and LaMer VK. The retention of aerosol particles in the human respiratory tract as a function of particle radius. J Ind Hyg Toxicol 1948; 30:265.

30. Herxheimer H. Atropine cigarettes in asthma and emphysema. Br Med J 1959;2:167.

31. Lowell FC. Experimentally induced asthma in man. Proc. 4th Conf. Res. in Emphysema. Aspen, Colorado, 1961.

32. Storms WW, Dopico GA, Reed CE. Aerosol Sch 1000, an anticholinergic bronchodilator. Am Rev Respir Dis 1975;111:419.

33. Gross NJ. Sch 1000: a new anticholinergic bronchodilator. Am Rev Respire Dis 1975;112:823.

34. Bordley JE, Harvey AMcG, Howard JE, Newman EV. Preliminary report on the use of ACTH in the hypersensitivity state. Proc Clin ACTH Conf 1949;1:469.

35. Randolph TG, Rollins JP. Relief of allergic diseases by ACTH therapy. Proc Clin ACTH Conf 1949;1:479.

36. Carryer HM, Koelsche GA, Prickman LE, Maytum CK, Lake CF, Williams HL. The effect of cortisone on bronchial asthma and hay fever occurring in subjects sensitive to ragweed pollen. J Allergy 1955;21:282.

37. Rose B. Asthma and rhinitis. In: Luken's medical uses of cortisone. New York: Blakiston, 1954:326.

38. Barach AL, Bickerman HA, Beck GJ. Clinical and physiological studies on the use of metacortandracin in respiratory disease. Bronchial Asthma Dis Chest 1955;28:515.

39. Thorn GW, Jenkins D, Laidlaw JC, et al. Pharmacologic aspects of adrencortical steroids and ACTH in man. N Engl J Med 1953;248:414, 588.

40. Harter JC, Reddy WJ, Thorn GW. Studies on an intermittent corticosteroid dosage regimen. N Engl J Med. 1963;269:591.

41. Howell JB, Altownyan RE. A double-blind trial of disodium cromoglycate in the treatment of allergic bronchial asthma. Lancet 1967;2:539.

42. Segal MS, Dulfano MJ. Chronic pulmonary emphysema: physiopathology and treatment. New York: Grune & Stratton, 1953.

43. Stalport J. Aerosols medicamenteux. VIII Nouvelles reserches sur quelques characteristiques physiochimiques des aerosols. Etude de leur absorption par les porimons. Actin chez l'hormone d'aerosols formes a patir de substances diuritiques. Arch Intern Pharmacodyn 1958;71:248.

44. Dautrebande L. Physiological and pharmacological characteristics of liquid aerosols. Physiol Rev 1952;32:214.

45. Miller WF. A consideration of improved methods of nebulization therapy. N Engl J Med 1954;251, 589.

46. Miller WF, Cade JR, Cushing IE. Preoperative recognition and treatment of bronchopulmonary disease. Anesthesiology 1957;18:483.

47. Reinarz JA, Pierce AK, Mays BB, Sanford JP. The potential role of inhalation therapy equipment in nosocomical pulmonary infections. J Clin Invest 1965;44:831.

48. Miller WF, Johnston FF, Tarkoff MP. Use of ultrasonic aerosols with ventilatory assistors. J Asthma Res 1968;5:335.

49. Sutton PP. Chest physiotherapy and cough. In: Clarke SW, Pavia D, eds. Aerosols and the lung: clinical and experimental aspects. London: Butterworths, 1984:156.

50. Wanner A, Ras A. Clinical indicators for and effects of bland, mucolytic and antimicrobial aerosols. Am Rev Respir Dis 1968;122:79.

51. Welch WH. Zur pathologie des lungenodems. Virchows Arch [A] 1878;72:375.

52. Norton NR. Forced respiration in a case of carbolic acid poisoning. Med Surg Rep Presby Hosp NY 1896;1:127.

53. Emerson H. Artificial respiration in the treatment of edema of the lungs. Arch Intern Med 1909;3:368.

54. Poulton EP. Left-sided heart failure with pulmonary edema treated with the pulmonary plus pressure machine. Lancet 1936;2:283.

55. Barach AL. The use of helium in the treatment of asthma and obstructive lesions of larynx and trachea. Ann Intern Med 1935;9:739.

56. Barach AL, Martin S, Eckman M. Positive pressure respiration and its application to the treatment of acute pulmonary edema and respiratory obstruction. Proc Am Soc Clin Invest 1937;6:664.

57. Segal MS. Inhalation therapy in the treatment of serious respiratory disease. N Engl J Med 1943;229:235.

58. Segal MS, Aisner M. Management of certain aspects of gas poisoning with particular reference to shock and pulmonary complications. Ann Intern Med 1944;20:219.

59. Ansbro FP. Positive pressure respiration in treatment of acute pulmonary edema. Am J Surg 1945;68:185.

60. Barach AL, Fenn WO, Ferris EB, Schmidt CF. The physiology of pressure breathing. A brief view of its status. J Aviat Med 1947;18:73.

61. Ashbaugh DG, Petty TL, Bigelow DB, Levine BE. Continuous positive pressure breathing (CPPB) in adult respiratory distress syndrome. J Thorac Cardiovasc Surg 1969;57:31.

62. Petty TL, Nett LM, Ashbaugh DG. Improvement in oxygenation in the adult respiratory distress syndrome by positive and expiratory pressure (PEEP). Resp Care 1971;16:173.

63. Gregory GA, Kitterman JA, Phibbs RH, Tooley WH, Hamilton WK. The treatment of the idiopathic respiratory distress syndrome with continuous positive airway pressure. N Engl J Med 1971;284:1333.

64. Bourtourline-Young HJ, Whittenberger JL. Use of artificial respiration in pulmonary emphysema accompanied by high carbon dioxide levels. J Clin Invest 1951;30:838.

65. Cournand A, Motley HL, Werko L, Richards DW Jr. Physiolological studies of effects of intermittent positive pressure breathing on cardiac output in man. Am J Physiol 1948;152:163.

66. Motley HL, Lang LP, Gordon B. Use of intermittent positive pressure breathing combined with nebulization in pulmonary disease. Am J Med 1948;5:853.

67. Fowler WS, Helmholtz HF, Miller RD. Treatment of emphysema with aerosolized bronchodilator drugs and intermittent positive pressure breathing. Proc Staff Mayo Clin 1953;28:741.

68. Wu N, Miller WF, Cade RF, Richburg PR. Intermittent positive pressure breathing in patients with chronic bronchopulmonary disease. Am Rev Tuberc 1955;71:693.

69. Chester EH, Racz I, Barlow PB, Baum GL. Bronchodilator therapy: comparison of acute response to three methods of administration. Chest 1972;62:394.

70. Goldberg I, Cherniack RM. The effects of nebulized bronchodilator delivered with and without IPPB on ventilatory function in obstructive emphysema. Am Rev Respir Dis 1965;91:13.

71. Curtis JK, Rasmussen HK, Cree EM. IPPB therapy in chronic airway obstructive pulmonary disease. JAMA 1968;206:1037.

72. Cherniack RM, Svanhill E. Long-term use of intermittent positive pressure breathing (IPPB) in chronic obstructive pulmonary disease. Am Rev Respir Dis 1976;113:721.

73. Intermittent positive pressure breathing trial group. Intermittent positive pressure breathing therapy of chronic obstructive pulmonary disease. Ann Intern Med 1983;99:612.

74. Jacobson E. Progressive relaxation: a physiological and clinical investigation of muscular states and their significance in psychology and medical practice, 2nd ed. Chicago: Chicago University Press, 1938.

75. Fink DH. Release from nervous tension. New York: Simon & Schuster, 1943.

76. Vachon L, Rich ES Jr. Visceral learning in asthma. Psychosom Med 1976;38:122.

77. Schultz J, Luthe W. Autogenic training: a psychophysiological approach in psychotherapy. New York: Grune & Stratton, 1959.

78. Green E, Green A. Beyond biofeedback. New York: Dell, 1977.

79. Hofbauer L. Pathologische physiologie der atmung. In: Bethe A, Bergmann GV, Emden G, Ellinger A, eds. Handbuch der normalen und pathologischen physiologie. Berlin: Julius Springer, 1925:337.

80. Cournard A, Brock HJ, Rappaport I, et al. Disturbances of the respiratory muscles as contributing cause of dyspnea. Arch Intern Med 1936;57:1008.

81. Dayman HG. Mechanics of airflow in health and emphysema. J Clin Invest 1951;30:1175.

82. Schutz K. Respiratory and physical exercises. Wein Klin Wochenschr 1935;48:392.

83. Livingston JL, Gillespie M. The value of breathing exercises in asthma. Lancet 1935;2:705.

84. Bolton JH, Gandevia B, Ross M. Rationale and results of breathing exercises in asthma. J Australasia 1956;2:675.

85. Dayman HG. Management of dyspnea in emphysema. NY J Med 1956;56:1585.

86. Williams MH Jr, Kane C. Effects of simulated breath sounds on ventilation. J Appl Physiol 1964;19:233.

87. Motley HL: Effects of slow deep breathing on the blood gas exchange in emphysema. Am Rev Respir Dis 1963;88:485.

88. Pfeiffer VR, Wilson NL, Wilson RL. Breathing patterns and gas mixing. J Am Phys Ther [A] 1964;44:331.

89. Thoman RL, Stoken GL, Ross JC. Effacy of pursed-lips breathing in patients with chronic obstructive pulmonary disease. Am Rev Respir Dis 1966;93:100.

90. Meuller RE, Petty TL, Filley GF. Ventilation and arterial blood gas exchanges induced by pursed lips breathing. J Appl Physiol 1970;28:784.

91. Barach AL. Breathing exercises in pulmonary emphysema and allied chronic respiratory disease. Arch Phys Med Rehabil 1955;36:379.

92. Barach AL. Breathing exercises and allied aids to breathing in the treatment of emphysema. Med Rec Ann 1952;46:323.

93. Reich L. Der einfluss des pneumoperitoneum auf das lungen emphysema. Wein Arch Inn Med 1924;8:245.

94. Gaensler EA, Carter MG. Ventilation measurements in pulmonary emphysema treated with pneumoperitoneum. J Lab Clin Med 1950;35:945.

95. Beck GJ, Eastlake C Jr, Barach AL. Venous pressure as a guide to pneumoperitoneum therapy in pulmonary emphysema. Dis Chest 1952;22:130.

96. Mendez C, Guerra F, trans; Kilgore FG, ed. Book of bodily exercise. New Haven: Elizabeth Glick, 1960 [Originally published 1953].

97. Miller WF, Taylor HF, Jasper L. Exercise training in the rehabilitation of patients with obstructive lung disease: the role of oxygen breathing. South Med J 1962;55:1216.

98. Miller WF, Talyor HD, Pierce AK. Rehabilitation of the disabled patient with chronic bronchitis and pulmonary emphysema. Am J Public Health 1963;53:18.

99. Pierce AK, Taylor HF, Archer RK, Miller WF. Responses to exercise training in patients with emphysema. Arch Intern Med 1964;113:28.

100. Donaldson A, Gandevia B. The physiotherapy of emphysema. Aust J Physiother 1962;8:55.

101. White A, Donaldson A, Gandevia B. A therapeutic regimen for the emphysematous patient in hospital. Aust J Physiother 1963;9:68.

102. Cotes JE, Gilson JC. Effect of oxygen on exercise ability in chronic respiratory insufficiency. Use of portable apparatus. Lancet 1956;1:872.

103. Pierce AK, Paez PN, Miller WF. Exercise training with the aid of portable oxygen supply in patients with emphysema. Am Rev Respir Dis 1965;91:653.

104. Paez PN, Phlllipson EA, Masangkay M, Sproule B. The physiologic basis of training patients with emphysema. Am Rev Respir Dis 1967;95:944.

105. Pierce AK, Luterman D, Loudermilk J, Blomqvist G, Johnson RL Jr. Exercise ventilatory patterns in normal subjects and patients with airway obstruction. J Appl Physiol 1968;25:249.

3

LAURA J. REISMAN BEYTAS

GERILYNN L. CONNORS

Organization and Management of a Pulmonary Rehabilitation Program

This chapter examines the ingredients necessary to organize, structure, and manage a new or existing pulmonary rehabilitation program. The planning, execution, and reevaluation of a pulmonary rehabilitation program will be discussed, emphasizing patient assessment through follow-up and determining patient outcomes through a continuous quality improvement management program. Basically, this chapter will cover the ABCs of pulmonary rehabilitation.

PLANNING A PULMONARY REHABILITATION PROGRAM

Laying of the groundwork for a new pulmonary rehabilitation program (PRP) or changing the program options offered by an existing program entails a specific plan of action. This plan must be outlined before approaching administration or the medical staff for support and approval of the program. Program failure occurs if patient resources, financial resources, or physical resources are not evaluated before implementation. Questions to be asked in planning a program can be seen in Table 3–1. A detailed analysis of program planning is outlined in Chapter 28. An investment of time and money to plan the program at this stage will avoid roadblocks or disaster later.

PROGRAM STRUCTURE

The organization and structure of a PRP may vary among facilities, but the *basic components* of pulmonary rehabilitation are the same.[1,2] By understanding the essential components of pulmonary rehabilitation, as seen in Figure 3–1, the implementation of a PRP will be successful. The components of team assessment, patient training, psychosocial intervention, exercise, and follow-up, all need to be carefully outlined for each rehabilitation patient.[3-7] Pulmonary rehabilitation is not just an education or exercise program, but a carefully integrated program that follows a logical sequence (see Fig. 3–1). In fact, pulmonary rehabilitation provides thorough, com-

TABLE   3-1.   **Questions to Be Asked in Planning a Pulmonary Rehabilitation Program**

Goals

What kind of patient population and how many do you want to serve at one time?

Who is the patient population we want to address?

What are the time restraints?

How often will the program meet?

What will the patient evaluation procedure be before, during, and after the program?

Expenses

What are the financial restraints to both the patient and facility?

What is the available personnel?

Is there an existing site or equipment already in use?

How will the program be marketed to the public?

Revenue

Do you have any competition?

How many pulmonary rehabilitation programs are in your area?

What services billed will be reimbursable?

Does the patient have "out-of-pocket" expenses?

Who are the third-party payors servicing your target patient population?

What volume and revenue is generated by your program from ancillary testing?

---

prehensive care for the lung-impaired patient. Pulmonary rehabilitation is individualized to meet the singular needs of each patient.

PATIENT SELECTION AND SEQUENCE

Chronic obstructive pulmonary disease (COPD) and allied conditions ranked as the fifth leading cause of death in the United States in 1988.[8] The challenge for the PRP in meeting the needs of this lung patient population is great and continually growing.[9] Pulmonary rehabilitation is no longer comprehensive care for just patients with COPD, it is appropriate for a wide variety of patients with other lung disorders (Table 3–2).[4,10–18] An individualized PRP can help lung transplant patients, both before and after surgery, those who require ventilator assistance, and occupationally lung-impaired persons. In selecting a potential patient for pulmonary rehabilitation, there are permanent or temporary conditions that may be considered contraindications to such rehabilitation, from severe psychiatric disturbances to other unstable medical conditions, as listed in Table 3–3. The patient may be considered for a pulmonary rehabilitation program in the future, once the "unstable" medical conditions have

(*Text continues on p. 36*).

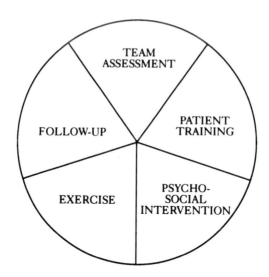

FIGURE 3-1 The essential components of a pulmonary rehabilitation program are team assessment, patient training, psychosocial intervention, exercise, and follow-up. Training or exercise alone does not constitute a pulmonary rehabilitation program.

*Team Assessment**
PR team medical director
Respiratory care practitioner
Nurse
Occupational therapist
Physical therapist
Exercise physiologist
Psychologist
Vocational counselor
Recreational therapist
Social worker
Nutritionist

Exercise
Exercise conditioning
Respiratory muscle strength
Upper extremity strength
Home program plan

Follow-up
Patient outcomes
Maintenance exercise group
Group meetings
Reevaluation as necessary

Patient Training
Breathing retraining
Bronchial hygiene
Medications
Proper nutrition
ADL training
Panic control/relaxation
Energy conservation
Warning signs of infection
Sexuality for COPD patient and others

Psychosocial Intervention
Support system and dependency issues
Anger management
Treatment of depression
Counseling
Self-efficacy for rehabilitation-related behaviors
Impact of role change
Coping styles

* An individualized pulmonary rehabilitation program will meet the specific needs of the patient. Not every member of the pulmonary rehabilitation program team may be involved with the patient.

TABLE 3-2. **Conditions Appropriate for Pulmonary Rehabilitation**

Obstructive pulmonary disease
Chronic obstructive pulmonary disease (COPD)
Asthma
Asthmatic bronchitis
Chronic bronchitis
Emphysema
Bronchiectasis
Cystic fibrosis

Restrictive pulmonary disease
Interstitial fibrosis
Rheumatoid pulmonary disease
Collagen vascular lung disorders
Pneumoconiosis
Sarcoidosis
Kyphoscoliosis
Rheumatoid spondylitis
Severe obesity
Poliomyelitis

Other conditions
Pulmonary vascular diseases
Lung resection
Lung transplantation
Occupational or environmental lung diseases

TABLE 3-3. **Permanent or Temporary Conditions that May Be Considered Contraindication to Pulmonary Rehabilitation**

Severe psychiatric disturbance
Dementia
Organic brain syndrome

Significant or unstable medical conditions
Congestive heart failure
Acute cor pulmonale
Substance abuse
Significant liver dysfunction
Metastatic cancer
Disabling stroke

been appropriately treated or stabilized. This table emphasizes the importance of an initial team assessment to determine patient appropriateness.

When evaluating patients for the PRP, the effect of the lung disease on the patient relative to such things as the basic activities of daily living (ADL), the use of medical resources, and occupational performance needs to be identified. Table 3–4 provides helpful criteria in selecting a patient for pulmonary rehabilitation. This selection process is just the first step of a comprehensive PRP. The issue of a pulmonary rehabilitation patient who smokes and accepting such a candidate for the program who continues to smoke is controversial.[19,20] Obviously, helping a patient quit smoking can be an important part of the pulmonary rehabilitation program. A consideration for allowing such a patient into a PRP may be to help the patient with smoking cessation through assistance by the team members.

Determining patient needs, developing an individualized treatment program, assessing the patient's progress throughout the PRP, and determining the patient's follow-up needs are an important sequence for the PRP patient. Table 3–5 summarizes the sequence of pulmonary rehabilitation. To initiate the process of pulmonary rehabilitation, the potential patient may be referred by a physician or be self-referred. Remember, it is always the responsibility of the PRP medical director to determine the patient's appropriateness for the program.

During the initial assessment component of the program, the patient should be asked about his or her expectations of the program, thereby enhancing program effectiveness and determining if the patient's goals are realistic. If a patient has a vested interest in the program through personal goals, then improved compliance is seen. See Chapter 6 for a detailed explanation of compliance. The assessment of the

---

TABLE 3-4. Criteria to Be Evaluated in Selecting a Patient for Pulmonary Rehabilitation*

- Disease effect on patient's quality of life
- A decrease in physical activity
- Changes in occupational performance
- Dependence vs independence in activities of daily living
- Disease effect on patient's psychosocial status (e.g., anxiety, depression, and such.)
- Use of medical resources (e.g., hospitalizations, emergency room visits, and such.)
- Presence of other medical problems
- Pulmonary function assessment
- Smoking history
- Patient motivation
- Patient commitment to time and active program participation
- Patient transportation needs
- Financial resources
- Patient's background

---

* Any patient with impairment due to lung disease who is motivated should be a candidate for pulmonary rehabilitation.

TABLE   3-5.   **Sequence of Pulmonary Rehabilitation**

1. Patient selection
2. Assess patient needs
3. Develop goals
4. Develop individualized treatment program
5. Assess the progress of goals achieved and the need for
   skilled level of care
6. Reassess the treatment program
7. Develop a home program plan for self-management and
   treatment
8. Determine patient follow-up needs and reassess for
   postprogram therapy

patient's progress during the program is accomplished with team conferences. This is discussed later in the chapter. Goals for home recommendations should be considered at the time of the initial assessment, since it is necessary for each team member to develop a treatment program to meet the patient's needs at home. Variations in the program sequence, as seen in Table 3–5, may occur, but a logical, straightforward process should be understood by every team member involved with the patient. This will enhance program effectiveness and documentation.

PROGRAM ORGANIZATION

The first component of a PRP is team assessment. This team may be the PRP medical director and program director, or a multidisciplinary team. The advantage of a multidisciplinary team approach is to allow each professional to assess, train, and advise the patient on areas of deficiency that fall into his or her specialty area. Regardless of the size of the PRP team, it is essential to have at least a designated program director and medical director to operate a program effectively.

The program director is responsible for the "ABCs of pulmonary rehabilitation." The director's role encompasses program development, management, and marketing. The director may function as a liaison with the team, facilitator of the patient's total treatment program, leader, educator, and communicator. The program director should be trained in a health-related profession, possess the clinical expertise in caring for the lung-impaired patient, and understand the philosophy and goals of pulmonary rehabilitation. The program director works under the guidance and supervision of the program medical director.

The medical director of a PRP should have knowledge in the areas of pulmonary function, exercise testing, acute and chronic pulmonary medicine, treatment of lung disease, along with a special interest in pulmonary rehabilitation. The medical director may function as an administrator, diagnostician, clinician, educator, and research coordinator, serving as a source of knowledge for the PRP team. The medical director should make certain that the PRP patient receives a complete examination to determine accurately the patient's diagnosis and treatment program. This evaluation should include pulmonary function testing, exercise testing, and laboratory testing as appropriate to determine the patient's functional limitations and potential for rehabilitation. See Chapter 4 for a thorough discussion of patient evaluation and testing prior to rehabilitation. After this initial evaluation, the PRP can then be tailored to the patient's needs. As a liaison between the team, the patient, and the patient's primary care physician, the medical director ensures the successful treatment of the patient (Fig. 3–2).

The need for other team members to evaluate the patient will be determined, based on the initial assessment and the patient's deficiencies. Each team member must possess the knowledge and skills to assess, treat, train, reevaluate, document, and determine home recommendations for the patient. In addition, they must be trained on basic life support should such an emergency arise. A list of the core members of the multidisciplinary team can be found in Figure 3–1, under Team Assessment. There are other allied health specialists who may also be considered important contributors to the patient and the program's success, such as the pulmonary function technologist, pharmacist, psychiatrist, chaplain, speech therapist, biofeedback technician, home care personnel, and a business office representative. The smooth working and flow of a PRP will depend on many people in the health care setting, their quality of communication and interaction with the patients and each other. This quality of interaction among the many potential team members during a program is known as the *team* or *family conference* and will determine program success.

It is important to allow each team member the freedom to approach the PRP patient in his or her unique way, yet always being aware of the other team members' contributions. In fact, a successful team member possesses the skills to enhance other team members' training. This is accomplished through regular team conferences (TC) on each patient during the program. The medical director or program director generally begins the TC with a short description of the history, physical examination findings, and test results obtained during the initial PRP assessment. The patient's

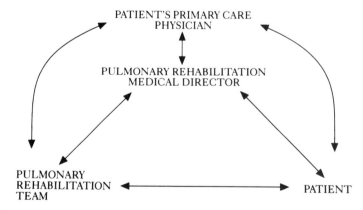

FIGURE   3-2   The medical director's role in a pulmonary rehabilitation program may be as an administrator, diagnostician, clinician, educator, or research coordinator. The medical director is an important liaison between the patient, the patient's primary care physician, and the pulmonary rehabilitation team, ensuring the successful treatment of the pulmonary rehabilitation patient.

stated goals are shared with all the team, so each discipline can direct their training to meet the patient's realistic goals. Then each team member lists the patient's problems and treatment plans in their specific area of expertise, with a discussion leading toward a home program plan. The TC enables the development of an individualized and integrated treatment program for each patient. Documentation of the TC— listing the specific patient problems, limiting factors, treatment plans, and goals for each patient—is important and may be signed by the medical director or program director. A family TC is indicated if the team feels it is necessary to invite family members to meet with them to discuss the patient's program and home goals. The family TC can optimize the patient's discharge plans by making the family aware of the patient's needs and giving the family an opportunity to voice their concerns. The format of the conference is informal, but organized and documented accordingly. In fact, each team member needs to possess the skills needed for documentation, as discussed in Chapter 30.

PROGRAM MANAGEMENT

The PRP must take exceptional care of its customers with superior service and quality of care. Sound budget and financial controls are essential, regardless of the program's operating budget. The PRP needs to be externally focused toward the publics that affect pulmonary rehabilitation, always sensing change and ready to alter the program's direction to adapt to the change (see Chapter 28 for a further explanation of the many publics of pulmonary rehabilitation).

Sound financial control and solid financial planning are necessary for a successful program, but superior customer service and constant program innovation are equally important; these are built on listening, trusting, and respecting the dignity and creative potential of each team member in pulmonary rehabilitation.[22] The difference between a good program and a great program is often the staff, the "turned-on people." The pulmonary patient has specialized needs that are best met by a special type of individual who is competent, often cross-trained, and able to handle emergency situations as they arise. The pulmonary rehabilitation team members must exude a positive attitude and belief in the goals and objectives of pulmonary rehabilitation.[21,23]

An investment of time to initially plan or reevaluate an existing pulmonary rehabilitation program will allow one to avoid roadblocks and prevent unnecessary problems. Specific areas to consider include knowing the program's financial restraints, available personnel, location site, equipment needs, time constraints, the patient population who the pulmonary rehabilitation program is serving, other pulmonary rehabilitation programs in the local area competing for the same patients, and what services provided by the program are reimbursable. This laundry list covers a wide range of topics, but program directors must be knowledgeable managers as well as pulmonary rehabilitation specialists. With a strong understanding of the management needs of a PRP, one can avoid managerial disasters.

In budgeting for a program, determine what are the most essential types of resources needed for the program; what mandates or requirements are imposed on the program through the parent organization, regulatory agencies, or third-party payers; and how best to develop the budget to permit program stability and growth. The budget process is actually a tool used for accomplishing the PRP objectives and looking at program accountability or "outcomes." This process entails budget planning, estimating, managing, coordinating, assessing, reporting, accounting, and projecting the program.[22]

In managing a PRP, the team must be focused, but yet flexible to change as the environment and patient population needs and desires change. External environmental forces that managers will face in the late 20th century and in the 21st century include personnel shortages, population changes, technology advances, increasing and changing government regulations, changes in third-party reimbursement, and increasing competition. Management of a PRP may be complicated and challenging, but it is vital to the successful growth of the program.

A model that Peters emphasizes to lead to business success is: care of the customer, constant innovation, "turned-on people," and leadership.[24] Figure 3–3 adapts this model of success to pulmonary rehabilitation programs. Constant program innovation, laced with team member enthusiasm plus a special caring for the pulmonary rehabilitation client, all overseen by leadership, will result in program success. Peters defines *leadership* as

> . . . vision, cheerleading, enthusiasm, love, trust, verve, passion, obsession, consistency, the use of symbols, paying attention as illustrated by the content of one's calendar, out-and-out drama (and the management thereof), creating heroes at all levels, coaching, effectively wandering around, and numerous other things.[24]

When leadership is present at all levels of a pulmonary rehabilitation program, the model can work and pulmonary rehabilitation will not be added to the "endangered species" list.

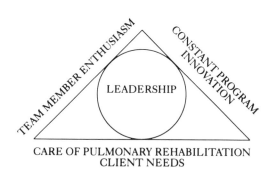

CARE OF PULMONARY REHABILITATION
CLIENT NEEDS

FIGURE   3-3   Program success is a goal every program aims for. Use of the management model for success (which entails constant program innovation coupled with team member enthusiasm), and demonstrating special care for the pulmonary rehabilitation patient, bonded together with strong leadership, results in program success. The ingredients are simple, but when used together will lead to success. (Adapted from Peters T, Austin N. A passion for excellence: The leadership difference. New York: Random House, 1985)

GOALS, OBJECTIVES, AND OUTCOMES

To assist with the direction of the pulmonary rehabilitation program, clear and concise goals and objectives need to be established.[2] In establishing these goals and objectives, keep in mind the mission statement of the "mother" facility from which your program will operate and the fact that pulmonary rehabilitation is not just therapeutic, but is also preventative.[21,25,26] Early screening for lung disease is essential to reach a younger population with less pulmonary disease ("the less–pulmonary-impaired cripple"), so decreases in the mortality rate of COPD and allied conditions can be documented after comprehensive pulmonary rehabilitation.

When the program director maps out the department's goals and objectives, it is important for the team members to be involved also as active participants in establishing these goals and objectives. The program goals are refinements of the mother facility mission statement, but are broadly stated. The goals may address key issues in the program, such as treatment of the client, efficiency, treatment of the team members, growth market standing, innovation, productivity, physical and financial resources, profitability, management performance and development, and team member performance and attitude.[27] The goals are not as specific as the objectives and are open-ended statements of purpose. The goals will describe the program's philosophy. The objectives of the program then become specific statements of the results anticipated. The objectives further define the program's goals. Objectives are important to the program for the following reasons: they provide a specific direction, an integration of team members' actions, a mechanism for control looking at standards of performance that hold the team members accountable for their decisions, to provide motivation to the team by channeling their energies, to help relieve boredom, and to provide feedback on accomplishments resulting in team recognition. Achievement of objectives helps raise team member self-esteem and, when achievement is coupled with feedback, an increase in team member performance may be seen.[27] The objectives should challenge the PRP team members, but not be so demanding that they discourage or create a fear of failure. The number of objectives that are manageable ranges from 6 to 12 for the program.[27] For objectives to be effective, they should be *specific* and not simply "do the best you can."

A pulmonary rehabilitation program is individually tailored to meet the needs of the patient. The setting of realistic patient goals and objectives is important and will allow the patient to know success and have a clear understanding of the target areas to be worked on during the pulmonary rehabilitation program. Another way of looking at objectives is to state them in terms of patient outcomes.[28] With the Joint Commission on Accreditation of Healthcare Organizations (JCAHO) in 1993 expecting outcome measurements in departments, it would be advisable for pulmonary rehabilitation programs to begin using this form of evaluation. The changes of exercise tolerance and symptoms are often looked at in terms of outcomes, but "other" areas of outcome evaluation are also important. Table 3–6 looks at the many areas of outcomes to be considered when evaluating a patient's progress during and after a pulmonary rehabilitation program, from changes in exercise and symptoms to return to work.

TABLE 3-6. Evaluating Patient Outcomes

Changes in exercise tolerance
Pre- and post 6- or 12-min walk
Pre- and postpulmonary exercise stress test
Review of patient home exercise training logs
Strength measurement
Flexibility and posture
Performance on specific exercise training modalities (e.g., ventilatory muscle, upper extremity)

Changes in symptoms
Dyspnea measurements comparison
Frequency of cough, sputum production, or wheezing
Weight gain or loss
Psychologic test instruments

Other changes
Activities of daily living changes
Postprogram follow-up questionnaires
Pre- and postprogram knowledge test
Compliance improvement with pulmonary rehabilitation medical regimen
Frequency and duration of respiratory exacerbations
Frequency and duration of hospitalizations
Frequency of emergency room visits
Return to productive employment

The areas of outcome will continue to be the buzzword of the 1990s as continuous quality improvement (CQI) takes over for quality assurance, and emphasis is placed on outcomes. The CQI idea was developed by W. Edwards Deming in the 1950s. In fact, Deming's ideas revolutionized the Japanese manufacturing industry, and today we see the Deming principles being applied to the health care industry.[29] Total quality management is the focus of the 1990s in the health care industry, and CQI leads to just this. In the past, health care evaluation was based on measuring the ability to provide the care and not on the outcome of the care. Now, with CQI, the end result of the care being rendered is assessed. The enhancement of understanding the effectiveness of different interventions and the promulgation of national practice guidelines for the care providers will result in a decreased variation in data generation, allowing better decision making by the patient, provider, and payor, which is the "outcome" movement. The forces of cost containment, health care restructuring to managed care, and ever-advancing technology promote the emphasis on outcomes. In fact, clinical indicators will measure outcomes.[30,31] The American Association for Respiratory Care is active in writing clinical practice guidelines for respiratory care practices that are a precursor to clinical indicators. Clinical indicators are on the agenda for change in the health care arena and pulmonary rehabilitation programs cannot be excluded from this reality.[31] Program directors, team members, and medical directors need to become familiar with the movement occurring in the health care industry.

POLICY AND PROCEDURE MANUAL

When writing the proposal or policy and procedure manual for the PRP, it should resemble a doctor's prescription. The documents should detail the who, what, why, when, where, and how of pulmonary rehabilitation. The purpose of the policy and procedure manual is to define the rules for program operation. Staff requirements, including the job descriptions, responsibilities, attendance, in-service, evaluation, dress code, and professional behavior need to be stipulated. The policy and procedure manual for the program should include the following areas: the criteria for patient selection and admission to the program; the process of evaluation; an outline of the basic components of pulmonary rehabilitation; hours of operation; a typical program schedule; protocols for exercise testing, training, and medication changes per physician orders; emergency procedures; documentation; continuous quality improvement procedures; and ethical issues to be addressed with the pulmonary rehabilitation patient. Elaboration on the basic components of pulmonary rehabilitation for the manual can be found in subsequent chapters.

Emergency procedures and equipment for the exercise or patient-training location should be described in detail so every team member is aware of the correct process. The mother facility's protocol will provide general emergency instructions, but specific pulmonary rehabilitation program procedures should be noted and understood by all team members.

THE PATIENT SCHEDULE

When organizing the patient's schedule, avoid over-scheduling on the orientation and evaluation days, so that the patient does not become overwhelmed and exhausted at the beginning of the program. Emphasize that the patient should make use of the evenings and scheduled days off by relaxing and practicing what they have learned thus far. The scheduling of exercise sessions between the didactic training sessions can break up the monotony of sitting in one room for 2 to 3 hours. Schedule additional evaluations and testing around the core schedule to avoid having the patient miss a training session. Allow enough time for each training session so the patient will not feel rushed. Vary the type of training used with the patient to meet the goals and objectives of the program (see Chapter 5 for a detailed discussion on the education and training of the PRP patient). Program length may vary depending on the individual patient's needs. Table 3–7 shows a sample 5-week outpatient pulmonary rehabilitation schedule.

PHYSICAL NEEDS

There are many locations from which to operate a PRP that may be considered.[23,32] The traditional outpatient hospital setting is just one example listed in Table 3–8. The inpatient, outpatient, and alternative site locations need to be taken into con-

TABLE   3-7.   Sample Schedule for a 5-wk Pulmonary Rehabilitation Program

Wk No.	*Day*		
1*	**Tuesday**	**Thursday**	**Friday**
1:00–2:00	Orientation	Inhaler training	Supervised exercise
2:00–3:30	Introduction to supervised exercise	Supervised exercise	
3:30–4:30	Breathing retraining	Anatomy and Physiology of disease process	
2			
1:00–2:00	Medication use, part 1	Importance of exercise	Supervised exercise
2:00–3:30	Supervised exercise	Supervised exercise	
3:30–4:30	Panic control	Relaxation training	
3			
1:00–2:00	Understanding tests results (e.g., pulmonary function test)	Group dynamics	Supervised exercise
2:00–3:30	Supervised exercise	Supervised exercise	
3:30–4:30	ADL and energy conservation	Intimate relations	
4			
1:00–2:00	Preventing infection	Nutrition and the lungs	Supervised exercise
2:00–3:30	Supervised exercise	Supervised exercise	
3:30–4:30	Medication use, part 2, oxygen as a medicine	Relaxation training	
5			
1:00–2:00	Travel tips	Environmental factors	Home recommendations (e.g., respiratory therapy, exercise, occupational therapy, etc.)
2:00–3:30	Supervised exercise	DC exercise evaluation	Graduation
3:30–4:30	Group dynamics	Community resources	

* The initial team assessments and medical testing may be performed prior to the program start or during the first week of the program.

TABLE 3-8. Location Options for Pulmonary Rehabilitation Programs

Inpatient care
Acute care during hospitalization
Transitional care unit
Rehabilitation hospital

Outpatient care
Outpatient hospital setting
Physician office
Clinic setting
Residential outpatient facility
Comprehensive outpatient rehabilitation facility (CORF)
Shared facility with other rehabilitation programs

Alternative sites
Storefront
Home residence
Fitness center or spa
Wellness center
Senior citizen center
Local high school or community college
Adult education center
Places of worship
Club meeting halls

sideration when trying to optimize the management and financial bottom lines of the PRP.

For an inpatient program location, the patient's room can be used to train in energy conservation with activities of daily living. A conference room on the patient care unit or the inpatient room may be used for pulmonary rehabilitation training sessions to prevent overtiring the patient. The patient's nurse can then readily find the patient if medications are to be given or if a test has been ordered. The hospital hallway can be used for a walking program, with distances marked off for an objective measurement of improvement.

The outpatient program location should have a central office. A teaching classroom or demonstration room should have easy access for the patient and should accommodate wheelchairs. Hallways, outside walkways, or gymnasiums can be used for exercise training sessions. Adequate parking and easy access to the PRP location are also necessary.

An emotional environment that promotes wellness, comfort, and a sense of caring is essential to the PRP patient, who is often angry or depressed and accustomed to acting out the "sick" role. The patient should be encouraged to communicate and interact with those around him or her. The PRP staff can enhance patient compliance and independence if they deal with the patient firmly, yet kindly, and are sensitive to the patient's needs. Adolescent or cardiac rehabilitation programs do not mix well with the end stage COPD patient, for these groups do not identify well with each other and will only lead to discouragement for the PRP patient.

Equipment needs will depend upon the services provided, staff used, and the program budget, but emergency equipment for cardiopulmonary resuscitation is always needed.[18,19] The team and program components, rather than elaborate equipment, are what make a good program. Program equipment may be divided into four general categories: exercise, training materials, respiratory care, and patient monitoring. Table 3–9 lists equipment considerations for a PRP. Not all the equipment listed in Table 3–9 is necessary, but specific equipment needs do exist in each area for every pulmonary rehabilitation program. The equipment budget for a PRP should take into consideration the equipment expenses in relation to its maintenance, depreciation, and purchase. Regardless of equipment or space used for a PRP, it must be safe and create a comfortable environment for the pulmonary rehabilitation patient.

TABLE 3-9. Equipment Considerations for Pulmonary Rehabilitation Programs

Exercise
Walking track or measured distance
Treadmill
Free weights (cuff weights, dumbbells)
Stationary bicycle
Ventilatory muscle trainer
Mats
Arm ergometer
Latex bands
Stair simulator
Rowing machine
Universal gym
Nautilus equipment
Swimming pool

Training materials
Patient manual
Chalk, marking pens, eraser
Chalkboard/whiteboard
VCR
Overhead projector
Slide projector
Flip charts
Models
Tape recorder
Paper, pencils, pens

Respiratory care
Oxygen source (e.g., cylinders, liquid, concentrators)
Oxygen tubing, cannulae, TTOs
Oxygen-conserving devices
Metered-dose inhalers
Nebulizers and setups
Oral medications
Tilt table

Patient monitoring
Pulse oximeter—portable and/or stationary
Blood pressure manometer
Stethoscope
Spirometer
Cardiac telemetry
Pedometer
Timers, second-hand watch
Data flow sheets, charting forms, pens
Patient chart

TABLE 3-10. Follow-up Options for Pulmonary Rehabilitation Programs

Regular physician visits

Maintenance exercise group

Program graduate group outings and trips

Program graduate group meetings

Referral to community groups (e.g., American Lung Association's "Better Breathers Club")

Phone follow-up by program staff

Newsletters

Postprogram questionnaires

Reevaluation as indicated

Home health referral

Home visits

Activities during National Pulmonary Rehabilitation Week (observed during the first week of spring)

PROGRAM FOLLOW-UP

The follow-up needs of a pulmonary rehabilitation graduate should be considered at program initiation. What needs the patient will have at the end of the program are based on the patient's achieved or open goals. The reason for program failure is often the lack of patient follow-through on home recommendations developed by the PRP team. The patient becomes skeptical of the progress potential he or she can attain if a system is not present to continually encourage the patient. Therefore, postprogram follow-up must be given a strong emphasis during the entire rehabilitation program. To assist with the patients follow-through of team home recommendations, the patient's primary care physician should receive specific patient records from the program. These records should include a cover letter from the program medical director or coordinator, all test results, consultation, the discharge team conference report, and outlined home recommendations the patient has been instructed to follow. Making an appointment for the patient's first follow-up visit during the admission may also emphasize to the patient that they will not be "dropped" after graduating from the program. This visit may include an interview concerning the patient's progress at home, actual demonstration of techniques learned, and a review of the patient's exercise and medication programs. The patient should feel they can always contact the PRP office if a question or concern arises and be assured there will always be a caring and interested team member to help them. The PRP staff office is a very good resource to the PRP graduate. Table 3–10 lists the various program follow-up options that may be considered. Remember, to evaluate patient outcomes, follow-up is necessary.

SUMMARY

The process of pulmonary rehabilitation program management is very specific. The potential customers, team members, and creative ideas of a pulmonary rehabilitation program will lead to program success or demise. An understanding that pulmonary rehabilitation is not just for the COPD patient is critical to expand the potential clients that may be helped by a comprehensive, individualized pulmonary rehabilitation program. The basic components of pulmonary rehabilitation from team assessment, patient training, psychosocial intervention, exercise, to follow-up must be understood by each team member. Documentation of patient outcomes will allow program growth and enhancement. The ABCs of pulmonary rehabilitation must be followed for program success.

Acknowledgment

We wish to thank Neil MacIntyre, M.D., for his review of this manuscript and for his helpful suggestions.

REFERENCES

1. Hodgkin JE. Organization of a pulmonary rehabilitation program. Clin Chest Med 1986;7:541.

2. Hodgkin JE, Farrell MJ, Gibson SR, et al. Pulmonary rehabilitation: official ATS statement. Am Rev Respir Dis 1981;124:663.

3. Butts JR. Pulmonary rehabilitation through exercise and education. Respir Ther 1981;37.

4. Ziment I. Helping asthma patients help themselves, improving treatment compliance among your respiratory patients. J Respir Dis 1980;2

5. Maddox SE. Planning, implementing, and managing a self-administration of medications program in the hospital. Unpublished manuscript given at pulmonary symposium at Hoag Memorial Hospital Presbyterian; Newport, CA, Dec 1981.

6. Kaplan RM, Reis A, Atkins, CJ. Area review: behavioral management of chronic obstructive pulmonary disease, behavioral issues in the management of chronic obstructive pulmonary disease. Ann Behav Med 1985;7(4):5.

7. McKay DA, Blake RL, Colwill JM, et al. Social supports and stress as predictors of illness. J Fam Pract 1985;20:575.

8. US Dept of Commerce, Bureau of the Census, 110th ed. Statistical abstract of the United States, 1990:79.

9. Tiep BL. Reversing disability of irreversible lung disease. In: Rehabilitation medicine: adding life to years [special issue]. West J Med 1991;154:591.

10. Lertzman MM, Cherniack DR. Rehabilitation of patients with chronic obstructive pulmonary disease. Am Rev Respir Dis 1976;114:1145.

11. Miller WF. Rehabilitation of patients with chronic obstructive lung disease. Med Clin North Am 1967;51:349.

12. Hazinski T. Bronchial hyperreactivity in infants. Respir Care 1991;36(7):735.

13. Orenstein DM. Cystic fibrosis. Respir Care 1991;36(7):746.

14. Martin RJ, Chatburn RL. Respiratory care of infants and children: conference summary. Respir Care 1991;36(7):757.

15. Squires RW, Allison TG, Miller TD, Gan GT. Cardiopulmonary exercise testing after unilateral lung transplantation: a case report. J Cardiopulm Rehabil 1991;11(3):192.

16. Owen RR. Postpolio syndrome and cardiopulmonary conditioning. In: Rehabilitation medicine: adding life to years [special issue]. West J Med, 1991;154:557.

17. Ries AL. Position paper of the American Association of Cardiovascular and Pulmonary Rehabilitation: Scientific basis of pulmonary rehabilitation. J Cardiopulm Rehabil 1990; 10(11):418.

18. Bickford LS, Hodgkin JE. National pulmonary rehabilitation survey. Respir Care 1988;33:1030.

19. Callahan M. A prudent pulmonary rehabilitative program. Am J Nurs 1985; 85(12):1368.

20. US Dept of Health and Human Services. How you can help patients stop smoking, opportunities for respiratory care practitioners. Public Health Service, National Institutes of Health, NIH Publ No. 89-2961; 1989.

21. Balchum OJ. What rehabilitation for COPD patients should entail. J Respir Dis 1986;7:68.

22. Vinter RD, Kish RK. Budgeting for not-for-profit organizations. London: Collier Macmillan Publishers, 1984.

23. Parham JD. Developing an integrated community-based system of extended rehabilitation services. J Rehabil 1989;55:64.

24. Peters TJ. A passion for excellence. New York: Random House, 1985.

25. Hudson LD, et al. Hospitalization needs during an outpatient rehabilitation program for severe chronic airway obstruction. Chest 1976;70:606.

26. Petty TL. Ambulatory care for emphysema and chronic bronchitis. Chest 1970;58 (suppl 2):441.

27. Higgins JM. The planning process and organization purpose. In: The management challenge. An introduction to management. New York: Macmillan Publishing, 1991:145.

28. Burns MR, Sherman B, Madison R, Kao D, Petty TL. Pulmonary rehabilitation outcomes. J Respir Care Pract 1989;2:25.

29. Lynn ML, Osborn DP. Deming's quality principles: a health care application. Hosp Health Serv Admin, 1991;36:1.

30. Audet A, Greenfield S, Field M. Medical practice guidelines: current activities and future directions. Ann Intern Med 1990;113:709.

31. Summary Second National Invitational Forum on Clinical Indicator Development, Joint Commission on Accreditation of Healthcare Organizations, 1989.

32. Nielsen-Tietsort J, Repsher LE: Storefront pulmonary rehabilitation. AARC Times, 1990;14(6):42.

GERILYNN L. CONNORS

LANA R. HILLING

KATHLEEN V. MORRIS

Assessment of the Pulmonary Rehabilitation Candidate

The initial assessment of a pulmonary rehabilitation candidate is one of the most critical components of a pulmonary rehabilitation program.[1] Its purpose is to determine the correct pulmonary diagnosis, to determine if there are problems with other organ systems that need to be considered, and to assess the patient's needs so that a comprehensive individualized program for the patient can be outlined.[2] Education, exercise, or psychosocial interventions alone or together do not constitute a pulmonary rehabilitation program. The program must incorporate a thorough assessment and appropriate follow-up for comprehensive pulmonary rehabilitation intervention to be carried out.[3] An understanding of this concept is important, since the pulmonary rehabilitation program needs to be individualized to meet each patient's needs. Only through appropriate team assessment can this be done. The foundation of the patient's individualized program is formulated from the goals and objectives established during the initial team assessment. Patient achievement of these personalized goals and objectives will result in program success. The initial team assessment is the precursor to patient training, psychosocial support, exercise, and follow-up that together formulate a comprehensive pulmonary rehabilitation program (Fig. 4–1).

Patient assessment is performed by those members of the pulmonary rehabilitation team, as warranted. A physical therapy assessment or occupational therapy assessment is considered important if deficits are noted in these areas, but an assessment by a physician oriented to pulmonary rehabilitation is often overlooked. The physician should be a vital member of the pulmonary rehabilitation team and assist in the assessment of the patient (Fig. 4–2). When program directors and staff members consider a physician as an essential member of the team, other physicians and medical staff will, in turn, recognize the importance of the physician's role. The pulmonary rehabilitation team physician's assessment does not diminish the role of the patient's primary care physician. It is simply one of the team assessments necessary for a thorough evaluation.

During the initial assessment, the pulmonary rehabilitation program director should consider the following areas as they relate to the pulmonary rehabilitation

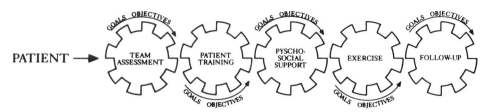

FIGURE 4-1 The essential components of pulmonary rehabilitation are very specific. Once the initial assessment is completed, the foundation of the patient's individualized program is developed from the goals and objectives established. It is essential for each component to be incorporated into a comprehensive pulmonary rehabilitation program.

patient: degree of motivation, financial limitations, pulmonary diagnosis, other concurrent medical problems or conditions, and the reasonableness of the patient's goals and expectations of the program.

THE ASSESSMENT

The initial assessment is the cornerstone of the pulmonary rehabilitation program's development for each patient. It is not only an invaluable tool for getting to know the patient; it is also an opportunity to ascertain the medical problems.[4,5] The assessment should be conducted in a comfortable and private setting to allow free and open discussion by the patient. The interviewer should allow ample time for the exchange so the patient does not feel hurried. A proper introduction with an explanation for the necessity of the assessment is a prerequisite. The attitude of the interviewer should be pleasant, demonstrating sincerity and warmth. Even with the difficult patient, it is

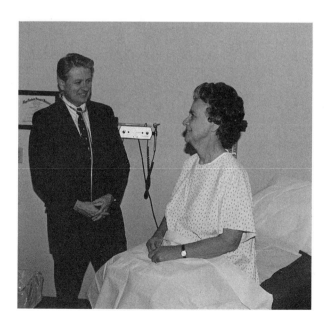

FIGURE 4-2 The physician, a vital member of the pulmonary rehabilitation team, is also involved in the assessment of the patient. This physician assessment does not diminish the role of the patient's primary care physician, but is simply one of the "team" assessments necessary for thorough evaluation and treatment of the pulmonary rehabilitation patient.

important that the interviewer remember that the anger often shown is due to the patient's physical limitations and disease, which can result in frustration and denial. Awareness of the patient's attitude is foremost in establishing an effective interchange of information. The recognition of fear, anger, denial, frustration, depression, intolerance, or low self-esteem displayed by the patient will assist the interviewer in guiding an informative discussion.

To assist the interviewer with the process, it is helpful to have a form specifically developed to cover the pertinent symptoms and areas of assessment. An example of this form is found in Table 4–1. Use of a similar form will ensure that the initial assessment is comprehensive and evaluates the needs of the pulmonary rehabilitation patient. Reasons for a poor assessment include the following: inadequate questions asked and responses given, failure to record the patient's negative responses or uneasiness at the start of the interview, an unstructured assessment process, repeated questioning resulting from failure to record the patient's responses, a sense of being rushed, lack of eye contact, communication errors (such as interrupting the patient or "putting words in the patient's mouth"), and the use of technical medical language.[4]

The assessment will be only as good as the interviewer.[6] The interviewer needs to take note of the potential errors and develop skills to achieve maximum results with accurate information. It is important to remember that the more organized the interviewer, the more accurate the data collected, and the more time-efficient the approach.

Besides using a standard pulmonary rehabilitation assessment form, it is also helpful to have the patient fill out a medical history questionnaire before the assessment. This questionnaire should have an area to list current medications used, including dosage, frequency of administration, and reason for medication use. Leading off the assessment with the medical history questionnaire will assist the process by decreasing the need to ask repetitive questions. Table 4–2 suggests questions to include on a medical history questionnaire.

Financial Status

Since most patients participating in a pulmonary rehabilitation program are older than 65, Medicare is their primary insurance. This means the patient population is probably on a fixed income and may or may not have secondary insurance. Potential patients are often reluctant to pursue pulmonary rehabilitation programs because of the cost, assuming they will not be able to afford it. Therefore, an understanding of a patient's financial concerns and how much money they will have to pay out-of-pocket for the program is key to their participation. If finances are of major concern to the patient, this could interfere with the rehabilitation process. The financial issue needs to be resolved before the patient begins the program (see Chapter 30 for more details).

Patient Motivation

Is the patient coming to the pulmonary rehabilitation program because his or her spouse insisted and made all the arrangements? Or is the patient coming because his or her physician ordered the program? Does the patient have a desire—a need—to do

TABLE 4-1. Pulmonary Rehabilitation Evaluation Form

Primary Diag: _____

_____

Chief complaint: _____

_____

Medical History

____ Cardiac complications
____ Hypertension
____ Diabetes
____ GI problems
____ Reflux/hiatal hernia
____ Orthopedic problems
____ PND/sinus problems
____ Vision/hearing
____ Childhood illnesses
____ Other _____

Symptoms

Y	N	Cough	Freq ____
Y	N	Sputum	
		Volume ____	Color ____
		Viscosity ____	Freq ____
Y	N	Wheeze	
		Onset/cause ____	
Y	N	Fluid retention	
		Where ____	When ____
Y	N	Dyspnea	
		Onset/Cause ____	
Y	N	Sleeping problems	#Hrs ____
Y	N	Extra pillows	# ____

Dyspnea Index (Circle one)

Class 1: If SOB, consistent with activity
Class 2: SOB climbing hills or stairs
Class 3: Can walk at own pace but not at normal pace without SOB
Class 4: SOB walking 100 yds on level ground, dressing, or talking

Metered-dose inhalers (MDI)

MDI 1 _____
  Prescription _____
MDI 2 _____
  Prescription _____
MDI 3 _____
  Prescription _____
MDI 4 _____
  Prescription _____

| Y | N | Needs spacer |
| Y | N | Needs training |

Allergies

Food: _____
Medications: _____
Other: _____

Occupation

Occupation _____
Retirement/disability date _____

Occupational Exposures:

____ Farm/ranch	____ Pottery
____ Welding	____ Gas/fumes
____ Mines/foundry	____ Chemicals
____ Sand blasting	____ Dust
____ Quarry	____ Asbestos

Respiratory infections/hospitalization

____ Infections/year (no.)
  Antibiotic use: _____
____ Hospitalizations/year (no.)
  When: _____
  Problem _____

Vaccines   Flu ____ (year)
     Pneumonia ____ (year)

| Y | N | Aware of warning signals? |

Smoking History

Y	N	Quit date _____
		____ Packs ____ Years
Y	N	Second-hand smoke

Breathing Retraining

Y	N	Pursed-lips breathing
Y	N	Diaphragm breathing
Y	N	Accessory muscle use

Objective

B/P ____	Br Sds ____
HR ____	Edema ____
RR ____	Other ____

Aerosol Therapy

| Y | N | Hand-held nebulizer |

Vendor: _____
Medication: Type   Dose

_____

Frequency prescribed vs use: _____

Oxygen therapy

| Y | N | Oxygen therapy |
| Y | N | Needs training |

System/vendor: _____

(*continued*)

TABLE 4-1. (*continued*)

Oral medications		Fluid intake (glasses/day)	
_____	_____	_____ Water	_____ Beer
_____	_____	_____ Soda	_____ Hard liquor
_____	_____	_____ Wine	_____ Coffee
_____	_____	_____ Juice	_____ Tea

Stress management   **Nutrition**

Stressors _____   Appetite _____

_____   Diet _____

Relaxation techniques _____   Restaurants/week _____

Current exercise program _____   Salt use (restriction) _____

Leisure activities _____   Vitamins _____

Assessment

1. Understanding of diagnosis _____

_____

2. Personal goals _____

_____

3. _____

Plan

1. _____
2. _____
3. _____

Staff   Date

(Courtesy of the Pulmonary Rehabilitation Department at St. Helena Hospital, Napa Valley, CA)

more for him- or herself, wish to live independently, improve the quality of life, and optimize the level of lung health? Knowing the patient's reasons for participating in a pulmonary rehabilitation program will help the interviewer understand the patient's motivational level and interest. However, just because a patient does not immediately express a desire to participate, does not rule him or her out. Many program directors relate stories of a patient who was most difficult at the beginning of a program, but completed the program as one of the most compliant. Team member intervention during a program can help identify the reasons for poor motivation, such as fear, low self-esteem, guilt, anger, or depression. Goals and objectives are then established by the team and the patient to address the issues related to motivation. The interviewer needs to discern the patient's perception of his or her disease so that the team will know where to start in helping the patient achieve better health through successful rehabilitation.

It is important for the interviewer to recognize that patients with severe lung disease have great difficulty believing that they will be able to cope with the pulmo-

TABLE 4–2. Sample Questions for a Medical History Questionnaire

- Please list the main problem or reason for which you are coming to pulmonary rehabilitation:
- How long ago did you first develop any problem with your lungs or breathing? Please describe what the problem was.
- Have you ever been told you have asthma? If yes, when?
- Have you every been told you have chronic bronchitis? If yes, when?
- Have you ever been told you have emphysema? If yes, when?
- Have you ever been told you have COPD? If yes, when?
- Do you have a cough? If yes, how long have you had it? If yes, how many days per month do you have a cough?
- Do you cough up phlegm or sputum? If yes, on the average, how much phlegm do you cough up per day? If yes, for how many years have you coughed up phlegm? If yes, what color is your phlegm?
- Do you become short of breath? If yes, what do you have to do to get short of breath? If yes, how far can you walk on a flat surface at a normal pace before you become short of breath?
- Do you ever become short of breath at night? If yes, how often? If yes, how long has this been happening? If yes, what do you do to relieve your shortness of breath?
- Have you ever been told you have an abnormal chest x-ray? If yes, when? If yes, what were you told?
- Does your nose plug up or get congested? If yes, how often? If yes, for how long has this been happening?
- Do you have postnasal drainage? If yes, how often? If yes, for how long has this been happening?
- Do you ever have heartburn? If yes, how often does this happen?
- Do you ever have regurgitation of food or fluid from your stomach back up into your mouth? If yes, how often does this happen?
- Have you ever been told you have a hiatal hernia? If yes, when?
- Do you ever have chest pain? If yes, answer the following: What brings on your chest pain? Where in your chest is the pain? What do you do to relieve your chest pain?
- Do your feet or ankles ever swell? If yes, how often?
- Please list all medications you are currently using, their dose, how many times each day you take them, and reason for medication use.
- Please list any medications you have tried in the past and quit using, and why you quit them.

nary rehabilitation team recommendations, especially in using exercise as a treatment for their conditions. Since shortness of breath increases with exercise in patients with severe lung disease, this commonly results in a fear of activity that not only limits traditional exercise, but daily-living activities as well.[7] A recognition of the patient's level of self-efficacy or perceived internal control can greatly assist the interviewer in enhancing motivational levels during the assessment.[8] The patient's perceived internal control has been described by Bandura as two distinct attributes.[8] The first is the belief that the recommended behavior will lead to a favorable outcome (*outcome expectation*), and the second is the belief that the behavior required to produce the outcome can be executed (*efficacy expectation*). Efficacy and outcome expectations need to be differentiated because ". . . individuals can come to believe that a particular course of action will result in certain outcomes, but question whether they can perform those actions."[8]

Although patients may have been referred to the pulmonary rehabilitation program by their physician, they may believe this recommendation will exceed their coping capability. Patients' judgment of self-efficacy can limit how much motivational intent they demonstrate and how long they will persist when their perceived lack of control, in the form of shortness of breath, presents itself as a limiting factor.

Pulmonary rehabilitation programs designed to provide mastery experiences in particular situations will stimulate the participants to increase their expectations for success in similar situations or future activities. The more successful they become at this kind of personal management, the better they are motivated to perform.[9]

The interviewer can assist in initially stimulating motivation by helping participants review their history, identifying situations where shortness of breath was not the limiting factor in performance. These efforts, complemented by reassurance that the participant's activities in the program will be modified to meet their tolerance levels, will reinforce their ability to believe they can participate and perform at a satisfactory level without embarrassment in an exercise–activity intervention.

Another adjunct to understanding a patient's motivational level is to assess how their lung disease has affected their quality of life.[10,11] Just the assessment of the patient's severity of airflow limitation (based on pulmonary function analysis) does not give an accurate basis for determining how this severity has affected their functional status and quality of life.[12] Pulmonary function analysis and impaired quality of life do not correlate well. Therefore, direct questioning is needed to assess the lung disease influence on the functions and quality-of-life issues.

Quality-of-life assessment in lung disease is not a simple issue. It includes several major areas of dysfunction: dyspnea, mastery, fatigue, sleep disturbances, and various aspects of emotional dysfunction (e.g., anxiety, depression, fear).[10] How best can we measure quality of life in the chronically ill patient? Illness is an intensely personal and unique experience; each patient perceives differently its threat to all that is meaningful.

Patients do not volunteer information readily, but need to be probed for answers, especially in the area of emotional dysfunction. The patient's perception of his or her disease is an important determining factor in how it will affect the quality of life. As the integrity of the body changes, so does one's sense of well-being. The interviewer must take into account all aspects of the participant's life-style: the physical, mental, emotional, and spiritual.[13] A knowledge of the impairments and limitations that exist will help the patient and pulmonary rehabilitation team develop appropriate goals and objectives. Specific areas to look at in assessing a patient's quality of life are listed in Table 4–3.[10] The interviewer needs to identify the areas of physical, social, or emotional dysfunction the patient is experiencing. Given a patient's individual needs, psychiatry, psychology, or a social service assessment and follow-up may be indicated.

TABLE 4–3.   Specific Areas of Quality-of-Life Impairment

Physical	Social and emotional
Dyspnea	Social limitations
Cough	Dependency issues
Sputum production	Embarrassment
Wheezing	Anger
Mastery*	Anxiety
Fatigue	Frustration
Sleep disturbances	Hostility
Depression	Fear
Cognitive impairment	Panic
Ambulation problems	Impatience
Mobility	Irritability

* The degree to which patient feels control over his disease or its manifestations.

History and Symptoms

The information gathered during the history should include the following: chief complaint, history of present problems, date of onset, nature of complaint, cause of complaint, location, exacerbations, previous hospitalizations, treatment, past medical history, childhood diseases, occupational history and exposures, smoking history, dietary habits, sleep habits, medications prescribed, and over-the-counter drugs used.[4] The form (see Table 4–1) discussed earlier covers these areas. As the interviewer progresses through the history, it is crucial to document the symptoms stated by the patient by obtaining very specific information on each. Table 4–4 describes how each symptom should be analyzed to ensure a comprehensive assessment.[14] The most common symptoms and signs considered for the lung patient are cough, sputum, wheezing, shortness of breath, hemoptysis, chest pain or tightness, and fluid retention.[6]

Symptoms associated with nasal, sinus, or gastrointestinal problems often go overlooked during the history. These "other" systems that need to be considered in evaluating the pulmonary rehabilitation patient are listed in Table 4–5. It is important to know if the patient has other aggravating factors that will limit achievement of optimum lung health and rehabilitation.[15] Only by questioning the patient during the history will this information be retrieved. If aspiration of nasal, sinus, or stomach secretions occurs, the airways will be constantly aggravated, worsening the symptoms. No matter how good a pulmonary rehabilitation program is, the patient will never reach his or her full rehabilitation potential unless these aggravating conditions are identified and treated.

Cough is one of the most common symptoms of lung disease. The patient often underestimates its frequency. Smokers will commonly minimize or deny the symptom

TABLE 4-4. Symptom Analysis of Cough—An Example

Interviewer questions	Patient response
Onset	About 1 yr ago
Location	Not applicable
Quality	Deep, productive cough
Quantity	2–3 tablespoons sputum
Frequency and duration	Daily, first few hours in the morning, for the past 12 mo
Aggravating factors	Sinus drainage
Alleviating factors	Nothing
Associated factors	Worsens with chest cold
Course	No change in frequency noticed, even with seasons

saying it is just a "smoker's cough." The interviewer needs to observe how many times a patient coughs during the interview. It is also recommended that the patient's significant other be asked how often the patient coughs to get a more accurate history, especially for evaluation of the patient's cough during the night.

Sputum production is socially unpleasant and often forces the patient to swallow or minimize its presence. The interviewer needs to question the patient to determine if the sputum is coming from the nasal area (postnasal drainage) or from the lungs, and document the specific characteristics of the sputum as stated by the patient, such as its color, volume, viscosity, and odor. When describing volume, it is often easier for patients to visualize how much sputum is produced by having them put it in terms of a teaspoon (5 mL) or a tablespoon (15 mL).

Dyspnea is a very subjective symptom that is based on perception, but the team needs to understand how the patient feels about his or her breathing.[16] When determining the extent of dyspnea, the interviewer should ascertain if the dyspnea occurs at rest, occurs with activity or exertion, awakens the patient at night, or is continuous. Dyspnea may be more profound with upper extremity activities, such as combing or shampooing the hair. The patient may have given up trying to shower, climb stairs, or go out with friends when keeping up with their friends' pace is too difficult. There is often great denial about dyspnea, since it has an insidious onset,

TABLE 4-5. "Other" Systems to Be Considered in Evaluating the Pulmonary Rehabilitation Candidate

Nasal/sinus
Gastrointestinal
Cardiovascular
Musculoskeletal

progresses slowly, and allows patients to adjust their life-style according to their breathing capacity. Patients will gradually avoid activities or outings during which they might experience dyspnea. An important point to remember is that dyspnea generally correlates well with the work of breathing, but not with the level of hypoxemia. Dyspnea occurs because of a disturbance in ventilatory function. The onset of dyspnea with exertion is a much earlier sign of physiologic impairment than dyspnea at rest.[17] Because the patient's report of dyspnea is very subjective, it is helpful to use some type of dyspnea scale that can give a degree of objectivity to this symptom. In evaluating dyspnea, the Baseline Dyspnea Index is one such scale that correlates well with physiologic measurements (Table 4–6).[18] The use of this scale can provide a quantification of dyspnea that looks at three areas: functional impairment, magnitude of task, and magnitude of effort effecting breathlessness. Other methods used to evaluate dyspnea are the Oxygen–Cost Diagram and the Medical Research Council Scale, but these are based on only the performance of physical tasks.

Wheezing means airway narrowing from such things as bronchospasm, edema, or mucus. The interviewer needs to elicit carefully what the term *wheezing* means to the patient. It is important to clarify if there is true wheezing or if the individual is just clearing the throat. The interviewer needs to determine when wheezing occurs and what the triggers may be (e.g., cold, humidity, molds, mildew, seasonal changes, allergies, or stress).

Chest pain may be esophageal, precordial, tracheobronchial, pleuritic, cardiac, or musculoskeletal. In characterizing chest pain, the interviewer should note the location, severity, setting, what relieves it, and what aggravates it. Chest pain most commonly arises from areas other than the lungs.

TABLE 4–6. Baseline Dyspnea Index

Functional impairment

_____ Grade 4: *No impairment.* Able to carry out usual activities* and occupation without shortness of breath.

_____ Grade 3: *Slight impairment.* Distinct impairment in at least one activity, but no activities completely abandoned. Reduction, in activity at work *or* in usual activities, that seems slight or not clearly caused by shortness of breath.

_____ Grade 2: *Moderate impairment.* Patient has changed jobs and/or has abandoned at least one usual activity due to shortness of breath.

_____ Grade 1: *Severe impairment.* Patient unable to work *or* has given up most or all usual activities due to shortness of breath.

_____ Grade 0: *Very severe impairment.* Unable to work *and* has given up most of all usual activities due to shortness of breath.

(continued)

* Usual activities refer to requirements of daily living, maintenance or upkeep of residence, yard work, gardening, shopping, etc. (Mahler DA, et al. The measurement of dyspnea: contents, interobserver, agreement, and physiologic correlates of two new clinical indexes. Chest 1984;45:751, with permission)

TABLE 4–6. (*continued*)

⎯⎯	W:	*Amount uncertain.* Patient is impaired due to shortness of breath, but amount cannot be specified. Details are not sufficient to allow impairment to be categorized.
⎯⎯	X:	*Unknown.* Information regarding impairment unavailable.
⎯⎯	Y:	*Impaired for reasons other than shortness of breath,* for example, musculoskeletal problem or chest pain.

Magnitude of task

⎯⎯	Grade 4:	*Extraordinary.* Becomes short of breath only with extraordinary activity such as carrying very heavy loads on the level, lighter loads uphill, or running. No shortness of breath with ordinary tasks.
⎯⎯	Grade 3:	*Major.* Becomes short of breath only with major activities as walking up a steep hill, climbing more than three flights of stairs, or carrying a moderate load on the level.
⎯⎯	Grade 2:	*Moderate.* Becomes short of breath with moderate or average tasks such as walking up a gradual hill, climbing less than three flights of stairs, or carrying a light load on the level.
⎯⎯	Grade 1:	*Light.* Becomes short of breath with light activities such as walking on the level, washing, or standing.
⎯⎯	Grade 0:	*No Task.* Becomes short of breath at rest, while sitting, or lying down.
⎯⎯	W:	*Amount uncertain.* Patient's ability to perform tasks is impaired due to shortness of breath, but amount cannot be specified. Details are not sufficient to allow impairment to be categorized.
⎯⎯	X:	*Unknown.* Information unavailable regarding limitation of magnitude or task.
⎯⎯	Y:	*Impaired for reasons other than shortness of breath.* For example, musculoskeletal problem or chest pain.

Magnitude of effort

⎯⎯	Grade 4:	*Extraordinary.* Becomes short of breath only with the greatest imaginable effort. No shortness of breath with ordinary effort.
⎯⎯	Grade 3:	*Major.* Becomes short of breath with effort distinctly submaximal, but of major proportion. Tasks performed without pause unless the task requires extraordinary effort that may be performed with pauses.
⎯⎯	Grade 2:	*Moderate.* Becomes short of breath with moderate effort. Tasks performed with occasional pauses and requiring longer to complete than the average person.
⎯⎯	Grade 1:	*Light.* Becomes short of breath with little effort. Tasks performed with little effort or more difficult tasks performed with frequent pauses and requiring 50% to 100% longer to complete than the average person might require.
⎯⎯	Grade 0:	*No effort.* Becomes short of breath at rest, while sitting, or lying down.
⎯⎯	W:	*Amount uncertain.* Patient's exertional ability is impaired due to shortness of breath, but amount cannot be specified. Details are not sufficient to allow impairment to be categorized.
⎯⎯	X:	*Unknown.* Information unavailable regarding limitation of effort.
⎯⎯	Y:	*Impaired for reasons other than shortness of breath.* For example, musculoskeletal problems or chest pain.

Fluid retention in the extremities may be a result of the chronic lung disease causing cor pulmonale. Long-term hypoxemia, caused by lung disease, places an extra burden on the right side of the heart, resulting in right ventricular hypertrophy and impedance of venous blood flow back to the heart. The peripheral blood vessels become engorged with fluid, resulting in leakage of this fluid into the subcutaneous tissue. Because of gravity, this fluid retention is seen in the ankle or pretibial area. When checking the patient for fluid retention, remember to evaluate both lower legs. An increase in weight over a short period is suggestive of fluid retention. It is important to note if the patient awakens with edema, or if it occurs predominantly toward evening. Checking for fluid retention is one way to evaluate right heart function.

Significant weight loss (below the ideal body weight) contributes to a decrease in the maximum respiratory muscle force, a decrease in the hypoxic ventilatory response, and a decrease in resistance to infection.[19] Loss of muscle mass, especially in the respiratory muscles, occurs in malnutrition. Malnutrition increases morbidity and mortality.[20] (See Chapter 17 for an extensive coverage of nutrition.)

The importance of assessing other systems was mentioned earlier and will now be expanded. Nasal symptoms from allergic rhinitis are caused by exposure to inhaled allergens. The symptoms may be categorized according to location: the nose, the paranasal sinuses, the middle ear, the eyes, or generalized.[21] Table 4–7 summarizes the symptoms associated with allergic rhinitis by location. Vasomotor rhinitis is another cause of excessive nasal secretions. The etiology is unclear, but the symptoms are described in Table 4–8.[22] Another cause for postnasal drainage of secretions is sinusitis. It results in swelling of the sinus mucosa and obstruction of the ostium, leading to retention of purulent secretions. The symptoms and signs associated with sinusitis are described in Table 4–9.[23]

TABLE 4–7.   The Symptoms of Allergic Rhinitis by Location

Nose	Paranasal sinuses	Middle ear	Eyes	Generalized
Rhinorrhea	Headache	Pressure	Redness	Fatigue
Sneezing	Facial pressure	Itching	Discharge	Malaise
Nasal itching	Congestion	Popping	Itching	
Nasal obstruction				
Increased nasal secretions				
Postnasal drainage stimulating cough reflex				

(Adapted from Druce HM, Kaliner MA. Allergic rhinitis. In: Cherniack RM, ed. Current therapy of respiratory disease—2. Toronto: BC Decker, 1986:7)

TABLE 4–8. Symptoms of Vasomotor Rhinitis

Swollen nasal mucosa

Ruddy red mucosa

Excess secretions

Postnasal drainage stimulating the cough reflex

(Adapted from Proctor DF. Vasomotor rhinitis. In: Cherniack RM, ed. Current therapy of respiratory disease—2. Toronto: BC Decker, 1986:7)

Exacerbations of asthma or bronchitis are commonly due to gastroesophageal reflux. It has been estimated that 45% to 65% of asthmatics have reflux.[24] Ten percent of the population in the United States have reflux daily.[24] In the person with twitchy airways, asthma, or bronchitis, this problem can be particularly troublesome. It is possible to have "silent reflux" in which no symptoms are present despite the reflux. Reflux may contribute to recurrent nocturnal cough, morning hoarseness, and recurrent pulmonary infiltrates.[25] Table 4–10 lists the signs and symptoms of gastroesophageal reflux.[26]

The cardiovascular system should be assessed to determine if arrhythmias, coronary artery disease, hypertension, or right ventricular failure may be of concern in the pulmonary rehabilitation patient. It has been reported that about 50% of patients with COPD who are older than 50 have some type of heart problem.[27] For the patient who has COPD pulmonary hypertension or right ventricular failure (cor pulmonale), a poor prognosis ensues. The abnormality of the cardiopulmonary and circulatory system in cor pulmonale is due to a disorder of tissue oxygenation caused by arterial hypoxemia, pulmonary vasoconstriction, right ventricular dysfunction, increased

TABLE 4–9. Symptoms of Sinusitis and Location of Sinus Pain

General symptoms of sinusitis

Fever

Malaise

Cough

Sore throat

Facial fullness

Purulent nasal discharge

Pain

Sinus pain

Maxillary: upper cheek, upper teeth

Frontal: forehead

Ethmoid: around eye or in the head

Sphenoid: retro-orbital

(Adapted from Brodovsky DM. Sinusitis. In: Cherniack RM, ed. Current therapy of respiratory disease—2. Toronto: BC Decker, 1986:9)

TABLE 4–10. Symptoms of Gastroesophageal Reflux

Digestive symptoms
Recurrent retrosternal burning
Burning radiates up and down the chest
Burning worsens on lying down or bending over
Acid or food/fluid regurgitation into the throat
Pain with swallowing

Pulmonary symptoms
Morning hoarseness
Nocturnal cough
Recurrent pneumonia (pulmonary infiltrates)
Asthma
Bronchitis

Cardiac symptom
Chest pain, suggesting angina

(Adapted from Nelson HS. Is gastroesophageal reflux worsening your patient's asthma? J Respir Dis 1990;11:827)

cardiac output, increased pulmonary blood volume, increased blood viscosity, and increased intrathoracic pressure.[28] Avoidance of nonselective β-blockers, such as propranolol (Inderal), that may provoke bronchospasm is recommended when treating the COPD patient for cardiac disease. In patients with an irritating cough, it should be determined if they are using angiotensin converting enzyme (ACE) inhibitors, since this group of antihypertensives has been reported to aggravate coughing.

Evaluation of the musculoskeletal system is necessary as it relates to the patient's ability to perform an effective cough technique and activity or exercise. Depending on the severity of the disorder—kyphoscoliosis, ankylosing spondylitis, pectus excavatum, skeletal muscle disorders and abdominal disorders—lung expansion, worsening dyspnea, or diaphragmatic movement may be affected. Arthritis and long-term use of steroids, leading to osteoporosis or muscle atrophy, may also interfere with the patient being able to reach his or her full exercise potential. Musculoskeletal pain from rib fracture or chest trauma will limit the pulmonary rehabilitation patient's exercise capacity. Careful evaluation will allow the pulmonary rehabilitation team to set realistic goals for the patient's bronchial hygiene, activity, and exercise program.

Asthma and Chronic Obstructive Pulmonary Disease

It is critical to correlate the symptoms with the disease.[29] This section will review the major chronic lung problems.[29,30] *Asthma* is characterized by recurrent episodes of wheezing, with symptom-free intervals. The predominant symptoms of asthma are wheezing, dyspnea, cough, and sometimes chest tightness or sputum production.[31] The symptom of cough cannot be overstressed since, in some asthmatics, this is the only symptom reported.[32] Children with a cough are often treated for recurrent respiratory infections because their persistent cough is not recognized as asthma. The following characteristics of cough need to be evaluated in asthma: nocturnal, exercise-induced, cold air-induced, seasonal recurrence, or recurrence with an upper respiratory infection. The body's natural circadian rhythm can sometimes worsen a person's asthma at night by changes in lung function. The lungs reach their lowest function at 3:00 AM then increase to peak values over the next 12 hours. Other triggers of asthma may be induced by aspirin, nonsteroidal anti-inflammatory agents, tartrazine, FD&C yellow dye 5, sulfites, and occupational exposures.[33,34] Occupational asthma is a recognized cause of disability resulting from the sensitization of the patient to a substance encountered at work.[35] All asthmatics may not present with symptoms in the presence of substantial airflow limitation. Therefore, the best tool for assessment at home is the measurement of peak expiratory flow.[36]

Chronic bronchitis is diagnosed by a history of cough and sputum for at least 3 months of the year, for at least 2 successive years. For patients who have these symptoms combined with airflow abnormalities, their morbidity and mortality is altered. When the patient presents with a combination of cough, sputum production, and intermittent wheezing, the term *asthmatic bronchitis* is commonly used.

Emphysema is a pathologic diagnosis, characterized by destruction of the alveolar septae and dilatation of the alveolar airspace. Emphysema is irreversible, is progressive, and is most often found in conjunction with chronic bronchitis. The term *chronic obstructive pulmonary disease* (COPD) usually refers to an individual with a combination of emphysema and chronic bronchitis. Symptoms associated with emphysema caused by α_1-antiproteinase (AAP) deficiency, begin before age 40 in 60% of reported cases and before age 50 in 90% of reported cases.[37]

Physical Examination

The extent of the physical examination during the initial assessment will be based upon the interviewer's personal preference and the needs of the pulmonary rehabilitation program. If the pulmonary rehabilitation team physician performs an assessment on the patient that includes a detailed physical examination, then the interviewer may need to cover only the basics: heart rate and rhythm, respiratory rate, blood pressure, breath sounds, weight, edema, and use of accessory muscles. Other physical findings of importance include the presence of neck vein distention, chest expansion, heart sounds, liver size, and carotid and extremity pulses. It can be useful to have the team member responsible for the pulmonary rehabilitation initial assessment present when the physician performs the assessment.

Medical Testing

The importance of medical testing in the initial assessment of the patient cannot be understated, since a clinical assessment alone is insufficient to detect, diagnose, or characterize lung disease.[38-41] Basic medical tests recommended for the initial assessment of the pulmonary rehabilitation candidate are described in Table 4–11.

TABLE 4–11. Basic Medical Tests Recommended for the Initial Assessment of the Pulmonary Rehabilitation Candidate

Pre- and postbronchodilator spirometry
Diffusing capacity
Lung volume study
Resting ECG
Resting ABG
PA and lateral chest x-ray films
Complete blood count
Blood chemistry profile
Theophylline level (if applicable)
Exercise test

If the patient brings recent medical test reports to the program, the pulmonary rehabilitation team physician can review the reports to determine if the results are acceptable or require further investigation. This should be taken into careful consideration to help curb extra costs to the patient. It is always recommended that patients bring past medical tests with them or have their primary care physician send records to the program office for comparison with current studies. Previous pulmonary function tests for comparison can help determine the course of the disease process. A description of each basic medical test is presented below.

Spirometry Before and After Use of a Bronchodilator

Pulmonary function studies are the best way to assess for the presence of lung impairment.[42] The simple spirogram should be considered for anyone with signs or symptoms of respiratory disease. The forced expiratory volume in 1 second (FEV_1) is often used as a predictor of prognosis, knowing that the normal decline in FEV_1 caused by the aging process is about -30 mL/year for persons over aged 30, and -60 to -120 mL/year for COPD patients.[42,43] Macklem and Permutt state:

> In considering the simplicity of determination of FEV_1 and its potential use in detecting individuals who are headed toward serious trouble at a time when intervention might have prevented a disastrous outcome, it is interesting to explore the reasons why the spirometer has not achieved a position comparable to the clinical thermometer, the sphygmomanometer, the opthhalmoscope, the chest x-ray and the EKG.[44]

Although the use of peak expiratory flow as a home self-monitoring technique is reported to be helpful in asthmatics, the total reliance on this maneuver can result in an unreliable estimate of airway patency in comparison with the FEV_1.[45] Measurement of the FEV_1 does have an important role in evaluating the lung status.

Diffusion Test

The measurement of carbon monoxide diffusion in the lungs is one of the most sensitive tests for detecting the presence of emphysema. The diffusing capacity may be significantly reduced, whereas there is no evidence for emphysema by physical examination or on chest x-ray films. The diffusing capacity is usually normal in asthma and normal or only mildly reduced in chronic bronchitis. Since emphysema destroys the alveolar walls, resulting in less surface area, a decrease in diffusion occurs. Interstitial diseases, such as pulmonary fibrosis, asbestosis, and sarcoidosis, also alter the alveolar–capillary membrane, resulting in a reduction in diffusion.

Lung Volumes

Lung volume tests are necessary to determine if a decrease in the forced vital capacity (FVC) in a patient with an obstructive defect is secondary to air-trapping from the obstructive disease or is indicative of a concomitant restrictive defect. An increased total lung capacity (TLC) may occur in asthma during an acute attack, but is usually normal with chronic bronchitis and with stable asthma. An increased TLC, in a stable patient, suggests the presence of emphysema.

Electrocardiogram

An electrocardiogram (ECG) should be performed to review the rate and rhythm, to detect any sign of right or left ventricular enlargement, and to detect any evidence of myocardial ischemia or injury. Approximately 50% of COPD patients older than 50 have either ischemic heart disease, hypertension, rhythm disturbances, or heart failure.[15]

Posteroanterior and Lateral Chest X-Ray Studies

The limitations of the chest x-ray film must be understood. Too much emphasis has been placed on the chest x-ray study, rather than pulmonary function tests, in determining the presence of lung disease. Asthma, chronic bronchitis, and emphysema, all can be present, but undetectable on a chest x-ray film. Emphysema is certainly suggested by the presence of flattened diaphragms, hyperinflation, or bullous changes. Thickening of the bronchial walls may be seen on the x-ray film with chronic bronchitis. Hyperinflation may be present during an acute asthmatic attack. Lung malignancy, congestive heart failure, or pneumonia may be detected by a x-ray examination. With mild chronic bronchitis and emphysema, the pulmonary function studies will commonly show abnormalities, whereas the chest roetgenogram is still normal.[46] In elderly patients, the chest radiograph is sometimes incorrectly interpreted as showing emphysema (because the lungs appear hyperinflated) when, in fact, the TLC and diffusing capacity are normal.

Arterial Blood Gas Values

The arterial blood gas (ABG) values at rest is an important test that assesses both the lungs' ability to oxygenate the blood and remove carbon dioxide, and the body's acid–base status. The PaO_2 at rest does not reflect the PaO_2 during exercise. Also, "awake" ABG results do not accurately predict nocturnal arterial oxygen desaturation, and further evaluation may be indicated.[47]

Complete Blood Count

The complete blood count should be checked for polycythemia, anemia, elevation in the number of white blood cells, and the eosinophil level. An increase in the number of eosinophils in the differential count suggests the presence of an allergy and will often predict a good response to corticosteroid therapy.

Blood Chemistry Profile

The basic electrolytes, glucose, magnesium, phosphate, and thyroid levels are important. Certain medications, such as diuretics or oral steroids, may produce hypokalemia, hypomagnesemia, and metabolic alkalosis. The assessment of thyroid function is useful, since patients with hyperthyroidism often complain of breathlessness caused by respiratory muscle weakness,[48] and hypothyroidism can lead to weakness and respiratory failure.

Theophylline Level

If the patient is taking a theophylline medication, it is important to evaluate the theophylline level in the blood. The optimal blood level is between 10 and 20 μg/mL for most individuals. Theophylline is metabolized by the liver, and various factors affect its metabolism. An increase in clearance occurs in young children, smokers, and from diets high in protein. A decrease in theophylline clearance is caused by liver disease, congestive heart failure, cor pulmonale, severe exacerbations of COPD, the aging process, pneumonia, influenza, and medications, such as cimetidine (Tagamet), erythromycin, and ciprofloxacin.

Exercise Test

Evaluation of the patient's current exercise tolerance will permit a realistic and safe exercise program to be developed for the patient. A simple test, such as the 6- or 12-minute walk, or an elaborate test, such as the pulmonary exercise stress test, can provide the pulmonary rehabilitation team with important information.[17] The spirogram cannot reliably predict exercise-induced hypoxemia in the COPD patient.[49] Exercise-induced hypoxemia is typical of interstitial pulmonary disease.[49] In the patient with moderate or severe COPD, exercise-induced hypoxemia is impossible to predict. The three most common reasons to perform exercise tests on the patient with lung disease are:

1. to determine the cause of the patient's shortness of breath
2. to evaluate a patient's potential for working as it relates to his or her current or future occupation
3. to outline a safe and realistic home exercise training program for the patient.

The exercise assessment can determine if a patient develops cardiac arrhythmias, angina pectoris, or if supplemental oxygen is needed during the training sessions.

The type of diagnostic exercise test done will vary between pulmonary rehabilitation programs, based upon the program's budget for equipment, staff or technician time, and what type of information is really needed to outline a safe home exercise program for the patient. An initial 6- or 12-minute walk test is helpful to give baseline information that can be used for determining the pulmonary exercise stress test protocol, if ordered. During the 6- or 12-minute walk test, oxygen saturation, blood pressure, respiratory rate, heart rate, and EKG tracing with three leads for the pre- and post-walk test all are helpful. Documenting the maximum heart rate and heart rate at which the patient became short of breath are also very useful.

During the exercise evaluation, it is important to document the patient's orthopedic problems. Pain in the hip, knee, or other joints, or shoulder stiffness should be noted to individualize the patient's exercise program. Exercise limitations will then determine the patient's realistic goals for the exercise program.

If a pulmonary exercise stress test (PEST) is ordered, it may be performed as a steady-state, progressive, symptom-limited, or maximal-level test. A maximal exercise test is often used to determine the cause of dyspnea (e.g., whether cardiac or pulmonary) or to determine a patient's ability to participate in various jobs. If the only reason for the PEST is to help outline a home exercise training program, then a submaximal stress test that correlates to the same energy expenditure as the level of intensity to be used in the exercise program would be appropriate.

The advantages of using a maximal PEST protocol include:

1. Arrhythmias or ischemic EKG changes can be documented at the higher work levels that may not be noted at submaximal levels.
2. An objective determination of the anaerobic threshold can help determine if a cardiovascular impairment is present in addition to the lung problem.
3. Determining the patient's maximal achievable heart rate can be helpful in selecting a target heart rate to be used in exercise training.
4. Detection of oxygen desaturation which may not be present at lower work levels.[50]

When selecting the mode of exercise to be used in testing, keep in mind the type of equipment the patient will use at home. Either a stationary bike or treadmill is reasonable. If exercise training is to be done with a walking program, then testing on a treadmill makes sense. (See Chapter 14 for a discussion of exercise training in the patient with lung disease.)

This covers a brief description of the basic medical tests. Other tests that may be considered, depending on the medical history and physical examination, may include a sputum evaluation, α_1-antiproteinase assay, skin tests, sleep evaluation, bronchial challenge test, postexercise spirometry, cardiovascular test, sinus x-ray studies, and upper gastrointestinal series.

SUMMARY

Severe lung disease is usually not diagnosed until the individual has advanced disease; hence, patients referred for pulmonary rehabilitation are commonly elderly and debilitated. Since the typical course of COPD is about 20 to 30 years, it would be more practical for pulmonary rehabilitation to be instituted earlier, when the course of the disease might still be altered favorably. Therefore, we challenge all pulmonary rehabilitation specialists to look toward prevention and early detection of lung disease when intervention may prevent a disastrous outcome.[2,51] Pulmonary rehabilitation programs need to be interested in prevention as well as treatment. Health professionals should understand that assessment of the pulmonary rehabilitation candidate is necessary for optimal pulmonary rehabilitation to be accomplished. Assessment is the key to prevention and early detection of lung disease. Now is the time for pulmonary rehabilitation specialists to lead the way to better lung health.

REFERENCES

1. Connors GA, Hodgkin JE, Asmus RM. A careful assessment is crucial to successful pulmonary rehabilitation. J Cardiopul Rehabil 1988;11:435.

2. Connors GA, Hodgkin JE. Pulmonary rehabilitation. In: Burton GG, Hodgkin JE, Ward JJ, eds. Respiratory care: a guide to clinical practice, 3rd ed. Philadelphia: JB Lippincott, 1991:655.

3. Ries AL. Position paper of the American Association of Cardiovascular and Pulmonary Rehabilitation, scientific basis of pulmonary rehabilitation. J Cardiopul Rehabil 1990;10:418.

4. Dixon RJ. The patient interview. In: Youtsey JW, ed. Assessment of the pulmonary patient. Denver: Multi-media Publ, 1985:3.

5. Wilkins RL, Hodgkin JE. History and physical examination of the respiratory patient. In: Burton GG, Hodgkin JE, Ward JJ, eds. Respiratory care: a guide to clinical practice, 3rd ed. Philadelphia: JB Lippincott, 1991:211.

6. Krider SJ. Interviewing and the respiratory history. In: Wilkins RL, Sheldon RL, Krider SJ, eds. Clinical assessment in respiratory care, 2nd ed. St Louis: CV Mosby, 1990:3.

7. Mertens PJ, et al. Long-term exercise therapy for chronic obstructive lung disease. Respiration 1978;35:96.

8. Bandura A. Self-efficacy: toward a unifying theory of behavior change. Psychol Rev 1977;84:191.

9. Morris K, Russo A. P.A.T.H. Positive Attitudes Toward Health: a handbook on pulmonary rehabilitation. Seton Medical Center, 1984:95.

10. Guyatt GH, Townsend M, Berman LB, Pugsley SO. Quality of life in patients with chronic airflow limitation. Br J Dis Chest 1987;81:45.

11. Kinsman RA, Yaroush RA, Fernandez E, Dirks JF, Schocket M, Fukuhara J. Symptoms and experiences in chronic bronchitis and emphysema. Chest 1983;83:755.

12. Kinsman RA, Fernandez E, Schocket M, Dirks JF, Covino NA. Multidimensional analysis of the symptoms of chronic bronchitis and emphysema. J Behav Med 1983;6:339.

13. Morris K, Russo A. P.A.T.H. Positive Attitudes Toward Health: a handbook on pulmonary rehabilitation. Seton Medical Center, 1984:1.

14. Fuller J, Schaller-Ayers J. Health assessment: a nursing approach. Philadelphia: JB Lippincott, 1990:22.

15. Branscomb BV. Aggravating factors and coexisting disorders. In: Hodgkin JE, Petty TL, eds. Chronic obstructive pulmonary disease, current concepts. Philadelphia: WB Saunders, 1987:183.

16. Sweer L, Zwillich CW. Dyspnea in the patient with chronic obstructive pulmonary disease: etiology and management. Clin Chest Med 1990;11:417.

17. Brown HV, Wasserman K. Exercise performance in chronic obstructive pulmonary diseases. Med Clin North Am 1981;65:525.

18. Mahler DA, Wells CK. Evaluation of clinical methods for rating dyspnea. Chest 1988;93:580.

19. Schols A, Monstert R, Soeters P, Greve L, Wouters E. Inventory of nutritional status in patients with COPD. Chest 1989;96:247.

20. Wilson DO, Rogers RM, Wright EC, Anthonisen NR. Body weight in chronic obstructive pulmonary disease. Am Rev Respir Dis 1989;139:1435.

21. Druce HM, Kaliner MA. Allergic rhinitis. In: Cherniack RM, ed. Current therapy of respiratory disease—2. Toronto: BC Decker, 1986:5.

22. Proctor DF. Vasomotor rhinitis. In: Cherniack RM, ed. Current therapy of respiratory disease—2. Toronto: BC Decker, 1986:7.

23. Brodovsky DM. Sinusitis. In: Cherniack RM, ed. Current therapy of respiratory disease—2. Toronto: BC Decker, 1986:9.

24. Castell DO. Asthma and gastroesophageal reflux. Chest 1989;96:2.

25. Ekstrom T, Lindgren BR, Tibbling L. Effects of ranitidine treatment on patients with asthma and a history of gastroesophageal reflux: a double-blind, cross-over study. Thorax 1989;44:19.

26. Nelson HS. Is gastroesophageal reflux worsening your patient's asthma? J Respir Dis 1990;11:827.

27. Reynolds RJ, Buford JG, George RB. Treating asthma and COPD in patients with heart disease. J Respir Dis 1982;3:41.

28. Wiedemann HP, Matthaz RA. Cor pulmonale in chronic obstructive pulmonary disease, circulatory pathophysiology and management. Clin Chest Med 1990;11:523.

29. Official statement of the American Thoracic Society. Standards for the diagnosis and care of patients with chronic obstructive pulmonary disease (COPD) and asthma. Am Rev Respir Dis 1987;136:225.

30. Petty TL. Definitions in chronic obstructive pulmonary disease. In: Hodgkin JE, guest ed. Chronic obstructive pulmonary disease. Clin Chest Med 1990;11:363.

31. Lopez M, Salvaggio J. Bronchial asthma. Asthma 1987;82:177.

32. Parrillo SJ. Cough variant asthma. Pediatr Emerg Care 1986;2:97.

33. Spector SL. Aspirin-induced asthma. In: Cherniack RM, ed. Current therapy of respiratory disease—2. Toronto: BC Decker, 1986:106.

34. Murlas C, Brooks SM. Occupational asthma. In: Cherniack RM, ed. Current therapy of respiratory disease—2. Toronto: BC Decker, 1986:110.

35. Canadian Thoracic Society, Ad Hoc Committee on Occupational Asthma of the Standards Committee. Occupational asthma: recommendations for diagnosis, management and assessment of impairment. Can Med Assoc J 1989;140:1029.

36. Beasley R, Cushley M, Holgate ST. A self management plan in the treatment of adult asthma. Thorax 1989;44:200.

37. Idell S, Cohen AB. The pathogenesis of emphysema. In: Hodgkin JE, Petty TL, eds. Chronic obstructive pulmonary disease, current concepts. Philadelphia: WB Saunders, 1987:7.

38. Habib MP, Klink ME, Knudson DE, Bloom JW, Kaltenborn WT, Knudson RJ. Physiologic characteristics of subjects exhibiting accelerated deterioration of ventilatory function. Am Rev Respir Dis 1987;136:638.

39. Chu LW, Wilkins RL. Clinical laboratory studies. In: Wilkins RL, Sheldon RL, Krider SJ, eds. Clinical assessment in respiratory care, 2nd ed. St Louis: CV Mosby, 1990:56.

40. George RB, Anderson WM. Laboratory evaluation of patients with COPD. In: Hodgkin JE, Petty TL, eds. Chronic obstructive pulmonary disease, current concepts. Philadelphia: WB Saunders, 1987:36.

41. Clausen JL. The diagnosis of emphysema, chronic bronchitis, and asthma. In: Hodgkin JE, guest ed. Chronic obstructive pulmonary disease. Clin Chest Med 1990;11:405.

42. Enright PL, Hodgkin JE. Pulmonary function tests. In: Burton GG, Hodgkin JE, Ward

JJ, eds. Respiratory care: a guide to clinical practice, 3rd ed. Philadelphia: JB Lippincott, 1991:157.

43. Hodgkin JE. Prognosis in chronic obstructive pulmonary disease. In: Hodgkin JE, guest ed. Chronic obstructive pulmonary disease. Clin Chest Med 1990;11:555.

44. Macklem PT, Permutt S. The lung in transition between health and disease. New York, Marcel Dekker, 1979.

45. Meltzer AA, Smolensky MH, D'Alonzo GE, Harrist RB, Scott PH. An assessment of peak expiratory flow as a surrogate measurement of FEV_1 in stable asthmatic children. Chest 1989;96:329.

46. Lillington GA. Roentgenographic diagnosis of pulmonary disease. In: Burton GG, Hodgkin JE, Ward JJ, eds. Respiratory care: a guide to clinical practice. 3rd ed. Philadelphia: JB Lippincott, 1991:233.

47. McKeon JL, Munee-Allen K, Saunders NA. Prediction of oxygenation during sleep in patients with chronic obstructive lung disease. Thorax 1988;43:312.

48. Mier A, Brophy C, Wass J, Besser G, Green M. Reversible respiratory muscle weakness in hyperthyroidism. Am Rev Respir Dis 1989;139:529.

49. Ries AL, Farrow JT, Clausen JL. Pulmonary function tests cannot predict exercise-induced hypoxemia in chronic obstructive pulmonary disease. Chest 1988;93:454.

50. Hodgkin JE. Exercise testing and training. In: Hodgkin JE, Petty TL, eds. Chronic obstructive pulmonary disease, current concepts. Philadelphia: WB Saunders, 1987:120.

51. Petty TL. The role of early identification of COPD. In: Hodgkin JE, Petty TL, eds. Chronic obstructive pulmonary disease, current concepts. Philadelphia: WB Saunders, 1987:263.

JOYCE W. HOPP

CHRISTINE M. NEISH

Patient and Family Education

Planning an educational intervention for patients follows the same protocol as does treatment of a chronic pulmonary disease: testing, diagnosis, a treatment regimen, and evaluation of the effectiveness of that regimen. Just as one would not prescribe the same medication for all patients and conditions, neither should one offer a stereotyped educational program. Although the diagnostic tools available in education currently may be more limited than the plethora of clinical tests, we should make full use of what is available, tailoring the educational program to fit patients and their disease conditions.

BENEFITS OF PATIENT EDUCATION

Among the benefits of integrating patient education into comprehensive rehabilitation programs are reduced days of hospitalization with corresponding reductions in costs,[1-5] increases in feelings of well-being and confidence, improvements in physical status known as "quality of life,"[2,4-11] and changes in knowledge and skill.[12]

Of particular interest is the influence of education on patient satisfaction, and patient satisfaction predicts compliance with medical regimens.[13,14] Variables frequently associated with patients' perceptions of health care quality and, hence, their satisfaction, are concern from staff,[15] practitioner warmth and concern,[16] sensitivity to patient's nonverbal behavior,[17] and using appropriate nonverbal cues to respond to the patient.[18] The degree of patient satisfaction with the provider's communication skills also influences compliance.[19,20] This is significant because approximately 50% of patients with a chronic disease fail to take their medications correctly.[21] Patient education seeks to meet the real and felt needs of persons who will ultimately be in charge of their own health care. Their perceptions of the caring nature of health providers are essential to the success of their efforts toward recovery or rehabilitation. The fact that three out of four illness events are handled by the patient without professional assistance suggests a need for total involvement of the patient in the rehabilitation process.[22] Training patients to more effectively use the health care system and interact with caregivers has been strongly suggested by several authors[23] and holds the key to effective rehabilitation. According to Fahrenfort, "Real education must entail emancipation: liberating people to make their own decisions on their own terms."[24]

MAKE AN EDUCATIONAL DIAGNOSIS

Table 5–1 outlines the protocol for making an educational diagnosis. Although you may not be able to elicit all of the information during one patient visit, a rehabilitation program offers the benefit of continued interaction over a time period. Be observant. *Listen* to your patient, being alert to cues concerning his or her beliefs, past experiences, and values, for a knowledge of these is essential to assist the patient in making behavioral changes.

Demographic data are the easist and most familiar to acquire. Our research reveals, however, that the area many persons older than aged 65 are reluctant to share is their level of education.[25] History of and current disease status are common features of referrals to rehabilitation programs.

Psychosocial characteristics can be categorized according to the areas of the health belief model[26] and locus of control theory.[27] Extensive research supports the notion that both of these models apply to patient education.[28–37]

Table 5–2 shows the categories of the health belief model, all of which lie in the perception of the participant, not the provider. Each of the five categories— seriousness, susceptibility, threat, benefits, and barriers—is viewed from the perspective of the patient. The health care provider may, or may not, view the categories in the same way. For example, if a patient feels that his or her disease condition is a normal sign of growing older and, therefore, of low seriousness, he or she may fail to see the importance of a rehabilitation program. Similarly, if the patient feels there is too much to learn in the rehabilitation program (high level of perceived barrier), he or she may put forth little effort to learn.

Listening is your best tool for identifying your patient's beliefs. When you hear statements such as those in Table 5–2, you can immediately recognize them as pertaining to the health belief model.

Likewise, a health care worker can pick up cues about a patient's locus of control. This construct developed by Rotter seeks to explain a person's world view by the degree of control a person has over events that occur.[38] A person who is more *internal* believes that a degree of control is possible, that if certain actions are taken, a measure of success can be achieved. Such a person is more likely to take preventive behaviors in areas of health, to seek information, and to use that information to control situations.

On the other end of the continuum of world view are those who are largely *external*, believing in fate, luck, or chance, or the control powerful others have over their lives. World view is shaped by the experiences of life, the culture, and situations in which a person is reared and lives. Individuals who are largely external believe that they are victims of fate or are controlled by events or persons, that there is little they can do to affect the course of their lives or health. Such patients may find it difficult to believe that their participation in a rehabilitation program will make any difference in the course of their disease. Expressions such as, "If it's going to happen, it's going to happen!" or "If the bullet's got my name on it . . ." are common to externals.

Wallston and Wallston have developed an instrument to measure a person's health locus of control (Table 5–3).[27] With it, one may ascertain how close a patient is to the population's mean. Individuals who score above the mean for externality,

TABLE 5–1. Protocol for Making an Educational Diagnosis of the Patient with Chronic Lung Disease

Assess learner characteristics	Demographic and disease data
	Age
	Sex
	Marital status
	Years of education completed
	Socioeconomic status
	Disease history
	Current disease status
	Sociopsychological status
	Locus of control
	Health beliefs
	Cultural beliefs
	Degree of acculturation
	Level of self-efficacy
Consider applicable learning theories	
	Behavior modification
	Cognitive learning theory
	Process of valuing
Assess patient deficits	**Knowledge deficits**
	Anatomy and physiology of cardiopulmonary system
	Pathophysiology
	Medications
	Nutrition
	Emergency care
	Sexual activity
	Recreation/travel
	Community resources
	Home care
	Skill deficits
	Pursed-lips breathing
	Postural drainage/clapping
	Use of inhalers
	Cleaning equipment
	Body mechanics
	Home modification

TABLE 5–2. Patient Statements and the Health Belief Model

Statement	Health Belief Model Category
"I had a friend with emphysema for years and he never had to go to a rehab program."	Perceived seriousness
"People die with heart attacks, not bronchitis."	Perceived seriousness
"I've been short of breath for years; just getting a little worse, that's all."	Perceived seriousness
"I don't know why the doctor thinks I've got lung disease. I'm just a little short of breath."	Perceived susceptibility
"This kind of cough runs in my family. No one has ever had lung disease from it."	Perceived susceptibility
"Everyone gets short of breath when he gets older."	Perceived susceptibility
"Nothing wrong with me now—that last medicine the doctor gave me took care of my problem."	Perceived threat (low)
"What good will going to this program do? I'm so bad now, nothing will help."	Perceived threat (high)
"I've been through a program like this before and it didn't help me much."	Perceived benefits
"It would take a miracle to make me feel better."	Perceived benefits
"I have no idea why the doctor thought I ought to come to this program."	Perceived benefits
"Do you think this program is going to be worth it?"	Perceived benefits
"I had to take time off work to come to this program; I'm not sure I can keep doing that."	Perceived barriers
"My daughter has to make a special trip to bring me here. She might not be able to do it very often."	Perceived barriers
"I am not sure that my insurance is going to cover this type of program."	Perceived barriers
"There is no way I'm going to be able to do all the things you've been teaching me."	Perceived barriers

appreciate information upon which they may base their own decisions. Externals, on the other hand, may benefit from firm direction from health professionals and will achieve target behaviors if given short-term goals.

Cultural beliefs and *degree of acculturation* affect the way in which people from one culture respond to a health provider of another culture. A patient from an Oriental culture may expect formal greetings and an exchange concerning family members, whereas a Western health provider brusquely addresses the health care needs. Definition of what constitutes disease varies widely according to culture. In the Hispanic culture, individuals are not "sick" unless they are unable to go to work. This often appears as a neglectful delay to an Anglo health provider. Recent immigrants from Southeast Asia often mix folk treatment with scientific medicine, using such treatments as "coining" for a chest cough or headache. Many fail to see the connection between years of smoking and chronic lung disease, or have little accurate record

TABLE   5–3.   The Multidimensional Health Belief Model

	Strongly Disagree	Moderately Disagree	Slightly Disagree	Slightly Agree	Moderately Agree	Strongly Agree
1. If I get sick, it is my own behavior that determines how soon I get well again.	1	2	3	4	5	6
2. Often I feel that no matter what I do, if I am going to get sick, I will get sick.	1	2	3	4	5	6
3. Having regular contact with my physician is the best way for me to avoid illness.	1	2	3	4	5	6
4. Most things that affect my health happen to me by accident.	1	2	3	4	5	6
5. Whenever I don't feel well, I should consult a medically trained professional.	1	2	3	4	5	6
6. I am directly responsible for my health.	1	2	3	4	5	6
7. Other people play a big part in whether I stay healthy or become sick.	1	2	3	4	5	6
8. Whatever goes wrong with my health is my own fault.	1	2	3	4	5	6
9. When I am sick, I just have to let nature run its course.	1	2	3	4	5	6
10. Health professionals keep me healthy.	1	2	3	4	5	6
11. My good health is largely a matter of good fortune.	1	2	3	4	5	6
12. My physical well-being depends on how well I take care of myself.	1	2	3	4	5	6
13. If I take care of myself, I can avoid illness.	1	2	3	4	5	6
14. When I recover from an illness, it's usually because other people (for example, doctors, nurses, family, friends) have been taking good care of me.	1	2	3	4	5	6
15. No matter what I do, I'm likely to get sick.	1	2	3	4	5	6
16. If it's meant to be, I will stay healthy.	1	2	3	4	5	6
17. I can pretty much stay healthy by taking good care of myself.	1	2	3	4	5	6
18. Following doctor's orders to the letter is the best way for me to stay healthy.	1	2	3	4	5	6

(continued)

TABLE 5–3. (*continued*)

Directions for Scoring Multidimensional Health Locus of Control Test

The person being tested will have circled a number (1–6) following each of a series of 18 statements. These numbers indicate how strongly he or she agrees or disagrees with the statement.

The test will produce three scores: Internality (IHLC); externality, powerful other (PHLC); and externality, fate, luck or chance (CHLC).

To obtain the IHLC score, add the numbers circled for questions

1 _____		
6 _____		
8 _____		
12 _____	Total _____	
13 _____	and	
17 _____		

If the score is above 25 (that is, 26 or more), the person is more internal than the average person.

To obtain the PHLC score, add the numbers circled for questions

3 _____		
5 _____		
7 _____		
10 _____	Total _____	
14 _____	and	
18 _____		

If the score is above 19 (that is, 20 or more), the person is more external in beliefs about powerful others than the average person.

To obtain the CHLC score, add the numbers circled for qeustions

2 _____		
4 _____		
9 _____		
11 _____	Total _____	
15 _____	and	
16 _____		

If the score is above 15 (that is, 16 or more), the person is more external in beliefs about fate, luck, and chance than the average person.

(Wallston K, Wallston BS. Development of the multidimensional health locus of control (MHLC) scales. Health Educ Monogr, 1978; [Spring]:160.)

of dates of past illnesses. Even though a person has not recently immigrated, he or she may be immersed in a cultural group that continues the habits, beliefs, and customs of the homeland, delaying the degree of acculturation.

Self-efficacy is a term developed by Bandura to denote a person's perception of his or her ability to accomplish a given behavior and is task-specific.[39] That is, a person may feel efficacious in one area of life, but not in another. For example, a retired businessman may feel that he can still handle business decisions, but perceive himself as incapable of performing postural drainage. Or a woman who has always managed her home to perfection may have low self-efficacy about planning a vacation trip that requires maintaining her supplemental oxygen supply en route.

Kaplan and Atkins found that specific efficacy expectations mediate exercise compliance in patients with chronic obstructive pulmonary disease (COPD).[40] Walking was the target behavior for the 60 patients in the study. Initially, perceived self-efficacy was highly dependent on lung status before entering the program. After participating in the rehabilitation program's walking education, however, efficacy judgments came to correspond more closely with exercise tolerance ($r = 0.47$). Walking efficacy is a function of successfully adhering to a regular exercise program. The researchers also reported a significant correlation with efficacy judgments on closely related behaviors, such as climbing, lifting, and pushing ($p < 0.05$).[40]

Most of these patient characteristics can be observed directly or elicited by questioning. Reading journal articles and attending workshops on dealing with specific ethnic groups are good ways to acquire information on cultural beliefs and behaviors. And, as mentioned earlier, there is no substitute for listening, with an awareness of the areas essential to making an educational diagnosis.

Learning theories abound, and continue to be developed and added to by psychologists as they study human behavior. We have selected three basic theories for their contribution to patient education: behavior modification, cognitive learning theory, and the process of valuing as it lends itself to values clarification. Each of these is supported by research and practice in patient education.

Behavior modification theory postulates that a person's behavior is shaped by environment, that target behaviors can be changed by appropriate rewards, and that, through systematic reinforcement, these behaviors become incorporated into a person's pattern of behavior. As most often practiced in health settings, the provider together with the patient selects the behaviors targeted for change, then develops a program designed to accomplish that change. The steps in behavior modification may be found later in this chapter.

Cognitive learning theory, formerly known as social learning theory, states that persons learn by watching others perform specific behaviors who, in turn, are rewarded for those behaviors. This process is labeled as *modeling,* and if a person identifies with that model, the theory holds that he or she will be encouraged to model his or her behavior after that which has been observed. Self-efficacy also comes from this learning theory and can be enhanced by watching a model with whom an individual identifies accomplish a given task. An important point to note is identification with the model. Patients may not identify with a health professional performing a certain procedure, but they may if a patient with a similar disease condition demonstrates this capability.

The process of valuing, as developed by Louis Raths, emphasizes the steps an individual goes through to arrive at a value (Table 5–4).[41] Raths indicates that adults do not achieve a lasting change of behavior until they have been reached at the value level. Facts, or knowledge, form the basis of change; these facts are brought together into concepts that can be applied in new situations, but do not result in behavioral change until they are taken to the value level, as indicated in Figure 5–1.

`An assessment of where a person is in this process provides insight into a patient's value status: Are some ideas only beliefs, or have they been embedded in the value structure? What is the potential for change? Simple teaching strategies can be developed from each of these steps, enabling patients to take those steps in an educational

TABLE 5–4.   Steps in the Valuing Process, According to Raths

Choosing

        Choosing freely

        Choosing from among alternatives

        Choosing after considering the consequences

Prizing and cherishing

        Prizing, or holding something important

        Publicly affirming when appropriate

Acting

        Acting on one's choices

        Acting repetitively, as part of a pattern of living

(Adapted from Raths LE, et al. Values and teaching. 2nd ed. Columbus, Ohio: Merrill Publishers, 1978.)

program. To do so greatly enhances the likelihood of reaching a person at the level of his or her values.

Assessment of patient deficits, both in the knowledge and skill areas, is a step frequently overlooked. "Canned programs" often assume that patients need to know everything, and proceed accordingly. A simple pretest of knowledge would help define the areas of need. Such a test has recently been developed and validated[42] and is available for use. Skill deficits listed in Table 5–1 should also be identified in advance to conserve time and effort of both patient and provider. Some patients may be excused from attending sessions that are concerned with something that is already familiar to them, or they can serve as "models" for demonstrating specific procedures in which they are already adept.

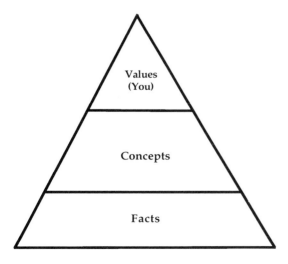

FIGURE 5-1 Levels of learning

SELECT APPROPRIATE
EDUCATIONAL METHODS

The making of an educational diagnosis facilitates selection of educational methods. Just as no two patients are alike in appearance and behaviors (unless they are identical twins!), so are few patients alike in learning style. They may share educational needs, the same diagnosis, even some of the same beliefs, but they may approach learning in a different manner. Some learn more readily in groups, whereas others prefer one-on-one instruction. The use of a variety of educational approaches enables all patients to find some meaningful learning environment in the program.

Educational methodology should be tailored insofar as possible to the characteristics of the patient: those characteristics identified in the educational diagnosis. For example, persons who are believers in fate, luck, or chance (external locus of control) appear to respond best to behavior modification regimens, so that they can perceive gaining control over some aspects of the progression of their disease. On the other hand, patients who are more internal locus of control (the information gatherers) respond best to a value-clarifying approach, in which they are encouraged to take an active role in goal-setting for their rehabilitation.

Practice in skills, both physical and behavioral, increases task-specific self-efficacy—the "I can do it" effect. If Joe has been having difficulty asking his old pals not to smoke around him, practicing with specific phrases he could use might enable him to be more assertive and tactful in securing a smoke-free environment. Or if Mabel feels reluctant to walk in the shopping mall carrying her portable oxygen pack, going with another patient who shares the same need may help lower the level of anxiety.

Training in behavioral skills also enhances a patient's sense of control. Teaching behavioral skills remains necessary even if only as a way of convincing a patient that he or she has some control.

To accommodate both internals and externals (locus of control) in one group, use the internals as group leaders or demonstrators of skills. Enlist their help in presenting areas with which they are already familiar.

Family members or close friends can be part of the methods you use for patient education. Even though they often must also be the target of the education, their support for behavioral change is essential. Social support is a powerful determinant of outcome in chronic diseases. Social support that is lacking in the family may be supplemented by support groups. Those who attend your rehabilitation program, or their families, may wish to form a support group in their local area or in your sponsoring institution.

Specific treatments or diets may need the collaborative efforts of family or friends. In such instances, education for the significant others must become part of your program. Face-to-face instruction, supplemented by written handouts, are best. Family members, too, may need guided practice in new skills (How do I help with postural drainage?).

Table 5–5 outlines the steps in using behavior modification. An illustration of one procedure necessary to many with chronic lung disease is given. This approach can be adapted for use with other desired behaviors.

TABLE 5–5.   Steps in Behavior Modification

Step	Example
Identify and define problem	Inadequate, regular exercise
Collect baseline data	Assess current exercise status (self-report or questionnaire listing daily activities for one week)
Specify goals and objectives	The patient will be able to establish a regular exercise program. By the end of week 1, I (the patient) will be able to select an activity in which I can participate. By the end of week 2, I shall have performed the activity at least twice. By the end of week 6, I shall perform the activity a minimum of 4 times per week.
Plan intervention	Review possibility of activity Facilities Location Equipment (e.g., walking shoes, portable oxygen) Determine time of day Select partner Determine appropriate reward Write self-contract (I will.)
Monitor and modify plan	Record sheets Self-reported improvement (e.g., ability to increase distance or time, less breathlessness) Revise contract, if necessary
Plan for termination	Acknowledge success Patient receives reward Reduce number of reporting contacts with health professional

Value-clarifying strategies, as mentioned earlier in the chapter, can be developed from the steps in the valuing process. For example, a strategy sheet considering the benefits of your rehabilitation program could include the following:

1. Select a cartoon that sets the stage for consideration of a patient's expectations. (*Example:* a patient sitting on the physician's examining table making the statement, "I thought the government was going to take care of me when I got to be 65!")
2. Ask the following questions, allowing time for the patient to respond in writing or orally:
   a. Whom did you think would take care of you when you got chronic lung disease?
   b. What do you expect to gain from this rehabilitation program?
   c. What did your doctor tell you to expect from this program?
   d. What, or whom, do you think will make this program a success for you?

Notice that there are no right or wrong answers in a value-clarifying strategy. The purpose of such strategies is to help a patient think through behavior patterns, their relations to things of value, and the willingness to do something about them.

Audiovisual materials, such as slides or videotapes, can be used to set the stage for value-clarifying strategies as well as to provide information.[25] For example, after viewing a video showing a person with chronic lung disease cope with the activities of daily living, you could ask a series of questions as follows (always allowing time for thought and exploration of responses):

- What could the patient have done differently? (looking at alternatives)
- What would you have done differently? How successful do you think you would have been? (looking at consequences)
- How important are some of these activities to you? (prizing)
- What new ideas have you gained that you are willing to try at home? (acting)

Both group and individual discussion can address the information you gathered about cultural beliefs, the areas of the health belief model, and the beliefs associated with locus of control theory. For example, it will do little good to insist that group members set goals for themselves if they do not believe they even have a chronic lung disease, or if they believe that their disease cannot be helped. Begin with the beliefs that will deter progress in a rehabilitation program.

Often health care providers feel that group discussion or strategies, such as those that are value-clarifying, takes valuable time away from their lectures. You may hear such comments as, "But I only have an hour to tell them about their nutritional needs." It comes down to achieving a balance between *content* and *process:* patients can only absorb so much content, and if they fail to process it because it runs counter to one of their beliefs, the information may flow in one ear and out the other. Better to lecture 40 minutes and allow 20 minutes to process it through group discussion or strategies than to pile in 60 minutes of content that evaporates as soon as the lecturer leaves the room.

A key element of any educational program is *involvement of the learner,* whether that be patient, family, or friends. Active involvement is better than passive; doing is better than listening. Create opportunities for direct involvement: discussion groups, strategies that call for thinking and responding, hands-on practice with real objects (better than with models), asking the patient to explain procedures in his or her own words.

According to Green, five conclusions have surfaced concerning the effectiveness of patient education programs.[43]

1. Specific instructions about a simple short-term regimen are usually sufficient for compliance.
2. Multiple strategies are required for long-term regimens, but no combination of interventions has demonstrated lasting effects.
3. Cueing is an effective strategy to increase compliance with medication taking and appointment attendance of persons who have chronic conditions.

4. Rewards help to sustain behavior change, but, when the rewards are removed, the behavior tapers off and eventually becomes extinguished.
5. Counseling, group discussions, social support, and self-monitoring have effectively increased compliance.

PLAN EVALUATION

Any evaluation must serve a purpose. Information gained from a well-planned evaluation is invaluable when anticipating program modifications or when seeking support. It is appropriate to design evaluation into any new or substantially modified program.

When planning an evaluation ask the following questions:

1. What are the programs's objectives? Did we intend to influence (a) professional practice; (b) patient attitudes, beliefs, knowledge, or skills; (c) patients' quality of life?
2. Whom, specifically, did we expect to influence in some way: staff, patients, family members, the community?
3. What instruments are available to measure success: written tests, questionnaires, observation, medical records, skill demonstrations?
4. What are our fiscal and personnel resources?
5. Who will need this information? How will the information be used?

Process Evaluation

The first level of evaluation is an examination of professional practice. Here we ask, "How'd we do?" You may address the physical arrangements, handouts, audiovisual presentations, quality of speakers, marketing, and inter- and intraagency support.

Information useful in process evaluations may be found in attendance records, minutes of planning meetings, financial statements, informal and formal feedback from participants and staff.

Impact Evaluation

This level of evaluation looks at changes in the learner's attitudes, beliefs, values, knowledge, and behaviors. We are most familiar with the use of quizzes or written tests and return demonstrations. Other tools may include notation of learners' comments about feelings and observation of affect. Valuable information on attitudes and feelings is often overlooked, since they are less quantifiable than data from a written test. Yet attitudes, beliefs, and values serve as the basis for the adoption of knowledge and implementation of new behaviors.

Outcome Evaluation

According to Bartlett, the evaluator should "designate quality of life the central outcome of medical care . . ."[23] Undoubtedly the most difficult, yet most meaningful, aspect of evaluation is examining the influence of education upon the patient's health and quality of life. Those who have the opportunity of working with individuals with chronic disease have occasions to observe the long-term effects of their efforts. Did symptoms subside? Can the patient more comfortably perform the activities of daily living?

REFERENCES

1. Hodgkin J, Balchaum O, Kass I, et al. Chronic obstructive airways disease: current concepts in diagnosis and comprehensive care. JAMA 1975;232:1243.

2. Hudson LD, Tyler ML, Petty TL. Hospitalization needs during an outpatient rehabilitation program for severe chronic airway obstruction. Chest 1976;70:606.

3. Lertzman MM, Cherniack RM. Rehabilitation of patients with chronic obstructive pulmonary disease. Am Rev Respir Dis 1976;114:1145.

4. Petty TL, Nett LM, Finigan MM, Brink GA, Corsello PR. A comprehensive care program for chronic airway obstruction. Ann Intern Med 1969;70:1109.

5. Wright RW, Larsen DF, Monie RG, Aldred RA. Benefits of a community-hospital pulmonary rehabilitation program. Respir Care 1983;28:1474.

6. Bebout DE, Hodgkin JE, Zorn EG, Yee AR, Sammer EA. Clinical and physiological outcomes of a university-hospital pulmonary rehabilitation program. Respir Care 1983; 28:1468.

7. Casciari RJ, Fairshter RD, Harrison AH, Morrisoon JT, Blackburn C, Wilson AF. Effects of breathing retraining in patients with chronic obstructive pulmonary disease. Chest 1981;79:393.

8. Elliot LS. Roundtable discussion: COPD patient rehabilitation. Respir Ther 1979;9:17.

9. Fishman D, Petty TL. Physical, symptomatic and psychological improvement in patients receiving comprehensive care for chronic airway obstruction. J Chronic Dis 1971; 24:775.

10. Miracle VA. Pulmonary exercise program: a model for pulmonary rehabilitation. J Cardiopul Rehabil 1986;6:368.

11. Moser K, Bokinsky G, Savage R, Archibald C, Hanser P. Results of a comprehensive rehabilitation program. Arch Intern Med 1980;140:1596.

12. Perry JA. Effectiveness of teaching in the rehabilitation of patients with chronic bronchitis and emphysema. Nurs Res 1981;30:219.

13. Ley P. Cognitive variables in noncompliance. J Compliance Health Care 1986;1:171.

14. Smith NA, Ldy P, Seale JP, Shaw J. Health beliefs, satisfaction, and compliance. Patient Educ Counsel 1987;10:279.

15. Steiber SR. How consumers perceive health care quality. Hospitals 1988;7:84.

16. Gerrard BA, Boniface WJ, Love BH. Interpersonal skills for health professionals. Reston, VA: Reston Publishing, 1980.

17. DiMatteo MR, Taranta A. Non-verbal communication and physician–patient rapport: an empirical study. Prof Psychol 1979;540.

18. DiMatter MR, DiNicola DD. Achieving patient compliance. New York: Pergamon Press, 1982.

19. Blackwell B. Drug therapy: patient compliance. N Engl J Med 1973;289:249.

20. Linn MW, Linn BS, Stein SR. Satisfaction with ambulatory care and compliance in older patients. Med Care 1982;20:606.

21. Dwyer MS, Levy, RA, Menander, KB. Improving medication compliance through the use of modern dosage forms. J Pharm Techol 1986;(Jul/Aug):166.

22. Pratt L. The significance of the family in medication. J Comp Fam Stud 1973;1:13.

23. Bartlett EE. Whither patient-centered care? Patient Educ Counsel 1989;14:97.

24. Fahrenfort M. Patient emancipation by health education: an impossible goal? Patient Educ Counsel 1987;10:25.

25. Cotunga N, Hopp JW, Lee JW. Predictors of nutrition supplement use in the elderly, part II: the role of beliefs, attitude and intention. J Nutr Elderly 1989;8:4.

26. Becker MH, ed. The health belief model and personal health behavior. New Jersey: Slack Publishers, 1974.

27. Wallston KA, Wallston BS. Health locus of control. Health Educ Monogr 1978;6:2 [whole issue].

28. Smith NA, Ley P, Seale JP, Shaw J. Health beliefs, satisfaction, and compliance. Patient Educ Counsel 1987;10:279.

29. Miller P, McMahan M, Garrett MG, Johnson NL. Values of regimen compliance as perceived by ischemic heart disease patients. Health Values 6:7.

30. King JB. Illness attributions and the health belief model. Health Educ Q 1984;3/4:287.

31. Gross PA, Bonwich E. Operationalizing the health belief model in a spinal cord injury prevention model. Health Educ 1982;(Sept/Oct):26.

32. Hershey JC, Morton BG, Davis JB, Reichgott MJ. Patient compliance with antihypertensive medication. Am J Public Health 1980;70:1081.

33. McCusker J, Morrow G. The relationship of health locus of control to preventive health behaviors and health beliefs. Patient Counsel Health Educ 1979;1:146.

34. Lau RR, Hartman KA. Health as a value: methodological and theoretical considerations. Health Psychol 1986;5:25.

35. Schlenkk EA, Hart LK. Relationship between health locus of control, health value, and social support and compliance of persons with diabetes mellitus. Diabetes Care 1984;7:566.

36. Lewis FM, Morisky DE, Flynn BS. A test of the construct validity of health locus of control: effects on self-reported compliance for hypertensive patients. Health Educ Monogr 1978;6:138.

37. Shillinger FL. Locus of control: implications for clinical nursing practice. J Nurs Scholarship 1983;15:58.

38. Rotter JB. Generalized expectancies for internal vs external control of reinforcement. Psychol Monogr 1966;609: [complete issue].

39. Bandura A. Self-efficacy: toward a unifying theory of behavioral change. Psychol Rev 1977;84:191.

40. Kaplan RM, Atkins CJ. Specific efficacy expectations mediate exercise compliance in patients with COPD. Health Psychol 1984;3:223.

41. Raths LE, Harmin M, Simon SM. Values and teaching. 2nd ed. Columbus, Ohio: Merrill Publishers, 1978.

42. Hopp JW, Lee JW, Hills R. Development and validation of a pulmonary rehabilitation knowledge test. J Cardiopulm Rehabil 1989;8:15.

43. Green CA. What can patient health education coordinators learn from their years of compliance research? Patient Educ Counsel 1987;10:167.

ROBERT M. KAPLAN

ANDREW L. RIES

Adherence in the Patient with Pulmonary Disease*

Medical encounters typically end with advice. Patients are told to take medication on a specific schedule, to exercise, or to engage in some other routine. Nonadherence occurs when this advice is not followed. Because of nonadherence, patients may not get the optimal benefits from therapy. In this chapter we will explore the issue of nonadherence for patients with pulmonary diseases. Some authors prefer the terms noncompliance, noncooperation, or patient resistance. The terms *adherence* or *cooperation* are often preferred over *compliance* because they give more emphasis to the patient's active role in the encounter. In this chapter we will use the terms adherence and compliance interchangeably.

THE EXTENT OF THE PROBLEM

Patient nonadherence is believed to be a common problem. For example, published figures suggest that nonadherence rates vary between 15% and 93%, depending on patient population and the definition of nonadherence.[1-3] Most estimates suggest that about one-third of patients fail to comply with any particular medical regimen.[4,5] Nonadherence for patients with chronic lung diseases may be higher. Studies that examine nonadherence rates by disease state have consistently shown that chronically ill individuals comply less than those with acute illnesses.[6,7]

In this chapter we will explore a variety of different adherence behaviors, ranging from keeping appointments to taking medication or complying with complex exercise regimens. Even behaviors as simple as keeping an appointment may have high nonadherence rates. It has been estimated that, in some settings, as many as 50% of scheduled appointments are missed.[7] However, this rate drops to about 20% if the patient makes his or her own appointment and may be reduced to as low as 10% if appointment reminders are used.[8] Long-term therapies, such as the use of antihypertensive medications, are associated with dropout rates as high as 50%.[9] In considering the adherence problem, it is important to recognize that many factors influence adherence behavior. Some regimens are easy to follow. Advice to take one

* Supported by Grant HL 34732 from the National Heart, Lung, and Blood Institute.

pill per day, for example, is not difficult to understand. Other treatments may be more complex if, for instance, they involve side effects or frequent dosing schedules for medications, or life-style changes that can be time-consuming and painful. Thus, adherence rates need to be estimated for specific regimens.

PHYSICIAN AWARENESS OF THE PROBLEM

Most physicians believe that their patients satisfactorily comply with prescribed treatments. However, the evidence does not support these beliefs. DiMatteo and DiNicola reviewed studies on physician accuracy in estimating nonadherence and reported that physicians typically overestimate adherence.[1] For example, Caron and Roth found that 22 of 27 medical residents overestimated the extent to which their patients followed instructions in the use of a prescribed liquid antacid.[10] In the same study, the correlations of senior attending physician estimates of patient adherence with actual adherence levels were near zero. Physicians typically overestimate the extent to which their patients comply and overstate the extent to which patient behaviors correspond with physician orders.[11]

It is difficult to assess nonadherence because physicians rarely have objective measures. Epstein and Cluss reviewed the studies comparing self-reports of adherence against some objective measure (pill count, biochemical tracer, or blood level of drug).[12] They found that patient reports of nonadherence tended to be accurate. There were few cases in which patients reported nonadherence and were actually taking the medication. Conversely, patient self-reports of high adherence tended to be less accurate. A more recent study provides other insights. Hillman and colleagues interviewed patients away from the medical setting.[13] Many of these patients acknowledged that they reported high adherence to their physician, even though their actual adherence rates were low.

In summary, then, nonadherence with medical recommendations is a common problem in health care, and physicians may be unaware of the extent of this problem. In part, this may be attributable to patient reluctance to fully divulge the extent of noncompliant behavior.

ADHERENCE IN CHRONIC OBSTRUCTIVE PULMONARY DISEASE

The medical regimen for patients with chronic obstructive pulmonary disease (COPD) is often complex. It is not uncommon for patients with COPD to be using several types of medications simultaneously. A common regimen might include bronchodilators, corticosteroids, antibiotics, and diuretics. Dosage schedules are typically complex. In addition, patients with more severe hypoxemia often use supplemental oxygen. Patients in rehabilitation may participate in a variety of behavioral programs. Ultimately, the determinants of adherence may be different for each of these varied regimens.

Adherence with various components of the medical regimen has not been well studied for patients with COPD. There has been considerable speculation that preparations of some medications may improve patient adherence. For example, newer theophylline products include slow-release anhydrous preparations that require fewer doses per day. These products are widely promoted to enhance patient adherence; yet, there are few studies specifically documenting these claims.

In the next sections we will consider adherence in three areas, taking medicine, cigarette use, and exercise.

Taking Medicine

Despite a large amount of literature on adherence to medical regimens, surprisingly little has been written about adherence in patients with chronic pulmonary disease. We recently reviewed the literature and found only a handful of published studies.[14]

Although some aspects of COPD are treatable, the medical regimen is extremely complex. Traditional medical management of patients with COPD relies heavily on pharmacologic intervention. However, treatment regimens may also include additional modalities such as chest physiotherapy, exercise, and smoking cessation. Most patients are confronted with complex combinations of treatment options.

To gain a better understanding of patient adherence with regimens for COPD, we conducted computer searches using the National Library of Medicine data bases. Reviews of the literature before 1980 did not identify studies on adherence to medical regimens for patients with COPD.[15,16] Haynes and associates' annotated bibliography, for example, did not list a single reference to a study limited to patients with COPD.[16] A new search, dated back to 1980, revealed few studies that have directly addressed the issue of adherence with traditional medical regimens for patients with COPD. The studies considered different treatments in diverse samples and employed various definitions of, and measurements for, adherence.

The traditional view of adherence or nonadherence in the literature, in which the patient either strictly follows or fails to follow a treatment recommendation, may no longer be the optimal direction of adherence research in the future. The degree of adherence required for the desired outcome, be it adherence to a prescribed regimen or maximizing quality of life, varies from treatment to treatment and should be considered. Few studies have yet systematically evaluated adherence with medical treatments for the patient with COPD, and in these few cases, the focus has been on drug and oxygen therapy. In the United Kingdom, for example, James and coworkers reported that only half of their patients took medicines regularly.[17] In one study of 78 patients with COPD, cared for at a southeastern medical center, the average patient received 6.26 medications. These prescriptions were for various dosage schedules and different modes of administration. More than half of the patients (54%) underused medications. However, during periods of respiratory distress, half of the patients overused their medications.[18] We found only one study evaluating interventions to improve adherence for patients with COPD. This report suggested that simple counseling interventions by pharmacists might increase adherence to prescriptions commonly used by patients with COPD.[19]

Patients with COPD with significant hypoxemia may be treated with oxygen. Two important clinical trials demonstrated the benefits of oxygen therapy. In the National Institutes of Health (NIH)-sponsored multicenter Nocturnal Oxygen Therapy Trial (NOTT), hypoxemic patients with COPD were randomly assigned to receive oxygen therapy for either 12 or 24 hours.[20] In the British Medical Research

Council study, hypoxemic patients with COPD received either no oxygen or 15 hours of therapy.[21] Both studies demonstrated a significant reduction in mortality associated with the use of oxygen. Patients receiving continuous oxygen therapy had significantly reduced mortality compared with patients receiving intermittent oxygen (12 or 15 hours). The highest mortality rate was seen in patients who received no oxygen. In addition, the 24-hour oxygen group experienced higher scores on general quality of life measures[22] and, after 1 year, on selected tests of cognitive function.[23]

Although oxygen is expensive and inconvenient for patients, several types of oxygen therapy systems are now available. These include portable units that allow continuous therapy for ambulatory patients. Therefore, with the use of oxygen, hypoxemic patients with COPD can remain active and engage in a variety of physical activities and beneficial exercises. Despite these advances, adherence rates remain low. Estimated or measured adherence values do not appear to converge on a specific rate or even a specific pattern. One British study, from the Liverpool district, indicated that only 55% of patients using oxygen therapy were using it correctly and had stopped smoking. However, those patients with most symptoms were also the most likely to comply.[24] Alternative methods for oxygen delivery may be useful for increasing compliance with therapy. For example, Heimlich and Carr demonstrated that transtracheal oxygen can increase the number of patients who use therapy 24 hours/day.[25] From the results of the NOTT estimate of the impact of improved adherence upon life expectancy, analysis suggests that transtracheal oxygen can improve life expectancy because it improves adherence.

Behavioral and Rehabilitation Programs in Chronic Obstructive Pulmonary Disease

Comprehensive pulmonary rehabilitation programs have been developed to provide a multidisciplinary therapeutic program tailored to the needs of the individual patient. As suggested in this volume and elsewhere, rehabilitation efforts are well justified.[26–28] Such programs may include several components, such as individual assessment, education, instruction in respiratory and chest physiotherapy techniques, psychosocial support, and supervised exercise training. The primary goal of pulmonary rehabilitation is to restore the patient to the highest possible level of independent function. Successful programs can help patients become better educated and more involved in their own care. In addition, patients may experience reduced symptoms,[29] improved exercise tolerance,[30] fewer hospitalizations and physician visits, and more gainful employment.[31] Pulmonary rehabilitation programs have expanded substantially in the last two decades and are now an accepted form of comprehensive therapy for many patients with COPD. The American Thoracic Society has recommended standards for pulmonary rehabilitation programs,[32] and the scientific basis for rehabilitation has been published.[33]

A regular exercise regimen is an important component of most pulmonary rehabilitation programs. Physical conditioning exercises, including walking, can maintain physical functioning as documented in several studies.[30,34–40] Several studies have shown that physical conditioning exercises can improve maximum exercise tolerance and endurance, reduce heart rate, and improve ventilatory and mechanical efficiency for exercise.[34–40]

There have been few controlled studies evaluating COPD rehabilitation programs or their components. Reports from nonrandomized studies typically suggest that the objectives can be achieved.[34–37] Recently, a few controlled trials documented the benefits of exercise programs for patients with COPD. Cockcroft and associates randomly assigned 39 patients to a 6-week exercise training program or to a no-treatment control group.[41] In comparison with the control group, patients in the exercise group experienced subjective benefits and increased the amount of distance they could walk in 12 minutes. However, the length of follow-up was only 2 months. McGavin and coworkers randomly allocated 24 patients with COPD to a 3-month unsupervised stairclimbing home exercise program or to a nonexercise control group.[42] The 12 patients in the exercise group noted subjective improvements and an increased sense of well-being and decreased breathlessness. They also reported an objective increase in the 12-minute walk distance and maximal level of exercise on a cycle ergometer. These changes did not occur in the control group. However, the length of follow-up was limited to 3 months. Ambrosino and coworkers randomly assigned 23 patients to a 1-month medical and rehabilitative therapy group and 28 patients to medical therapy alone (without exercise training).[43] The experimental group improved in exercise tolerance and ventilatory pattern (as evidenced by decrease in respiratory rate and increase in tidal volume). Again, these changes were not present in the control group.

Development of exercise programs for patients with COPD is difficult for several reasons. First, principles of training that have been well studied for normal persons or for cardiac patients do not necessarily apply for patients with COPD.[44] Adherence is often a major problem for the patient with COPD. Some studies suggest that the degree of benefit is associated with compliance to the exercise regimen.[45] Although patients can benefit from exercise, the routine is typically uncomfortable for them. Many participants in rehabilitation programs have become physically deconditioned over a long period. Exertion may be uncomfortable and commonly leads to the frightening symptom of breathlessness (dyspnea). Because of these problems, discontinuation of the exercise regimen is common.

Remarkably few studies have evaluated methods to improve adherence to an exercise regimen. In one experimental trial, patients with COPD underwent exercise testing and were given an exercise prescription.[46] They were then randomly assigned to one of five experimental or control groups. The experimental groups were based on the principles of behavior modification or a variant of behavior modification known as cognitive-behavior modification. These methods involve setting goals, analyzing the reinforcers for walking, and the use of behavioral contracts. The experimental programs included six weekly sessions in the patient's home. One control group received attention, but did not have the behaviorally based sessions, whereas the other control group received no treatment. After 3 months, there was greater compliance with the exercise program for the experimental groups in comparison with the two control groups. These changes were reflected in changes in exercise tolerance measured 1 month after the treatment. However, there were no significant changes in spirometric parameters.[46]

Several additional analyses were performed using a general quality-of-life measure[47] and a general health policy model.[48] Over the course of 18 months, the experimental and control groups showed significant differences on a quality-of-life index. These differences were used to calculate quality adjusted life years and perform cost–effectiveness studies. There is considerable debate about the economic value of behavioral and rehabilitation programs. The cost–effectiveness analyses suggested that behavioral programs designed to increase adherence for patients with COPD produce an equivalent of a well-year for approximately 23,000 dollars. This is comparable with other widely advocated health care programs.[49]

These same patients were studied again 3 years after the beginning of the program. At this time, observed differences between the experimental and control groups remained for quality of life as measured by the quality of well-being scale,[50] yet substantial increases in variability precluded the detection of statistically significant effects. Analysis of the data using concepts derived from social learning theory[51] suggested that perceived self–efficacy-mediated changes in behavior and function.[52]

Cigarette Smoking

Because of the well-documented association between smoking and COPD, successful smoking prevention programs are expected to reduce the incidence of these diseases. Smoking cessation programs are also valuable. There is considerable interest in the effects of smoking cessation for smokers with mild airway obstruction who may be at risk for COPD. The NIH is currently conducting an experimental trial to evaluate the benefits of smoking cessation for these high-risk individuals.

In addition to the role of smoking as a cause of COPD, active cigarette smoking also affects the course of the illness. For example, cigarette smoking is associated with mucous hypersecretion, acute respiratory illnesses, altered airway reactivity, and increased risk of mortality from other causes, including coronary heart disease. Some of the relations between smoking and problems in the airways have been reviewed elsewhere.[53] A variety of studies have suggested that loss in lung function is associated with total duration of cigarette use.[54] Longitudinal studies indicate that there is a progressive loss of pulmonary function with continued cigarette smoking. However, there is at least some evidence that there is partial recovery of lung function for those who cease cigarette smoking, particularly for those who do so early in life.[55]

Because of the potential benefits of smoking cessation, efforts to improve adherence to smoking cessation programs are of great importance. Evidence has accumulated suggesting that the physician may play a critical role in helping patients stop smoking and maintain this behavioral change.[56] Several experimental trials have trained physicians to deliver a smoking cessation intervention. The components of the intervention include approaches for taking a smoking history, personalizing the health risks, setting a quit date, prescribing nicotine chewing gum, and counseling techniques for follow-up. In one study, Ockene and associates assigned physicians to receive training in behaviorally oriented counseling techniques or to a control group in which patients were provided with only brief advice to stop smoking. Some of the interventions involved the use of nicotine gum, whereas others did not. The results suggested that the behavioral intervention, with or without the use of nicotine gum, resulted in greater reductions in cigarette use among patients. Further, differences between these groups remained at 6-month follow-up.[57]

It is important to emphasize that not all studies on physician interventions have shown significant effect upon patient smoking rates. For example, two recent studies failed to demonstrate significant benefits of physician training.[58,59] However, in each of these programs, the comparison was between patients of physicians who had attended a continuing medical education (CME) course on smoking cessation and patients of physicians who had not taken the course. Each of these studies demonstrated little impact of the CME course upon the likelihood that the physicians would even discuss smoking with their patients. We suggest that CME courses are a minimal intervention and may not produce enough change in physician behavior to ultimately result in changes in patient smoking behavior.

OVERADHERENCE

Most of the literature on adherence behaviors focuses on the extent to which patients underuse medications. A less common, but perhaps equally important problem involves the overuse of medication. Overadherence is a more common problem when medications provide prompt symptomatic relief. In the study by Chryssidis and coworkers, for example, the use of high doses of aerosol therapy often exceeded prescription rates.[60] The mean percentage of prescribed dose actually used was 98.5% at 1-month follow-up and 110.8% at 2-month follow-up. Since there was variability for each of these estimates, it appears that some portion of the patients took considerably more medication than was prescribed. This finding has been confirmed by more recent investigations.[18] It is not surprising that patients suffering from COPD, a highly symptomatic disorder, would overuse a medication that provides rapid symptomatic relief.

Some of the evidence for patient overcompliance comes from innovative studies on the assessment of adherence. For example, in one clinical trial on antihypertensive medications, patients were asked to bring their medications with them for follow-up visits. Adherence rates were remarkably high—sometimes approaching 100%. However, there was considerable variability among subjects, and those at higher adherence levels did not necessarily obtain the best clinical results. Technological advances have allowed the placement of microprocessors on pill blister packs or on the caps of standard pill bottles. With these methods it is possible to estimate not only how many of the pills were removed from the packages, but also specifically when they were removed. One device, known as the Medication Event Monitoring System (MEMS), uses a microprocessor in the cap of a pill bottle to monitor the time at which the bottle was opened. These studies using such methods suggest that patients often have lapses in adherence in periods between visits or that medicine taking is erratic.[61] Also, they may overuse medication or engage in "pill dumping" just before a clinic visit. These findings imply that medications may not be used as prescribed. This may substantially bias estimates of dose–response in clinical trials as well as provide an inaccurate measure of treatment side effects.[62,63]

RATIONAL NONADHERENCE

There are at least three explanations for why patients fail to adhere: those that focus on the patient, those that focus on the patient's environment, and those in which there is a problem in the interaction between the patient and the provider. Patient-oriented explanations suggest that certain personalities fail to adhere to medical treatments or that patients intentionally reject therapy because of some flaw in their personality.[64] These explanations have failed to gain empirical support. There is some evidence that patients misunderstand instructions,[65] but relatively little evidence that patients intentionally try to harm themselves by ignoring advice.

Environmental explanations suggest that elements in the patient's environment, such as family variables, reminders, or other environmental stimuli, influence adherence behavior.[66] Evidence for this view of adherence is suggested by studies demonstrating that reminders and simple environmental cues increase adherence behavior.[67] These simple reminders might be notes attached to a refrigerator, or an electronic device that beeps when a dose of medication is indicated. In one study, it was shown that individual rather than block appointments and simple appointment reminders significantly improved adherence.[68]

The third view of adherence emphasizes the role of the patient–provider relation. Although the evidence cannot be reviewed in detail here, suffice it to say that there is a substantial literature demonstrating that information exchanged between patients and providers is often poor.[1,69] This view of adherence suggests that the remedy for the problem is to improve communication between patients and their physicians.

In considering the three views of noncompliant behavior, we find little evidence that patient personality variables explain much of the variability in nonadherence.[5] The environmental view is valuable in identifying simple manipulations that may enhance adherence behavior in some settings. However, the environmental view is not a comprehensive explanation that considers the patient's role in the choice to use or not use medications. The patient–provider interaction view comes closest to dealing with the realities of the problem. Substantial evidence suggests that patients often do not comprehend instructions offered them by their providers.[1] Conversely, providers often have an inadequate picture of the responses their patients have to treatment recommendations. In the following sections, we will explore this issue in more detail.

Liang offered reasons why his chronically ill patients failed to take their medications.[70] Common explanations were, "I forgot," "too expensive," "felt dopey," "felt constipated," and "didn't work." Patients often have poor responses to medications, find that the medications are not providing the expected benefit, or cannot afford to purchase the medications. However, this may not be deviant behavior because patients are taking several factors into consideration in their decision to use or not use a product. Kaplan and Simon suggested that patients are more likely to comply with treatment when they perceive a net health benefit.[5] Nonadherence occurs when the perceived consequences outweigh expected benefits. In this decision process, patients may discount future benefits because of current side effects. A corollary of the theory is that treatments that produce a short-term benefit may evoke better adherence than those that produce a delayed benefit. For example, treatments that provide immediate symptomatic relief, such as inhalers, may be associated with higher adherence than those, such as antihypertensive therapies, that exchange current inconvenience for future benefit.

One major reason for nonadherence is that patients experience treatment side effects and, therefore, increased medicine use results in increased discomfort.[71] In one study, 36% of patients in a large tertiary care hospital had some iatrogenic disease.[72] Older individuals may experience a sevenfold increase in adverse reactions in comparison with those aged 20 to 29.[70] Evidence from the United Kingdom indicates that as many as 10% of admissions in geriatric units result from adverse reactions attributable to drug interactions.[71] Observed nonadherence might reflect patient feedback about bad experiences with the regimen. Although patients may be less direct about their decision not to adhere, observations of nonadherence may be a stimulus for discussion of treatment side effects.

Several authors have argued that nonadherence can be rational.[3] Patients may adhere to a regimen, but fail to obtain the desired benefit. If the probability of an expected benefit is low and there are undesirable side effects, nonadherence may be rational. For example, a patient with streptococcal pharyngitis who discontinues an antibiotic on the eighth day of a 10-day course might be regarded as a noncomplier. However, if the patient decides that the inconvenience and side effects associated with the medication are a greater concern than the low probability of developing rheumatic fever, the decision may be regarded as rational. Nonadherence might also be regarded as rational when the patient achieves the desired result, despite nonadherence. Indeed, studies in many areas do not show a systematic relation between adherence and health outcome.[67] Many studies in the adherence literature fail to take health outcomes into consideration.

SUGGESTIONS FOR IMPROVING PATIENT ADHERENCE

Patients with COPD are required to adhere to several different and often complex regimens. Some evidence suggests that adherence behaviors are not related to one another. Patients may comply with their antibiotic regimens, but fail to comply with exercise or oxygen therapies. Thus, a successful program must take into consideration the demands of each regimen.

Taking Medicine

Several practical suggestions emerge from the review of research on adherence to medical regimens. These suggestions parallel discussions on the locus of the problem. First, alterations in the patient's environment may increase adherence behavior. Simple techniques, such as using mailed reminders, placing reminder magnets on refrigerators, or phone call reminders, have been successful in several studies. Some new products provide auditory cues as reminders. Patients might also purchase digital watches that beep according to their medical regimen schedule.

Behavioral contracts have also been used with some success. These contracts specify precise regimens and often require the patient to make some desired event or activity contingent upon medicine use. For example, the contract might make some highly probable behavior, such as watching television, contingent upon medicine use.

A second approach to increasing medicine taking compliance requires enhanced physician–patient communication. A major focus of pulmonary rehabilitation programs is in educating patients and family members about their disease and treatments and in enhancing their ability to communicate with their physicians. Several studies have shown that patients often have misconceptions about their illness and about the expected effects of medications.[75] Furthermore, patients often experience side effects of medication. Rarely is this information fully communicated to the provider.[5] Physicians should ask about all reactions to medication, barriers to taking medication in the patient's environment, and should clarify the patient's view of why the medications may or may not be effective.

Finally, several recent papers have suggested that interventions designed to increase patient's involvement might increase adherence and ultimately affect patient outcome. In one experiment, patients were coached on which questions to ask their provider before their encounter. In comparison with a group that received traditional patient education, those in the coaching group had actually achieved better health outcomes. Analysis of audio tapes of these physician–patient interactions demonstrated that those in the experimental group were twice as effective as those in the control group in obtaining appropriate information from their physician.[76] The patient-counseling sessions involved the use of a disease-specific algorithm and a set of diagnostic and therapeutic guidelines presented in the branching logic format. The purpose of the session was to identify important components of medical decisions and to increase the patient involvement at each decision point. Other algorithms have now been developed for several chronic disease conditions.

Smoking

Practical guidelines for helping patients to stop smoking have been well described in the literature. Despite the well-established health consequences of cigarette smoking, less than one-half of physicians commonly advise their patients to give up cigarettes.[77] Among those who discuss smoking with their patients, few go much further. For example, only about one in four physicians makes any effort beyond simply stating that the patient should quit smoking.[78]

One of the most important and simple components of a smoking cessation program is to set a specific quit date. Beyond this, patients also need specific instructions in how to prepare for potential relapse situations. For example, weight gain following smoking cessation is common, particularly among women. Counseling relative to these issues is important.

A variety of excellent materials are available to help the patient through the cessation process. Some of these are described in Table 6–1. We prefer the American Lung Association programs because they have been widely disseminated and well tested. However, many of the other programs are equally effective.

TABLE   6–1.   Self-Help Smoking Cessation Programs
Available to Physicians

Name of Program	Materials	Available From
Stop Smoking Kit	Guidebooks, posters, audio tapes, behavioral contracts, and other	American Academy of Family Practice
Heart Rx	Guidebooks, posters, outreach materials, pearl forms, and other	American Heart Association
University of Massachusetts Program	Slides, manual, video tapes	Department of Preventive Medicine University of Massachusetts
Quit for Good	Guidebook, posters, and program, "Let's help smokers quit"	Office of Cancer Communication— American Cancer Society
Freedom From Smoking	Individual self-help program	American Lung Association
Cool-Turkey Kit	Self-help manual with behavior modification instructions	Center for Disease Prevention Stanford University

Exercise

Patient adherence to exercise is perhaps the most difficult and least studied of problems. Exercise requires alteration in life-style, coping with uncomfortable sensations, and changes in daily schedules. To improve adherence with an exercise program, we recommend the following:

1. *Set realistic goals.* Patients who set goals too high become discouraged.
2. *Perform a functional analysis.* This involves identifying highly probable enjoyable behaviors such as watching television, reading a novel, or having a cup of coffee. These activities will differ from patient to patient. Once identified, the highly probable behaviors can be used as reinforcers for the exercise activity. The patient might be asked to sign a contract in which he or she agrees to make enjoyable activities contingent upon completion of an exercise session.
3. *Use cognitive techniques.* Identify negative things a patient may say to himself or herself during an exercise session. Then teach the patient to use realistic, but positive, self-talk. For example, for a person who says to himself or herself, "This is painful, I can't stand this," the positive coping self-statements of, "Although this is painful, I know it will be good for me in the end," might be substituted. These statements must be rehearsed and practiced. Techniques for developing these statements have been described elsewhere.[79]

SUMMARY

Given the importance of COPD in terms of death, disability, and medical expense, it is surprising that so little attention has been devoted to adherence with common regimens. In contrast to nearly every other major medical condition, there are few published studies evaluating the benefits of behavioral interventions to improve adherence. In addition, there are no population-based studies on adherence; hence, we cannot estimate the magnitude of the problem with much certainty. We also do not know the extent to which problems, such as overcompliance, affect detrimental outcomes for patients with COPD. At present, the measures of adherence used, such as the mean number of pills consumed, self-report of regimen adherence, or percentages of patients who complied with "all recommendations," no longer provide sufficient information. Newer techniques, such as those that attach microprocessors to pill bottle caps, may soon provide important new insights.

Directions for Future Research

The typical regimen for patients with COPD requires many different behaviors. These might include the use of several different medications, exercise, oxygen, respiratory and physiotherapy techniques, and other aspects of self-care. It is unknown whether or not these different behaviors are intercorrelated. In other chronic illnesses, such as hypertension and diabetes, adherence with one aspect of the regimen is often not correlated with adherence to other components. More research is necessary to define the interrelations between behaviors relevant to the management of patients with COPD.

A second direction for future research concerns overcompliance. This is a particular concern for inhaled medications that provide symptomatic relief and have potential toxic side effects. More research is necessary to document overcompliance and evaluate effects upon health outcome.

More research is also needed to link adherence with measurable health outcomes. Currently, we know very little about how to improve adherence for patients with COPD. There are only a few published studies on increasing adherence to prescribed medications. The problem of smoking cessation has been well studied, but has received insufficient attention in some groups such as the elderly. These problems require further systematic investigation.

In summary, COPD is an important health problem that requires further systematic investigation. There has been very little behavioral research relevant to COPD. Yet, behavior change, in the form of adherence to various recommendations, may be essential for obtaining optimal patient outcomes. We strongly encourage further research relevant to the clinical management of patients with COPD.

REFERENCES

1. DiMatteo MR, DiNicola D. Achieving patient compliance. New York: Pergamon, 1982.
2. Becker MH, Maiman LA. Strategies for enhancing patient compliance. J Commun Health 1980;6:113.
3. Becker MH. Patient adherence to prescribed therapies. Med Care 1985;23:539.

4. Blackwell B. Patient compliance. N Engl J Med 1973;289:249.

5. Kaplan RM, Simon HJ. Compliance in medical care: reconsideration of self-prediction. Ann Behav Med 1990;12:2.

6. Sackett DL. A compliance practicum for the busy practitioner. In: Haynes RB, Taylor DW, Sackett DL, eds. Compliance in health care. Baltimore: Johns Hopkins University Press, 1979.

7. Sackett DL, Snow JC. The magnitude and measurement of compliance. In: Haynes RB, Taylor DW, Sackett DL, eds. Compliance in health care. Baltimore: Johns Hopkins University Press, 1979.

8. Gates SJ, Colborn DK. Lowering appointment failures in a neighborhood health center. Med Care 1976;14:263.

9. Caldwell JR, Cobb S, Dowling MD, DeJongh D. The dropout problem in antihypertensive treatment: a pilot study of social and emotional factors influencing a patient's ability to follow antihypertensive treatment. J Chronic Dis 1971;22:579.

10. Caron HS, Roth HP. Objective assessment of cooperation with an ulcer diet: relation to antacid intake and to assigned physician. Am J Med Sci 1971;261:61.

11. Norell SE. Accuracy of patient interviews and estimates by clinical staff determining medication compliance. Soc Sci Med 1981;15:57.

12. Epstein LH, Cluss PA. A behavioral medicine perspective on adherence to long-term medical regimens. J Consult Clin Psychol 1982;50:950.

13. Hillman E, Huffmann K, Harari H, Yaremko RM. Deliberate noncompliance, client improvement and feedback to physicians. Presented at the Western Psychological Association, Reno, April, 1988.

14. Kaplan RM, Toshima MT, Atkins CJ, Ries AL. Adherence to prescribed regimens for patients with chronic obstructive pulmonary disease. In Shumaker, SA, Shron EB, Ockene JK, eds. The handbook of health behavior change. New York: Springer, 1990;126.

15. Atkins CJ. A randomized clinical trial comparing cognitive and behavioral strategies for exercise compliance among chronic obstructive pulmonary disease patients [Dissertation]. Riverside: University of California, 1981.

16. Haynes RB, Taylor DW, Sackett DL. Compliance in health care. Baltimore: John Hopkins University Press, 1979.

17. James PNE, Anderson JB, Priar JG, White JP, Henry JA, Cochrane GM. Patterns of drug taking in patients with chronic airflow obstruction. Postgrad Med J 1985;61:7.

18. Dolce JJ, Crips C, Manzella B, Richards JM, Hardin JM, Bailey WC. Medication adherence patterns in chronic obstructive pulmonary disease. Chest 1991;99:837.

19. DeTullio PL, Kirkling DM, Arslanian C, Olson DE. Compliance measure development and assessment of theophylline therapy in ambulatory patients. J Clin Pharm Ther 1987;12:19.

20. Nocturnal Oxygen Therapy Trial Group. Continuous or nocturnal oxygen therapy in hypoxemic chronic obstructive lung disease: a clinical trial. Ann Intern Med 1980;93:391.

21. Medical Research Council Working Party. Long term domiciliary oxygen therapy in chronic hypoxic cor pulmonale complicating chronic bronchitis and emphysema. Lancet 1981;1:681.

22. McSweeney AJ, Grant I, Heaton RK, Adams KM, Timms RM. Life quality of patients with chronic obstructive pulmonary disease. Arch Intern Med 1982;142:473.

23. Heaton RK, Grant I, McSweeney AJ, Adams KM, Petty TL. Psychologic effects of continuous and nocturnal oxygen therapy in hypoxemic chronic obstructive pulmonary disease. Arch Intern Med 1983;143:1941.

24. Walshaw MJ, Lim R, Evans CC, Hind CR. Factors influencing the compliance of patients using oxygen concentrators for long-term home oxygen therapy. Respir Med 1990;84:331.

25. Heimlich HJ, Carr GC. The micro-trach. A seven-year experience with transtracheal oxygen therapy. Chest 1989;95:1008.

26. American Thoracic Society. Standards for the diagnosis and care of patients with chronic obstructive pulmonary disease (COPD) and asthma. Am Rev Respir Dis 1987; 136:225.

27. Hodgkin JE. Pulmonary rehabilitation: structure, components, and benefits. J Cardiopulm Rehabil 1988;11:423.

28. Hodgkin JE, Zorn EG, Connors GL, eds. Pulmonary rehabilitation: guidelines to success. Boston: Butterworth Publishers, 1984.

29. Guyatt GH, Berman LB, Townsend M. Long-term outcome after respiratory rehabilitation. Can Med Assoc J 1987;137:1089.

30. Belman MJ. Exercise in chronic obstructive pulmonary disease. Clin Chest Med 1986;7:585.

31. Petty TL, Nett LM, Finigan MM, Brink GA, Corsello PR. A comprehensive care program for chronic airway obstruction: methods and preliminary evaluation of symptomatic and functional improvement. Ann Intern Med 1969;70:1109.

32. American Thoracic Society. Pulmonary rehabilitation. Am Rev Respir Dis 1981; 124:663.

33. Ries AL. Position paper of the American Association of Cardiovascular and Pulmonary Rehabilitation: scientific basis of pulmonary rehabilitation. J Cardiopulm Rehabil 1990;10:418–441.

34. Bell CW, Jensen RH. Physical conditioning. In: Jensen RH, Kass I, eds. Pulmonary rehabilitation home programs. Omaha: University of Nebraska Medical Center, 1977.

35. Unger K, Moser K, Hansen P. Selection of an exercise program for patients with chronic obstructive pulmonary disease. Heart Lung 1980;9:68.

36. Moser KM, Bokinsky GE, Savage RT, Archibald CJ, Hansen PR. Results of a comprehensive rehabilitation program: physiologic and functional effects on patients with chronic obstructive pulmonary disease. Arch Intern Med 1980;140:1596.

37. Bass H, Whitcomb JF, Forman R. Exercise training: therapy for patients with chronic obstructive pulmonary disease. Chest 1970;57:116.

38. Fishmen DB, Petty TL. Physical, symptomatic and psychological improvement in patients receiving comprehensive care for chronic airway obstruction. J Chronic Dis 1971;24:775.

39. Pierce AK, Paez PN, Miller WF. Exercise training with the aid of a portable oxygen supply in patients with emphysema. Am Rev Respir Dis 1965;91:653.

40. Shephard RJ. On the design and effectiveness of training regimens in chronic obstructive lung disease. Bull Eur Physiopathol Respir 1977;13:457.

41. Cockcroft AE, Saunders MT, Berry G. Randomized controlled trial of rehabilitation in chronic respiratory disability. Thorax 1981;36:200.

42. McGavin CR, Gupta SP, Lloyd EL, McHardy JR. Physical rehabilitation of chronic bronchitis: results of a controlled trial of exercises in the home. Thorax 1977;32:307.

43. Ambrosino N, Paggiaro PL, Macchi M, et al. A study of short-term effect of rehabilitative therapy in chronic obstructive pulmonary disease. Respiration 1981;41:40.

44. Belman MJ, Wasserman K. Exercise training and testing in patients with chronic obstructive pulmonary disease. Basics RD 1981;10:1.

45. Mertens DJ, Shephard RJ, Kavanagh T. Long-term exercise therapy for chronic obstructive lung disease. Respiration 1978;35:96.

46. Atkins CJ, Kaplan RM, Timms RM, Reinsch S, Lofback K. Behavioral programs for exercise compliance in COPD. J Consult Clin Psychol 1984;52:591.

47. Kaplan RM. Quality-of-life measurement. In: Karoly P, ed. Measurement strategies in health psychology. New York: Wiley-Interscience, 1985:115.

48. Kaplan RM, Anderson JP. The general health policy model: an integrated approach. In: Spilker B, ed. Quality of life assessment in clinical trials. New York: Raven Press, 1990:131.

49. Toevs CT, Kaplan RM, Atkins CJ. The costs and effects of behavioral programs in chronic obstructive pulmonary disease. Med Care 1984;22:1088.

50. Atkins CJ, Hayes J, Kaplan RM. Four year follow-up of behavioral programs in COPD. University of California Health Psychology Conference. Lake Arrowhead, CA: June 1984.

51. Bandura A. Self-efficacy: toward a unifying theory of behavior change. Psychol Rev 1977;84:191.

52. Kaplan RM, Atkins CJ, Reinsch S. Specific efficacy expectations mediate exercise compliance in patients with COPD. Health Psychol 1984;3:223.

53. Redline S, Tager IB. The relationship of airway reactivity to the occurrence of chronic obstructive pulmonary disease: an epidemiological assessment. In: Hensley NJ, Saunder NA, eds. Clinical epidemiology of chronic obstructive pulmonary disease. New York: Marcel Dekker, 1989:169.

54. Dockery DW, Speizer FE, Ferris BG, Ware JH, Louis TA, Spiro A. Cumulative and reversible effects of lifetime smoking on simple tests of lung function in adults. Am Rev Respir Dis 1988;137:286.

55. Camilli AE, Burrows B, Knudson RJ, Lyle SK, Lebowitz MD. Longitudinal changes in forced expiratory volume in one second in adults. Effects of smoking and smoking cessation. Am Rev Respir Dis 1987;135:794.

56. Ockene JK. Physician-delivered intervention for smoking cessation: strategies for increasing effectiveness Prev Med 1987;16:723.

57. Ockene JK, Kristeller J, Goldberg R, et al. Increasing the efficacy of physician-delivered smoking intervention: a randomized clinical trial. J Gen Intern Med 1991;6:1.

58. Kottke TE, Brekke ML, Solberg LI, Hughes JR. A randomized trial to increase smoking intervention by physicians. JAMA 1989;261:2101.

59. Cummings SR, Coates TJ, Richard RJ, et al. Training physicians in counseling about smoking cessation. A randomized trial of the "Quit for Life" program. Ann Intern Med 1989;110:640.

60. Chryssidis E, Frewin DB, Frith PA, Dawes ER. Compliance with aerosol therapy in chronic obstructive lung disease. N Z Med J 1981;94:375.

61. Cramer JA, Mattson RH, Prevey ML, Scheyer RD, Ouellette VL. How often is medication taken as prescribed? A novel assessment technique. JAMA 1989;261:3273.

62. Rudd P, Dyyny RL, Zachary V, et al. Pill count measures of compliance in a drug trial: variability and suitability. Am J Hypertens 1988;3(part 1):309.

63. Rudd P, Dyyny RL, Zachary V, et al. The natural history of medication compliance in a drug trail: limitations of pill counts. J Clin Pharm Ther 1989;46:176.

64. Appelbaum SA. The refusal to take one's medicine. Bull Menninger Clin 1977;41:511.

65. Stone GC. Patient compliance and the role of the expert. J Soc Issues 1979;35:34.

66. Corish CD, Richard B, Brown S. Missed medication doses in rheumatoid arthritis patients: intentional and unintentional reasons. Arthritis Care Res 1989;2:3.

67. Agras WS. Understanding compliance with the medical regimen: the scope of the problem and a theoretical perspective. Arthritis Care Res 1989;2:S2.

68. Stamler R, Stamler J, Civinelli J, et al. Adherence and blood pressure response to hypertension treatment. Lancet 1975;2:1227.

69. Inui TS, Carter WB. Problems and prospects for health services research on provider–patient communication. Med Care 1985;23:521.

70. Liang MH. Compliance and quality of life: confessions of a difficult patient. Arthritis Care Res 1989;2:S71.

71. Green LW, Mullen PD, Stainbrook GL. Programs to reduce drug errors in the elderly: direct and indirect evidence from patient education. J Geriat Drug Ther 1986;1:3.

72. Steel K, Gertman P, Crescenzi C, Anderson J. Iatrogenic illness on a general medicine service at a university hospital. N Engl J Med 1981;304:638.

73. Hurwitz N. Predisposing factors in adverse reactions to drugs. Br Med J 1969;1:536.

74. Williamson J, Chapin JM. Adverse reactions to prescribed drugs in the elderly: a multicare investigation. Age Ageing 1980;9:73.

75. Leventhal H. The role of theory in the study of adherence to treatment and doctor–patient interactions. Med Care 1985;23:556.

76. Greenfield S, Kaplan S, Ware JE. Expanding patient involvement in care: effects on patient outcomes. Ann Intern Med 1985;102:520.

77. Ockene JK, Aney J, Goldberg RJ, Klar JM, Williams JW. A survey of Massachusetts physicians for the possibility of preventing smoking practices. Am J Prev Med 1988;4:14.

78. Rose G, Hamilton PJS. A randomized controled trial of the effects on middle-aged men of advice to stop smoking. J Epidemiol Community Health 1982;36:102.

79. Kaplan RM, Atkins CJ. Interventions for patients with COPD. In: McSweeney AJ, Grant I, eds. Chronic obstructive pulmonary disease: a behavioral perspective. New York: Marcel Dekker, 1988:123.

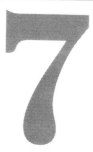

JAMES A. PETERS

Preventive Care in Pulmonary Rehabilitation

LEADING CAUSES OF MORBIDITY AND MORTALITY

Each year in the United States there are over 2 million people who die of all causes. Chronic diseases are the major contributing factors to about 75% of these deaths. Chronic obstructive pulmonary disease (COPD) makes up one category of these chronic diseases and ranks as the fifth leading cause of death, with approximately 79,000 deaths in 1989. It is also responsible for a disporportionate amount of morbidity. With a current COPD prevalence of 10 million Americans and with indications that it is continuing to increase, the impact on daily living is significant.[1] Patients with chronic lung disease are twice as likely to rate their health as being poor, and they experience twice as many restricted activity days and days spent in bed because of illness than do the general population. It is calculated that, for 1989, over 140,000 years of productive life were lost secondary to COPD.[2] Additionally, patients with COPD make up 5% of physician office visits and 13% of hospital admissions each year.[3] The leading causes of morbidity in the United States are respiratory problems. This accounts for the most days off from work. In a patient population with severely compromised lung function, respiratory infections, such as pneumonia or influenza, can be life-threatening.

Chronic diseases typically have long incubation periods before symptoms become discernible or the disease diagnosable. Because of the long incubation period, which can be measured in decades, there is opportunity for preventive medicine to alter the course, and possibly the outcome, of the disease process. When rehabilitation is instituted, there is already presumption of disease; however, since pulmonary disease is a continuous progressive process, preventive interventions can be of benefit at any point along the way.

Since pulmonary disease becomes manifest preponderantly in older persons, there is an increased likelihood that other chronic diseases may also be present. The coexisting chronic diseases must be addressed in the rehabilitation process. One must be aware of the other leading causes of death that are of high prevalence in this aged group: heart disease, cancers, stroke, pneumonia and influenza, accidents, and suicide.[4]

Many pulmonary patients may have complicating factors from coexisting cardiovascular disease which, by itself, remains the single leading cause of mortality in the United States. Evidence suggests that heart patients with diminished lung function have a poorer prognosis, and poor lung function appears to be an independent risk factor.[5,6] Some level of airway obstruction, whether identified or not, might be a contributing cause of cardiac mortality. Lung mechanics appears to be an independent predictor of mortality for patients with coronary disease, for patients with COPD, and for the population in general. The pathophysiologic relation is unclear, but the forced expiratory volume in 1 second (FEV_1) is inversely related to mortality.[7,8]

Cancer mortality is additionally higher in the pulmonary patient age group. The leading cause of cancer mortality is cancer of the lung, which has been on the increase. In fact, there appears to be a consistent relation between obstructive airway disease and increased risk of lung cancer.[8,9] Therefore, recognizing this and implementing appropriate screening are indicated.

Rehabilitation and prevention, to have a real effect, must deal with all of the factors that affect a patient's life, not just their primary disease.[10,11] Therapeutic preventive interventions require the support of all members of the rehabilitation team, owing to the multiple components that affect one's health.

REHABILITATION AND PREVENTIVE MEDICINE DEFINED

Rehabilitation is the process of restoring a person to a maximal degree of functioning. Rehabilitation is actually on the opposite end of the health care spectrum from prevention. Whereas *prevention* tries to keep one from harm, rehabilitation tries to restore one to health *after* being harmed. However, preventive medicine remains applicable throughout the health spectrum as long as someone is alive. No matter how sick one is, there is always some further complication that can be prevented. The primary goal of pulmonary rehabilitation is to return the patient to the highest level of function possible. The role of preventive care in pulmonary rehabilitation is to prospectively protect one's health. This is accomplished through health education, selected medical interventions, proper nutrition, specific physical exercises, abstaining from breathing harmful fumes, and improving one's respiratory living environment.

Preventive medicine has two major thrusts: health promotion and disease prevention. Health promotion requires the active participation of the patient. One must pursue healthy activities and not merely avoid harmful habits. It is the patients who are responsible for their own health, and it is their choices that ultimately determine the health outcome. Patients must become active in the treatment determine the health outcome. Patients must become active in the treatment process.

Prevention is vitally important, but often carries a negative connotation—one of avoiding disease or behaviors that are harmful. Avoidance of unhealthy items or activities is certainly necessary, but this should not be the focus. Avoidance is best accomplished by substituting new behaviors to replace the old. One must "overcome evil with good" (Romans 12:21).[12] Prevention is more secure when one actively pursues the desired behaviors, as opposed to simply trying to stop the undesired ones.

Prevention is defined in three levels: primary, secondary, and tertiary prevention. *Primary prevention* is similar to health promotion in that it deals with "riskness" instead of sickness; intervention with life-style change to decrease one's risk while there is still no evidence of disease. The prevention of smoking behaviors, therefore, of smoking, results in avoidance of smoking-related diseases. *Secondary prevention* begins after there is disease already present, but symptoms are not readily apparent. Here, a patient with an abnormal expiratory flow rate on a spirometry test who currently feels fine is encouraged to alter or cease his or her smoking. This is secondary prevention. This usually requires some type of screening or physical examination so that altered function can be detected. This is the purpose of regular or periodic health screens in populations at elevated risk. *Tertiary prevention* is what primarily occurs during pulmonary rehabilitation. Here, a patient already has an established disease with symptoms, and treatment is geared toward slowing down the progression and complications to minimize the disability.

The foregoing distinctions are classic definitions of prevention, but in clinical practice they are not mutually exclusive. All three components often occur simultaneously. Chronic hypoxemia secondary to chronic lung disease can eventually lead to cor pulmonale and subsequent worsening disability. The use of continuous low-flow oxygen can help prevent this from occurring, and this is primary prevention in an established disease process, since it prevents a new disorder from developing.[13] No matter what level of functioning, or what disease a patient has, preventive interventions can be efficacious.

Prevention is in essence a philosophy or attitude toward health wherein one pays attention to unhealthy behaviors, to environmental and hereditary factors that predispose a patient towards sickness, or to compromised function. These factors are termed *risk factors,* since they place a person at risk for illness. Special emphasis is placed on those risk factors that are modifiable. The major risk factors for the top six causes of death in the United States are tobacco use, hypertension, elevated blood cholesterol, poor nutrition, physical inactivity, and heavy alcohol use.[14] Recent estimates suggest that if only one risk factor is eliminated from each of the six major chronic diseases, mortality could be reduced by 47%.[15] Modest changes in life-style could result in significant decreases in health care expenditures and improvement in quantity and quality of life. Since prevention is focused on things that have not yet happened—but could—one could think of this as prospective health care.

Preventive medicine has traditionally emphasized interventions in the public health arena through education and legislation. Public health policies influence such basics as food safety and availability (for some), clean water, clean air, sanitation, housing, immunizations, and tuberculosis screening. These services definitely have an effect on pulmonary rehabilitation patients.

Pulmonary rehabilitation programs, however, make the most use of the emerging area of clinical preventive medicine. In clinical preventive medicine, conclusions from epidemiologic population-based studies are applied to the individual, with the purpose of individualizing a prospective plan for wellness. Clinical preventive medicine begins with careful assessment of an individual patient to determine current health status and functional capacities. Then a careful inventory is made of health behaviors, habits, addictions, nutritional intake, activities, and hereditary factors, along with the patient's personal health goals. Health risks are subsequently identified, specific educational interventions are implemented that target high-risk behaviors, and reinforcement is given to encourage healthy habits that the patient is already practicing. A health plan is outlined and prioritized, such that the most crucial health changes are given the most attention. If a patient smokes, there are few other behaviors that are as important—especially for patients with pulmonary disorders. Breathing fresh air on a 24-hour basis is always the first goal. If a patient does not smoke, but is exposed to second-hand smoke, fumes, dusts, or even poorly ventilated homes in which gas is used for cooking, fresh air remains a priority. In each instance, the health factors that affect the quality of the air breathed or the respiratory system itself, become one of the first priorities for preventive therapies. Reversible airway obstruction needs to receive appropriate pharmacologic treatments on a regular basis. Prompt treatment of respiratory tract infections is crucial to help prevent pneumonia and minimize further compromised lung function. Immunization for pneumococcal pneumonia, the most frequent community-acquired pneumonia, is prudent. Yearly vaccination against influenza is also recommended, as influenza can be life-threatening for the elderly, chronically ill and, especially, for those with diminished pulmonary reserves.[16] November is the best month for influenza immunizations so that immune titers are optimal during the peak of the season. Those with significant sensitivity to eggs should not be vaccinated.

Preventive medicine's role is to educate, motivate, and then assist the patient in achieving the level of health that he or she chooses. At times, patients will not choose to be as healthy as the physician or other health professionals feel they can be, but ultimately, each person is responsible for his or her own health. It would be unethical to "force" one's concept of health onto another person. The methods of intervention are through education, encouragement, and motivation, as well as creating an environment in which new healthy behaviors can be tried. The purpose of health education is to help people understand how their body and lungs function. They must also be taught the basics of pulmonary pathophysiology so that they can better deal with their disease. Compliance with therapy is enhanced when patients have a better understanding about what is going on.

DEFINITIONS OF HEALTH

It is worthwhile to define health, since this is what treatment or rehabilitation programs aim to achieve. The World Health Organization (WHO) has one of the best definitions of *health*: "Health is a state of complete physical, mental, and social well-being and not merely the absence of disease or infirmity."[17] Many would add to this definition of health a spiritual component that would encompass one's relation with God or a "higher power," self-worth, morals, higher values, and purpose. Figure 7–1 encompasses what is referred to as *(w)holistic medicine*, since the concept of health includes the "whole" person: physical, mental, social, and spiritual. Because of

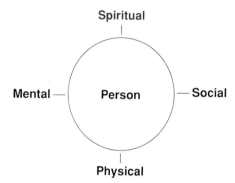

FIGURE 7-1 To be healthy requires a balanced interaction among the physical, social, mental, and spiritual aspects of life. All areas impinge on health, and each of these must be addressed.

the intimate interaction among each of these components, optimal health can be achieved only when a balance is realized among these areas. Physical health will affect how one thinks or relates with other people, as well as determining the amount of energy that is available to be spent on the other areas. Mental health affects how one feels and influences one's relationships. One's spiritual concepts will influence one's social life and mental aspects. In the true sense, health is not simply achieving some yet-to-be defined optimal state, but it is a way of living. Health is an attitude toward life that encourages the best physical, mental, social, and spiritual well-being. This process of being healthy requires choosing the best air to breath, the best fluids to drink, the best foods to eat, as well as planning for the appropriate exercise, rest, and social interactions.

THERAPEUTIC AGENTS OF PREVENTIVE MEDICINE

The therapeutic modalities of preventive medicine are outlined in Table 7–1. Unlike medicines, these agents are absolutely essential, whether in health or sickness. It can also be observed that these elements are subcomponents of the physical, mental, social, and spiritual aspects of people. Some of the elements are things that must be taken in; others are things which must be done by a person; and still other items represent things that take place within the person. Any therapeutic intervention—no matter what discipline—is achieved by influencing one or more of these elements.

The physical elements are self-selected, self-dosed, and consumed at will, by the patient. In moderation, adverse effects are rare. Because of the variety of options, and the uniqueness of some diseases, education concerning quantity, quality, and type of the consumable elements becomes important. In the proper amounts the body uses these essential elements for both energy and growth as well as healing. The most important item on the list is air, which is listed under *physical*. Air is the most urgent of the many listed, since it is the item that can most quickly affect a person's health if it is in insufficient supply or is contaminated. Provided good air is available, many patients must be taught more efficient ways of breathing. Respiratory mechanics are often less than efficient, use of accessory muscles of breathing are common, poor use of the diaphragm is frequent, minimal breathing endurance often exists, and poor posture often further limits respiratory activities. For some, altered chemosensor

TABLE 7–1. Primary Therapeutic Modalities of Preventive Medicine

Physical	Air
	Water
	Nutrition
	Exercise
	Rest
	Senses
	Hygiene
	Sunlight
Mental	Motivation
	Power of choice
	Positive self-concept
	Values
	Trust
Social	Positive relationships
	Love
	To care and be cared for
Spiritual	Meditation
	Concept of God
	Morality
	Ethics
	Love
	Beliefs

function can compromise respiratory drive and result in persistently elevated carbon dioxide (CO_2) and low oxygen (O_2) levels in the blood. Rehabilitation must assess all of these factors and aggressively assist the patient in the optimal exchange of gases from the lungs. This often involves first assessing, and then supplying, appropriate levels of supplemental oxygen. Morbidity and mortality improve with continuous use of supplemental oxygen in patients who are hypoxemic.[18] Unfortunately, the documentation for third-party reimbursement necessary to support oxygen therapy is becoming more burdensome. Breathing retraining with careful attention to muscle mechanics and posture is basic. Correct use of bronchodilator and steroid inhalers to facilitate improved airflow and decrease inflammation of the airways will help decrease the oxygen cost of breathing. Active avoidance of dusts, of airway irritants, and of extreme or abrupt temperature or humidity changes, as well as cessation of smoking, are vital tasks of preventive education in the rehabilitation process.

Second in importance is fluid intake. About two-thirds of a person's weight is water. Water is the medium in which all biochemical metabolic activities occur and is necessary to bring nutrients to the tissues as well as washing waste products away.

Adequate fluid intake is vital for lung function. Respiratory airways are at 100% relative humidity at body temperature, and proper viscosity of phlegm and enhancement of expectoration requires adequate water intake. Whether sufficient water is being consumed can be estimated by observing how clear the urine is. The urine should be clear in appearance at least one or more times in a day. Water applied externally is necessary for hygiene and, when experienced at differing temperatures, it can be either stimulating or relaxing without any untoward side effects.

Nutrition is an important consideration in patients with COPD.[19] The first concern of the body is meeting its energy requirements. There is a measured increase in metabolic rate in malnourished patients who have COPD, that is thought to be due to an increased work of breathing, but there may be other factors.[20] For bronchitic patients, weight loss may be in order. For emphysema patients, being underweight is more likely, and the challenge is in maintaining sufficient caloric intake. In fact, some patients with severe COPD continue to lose weight, even after caloric intake has been increased.[21]

The quality of the foods consumed has been receiving more attention, with special concern for carbohydrate and fat intake. Excess consumption of carbohydrates can result in increased carbon dioxide production and result in ventilatory problems if a patient's respiratory reserve is limited. It appears, however, that the problem lies in the *excessive* use of carbohydrates and not simply in their use in general. Carbohydrate foods remain one of the primary and important fuel sources. Problems associated with carbohydrate foods have largely been with excess parental use of carbohydrates, but can occur with enteral use. This being said, one should also note that there are definite advantages to the use of carbohydrates, and the appropriate use of these foods should not be discouraged. Carbohydrates can improve oxygenation, endurance performance, lower blood cholesterol, and decrease risk for heart disease and stroke. They can elevate partial pressure of arterial oxygen (PaO_2), which can significantly improve oxygen saturation when a patient's PaO_2 is low and, therefore, on the steep portion of the oxygen dissociation curve.[22] In fact, this advantage can also be seen in COPD carbon dioxide-retaining subjects without an additonal increase in $PaCO_2$.[23] On the other hand, increased fat in the diet tends to lower the oxygen saturation.[24,25] But then fat also contains the greatest number of calories for the volume consumed and, therefore, is an excellent source of extra calories for patients who are underweight. Fats also result in a lower carbon dioxide production with their metabolism, when compared with carbohydrates. Protein, like carbohydrate and fat, requires planning to help the patient obtain the appropriate quantity and quality. Not enough protein results in increased infections and edema, whereas too much increases stress on the kidneys, can alter acid–base balance (acidic residue of proteins), and increase ventilatory drive. Patients with limited respiratory reserve cannot tolerate an increased ventilatory drive for any prolonged period. The process of eating can also drop oxygen saturation.[26] Supplemental oxygen during meal times may be necessary for some; however, nasal cannula use diminishes the sense of smell, and this makes eating less enjoyable. Dietitians must be alert to the advantages and disadvantages of various dietaries and ultimately adjust the diet to best suit the patient, regardless of the theoretical arguments of one type of diet over another.

There appears to be benefits derived from the consumption of foods high in antioxidants, such as beta-carotene, vitamins C and E, selenium, and glutathione. There is a suggested decrease in various cancers—including some cancers of the lung—in those people who consume greater quantities of vegetables and fruits higher in these nutrients.[27] Vitamin C might help decrease lung emphysema development. Experimentally, vitamin C can decrease migration of polymorphonuclear leukocytes into lung tissue, in addition to its protective effects against lung oxidant injury.[28] Glutathione, a sulfhydryl compound, is an important endogenous antioxidant, and it plays an important role in the maintenance of cellular proteins and lipids in their functional state.[29] Research in these areas is ongoing and may provide exciting new therapeutic and preventive approaches.

Another preventive agent is exercise. Patients with disorders who engage in regular exercise, including those with marked hypercapnia, experience increased endurance and higher levels of functioning.[30] Typically, aerobic exercises, such as walking or use of a bicycle ergometer, are the major exercises prescribed for patients with COPD. However, specific training for respiratory muscles can improve maximal sustained ventilation, increase maximal inspiratory and expiratory pressures, and increase peak flow rates.[31–33] Regular upper body exercises for COPD patients are reported to decrease perceived breathlessness and fatigue.[34] A carefully designed and progressive exercise program that involves both upper and lower body exercises is of great benefit and can decrease hospitalizations and improve quality of living.[35,36] Prescribed exercise intensities should be derived from actual pulmonary exercise stress testing.[37] Some patients will be found to require supplemental oxygen with increased metabolic work, whereas others actually improve their oxygen saturation with light-to-moderate activity. The resting diffusing lung capacity for carbon monoxide (DLCO) and oxygen saturation have some predictive value for which patients might need supplemental oxygen during exercise.[38] The need for oxygen should not be a limiting factor to prevent one from exercise. Exercise is also a natural mood elevator and counteracts depression. Exercise will also help promote relaxation, improved high-density lipoprotein (HDL) cholesterol levels, better blood sugar regulation, improved performance of activities of daily living, better sleep, and faster emptying of the stomach. For those patients with symptoms of belching, indigestion, constipation, or acid reflux, light-to-moderate exercise helps speed up motility and can help decrease some of their symptoms without the use of medications.[39,40]

The full health benefits of sunlight are still to be elucidated. Sunlight has antimicrobial action, influences the circadian rhythm, contributes to vitamin D conversion in the skin, and lifts the spirits. Excess sunlight is to be avoided because of the damaging effects to the skin and the increased risk of melanoma.

The mental component of one's health is extremely important and influences the overall health to a major extent. A positive mental attitude and a good sense of humor appear to fortify against disease and help a person better deal with his or her disability. ("A merry heart doeth good like a medicine." Proverbs 17:22.[12]) Patients who keep their minds productive and active are observed to have fewer somatic complaints. Encouragement of their value as persons and attention to building patients' self-worth takes on increasing importance as their physical capabilities diminish.

Team members should help clarify a patient's health values. Compliance with healthy behaviors are more likely when a patient values the anticipated outcome. *Motivation* is defined as a driving force or a desire that is often triggered by an event that gets a person's attention. Some of the strongest motivating factors arise from the possibility of improved function, whereas other important motivation factors occur from the discovery of an abnormal test result. The motivation leads to efforts to change behavior to improve one's health or avoid an uncomfortable situation. Despite values or motivation, a person ultimately must *choose* to make a change. The decision to alter behavior requires effort. The more decisive a patient is in making the decision, then, the more energy he or she can focus on the new behavior. The rehabilitation team must help motivate and encourage positive choices by the patients that will support their health values. The mere decision to make a change does not immediately result in perceptible improvement. Consistent application of healthy choices and actions is necessary before improvement in health can be realized. During the early phases of behavioral change, patients need positive feedback to help reinforce the new behaviors. In time, the benefits inherent in the new behaviors will be self-reinforcing, and little or no outside feedback should be necessary. Motivating patient responsibility is a major task for the rehabilitation team. It is important for the patient to become responsible for his or her own health—no one else can provide as good care. The success of any health program or rehabilitation clinic is ultimately dependent on the patient, who finally must comply with treatment recommendations. Close cooperation between patient and rehabilitation team members is important so that the treatment plans developed are ones the patient is willing to follow.

Social interaction provides for love, companionship, and other social interactions. To care and be cared for is therapeutic and, in the right balance, enhances health. Chronic lung disease diminishes social interactions and produces difficulties in the management of home affairs.[41] Strategies for preventing increasing social isolation are necessary. Chronic lung disease in a family affects more than just the patient. The social unit—involving the spouse or significant other—should be involved in the rehabilitation process so that optimal relationships can be promoted.[42] Patients should also have the opportunity to discuss the implications of dyspnea on sexual activity with a qualified rehabilitation team member.[43–45] Maintenance of quality personal and intimate relationships are basic to good health.

The spiritual aspect adds another dimension of meaning and purpose to life. It provides a philosophy of life and system of beliefs that can help sustain one in daily pursuits. The concept of meditation and being at peace with oneself and others is proving to be beneficial to overall health.

People are complex, and to be healthy requires caring for the different elements that make up a person. Although separated out for analysis, the foregoing components are integrated into one continuous fabric that cannot be easily teased apart, and the whole of the spectrum of health must be addressed for wellness to be possible.

ASSESSMENT OF RISK FACTORS

One of the tasks of preventive medicine is to identify individual factors that may jeopardize health. Risk factors can be classified into *fixed* (nonmodifiable) and *modifiable* factors. Identifying the fixed factors will help determine the course and severity of the disease. Although there is nothing that can be done to alter these factors, identifying them does allow one to know with what type of patient they are dealing and can suggest how aggressive one needs to be in altering those factors that are modifiable. Examples of these factors are gender, heredity, previous disease history, past lung irritant exposure history, ciliary problems, α_1-antitrypsin deficiency, and developmental anomalies. By specific therapies, some of these factors' adverse influence might be lessened or even partially corrected.

Modifiable factors are those for which intervention can influence the health outcome of the patient, such as smoking, activity level, diet, and geographic factors. Geographic factors include altitude, climate, humidity, dusts, and pollens. Altitude is an important consideration for some. Living at a high altitude can certainly exacerbate hypoxemia and make underlying respiratory difficulties much more pronounced. For others it may be a damp climate. For some it may be living in an area where there is a lot of pollen and seasonal allergy potential. Air pollution is an important factor in cities and is being shown to exacerbate COPD as well as increase the prevalence of obstructive lung disease.[46] Dwellings that are in close proximity to congested or major highways are exposed to increased levels of carbon monoxide and other pollutants. Occupational exposure to dusts and fumes appear to be capable of inducing obstructive lung disease over time.[47,48] Certain mineral dusts contain oxygen radicals, which are suspected to predispose to emphysema.[49] Limiting occupational exposure is important, especially for those with overt disease, since they are obviously susceptible to these irritants.

The home environment contains many modifiable factors, some more difficult to alter than others. Radon in the home may be a long-term factor to consider.[50,51] Radon has been associated with lung cancer, although more recent studies suggest that the health problems associated with it may be less than previously thought, but, nonetheless, important.[52,53] Testing of the house or basement can be done, and kits are available for doing this. The Environmental Protection Agency (EPA) recommends that annual average radon levels be lower than 4 pCi/L (picocuries per liter of air).[54] How air-tight a house is can be an important factor in lung health. The more airtight the home, the greater the vapor pressure from synthetic materials as well as radon and, therefore, the higher the indoor air pollution. Plywood or particle board materials contribute formaldehyde to the indoor air, which is a known respiratory irritant. This has been especially noticed in new mobile homes. Aerosols and vapors from cleaning fluids can also contaminate the indoor air. Dusts, molds, and various pathogens can exist in the right conditions and, for some, adverse respiratory reactions can occur. Second-hand smoke is the most serious problem, since this is known to be one of the worst lung irritants.[55,56] Smoking outdoors or on the porch should be the rule, especially when there are residents who have chronic lung disease (and even for those who do not). Gas stoves in the house for cooking are associated with a greater incidence of lung problems, and people with pulmonary compromise are at greater risk. This may not be as large a problem if there is good ventilation in the kitchen area. Wood stoves and fireplaces are another source of respiratory irritation because of the fumes and smoke that escape into the house, which can linger.[57,58]

One can modify some of the home atmosphere by increasing home ventilation with fresh air—often accomplished by opening a window—or by use of air filters to remove particulate matter in the air. Indoor plants may help to clean the air of some gaseous vapors, formaldehyde being shown to decrease in concentration in the presence of some plants. High-efficiency particulate air (HEPA) filters can be purchased for the home and can provide effective filtering of particulate matter from the room.[59] This can help decrease pollen and dust exposure for those with sensitive airways. Air filters in a living room or bedroom can be helpful for some. There are electrostatic-type filters that can also work,[60] but some models may release ozone into the air and result in more airway irritation.

There are many personal factors that are modifiable. The categories with the greatest health impact involve what a patient breathes, eats, and does. To be healthy requires not only the pursuit of positive activities, but also the avoidance of harmful behaviors. Avoidance of tobacco smoke is one of the most important changes a patient can make. In fact, smoking is the major contributing cause of obstructive lung disease.[61] Addictions to nicotine and alcohol take a heavy toll on pulmonary patients.

Addiction can be defined as a continued, compulsive use of a substance or a behavior despite it having detrimental effects physically, mentally, socially, or spiritually. Addictions are permanent, and this makes relapse likely. Factors that increase the likelihood of relapse include hunger, anger, loneliness, or being tired or depressed, and not dealing with the craving or other behavioral cues. Nicotine addiction is clearly the most troublesome in the patient population with lung disorders. Long-term success rates range from 15% to 30% after 1 year; therefore, continued attention to a patient's smoking behavior must be an integral part of patient care. Nicotine addiction is one of the most difficult and insidious addictions to treat. It offers both stimulant and sedative effects, depending on the dose inhaled. Despite the many known harmful effects and over 400,000 American deaths per year, 50 million Americans still smoke. Patients must make a decision to stop. This is facilitated by having them select a date in the near future as opposed to making them decide on the spot. Helping the patient identify the reasons they smoke, as well as the benefits they personally could realize by breathing only fresh air, is a helpful preliminary task. The reasons patients cite for the advantages they receive from smoking—relaxation, stimulation, enjoyment, or habit—are important starting points for rehabilitation team members to help in the cessation process. Alternative activities, that can potentially satisfy their reasons for smoking, should be outlined, with the patients' input. A multifaceted intervention and treatment for smoking is necessary.[62] The use of nicotine replacement therapies can be beneficial.[63] Proper use of nicotine polacrilex (Nicorette), or use of a transdermal nicotine patch, along with a structured interaction, including counseling, can be quite effective for strongly addicted smokers.

Alcohol is probably a poorly recognized addiction in the pulmonary patient population. Since alcohol has strong mood-altering and sedative effects, it is often used to self-medicate for stress, pain, and overall discomfort. Although alcohol is used by many persons, its effects are not always benign. Over 10 million Americans are alcoholics, and few, if any, intended to become this way when they started to drink. Alcohol is a sedative, and for those with depressed respiratory drives, the effect is additive. The use of any sedatives, alcohol or benzodiazepine medications, are best avoided in patients with COPD.[64] Since most of these patients are receiving multiple medications, there is an increased risk of undesired drug interactions with the addition of alcohol to the mix. There are also epidemiologic suggestions that alcohol may contribute etiologically to some forms of obstructive lung disease. Alcohol can also alter ciliary function and impair immune capabilities. This combination is especially detrimental for patients with poor pulmonary function. Treatment for alcohol addiction is important to address in patients who have problems with alcohol. Getting a patient to realize they need treatment is often one of the more difficult tasks. Consultation with an alcohol counselor may be necessary. Pulmonary rehabilitation programs should incorporate at least a simple questionnaire, such as the CAGE or Michigan Alcoholism Screening Test (MAST) questionnaires, to assess for alcohol problems.[65] The CAGE questionnaire is composed of four questions (. . . feel you should *cut* down on drinking? . . . *annoyed* you by criticizing about your drinking? . . . *guilty* about your drinking? . . . drink first thing in the morning—*eye* opener?) and has been shown to have a high sensitivity for detecting those who have a problem with alcohol.[66]

Caffeine is a mild stimulant that generally has a larger threshold of safety when compared with other addictive substances. However, it produces dependence in many and can be a difficult addiction to break for some people. Since caffeine is a xanthine, it can interact with other xanthines, such as theophylline medications. In fact, caffeine does have some bronchodilator effects. It is important to know a patient's caffeine consumption, since it does interact with other medications.

Drugs that are nonaddictive should be carefully selected. β-Blockers should be avoided in patients with obstructive lung disease, since they are likely to exacerbate bronchospasm. Narcotic pain medications can have respiratory depressant effects and are best avoided in those with respiratory difficulties. Sleep medicines might not be tolerated by some, owing to their sedative effects and influence on respiratory centers. They also have addictive potential. Since every medication has side effects, it is important to frequently evaluate the continued necessity for the medicines patients are using.

PREVENTIVE CARE TREATMENT PLAN

Consistent evaluation and follow-up care are necessary for patients with chronic lung disease. This type of care may be initiated during a hospitalization; however, subsequent care in an outpatient pulmonary clinic is usually adequate for follow-up care. Attention to the needs of pulmonary patients does improve survival.[67] General health concerns appropriate to their age and gender group as well as specific concerns unique to pulmonary patients must be periodically checked. A suggested preventive care flow chart is shown in Table 7–2. The parameters listed are helpful to monitor periodically so that health trends can be seen and timely intervention can occur when needed. Follow-up visits are determined by the clinical condition of the patient and his or her compliance with treatments outlined. Individualized preventive measures for each patient should be part of his or her chart. A patient's risk factors should also be in a prominent place on the chart so each one's unique preventive tasks can be reviewed and monitored. Are immunizations current? Does the patient still smoke? How is the nonsmoking status going? Are medications being taken properly? Is weight stable? Does the patient wear seatbelts in the car? Are pulmonary mechanics and oxygenation status stable? Have there been any major changes in jobs, relation-

TABLE 7-2. Pulmonary Rehabilitation General Preventive Medicine Flowsheet

Name: _____ *Birthdate:* _____

Date										
Weight										
Guaiac										
Prostate										
PAP										
Mammogram										
PPD										
Flu Shot										
Glaucoma										
Seatbelt use										
Smoke										
Cotinine										
Alcohol										
Caffeine										
Theophylline										
Theo dose										
Digoxin										
Pro-time										
Warfarin dose										
Pneumovax										
O_2 Sat										
PaO_2										
$PaCO_2$										
O_2 LPM										
VO_2 max										
Dist. walk										
FVC										
FEV_1										
RV										
TLC										
D_LCO										
CXR										

ships, or geographic moves? A systematic plan for follow-up in pertinent health-related areas has to be in place and practiced or else important early preventive intervention opportunities will be lost.

Does the patient have questions about his or her medications? Are the medications being taken as prescribed and are the blood levels therapeutic for the appropriate medications? Patients should be trained in recognizing early signs of respiratory infections so that early treatment can be initiated. For many patients, a standby prescription for an antibiotic can be given with instructions about when to use it. Since compromised pulmonary function leads to greater susceptibility to infections, respiratory tract infections must be treated aggressively. Those with little or no lung reserve remaining cannot tolerate any additional work of breathing, such as would be imposed by an acute infection. Training of the patients helps foster independence and a sense of control over their condition. Clear guidelines for when to call the physician should be given to each patient.

A clear diet plan should be given to each patient with his or her personal target goals. Involvement of the spouse who does the cooking is essential for best compliance. Dietary rules should be simple and take into account the patient's personal food preferences.

Exercise prescription with duration, intensity, frequency, and type of exercises should be given to each patient. The patient should be able to demonstrate the prescribed exercises and methods for self-monitoring. Review of symptoms or signs of when exercise should be terminated should occur with each patient. Periodic assessment by exercise stress testing is necessary for objective evaluation of progress.

Periodic pulmonary function testing provides important data on lung capabilities over time and indicates whether the overall treatment plan is working. For asthmatics, a peak flowmeter is a useful device that the patient can use at home to monitor his or her condition and be alerted as to when to seek professional help. For some, lung diffusion studies (DLCO), are useful assessments for progression of emphysema or interstitial lung diseases. This can alert the team or a patient's physician whether alternate therapies should be introduced.

For patients who will be traveling, education about how to obtain necessary care when away from their usual care givers is of value. It is helpful for some patients to carry a list of their current medical problems and medications they are taking. Some may encounter problems with geographic areas that might be at higher altitudes. For those planning to travel by airplane, assessment of their potential need for oxygen should be addressed. Cabin pressure in commercial airliners range between equivalent altitudes from 4000 to 8000 ft (barometric 560 mmHg or greater). Pulmonary laboratory pretesting with hypoxic gas mixture (approximately 17% FiO_2) with measurement of oxygen saturation can determine if supplemental oxygen will be needed.[68] Some patients will require oxygen for air travel, and necessary arrangement ahead of time would have to be planned for.

SUMMARY

Careful attention to all aspects of the physical, mental, social, and spiritual components of our patients, along with a thorough knowledge of respiratory disease, will make possible improved health and well-being, despite disability.

REFERENCES

1. Thom TJ. International comparisons in COPD mortality. Am Rev Respir Dis 1989;140(3pt2):S27.

2. Roper WL, Thacker SB, Goodman RA, Foster KL, eds. Update: years of potential life lost before age 65—United States, 1988 and 1989. MMWR 1991;40:60.

3. Feinleib M, Rosenberg HM, Collins JG, Delozier JE, Pokras R, Chevarley FM. Trends in COPD morbidity and mortality in the United States. Am Rev Respir Dis 1989;140:S9.

4. Vital statistics. Vital statistics of the United States: 1987. CA 1991;41.

5. Kuller LH, Ockene JK, Townsend M, Browner W, Meilahn E, Wentworth DN. The epidemiology of pulmonary function and COPD mortality in the multiple risk factor intervention trial. Am Rev Respir Dis 1989;140(3pt2):S76.

6. Tockman MS, Comstock GW. Respiratory risk factors and mortality: longitudinal studies in Washington County, Maryland. Am Rev Respir Dis 1989;140(3pt2):S56.

7. Speizer FE, Fay ME, Dockery DW, Ferris BGJ. Chronic obstructive pulmonary disease mortality in six U.S. cities. Am Rev Respir Dis 1989;140(3pt2):S49.

8. Anthonisen NR. Prognosis in chronic obstructive pulmonary disease: results from muticenter clinical trials. Am Rev Respir Dis 1989;140(3pt2):S95.

9. Epler GR. Screening for lung cancer. Is it worthwhile? Postgrad Med 1990;87:181.

10. Kesten S, Rebuck AS. Management of chronic obstructive pulmonary disease. Drugs 1989;38:160.

11. Hodgkin JE. Pulmonary rehabilitation. In: Hodgkin JE, Petty TL, eds. Chronic obstructive pulmonary disease: current concepts. Philadelphia: WB Saunders, 1987:154.

12. The Holy Bible. Authorized King James Version. Grand Rapids, MI: Zondervan Publishing House, 1975.

13. Wiedemann HP, Matthay RA. Cor pulmonale in chronic obstructive pulmonary disease: circulatory pathophysiology and management [review]. In: Hodgkin JE, guest ed. Chronic obstructive pulmonary disease. Clin Chest Med 1990;11:523.

14. Goodman RA. Chronic disease prevention and control activities—United States, 1989 [Editor's Note]. MMWR 1991;40:697.

15. Hahn RA, Teutsch SM, Rothenberg RB, Marks JS. Excess deaths from nine chronic diseases in the United States. JAMA 1990;264:2654.

16. Murphy FA, Mahy BWJ, Kendal AP, Schonberger LB. Prevention and control of influenza: recommendations of the immunization practices advisory committee (ACIP). MMWR 1991;40(RR-6):1.

17. Last JM. A dictionary of epidemiology. 2nd ed. New York: Oxford University Press, 1988:57.

18. Tiep BL. Long-term home oxygen therapy. In: Hodgkin JE, guest ed. Chronic obstructive pulmonary disease. Clin Chest Med 1990;11:505.

19. Peters JA, Burke K, White D. Nutrition and the pulmonary patient. In: Hodgkin JE, Zorn E, Connors GL, eds. Pulmonary rehabilitation: guidelines to success. Boston: Butterworth Publishers, 1984:263.

20. Donahoe M, Rogers RM, Wilson DO, Pennock BE. Oxygen consumption of the respiratory muscles in normal and in malnourished patients with chronic obstructive pulmonary disease. Am Rev Respir Dis 1989;140:385.

21. Fiaccadori E, Del CS, Coffrini E, et al. Hypercapnic–hypoxemic chronic obstructive pulmonary disease (COPD): influence of severity of COPD on nutritional status. Am J Clin Nutr 1988;48:680.

22. Saltzman HA, Salzano JV. Effects of carbohydrate metabolism upon respiratory gas exchange in normal men. J Appl Physiol 1971; 30:228.

23. Gieseke T, Gurushanthaiah G, Glauser FL. Effects of carbohydrates on carbon dioxide excretion in patients with airway disease. Chest 1977;71:55.

24. Talbott GD, Frayser R. Hyperlipidemia, a cause of decreased oxygen saturation. Nature 1963;200:684.

25. Swank RL, Nakamura H. Oxygen availability in brain tissues after lipid meals. Am J Physiol 1960;198:217.

26. Brandstetter RD, Zakkay Y, Gutherz P, Goldberg RJ. Effect of nasogastric feedings on arterial oxygen tension in patients with symptomatic chronic obstructive pulmonary disease. Heart Lung 1988;17:170.

27. Committee on Diet and Health, NRC. Cancer. In: Diet and health: implications for reducing chronic disease risk. Washington, DC: National Academy Press, 1989:593.

28. Nowak D, Ruta U, Piasecka G. Ascorbic acid inhibits polymorphonuclear leukocytes influx to the place of inflammation—possible protection of lung from phagocyte-mediated injury. Arch Immunol Ther Exp (Warsz) 1989;37:213.

29. Patterson CE, Rhoades RA. Protective role of sulfhydryl reagents in oxidant lung injury. Exp Lung Res 1988;14:1005.

30. Foster S, Lopez D, Thomas HM 3rd. Pulmonary rehabilitation in COPD patients with elevated Pco_2. Am Rev Respir Dis 1988;138:1519.

31. Belman MJ, Shadmehr R. Targeted resistive ventilatory muscle training in chronic obstructive pulmonary disease. J Appl Physiol 1988;65:2726.

32. Mahler DA, Belman MJ. Controversies in pulmonary medicine. Respiratory muscle training should be instituted in all COPD patients. Am Rev Respir Dis 1988;138:1072.

33. Sharp JT. Therapeutic considerations in respiratory muscle function. Chest 1985;88:118S.

34. Ries AL, Ellis B, Hawkins RW. Upper extremity exercise training in chronic obstructive pulmonary disease. Chest 1988;93:688.

35. Weg JG. Therapeutic exercise in patients with chronic obstructive pulmonary disease. Cardiovasc Clin 1985;15:261.

36. Shephard R. Training and the respiratory system—therapy for asthma and other obstructive lung diseases? Ann Clin Res 1982;14(suppl 34):86.

37. Braun SR, Fregosi R, Reddan WG. Exercise training in patients with COPD. Postgrad Med 1982;71:163.

38. D'Urzo AD, Mateika J, Bradley DT, Li D, Contreras MA, Goldstein, RS. Correlates of arterial oxygenation during exercise in severe chronic obstructive pulmonary disease. Chest 1989;95:13.

39. Moore JG, Datz FL, Christian PE. Exercise increases solid meal gastric emptying rates in men. Dig Dis Sci 1990;35:428.

40. Keeling WF, Martin BJ. Gastrointestinal transit during mild exercise. J Appl Physiol 1987;63:978.

41. McSweeny AJ, Grant I, Heaton RK, Adams KM, Timms RM. Life quality of patients with chronic obstructive pulmonary disease. Arch Intern Med 1982;142:473.

42. Sexton DL, Munro BH. Impact of a husband's chronic illness (COPD) on the spouse's life. Res Nurs Health 1985;8(1):83.

43. Curgian LM, Gronkiewicz CA. Enhancing sexual performance in COPD. Nurse Pract 1988;13(2):34.

44. Hahn K. Sexuality and COPD. Rehabil Nurs 1989:14(4):191.

45. Stockdale WR. Sexual dysfunction and COPD: problems and management. Nurse Pract 1983;8(2):16.

46. Hodgkin JE, Abbey DE, Euler GL, Magie AR. Comparison of chronic obstructive

pulmonary disease prevalence in nonsmokers in high and low photochemical air pollution areas. Chest 1984;86:830.

47. Becklake MR. Occupational exposures: evidence for a causal association with chronic obstructive pulmonary disease. Am Rev Respir Dis 1989;140:S85.

48. Goren AI, Bruderman I. Effects of occupational exposure and smoking on respiratory symptomatology and PFT in healthy panelists and COPD patients. Eur J Epidemiol 1989;5:58.

49. Doelman CJ, Leurs R, Oosterom WC, Bast A. Mineral dust exposure and free radical-mediated lung damage. Exp Lung Res 1990;16:41.

50. Harley NH, Harley JH. Potential lung cancer risk from indoor radon exposure. CA 1990;40:265.

51. Council on Scientific Affairs. Radon in homes. [published erratum appears in JAMA 1988;259:47]. JAMA 1987;258:668.

52. Birrer RB. Radon: counseling patients about risk. Am Fam Physician 1990;42:711.

53. Blot WJ, Xu ZY, Boice JJ, et al. Indoor radon and lung cancer in China. JNCI 1990;82:1025.

54. Williams A. Radon fact sheet for California. American Lung Association of California, 1991.

55. Eriksen MP, LeMaistre CA, Newell GR. Health hazards of passive smoking. Annu Rev Public Health 1988;9:47.

56. Masi MA, Hanley JA, Ernst P, Becklake MR. Environmental exposure to tobacco smoke and lung function in young adults. Am Rev Respir Dis 1988;138:296.

57. Samet JM, Marbury MC, Spengler JD. Health effects and sources of indoor air pollution. Part I. Am Rev Respir Dis 1987;136:1486.

58. Utell MJ, Samet JM. Environmentally mediated disorders of the respiratory tract. Med Clin North Am 1990;74:291.

59. Reisman RE, Mauriello PM, Davis GB, Georgitis JW, DeMasi JM. A double-blind study of the effectiveness of a high-efficiency particulate air (HEPA) filter in the treatment of patients with perennial allergic rhinitis and asthma. J Allergy Clin Immunol 1990;85:1050.

60. Maloney MJ, Wray BB, DuRant RH, Smith L, Smith L. Effect of an electronic air cleaner and negative ionizer on the population of indoor mold spores. Ann Allergy 1987;59:192.

61. Davis RM, Novotny TE. The epidemiology of cigarette smoking and its impact on chronic obstructive pulmonary disease. Am Rev Respir Dis 1989;140:S82.

62. Peters JA, Lim V. Smoking cessation techniques. In: Hodgkin JE, Zorn E, Connors GL, eds. Pulmonary rehabilitation: guidelines to success. Boston: Butterworth Publishers, 1984:91.

63. Peters JA. Nicotine-replacement therapy in cessation of smoking. Mayo Clin Proc 1990;65:1619.

64. Gross NJ. Chronic obstructive pulmonary disease. Current concepts and therapeutic approaches. Chest 1990;97(suppl 2):19s.

65. Hays JT, Spickard WJ. Alcoholism: early diagnosis and intervention. J Gen Intern Med 1987;2:420.

66. Beresford TP, Blow FC, Hill E, Singer K, Lucey MR. Comparison of CAGE questionnaire and computer-assisted laboratory profiles in screening for covert alcoholism. Lancet 1990;336:482.

67. Foster S, Thomas HM 3rd. Pulmonary rehabilitation in lung disease other than chronic obstructive pulmonary disease. Am Rev Respir Dis 1990;141:601.

68. Schwartz JS, Bencowitz HZ, Moser KM. Air travel hypoxemia with chronic obstructive pulmonary disease. Ann Intern Med 1984;100:473.

DAVID DAUGHTON

A. JAMES FIX

8

Smoking Intervention Techniques: Historical and Practical Applications

There is substantial evidence suggesting that smoking cessation early in adult life may prevent severe, disabling chronic obstructive pulmonary disease (COPD). This optimistic viewpoint is based on three factors. First, smoking cessation appears to slow the rapid, downhill decline in pulmonary function common to susceptible smokers. With cessation of smoking, the decrease of lung function with aging appears to become similar to that of nonsmokers.[1] Thus, if a person quits smoking early in adulthood, his or her likelihood of developing COPD later in life should be low. Second, smoking cessation may produce an actual improvement in several pulmonary function assessments.[1,2-4]

The third, and perhaps the most critical factor, is the nature of COPD itself. Current evidence indicates that it may take a decade for the susceptible smoker to develop overt symptomatic airway disease. In this light, a decade of cigarette smoking may not cause a significant level of pulmonary dysfunction, whereas a decade of abstinence may offer former smokers some protection against COPD. At least one study supports these assumptions. Doll and Peto's massive study of 34,000 British physicians over a 20-year period found that the death rate from chronic bronchitis and emphysema fell significantly after 10 years of smoking abstinence.[5] They also observed that, in general, the mortality rate of those persons who quit smoking between 30 and 54 years of age was significantly less than those who continued to smoke.[5]

These findings are consistent with our own unpublished observations, and with the findings of the American Lung Association, who finally questioned the use of pulmonary function tests at open public screening sites. It was found that smokers often reacted with relief to findings of normal-range pulmonary function test results. Many times the results seemed to reassure them that their smoking was not hurting them when, in actuality, it takes many years for lung damage from smoking to show up in screening pulmonary function examinations.

Our work, using the Human Activity Profile, found that smokers' average activity levels continues essentially equal to that of nonsmokers' (when corrected for age and other demographic variables), until aged 50; after that, smokers' average daily energy expenditure slowly, but progressively, falls behind that of nonsmokers.

Medical evidence clearly offers hope for smokers who quit early in life. The data also suggest that smoking cessation can slow the rate of pulmonary function decline in patients with mild to moderate COPD. If cigarette abstinence occurs early enough, COPD patients with mild dysfunction may delay or perhaps eliminate their predicted encounter with severe pulmonary impairment. The literature provides little consolation, however, for those smokers with extremely severe emphysema.[6,7] For them, smoking cessation may be a case of too little, too late.

SMOKING CESSATION AND CHRONIC OBSTRUCTIVE PULMONARY DISEASE

Perhaps nothing can illustrate the intensity of the cigarette habit as well as one bedridden, oxygen-dependent, COPD patient who continues to smoke, even when he or she is a living example of why no one should smoke. To realize that some COPD patients smoke until the day they die is to gain a sense of the strength of the cigarette addiction. Most smokers become very dependent not only on the physical effects of nicotine, but also on the various ways smoking becomes linked to how they live their lives. A smoker's dependence on nicotine can develop to a degree at which abrupt abstinence is followed within 24 hours by such symptoms as headache, irritability, anxiety, problems with concentrating, craving for tobacco, anger, restlessness, frustration, drowsiness, and gastrointestinal disturbances. These withdrawal symptoms can become so unbearable that they can virtually destroy a smoker's resolve to quit. Although healthy smokers may have the physical and psychological resources required to help them quit, patients with COPD often do not. For impaired COPD patients, quitting smoking can represent not only an intensive physical and psychological battle they are ill prepared to fight, but also the act of giving up one of the few pleasures they can still enjoy.

Yet, patients with COPD do quit, and they generally have slightly higher rates of smoking cessation than the rest of the population.[8,9] Much of the impetus toward smoking cessation, however, appears to happen within the first years after the disease or spirometric abnormalities are detected. Petty and his colleagues reported that 18% of their subjects with abnormal pulmonary function tests achieved abstinence at 1 year, a rate that was 50% higher than that achieved by smokers with normal lung functions.[10] Hepper and coworkers found that smoking cessation rates in smokers with abnormal pulmonary functions was 21%, compared with a 12% rate in normals.[11]

Most patients with COPD quit smoking before they enter a pulmonary rehabilitation program. Daughton and his colleagues reported that two of every three COPD patients (67%) were former smokers at the time of admission to a pulmonary rehabilitation project.[9] Interestingly, the preadmission smoking cessation rate in a second rehabilitation study was a remarkably similar 68%.[12] In both rehabilitation projects, having psychosocial assets (being married, well employed, and such) were associated with smoking cessation. In the latter study, our findings indicated that the same psychosocial assets were related to the COPD patients' ability to quit smoking before hospitalization. In addition, the COPD patients who quit smoking before hospitalization were also older and more impaired in their diffusion capacity for carbon monoxide (DLCO) than those who continued to smoke.

In both rehabilitation studies, the hospital program for all smokers contained a smoking education component and maintained a heavy emphasis on the need to stop smoking. In the most recent project, only 26 of 80 patients with a smoking history were smoking on admission. Of the 26 patients, 4 died during the first year. Five of the remaining 22 patients quit smoking, which represents a 1-year cessation rate of 23%. Three of the 5 patients who were successful abstainers at 1 year gave up smoking during their stay in the hospital. This success rate may be discouraging to clinicians and rehabilitation workers, but it compares favorably with cessation rates attributed to several programs among other populations of smokers.

SMOKING CESSATION: BACKGROUND INFORMATION

In 1964, Dr. Luther Terry released *Smoking and Health: The Report of the Advisory Committee to the Surgeon General.*[13] The intent of the report was to single out cigarette smoking as a major health risk with the hope of encouraging smokers to break their cigarette addiction. The message got through to millions of smokers. Since 1964, the prevalence of smokers in the adult population declined from 40% to 29%; the lowest level in the United States since World War II.[14] In addition, surveys suggest that perhaps as many as 70% of the 50 million Americans who do smoke would like to quit (down from the 90% of earlier surveys—possibly indicating some reactionary entrenchment of people who have continued to smoke during increasing antismoking sentiment in the public at large).[14]

Since the first Surgeon General's report on smoking and health in 1964, society's antismoking message has grown stronger and louder. Increasingly, smoking is banned in public places, on buses, and on commercial airlines. It is now common for smoking to be prohibited or severely restricted in governmental offices, theaters, restaurants, retail stores, clinics, and hospitals, as well as many other locations. In some parts of the United States, cigarette smokers are not eligible for employment as a police officer or a firefighter. The antismoking message is being heard throughout the country. On May 20, 1984, Surgeon General C. Everett Koop declared the country's number 1 health goal to be a "smoke-free society by the year 2000."[15]

Such a goal will not be easy, or perhaps even attainable. Since 1964, when Dr. Terry's report was released, there has been a dramatic decrease in the number of smokers in the population. But, viewed on a year-to-year basis, the percentage impact is relatively small. At the current rate, by the year 2000, smoking in the United States is projected to decline to roughly 15% of the total population in this country, an impressive reduction, but a far cry from a smoke-free society.

SMOKING CESSATION: DEMOGRAPHIC FACTORS

Considerable evidence suggests that sociocultural factors play an important role in the success of quitting smoking. These factors include age, gender, cigarette consumption, marital status, health status, and socieconomic position:

1. *Age.* Smokers over aged 55 are more likely to quit permanently than younger smokers.[16]
2. *Gender.* Men, surprisingly, have better success in quitting permanently than women.[17] Although many reasearchers recognize that there is a gender factor associated with smoking cessation, no one has yet offered an adequate explanation of this in the literature.
3. *Cigarette consumption.* Lighter smokers tend to be more successful at quitting than heavier smokers.[18]
4. *Marital Status.* Persons with stable marriages seem notably more successful in smoking cessation than others.[16]
5. *Health.* Smokers with chronic disease are more likely to quit permanently than healthy smokers.[8,9]
6. *Occupational.* Smokers in higher-level occupations and in the upper socioeconomical strata are more successful at quitting than those in lower positions.[16] This is true for both unimpaired smokers and, as mentioned earlier, for COPD patients as well.
7. *The presence of other smokers in the home.* The presence of other smokers diminishes a person's long-term chances of quitting.[19]

Thus, the composite profile of the person least likely to give up smoking could look like this:

- Middle-aged
- Female
- Heavy smoker
- Unmarried, divorced, or separated
- Physically healthy, or at least having no recognized chronic disease
- Low level of employment or low socioeconomic status
- Living with a smoker or smokers

SMOKING CESSATION TECHNIQUES

Educational Techniques

For years, the cigarette addiction was seen largely as a psychological habit. As such, it was believed that smokers could quit—if they only wanted to quit and could muster sufficient psychological resources to do so. The earliest solution, then, seemed simple: Inform smokers about the dangers and hazards of cigarette smoking and they will quit. The Surgeon General's reports on smoking and health provide a good illustration of this philosophy. Although there is no doubt that these reports have prompted millions of Americans to break their cigarette addiction, the process has been tortuously slow.

Measured on a year-to-year basis, smoking cessation programs that relied heavily on providing smokers information about the dangers and hazards of cigarette smoking have provided disappointing results. Roughly 85% to 90% of smokers who participated in educational programs are still smoking 1 year later.[20]

Group-Counseling Programs

Several national voluntary health organizations, a few profit-making corporations, and the Seventh-Day Adventist Church (SDA) offer group smoking cessation programs. Although the programs differ in many respects, each usually includes lectures, films, group interaction, and recommendations on diet, on exercise, and on keeping personal records of current smoking behavior. These programs are similar in content and also in the results they achieve. Although the commercial smoking cessation programs may claim that 80% or more of their participants quit, at least one study suggests that the actual abstinence rate is much lower.[21] Schwartz and Rider found that 39% of "successful" graduates of one commercial smoking cessation program were abstinent at 4 years.[21] To achieve this percentage, the researchers examined only the success rates of smokers who quit during the program and assumed that the people who did not respond to their survey had the same quit rate as those who did answer. Had they included the total number of all program registrants and counted all nonrespondents as still smoking, the abstinence rate would have dropped to roughly 12%.

By comparison, a 19-month follow-up evaluation of 18 American Cancer Society (ACS) programs found that 18% of the participants had maintained their abstinence since the end of the ACS programs.[21] A review of the American Lung Association's (ALA) Freedom From Smoking (FFS) clinic suggests that 80% to 90% of smokers quit during the clinic and 19% remain abstinent for at least 1 year.[21] The Seventh-Day Adventist Five-Day Plan achieved end-of-clinic success rates as high as 97% and 1-year abstinent rates of 16% to 27%.[22] Although the 1-year abstinence rates achieved by group counseling are not impressive, the advantages of the clinics are that they are safe, and they do help roughly one of every five participants quit.

In terms of costs, the group-counseling programs sponsored by the ALA, ACS, and SDA clearly offer the best value to the smokers. However, these programs are conducted sporadically and may not be available at the time the smoker wants to quit. In the major cities, the commercial programs are more readily accessible, giving the smoker another, more costly group-counseling alternative.

Hypnosis

Hypnosis is among the oldest of the psychotherapeutic techniques. It has been used as a cure for a variety of psychological problems, including the treatment of cigarette addiction. The efficacy of hypnosis in helping people stop smoking appears to depend on the skill of the hypnotist, as 1-year abstinence rates range from zero to nearly 100%.[23] Self-hypnosis is associated with a 6-month smoking cessation rate of 20%,[24] whereas group hypnosis appears to achieve 1-year abstinence rates of roughly 14%.[25]

Some research investigators suggest that hypnosis plus counseling may yield higher smoking cessation rates than either hypnosis or counseling alone.[26,27] In an investigation by Peterson and her colleagues, 50% (8 of 16) of smokers receiving a combination of hypnotism and counseling achieved successful abstinence at 10 months, a rate that was much higher than either technique used alone.[27] Interestingly, the waiting list control group in Peterson's study achieved a higher 10-month abstinence rate than either the hypnosis-only or counseling-only groups.

Special Filters

Special commercial filters are advertised as smoking cessations aids. At least two studies suggest that these special filters are not an effective stop-smoking method.[28,29] In one study, comparing the efficacy of a special filter with quitting on your own, the latter achieved 1-year abstinence rates of 33%; the special filter group, 22%.[28] In a second study, no one on the filter system stopped smoking by the scheduled quit date, and the 10% that eventually achieved abstinence did so after they discarded their device.[29]

Chemical Approaches

During the last half-century, a vast and varied number of chemical remedies have been tried as smoking cessation agents. These include meprobamate, lobeline, doxepin, corticotropin, clonidine hydrochloride, tranquilizers, anticholinergics, amphetamines, silver acetate, quinine sulfate, garlic, mouth washes, and local anesthetics.[20,30-34] In the early studies on smoking cessation, many of these agents were used in combination with the central focus placed on various lobeline preparations. Since the chemical structure of lobeline is apparently very similar to nicotine, lobeline was once believed capable of serving as a nicotine substitute. The idea seemed promising until a British Tuberculosis Association study found that the 6-week success rates with lobeline were only 7% compared to a placebo rate of 10.5%.[34] For several years, some physicians prescribed tranquilizers as a smoking cessation aid—especially for patients who suffered acute anxiety when trying to quit. The tranquilizer therapy for smoking cessation proved inefficient.[20] Amphetamine compounds are contraindicated, as they not only have potential risks, but also appear to lessen, rather than improve, a smoker's capacity to quit.[20]

Of the chemical intervention techniques, clonidine hydrochloride (Catapres) has arguably shown the most promise as a smoking cessation aid. Clonidine, in both the tablet and patch form, has decreased tobacco withdrawal symptoms and enhanced smoking cessation rates.[35-37] It has not been approved as yet as a stop-smoking aid, but is available as an antihypertensive agent. Because of its availability, many physicians are now prescribing clonidine to help their patients quit smoking. Clonidine may indeed work to help *some* smokers quit and *may* someday be an effective second-line therapy for treating nicotine dependence. However, until clonidine receives FDA approval as a smoking cessation agent, its use as a stop-smoking aid is questionable.

Acupuncture

In some commercial programs, therapists claim that acupuncture is an incredible breakthrough in the treatment of the cigarette addiction. The data, however, suggest that the role of acupuncture in smoking cessation is vastly oversold. In a 1980 study, LaMontage compared the smoking cessation efficacy of acupuncture at "correct" and "incorrect" sites. At 6 months, the incorrect site was achieving a 16% cessation rate versus 8% for correct site therapy.[38] The overall failure rate for acupunctrure therapy was 88%.

Aversive Conditioning

According to some schools of thought, cigarette smoking is a learned response to positive stimuli. As such, some researchers believed that smoking behavior could be extinguished by aversive-conditioning techniques capable of creating a strong association in the smoker's mind between smoking and unpleasant sensation. Among the aversive techniques that have been tried are electroshock; breath holding; hot, smoky air; nausea-inducing drugs; and extensive or rapid smoking to the degree that smokers frequently become nauseated or sick.[20] Among the most creative of the aversive conditioning investigations was a researcher who fired a 0.22-caliber rifle over the head of a cigarette-puffing subject 100 times a week for 5 weeks.[20]

To some, these techniques represent nothing more than an unwarranted form of 20th century torture. Clearly, the use of these aversive-conditioning methods could be justified only by research data showing that their techniques are unequivocally superior to any other known nonaversive smoking cessation techniques. That is definitely not true, although for a while in 1972 and 1973, it seemed that it might be. In 1972 and 1973, Lichtenstein and his colleagues reported that smoking cessation techniques achieved 6-month abstinence rates of 53% or more.[39,40] Later studies on the use of rapid smoking, however, cast considerable doubt on both efficacy[41,42] and safety of this method.[43] Russell and his coworkers concluded that rapid smoking was a risk to all but the younger smokers.[43] For COPD and cardiac patients, such a technique could be extremely dangerous. Currently, there is no conclusive evidence to justify the use of aversive-conditioning techniques. Studies suggest that rapid-smoking techniques have questionable efficacy and safety, and electroshock aversion therapy appears to be of no more benefit than that obtained by simple support and attention from a therapist.[44]

Switching to Low-Nicotine Cigarettes

Smokers who switch to low-nicotine cigarettes do precious little to help their chances of breaking the cigarette habit. Research data suggest that smokers regulate their nicotine dosage to such an extent that when they switch from a high-nicotine to low-nicotine cigarette, they continue to maintain their same levels of nicotine. To compensate for the lower-nicotine levels, smokers appear to inhale the smoke of cigarettes more rapidly and more deeply, and smoke more cigarettes.[13] Thus, for many smokers, switching to low-nicotine cigarettes is countertherapeutic. There is, however, one major advantage commonly associated with low-nicotine cigarettes: low tar. Smokers of low-tar cigarettes are less likely to develop lung cancer than smokers of the high-tar cigarettes. In a 12-year study of more than 1 million smokers, the smokers using low-tar cigarettes had a 12% lower incidence of lung cancer mortality than those smoking high-tar cigarettes.[45]

Monetary Gain or Loss

Both the hope of monetary gain and the threat of financial loss have been used to help motivate smokers to quit. On an informal basis, some smokers have literally bet themselves off the cigarette habit. Others have tried to motivate themselves to stay off cigarettes by daily setting aside the monies formerly used to purchase cigarettes and then watching their savings grow. Several companies have tried employee incentive programs, encouraging cigarette abstinence with incentive programs, encouraging cigarette abstinence with monetary rewards. So far, the results of these programs are mixed, ranging from very high to mild success rates.[46] On the other side of the ledger sheet, Elliot and Tighe found that threat of monetary loss is an effective smoking cessation technique, achieving a 15-month success rate of 38.4%.[47]

Tapering and Cold Turkey

Tapering appears to make sense. By gradually reducing daily cigarette consumption, a smoker should, it seems, be able to reduce his or her physical dependence on nicotine to a point at which total cessation would produce a minimum of withdrawal symptoms. While logical, gradual quitting toward some unknown date does not work,[48,49] tapering appears to fail because most smokers stall between 5 and 15 cigarettes per day. Without a firm quit date, the smoker then generally returns to his or her original cigarette consumption level within a few weeks.

In comparison with gradual reduction techniques, smokers appear to have more success quitting with the cold turkey method. Smokers who set a target date for quitting are significantly more likely to quit than those who gradually taper toward an unknown date. Setting a firm target date for quitting is the key element for success. Once the target date is set, both abrupt quitting and gradual quitting appear to work.[50]

Physician Advice

Early studies on the efficacy of physician counseling as a smoking cessation aid were generally disappointing.[51,52] In one particular study, all 93 patients advised by physicians to quit were still smoking 6 months later.[52] It is now generally accepted that the influence of physician advice and pamphlets on enhancing smoking cessation is relatively small (approximately 5% abstinence rates at 1 year). However, physician advice to quit is clearly superior to nonintervention.[53]

Self-Help Manuals

Survey data suggest that the self-help manual approach to smoking cessation is much more appealing to smokers than are stop-smoking clinics.[54] Accordingly, the American Cancer Society (ACS) and the American Lung Association (ALS) have developed self-help smoking cessation manuals. The ACS manual can be obtained at no cost, while the ATS will provide the smoker with two glossy manuals for a modest fee. The abstinence yield associated with the ALA manuals at 1 year is about 5%.[55] Generally speaking, self-help manuals are not particularly effective by themselves,[56-59] but may serve as a helpful adjunct to a core program.[53,59]

Nicotine Polacrilex and Transdermal Nicotine Delivery

Increasingly, it is becoming widely accepted that nicotine is an addictive drug that plays a major role in maintaining the smoking habits of numerous persons.[60,61] In fact, evidence suggests that nicotine addiction is as difficult a habit to break as other forms of drug dependencies.[62,63] Hunt and his colleagues observed that the relapse rates for heroin, alcohol, and smoking were virtually identical, with two-thirds of those treated resuming the habit within 3 months.[63]

What makes the cigarette habit so addictive? Most of the answers seem to point to the pharmacologic properties of nicotine. Nicotine can become highly reinforcing to the cigarette user, as it has the unusual capacity to stimulate the brain's level of arousal[64,65] as well as relax muscle tension.[66,67] Thus, a smoker can use cigarettes literally to stimulate the body's system in the morning or when trying to stay awake at night, as well as provide the smoker with needed muscle tension reduction during times of stress. Nicotine's capacity to stimulate when a smoker wants stimulation and relax muscle tension when a smoker wants tension reduction makes it not only a pharmaceutical wonder, but highly addictive. In addition, not only does cigarette smoking help the smoker get *what* he or she wants from a cigarette, but delivers it *when* the smoker wants it. It takes less than 8 seconds for nicotine to travel from the lung to the brain.[66] Finally, nicotine dependence often reaches a level at which abrupt abstinence from cigarettes for 24 hours can produce such symptoms as irritability, anxiety, difficulty concentrating, restlessness, headache, dizziness, and gastrointestinal distress.[68] Thus, when a smoker wants to quit, he or she not only has to do without the pleasurable aspects of smoking (stimulation and tension reduction) but, at the same time, attempt to deal with the misery of withdrawal effects.

To combat this twofold problem, nicotine polacrilex (nicotine gum) and, more recently, transdermal nicotine systems (nicotine patches) were developed to help smokers break their cigarette addiction in stages. For the first time, the addicted smoker has the opportunity of giving up cigarettes without suffering disabling withdrawal symptoms. Both medically prescribed nicotine gum and transdermal nicotine systems can provide plasma nicotine at a level that reduces withdrawal symptoms, but does not attain the peak levels that appear to reinforce the smoking habit.

When persons smoke, large doses of nicotine enter the blood stream rapidly from the lungs. It appears that when these "nicotine boli" reach the brain, they produce a highly reinforcing sensation that helps perpetuate the smoking habit. The nicotine from nicotine polacrilex and transdermal nicotine systems, on the other hand, enters the blood stream more slowly to produce a level that approximates the hourly low points achieved by cigarette smoking.[69] This plasma nicotine level is not as high as smokers commonly reach, but it is sufficient to reduce withdrawal symptoms. Thus, a smoker who wants to quit can switch from cigarettes to nicotine gum or nicotine patches without suffering discomforting withdrawal symptoms. Both appear to help reduce nicotine dependence in two ways: prevent major physiologic withdrawal symptoms and avoid the pleasure-inducing nicotine peak blood levels.

Nicotine Polacrilex

Currently, research results would recommend the use of nicotine polacrilex with general populations of smokers.[70–75] Russell and his coworkers found that *just offering* the gum to smoking patients more than doubled the smoking cessation effects of pamphlets coupled with physician advice against smoking.[74] Several other general population studies have shown that the use of nicotine gum, when compared with a control group, achieves significantly higher smoking cessation rates.

Transdermal Nicotine Delivery (Nicotine Patches)

Transdermal nicotine delivery may represent the greatest advance yet in treating cigarette dependence. In a recent study, Daughton and his colleagues found that transdermal nicotine delivery, when used as an adjunct to low-intervention therapy, significantly decreased nicotine withdrawal symptoms and improved quit rates.[76] Transdermal nicotine patches are very convenient to use. The patches can be applied in a few minutes, as the patient attaches them to the upper outer arms or upper torso once a day. Unlike nicotine gum, the nicotine patches are not associated with hiccups, bad taste, heartburn, nausea, or sore jaws. Primary adverse events associated with transdermal nicotine delivery are temporary itching of the skin after application and erythema of the patch site persisting for a few minutes after removal. Most important, the nicotine patch users can achieve therapeutic blood nicotine levels with little or no effort. Moreover, with certain transdermal nicotine systems, individuals can wear their patches at night, thereby theoretically reducing early morning nicotine withdrawal symptoms.

Although transdermal nicotine delivery is a promising smoking cessation therapy, it is not a cure-all. Most smokers will experience tobacco withdrawal symptoms during the first few days of quitting—even if they are wearing a transdermal nicotine system. The system will only reduce the severity of the withdrawal symptoms.[76] Consequently, the temptation to smoke *and* wear the patches will be strong. However, most of those who do smoke while wearing the transdermal nicotine systems will ultimately fail in their stop-smoking efforts. Thus, it is extremely important to emphasize patch use as an adjunct to total cessation.

As a general rule, smokers who successfully quit on transdermal nicotine therapy will achieve total or near-abstinence within the first few days. Once smoke-free, recent quitters will probably need to stabilize themselves on a nicotine patch regimen for several weeks before discontinuing treatment. Because abrupt termination of a transdermal nicotine therapy may cause increased craving for cigarettes in some individuals, a weaning strategy is an important consideration. There are a variety of possible weaning techniques, most of which have not been adequately studied:

- Once stabilized in a 24-hour dosage regimen, remove the patches at bedtime. This technique is probably the least traumatic way of reducing daily nicotine exposure.
- Use on an as-needed basis, for as long as required. Currently, the problem with this is that the health risk of long-term transdermal nicotine use is not well defined.
- When you discontinue patch therapy, have a prescription of nicotine gum ready. The idea here is that it is better to relapse to nicotine gum than to return to smoking.
- Use a transdermal nicotine system that is designed to wean individuals off the patches by following a specific patch-wearing schedule. With this system, smokers will taper gradually from large, to medium, to small patches before discontinuing treatment. Evidence clearly indicates that this method is an effective stop-smoking technique.

Currently, the *best* weaning strategy is unknown, but current research could support the use of the patch-reducing method. Regardless of what technique is used, some persons may experience withdrawal symptoms when their nicotine blood levels fall below their comfort zone. As former smokers discontinue patch therapy, they would be well advised to again use stop-smoking techniques. The good news is that withdrawal from transdermal nicotine therapy is generally less traumatic and more transient than quitting cigarettes.

PREPARING SMOKERS FOR THE QUITTING PROCESS

There are several pitfalls that await smokers during the first year of quitting. Perhaps the greatest service that smoking cessation counselors can do is to anticipate for smokers the various problems they will likely encounter with quitting. These problems vary somewhat from smoker to smoker, but are so similar that we use the diagram of Quit Mountain (Fig. 8–1) to illustrate them.

Guide to Quit Mountain

1. Represents the start of the Quit Mountain climb. One advantage of using the Quit Mountain diagram is it can readily show smokers the tremendous amount of energy it will take them to make the climb toward quitting. We emphasize to smokers that

(continued)

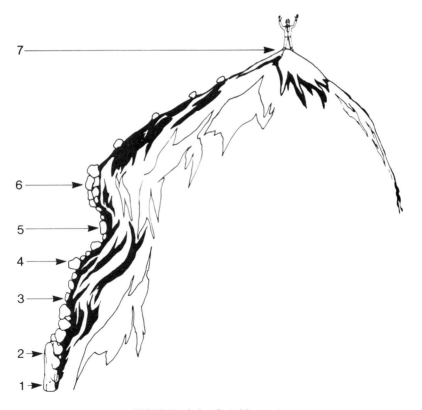

FIGURE 8-1   Quit Mountain

only a few smokers who will try to climb Quit Mountain this year will succeed, so they need to be prepared for the challenge.

2. The first 3 days of climbing Quit Mountain are the most difficult. Abrupt abstinence from cigarettes will require the same type of single-mindedness and persistent effort as climbing hand-over-hand a steep mountain wall. Most smokers hate the early climb, but realize that coping with these few days are a necessary part of conquering the mountain. During the first few days of quitting, smokers may feel many of these symptoms: anxiety, restlessness, difficulty concentrating, headaches, upset stomach, irritability, frustration, drowsiness, insomnia, and an almost unrelenting craving for cigarettes. For heavily addicted smokers (those who require cigarettes soon after awakening and regular nicotine dosing every 45 minutes during daytime hours), nicotine polacrilex or transdermal nicotine systems may be critical to the success of the early climb.

   Here are some common guidelines we provide all smokers with to help them cope with the early stages of quitting:

- Craving for nicotine will engulf you like a series of waves during your first few days of quitting. Like a wave, the craving sensation will fade whether *you smoke or not*.
- Use plenty of cinnamon gum. When you feel that you can no longer resist a cigarette, chew a piece of cinnamon gum. Often, the gum will provide a sufficient zing to get you over a craving hump.
- Be active. Do not become overwhelmed by the feelings of anxiety and restlessness. Get up, move around, stay active. Put the energy to good use. In a recent study, one woman volunteered to help her neighbor roof a house during the first 3 days of quitting. Some plan their quit days around golf, tennis, or long walks.
- Use deep-breathing techniques. Deep-breathing techniques are recommended for those occasions when you want to smoke, but cannot be active: driving a car, working at a desk, attending a meeting. The technique is simple: Hold your breath for as long as you can, then exhale *very* slowly through pursed lips.
- Avoid high-risk situations. During the first week of quitting, smokers are directed to avoid certain high-risk occasions. These can include any place there are other smokers *and* alcohol: bars, parties, and bowling alleys are to be avoided if possible; extended periods of being alone in the evening; heavy meals often trigger the cigarette habit—eat lightly and frequently. (After 1 week of quitting, smokers are encouraged to resume normal activity, but to be wary of these situations.)
- Monitor your caffeine intake according to how you feel. If you feel anxious, restless, and have insomnia, cut back on your caffeine. If, on the other hand, you feel drowsy (about 10% of early quitters complain about being tired or sleepy), increase your caffeine intake accordingly.

3. After 1 week of total abstinence, smokers have mastered roughly 25% of the mountain. "Craving waves" for cigarettes are still intense, but are becoming less frequent.

4. During the second and third weeks of abstinence, many recent quitters have a growing sense of satisfaction as they are becoming increasingly comfortable with being former smokers. Withdrawal symptoms have either vanished or have become more manageable. However, craving for cigarettes, while less frequent, can be as intense as during the first few days. We emphasize to smokers that as they progress up the mountain, the craving waves will be spaced further and further apart.

5. It is not unusual for people to become depressed or feel down at some time during the climb (note depression in mountain). We are not certain why, but this seems to occur most often between weeks 3 and 5 after quitting. Crying outbursts, a deep sense of loss (some smokers feel that they have lost their best friend—the cigarette), and

general malaise or tiredness are common. Some smokers return to smoking as they convince themselves that there is something wrong with them and their lives were better off as a smoker. Reassuring smokers that this down-stage may be a normal part of quitting for them probably reduces the likelihood of relapse. Severe cases of depression, however, may require medical intervention.

6. One of the final major battles is with weight gain, symbolized by the bulge on the mountain. Many quitters gain nearly 1 lb (0.45 kg)/week during the first 8 to 12 weeks of quitting. For some, this is the most disheartening and most difficult segment of the stop-smoking battle. Some choose of their own volition to return to smoking during this stage. They decide that they would rather be thin smokers than fat former smokers. Key information about smoking and weight control should be dispensed at this stage. First, reassure the quitter that the weight gain will soon stabilize and may, in fact, begin to decline. Fully one-fifth of quitters do not gain weight long-term. Emphasize that as the smoker gets more comfortable with being smoke-free, the "feeding frenzy" will end. Most, at this stage, will be able to recognize that they are no longer consuming as much food as they did during the early days of quitting. Second, emphasize the effects that smoking has on a person's appearance, particularly where nicotine-constricted blood vessels lead to increased wrinkles and a paler complexion. Thus, many quitters, despite adding a few pounds, may actually look better.

7. The smoker in Figure 8–1 has achieved a noteworthy goal, smoke-free for 1 year. Most former smokers are very comfortable here. Please note, however, that our happy quitter is standing on a sheet of ice and snow to symbolize that a person at this stage still may be just one cigarette away from sliding off the mountain.

The last stage of quitting actually extends beyond the first year—fighting the desire to have an occasional cigarette. Years after people quit, they may be reminded that a cigarette would be enjoyable after a heavy meal, during times of stress, or while drinking alcohol with friends who smoke.

We drill smokers repeatedly that they are "smoke-o-holics," or probably more accurately, "nicotinics." They cannot have just one cigarette. When a two–pack-a-day smoker smokes a single cigarette, he or she will likely return to the two–pack-a-day habit within a few weeks. We tell our quitters, "Never bum a cigarette. Go out and buy a carton instead."

REFERENCES

1. Fletcher CM, Peto R, Tinker CM, Speizer FE. The natural history of chronic bronchitis and emphysema. Oxford: Oxford University Press, 1976.

2. Buist AS, Nagy JM, Sexton GJ. Effect of smoking cessation on pulmonary function: a 30-month follow-up to two smoking cessation clinics. Am Rev Respir Dis 1979;120:953.

3. Bake B, Oxhoj H, Sixt R, Wilhelmsen L. Ventilatory lung function following two years of tobacco abstinence. Scand J Respir Dis 1977;58:311.

4. Bosse R, Sparrow D, Rose CC, Weiss ST. Longitudinal effect of age and smoking cessation on pulmonary function. Am Rev Respir Dis 1981;123:378.

5. Doll R, Peta R. Mortality in relation to smoking; 20 years' observation in male British doctors. Br Med J 1976;2:1525.

6. Burrows B, Earle RH. Course and prognosis of chronic obstructive lung disease: a prospective study of 200 patients. N Engl J Med 1969;280:397.

7. Daughton DM, Fix AJ, Kass I, Patil KD. Three-year survival rates of pulmonary rehabilitation patients with chronic obstructive pulmonary disease. J Natl Med Assoc. 1984;76:265.

8. Dudley DL, Aickin M, Martin CV. Cigarette smoking in a chest clinic population—psychophysiologic variables. J Psychosom Res 1977;21:367.

9. Daughton DM, Fix AJ, Kass I, Patil KD. Smoking cessation among patients with chronic obstructive pulmonary disease (COPD). Addict Behav 1980;5:125.

10. Petty TL, Pierson DJ, Dick NP, et al. Follow-up evaluation of a prevalence study for chronic bronchitis and chronic airway obstruction. Am Rev Respir Dis 1976;114:881.

11. Hepper NGG, Drage CW, Davies SF, et al. Chronic obstructive pulmonary disease: a community-oriented program including professional education and screening by a voluntary health agency. Am Rev Respir Dis 1980;121:97.

12. Kass I, Daughton DM, Fix AJ, Bell CW, Patil KD. The Nebraska COPD Rehabilitation Project II: A program to identify the predictive criteria involved in the rehabilitation of patients with chronic pulmonary disease. Final report. Special Education and Rehabilitation Services, 1982:20–23.

13. US Public Health Service. Smoking and health: report of the Advisory Committee to the Surgeon General of the Public Health Service. Bethesda, MD: US Department of Health, Education and Welfare; Public Health Service; Centers for Disease Control; PHS Publication No. 1103, 1964.

14. US Public Health Service. The health benefits of smoking cessation. Report of the Surgeon General. Bethesda, MD: Department of Health and Human Services, Public Health and Human Services, Office on Smoking and Health, 1990.

15. Koop EC. Julia M. Jones Lecture, annual meeting of the American Lung Association, Miami Beach, Florida, May 20, 1984.

16. Rustin RM, Kittel F, Dramaix M, et al. Smoking habits and psycho–socio–biological factors. J Psychosom Res 1978;22:89.

17. US Public Health Service. The smoking digest. Bethesda, MD: US Dept of Health, Education and Welfare, 1977:54.

18. Brantmark B, Ohlin P, Westling H. Nicotine-containing chewing gum as an anti-smoking aid. Psychopharmacologia 1973;31:191.

19. Daughton DM, Fix AJ, Roberts DE, Rennard SI. Evaluation of a worksite smoking cessation program: results and implications. Am Rev Respir Dis 1988;137:159.

20. Schwartz JL. A critical review and evaluation of smoking control methods. Public Health Rep 1969;84:483.

21. Schwartz JL, Rider G. Smoking cessation methods in the United States and Canada, 1969–1974. Proceedings of the third world conference on smoking and health, workshop on cessation methods. New York: June 3, 1975.

22. Thompson EL. Smoking education programs 1960–1976. Am J Public Health 1978;68:250.

23. Katz NW. Hypnosis and the addiction. Addict Behav 1980;5:41.

24. Spiegel H. A single-treatment method to stop smoking using ancillary self-hypnosis. Int J Clin Exp Hypn 1970;18:235.

25. Moses FM. Treating smoking habit by discussion and hypnosis. Dis Neurol Syst 1967;125:184.

26. Peterson LL, Scrimgeour WG, Lefcoe NM. Comparison of hypnosis plus counseling, counseling alone, and hypnosis alone in a community service smoking withdrawal program. J Consult Clin Psychol 1975;43:920.

27. Peterson LL, Scrimgeour WG, Lefcoe NM. Variables of hypnosis which are related to success in a smoking withdrawal program. Int J Clin Exp Hypn 1979;1:14.

28. Hymowitz N, Lasser NL, Safirstein BH. Effects of graduated external filters on smoking cessation. Prev Med 1982;11:85.

29. Miller GH. Devices to help smokers stop don't. Am Pharm 1980;20:53.

30. Ejrup B. Follow-up of the material of smokers difficult to treat. Sven Iakartidin 1959;56:1975.

31. Ejrup B. A proposed medical regimen to stop smoking: the follow-up results. Swed Cancer Soc Yearb 1963;3:468.

32. Rosenberg A. An attempt to break the smoking habit. Appl Ther 1962;4:1029.

33. Blum A. Nicotine chewing gum and the medicalization of smoking. Ann Intern Med 1984;101:121.

34. Research Committee of the British Tuberculosis Association. Smoking deterrent study. Br Med J 1963;2:486.

35. Glassman AH, Jackson WK, Walsh BT, et al. Cigarette craving, smoking withdrawal and clonidine. Science 1984;10:864.

36. Glassman AH, et al. Heavy smokers, smoking cessation and clonidine. Results of a double-blind, randomized trial. JAMA 1988;259:2863.

37. Ornish SA, et al. Effects of transdermal clonidine treatment on withdrawal symptoms associated with smoking cessation. Arch Intern Med 1988;148:2027.

38. Lamontage Y, Annable L, Gagnon MA. Acupuncture for smokers: lack of long-term therapeutic effect in a controlled study. Can Med Assoc J 1980;122:787.

39. Schmahl DP, Lichtenstein E, Harris DE. Successful treatment of habitual smokers with warm, smoky air and rapid smoking. J Consult Clin Psychol 1972;38:105.

40. Lichtenstein E, Harris DE, Birchler GR, Wahl JM, Schmahl DP. Comparison of rapid smoking, warm, smoky air, and attention-placebo in the modification of smoking behavior. J Consult Clin Psychol 1973;40:92.

41. Lando HA. Aversive conditioning and contingency management in the treatment of smoking. J Consult Clin Psychol 1976;44:312.

42. Raw M, Russell MAH. Rapid smoking, cue exposure and support in the modification of smoking. Behav Res Ther 1980;18:363.

43. Russell MAH, Raw M, Taylor C, Feyerabend C, Saloojee Y. Blood nicotine and carboxyhemoglobin levels after rapid-smoking aversion therapy. J Consult Clin Psychol 1978;46:1423.

44. Russell MAH, Armstrong E, Patel UA. Temporal contiguity in electric aversion therapy for cigarette smoking. Behav Res Ther 1976;14:103.

45. Hammond EC, Garfinkel C, Seidman H, Lee EA. Tar and nicotine content of cigarette smoke in relation to death rates. Environ Res 1976;12:263.

46. Rosen GM, Lichtenstein E. An employee preventative program to reduce cigarette smoking. J Consult Clin Psychol 1977;45:957.

47. Elliott R, Tight T. Breaking the cigarette habit: effects of a technique involving threat of loss of money [Mimeograph]. Hanover, NH: Dartmouth College, 1967.

48. Bernard HS, Efran JS. Eliminating versus reducing smoking using pocket timers. Behav Res Ther 1972;10:399–401.

49. Sachs LB, Bena H, Morrow JE. Comparison of smoking treatments. Behav Ther 1970;1:465.

50. Flaxman J. Quitting smoking now or later: gradual, abrupt, immediate or delayed quitting. Behav Ther 1978;9:260.

51. Mausner B. Mausner J, Rial W. The influence of the physician on the smoking behavior of his patients. In: Zagone SV, ed. Studies and issues in smoking behavior. Tucson: University of Arizona Press, 1967:103.

52. Mausner B. Report on a smoking clinic. Am Psychol 1986;21:251.

53. Russell MAH, Wilson C, Taylor C, Baker CD. Effect of general practitioners' advice against smoking. Br Med J 1979;2:231.

54. McAlister A. Helping people quit smoking: current progress. In: Enclow SJ, Hender-

son JB, eds. Applying behavioral sciences to cardiovascular risk. New York: American Heart Association, 1975.

55. Davis AL, Faust R, Ordentlich B. Self-help smoking cessation and maintenance program: a comparative study with 12-month follow-up by the American Lung Association. Am J Public Health 1987;74:1212.

56. Harris MB, Ruthburg C. A self-control approach to reducing smoking. Psychol Rep 1972;31:165.

57. Ober DC. Modification of smoking behavior. J Consult Clin Psychol 1971;37:80.

58. Glasgow RE, Rosen GM. Behavioral bibliotherapy: a review of self-help behavior therapy manuals. Psychol Bull 1978;85:1.

59. Glasgow RE. Effects of a self-control manual, rapid smoking, and amount of therapist contact on smoking reduction. J Consult Clin Psychol 1978;46:1439.

60. Kozlowski CT, Jarvik ME, Gritz ER. Nicotine regulation and cigarette smoking. Clin Pharmacol Ther 1975;17:93.

61. Knapp PH, Bliss CM, Wells C. Addictive aspects of heavy cigarette smoking. Am J Psychiatry 1963;119:966.

62. Russell MAH. Cigarette smoking: natural history of a dependence disorder. Br Med Psychol 1971;44:1.

63. Hunt WA, Barnett LW, Branch LG. Relapse rates in addiction programs. J Clin Psychol 1971;27:455.

64. Phillips C. The EEG change associated with smoking. Psychophysiology 1971;8:64.

65. Hall GH. Effects of nicotine and tobacco smoke on the electrical activity of the cerebral cortex and olfactory bulb. Br J Pharmacol 1970;38:271.

66. Domino EF. Neuropsychopharmacology of nicotine and tobacco smoke. In: Dunn WL, ed. Smoking behavior, motives and incentives. Washington, DC: Winston, 1973:531.

67. Domino EF, VonBaumgarten AM. Tobacco, cigarette smoking and patella reflex depression. Clin Pharmacol Ther 1969;10:72.

68. Diagnostic and statistical manual of mental disorders (DSM-III). Washington, DC: The American Psychiatric Association, 1980:159.

69. McNabb ME, Ebert RV, McCusker K. Plasma nicotine levels produced by chewing nicotine gum. JAMA 1982;248:865.

70. Fagerstrom K-O. A comparison of psychological and pharmacological treatment in smoking cessation. J Behav Med 1982;5:343.

71. Karvis MJ, Raw M, Russell MAH, Feyerabend C. Randomized controlled trial of nicotine chewing gum. Br Med J 1982;285:537.

72. Raw M, Jarvis MJ, Feyerabend C, Russell MAH. Comparison of nicotine chewing gum and psychological treatments of dependent smokers. Br Med J 1980;281:481.

73. Schneider NG, Jarvik MF, Forsythe AB, Read CC, Elliott ML, Schweiger A. Nicotine gum in smoking cessation: a placebo-controlled, double-blind trail. J Addict Behav 1983;8:253.

74. Russell MAH, Merriman R, Stapleton J, Taylor W. Effect of nicotine chewing gum as an adjunct to general practitioners' advice against smoking. Br Med J 1983;287:1782.

75. Daughton DM, Kass I, Fix AJ, Ahrens K, Rennard SI. Smoking intervention: combination therapy using nicotine chewing gum and the American Lung Association's "Freedom from Smoking" manuals. Prev Med 1986;15:432.

76. Daughton DM, Heatley S, Prendergast J, et al. Effect of transdermal nicotine delivery as an adjunct to low-intervention smoking cessation therapy. A randomized, placebo-controlled, double-blind study. Arch Intern Med 1991;151:749.

JOHN W. JENNE

Pharmacology in the Respiratory Patient

What do asthmatics and patients with COPD expect from us? They are interested in maintaining comfortable breathing at rest and in their necessary activities, the ability to withstand provocative stimuli, and the ability to weather acute exacerbations with minimum risk and discomfort.

Adequate drug therapy of these patients requires an understanding of the various bronchodilators and anti-inflammatory agents, along with the knowledge to individualize their use. This even extends to the patient with so-called fixed obstruction. Most of the latter have a reversible element that can be optimally treated to the considerable relief of the patient. But the greatest advances in therapy are in the management of asthma, particularly as we have come to appreciate the central role of inflammation in this disease and have become able to control it through drug therapy.

The aims of this chapter are to develop an appreciation of the pathophysiology and host pharmacology underlying drug therapy, to offer guidelines for manipulating drugs according to the clinical state of the patient, and to supply the minimum commonly needed information of the products used. An excellent and convenient general review has appeared by Barnes.[1]

ROLE OF INFLAMMATION IN ASTHMA

Certain mileposts can be cited leading to our present appreciation of the role of inflammation in asthma and its influence on therapy. These are core concepts for the practitioner.

Importance of Wall Thickness to Airway Resistance

We sometimes encounter patients with severe asthma or COPD who seem relatively comfortable one minute, and over the next few minutes or hours progress so rapidly downhill that they must be aggressively treated in an emergency room. Many times these patients are chronically coping with severe airway obstruction and have adapted to it. But they live on a precarious edge. Figure 9–1 illustrates how any inflammatory thickening of the bronchial wall leads to an exaggeration of luminal

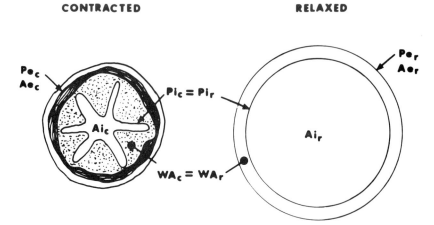

FIGURE 9-1   Relaxed (*r*) and contracted (*c*) membranous bronchiole, illustrating that the wall contents must be accommodated during contraction, and any inflammatory thickening accentuates luminal narrowing. *Pi,* internal perimeter; *Ai,* internal area; *Pe,* external perimeter; *Ae,* external area. (James AL, Pare PD, Hogg, JC. The mechanics of airway narrowing in asthma. Am Rev Respir Dis 1989;139:242, with permission)

narrowing created by bronchospasm.[2] The task of the physician is to maximize resting internal caliber, using bronchodilators and anti-inflammatory agents and, once an exacerbation occurs, to accelerate drug therapy within safe limits to minimize further encroachment.

Bronchial Hyperreactivity of Hyperresponsiveness

In 1933, Samter first observed that asthmatics react excessively to inhaled histamine.[3] Measurement of the threshold concentration of histamine or methacholine required to produce a fall of 20% in 1-second forced expiratory volume (FEV_1), the PC_{20} or PD_{20}, has become the standard method for detecting the otherwise inapparent mild asthmatic, and sometimes for following the results of various interventions.[4] This nonspecific reactivity correlates roughly with reactivity to cold air, exercise, diurnal variation in flow, and osmotic challenge, either hypo- or hyperosmotic.[5] There may be discrepancies in the individual case. Although measurement of the PC_{20} is most often applied to the asthmatic, some patients with COPD are also hyperresponsive, overlapping with asthmatics.[6] A PC_{20} under 8 mg/mL is considered abnormal. Severe asthmatics will have a PC_{20} well under 1.0 mg/mL.

Immediate, Late, and Chronic Phases of Reaction to Antigen Challenge

Responses to antigen challenge, and to certain small-molecular-weight substances, cause an *early* or immediate fall in FEV_1, and in a large proportion a *late* or delayed response.[7] The last response may last up to 12 hours, and is generally followed by a state of heightened nonspecific reactivity, which may last up to several weeks, contributing to the chronic state of inflammation.[8] The early obstruction is largely due to bronchospasm caused by release of preformed mediators, such as histamine, and the immediate generation of other contractile mediators from arachidonic acid, synthesized within minutes from IgE-bearing mast cells. The late-phase obstruction is thought to be principally due to inflammatory events (cells, edema, congestion) in response to mediators and cytokines. Bronchoalveolar lavage (BAL) studies at 48 and 96 hours following antigen challenge with a late phase show persistence of activated macrophages and eosinophils and helper T lymphocytes.[9] Whereas antispasmodics block the immediate phase obstruction, they have less effect when taken during or just before the late phase. Corticosteroids block the late phase, undoubtedly through suppression of many steps in the inflammatory response. Cromolyn can block both phases.

Asthma Triggers and Fluctuating Hyperreactivity

A major advance in understanding airway hyperreactivity was the demonstration that those asthmatics undergoing a late response to antigen could develop an exaggerated reactivity to nonspecific stimuli that could linger for weeks, as shown by a reduced PC_{20} to histamine.[8] Although this did not explain the presence of the original hyperreactivity, it did provide a mechanism whereby reactivity and asthma could become worse. Cockcroft has classified such challenges, or "triggers," according to whether they lead to further reactivity.[10] Those that do involve an element of inflammation, or complexity, not present with histamine or methacholine.

Morphologic Evidence of Chronic Inflammation in Asthma

Another major advance was the stunning demonstration by Laitenan that even mild asthmatics had inflammatory changes on bronchial biopsy.[11] Their extent had never been realized. In moderate asthmatics, shedding of the epithelium is common. Electron microscopy and special immunostaining techniques have further delineated these changes.[12] Even mild asthmatics have excessive collagen deposition in the lamina propria. Treatment that minimizes inflammation might prevent permanent alteration.

Long-Term Deterioration of the Chronic Asthmatic

Chronic asthmatics may develop an element of fixed obstruction, probably as a result of chronic inflammation, which occurs more commonly in cigarette smokers.[13] Their response to maximum bronchodilation and corticosteroids shows an overall decline. Consequently, it behooves clinicians to minimize inflammation and attempt to reduce allergen exposure in the home and workplace.

Muscular Control of Airway Caliber

The cholinergic nervous system dominates in the control of airway caliber (Fig. 9–2). Adrenergic fibers in direct contact with smooth muscle are too sparse to directly influence the airway, but they do inhibit cholinergic traffic through β_2-receptors at the ganglia. Sympathomimetic amines and circulating catecholamines directly influence airway smooth muscle through membrane receptors with β_2-specificity. Nonadrenergic, noncholinergic fibers traveling in the vagus are the principal inhibitory

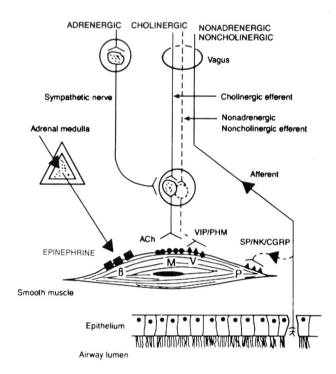

FIGURE 9-2 Elements of autonomic control of airways in humans. Cholinergic nerves travel down the vagus to release acetylcholine at muscarinic receptors (M_3 subtype) on the smooth muscle. Adrenergic fibers terminate at β_2-adrenoceptors on the ganglia inhibiting cholinergic traffic. Nonadrenergic noncholinergic fibers descend in the vagus nerve to relax smooth muscle through neuropeptides such as vasoactive intestinal peptide (VIP) and peptide histidine methionine (PHM). Reflexes from airways provoke cholinergic responses and are postulated to activate axon reflexes with release of inflammatory peptides substance P (SP), neurokinin (NK), and calcitonin gene-related peptide (cGRP). (Barnes PJ. The third nervous system in the lung. Thorax 1984; 39:561, with permission)

system to the airways in humans.[14] Their transmitter has been postulated to be vasoactive intestinal peptide (VIP) and peptide histidine methionine (PHM), but there is evidence to the contrary as well. Stimulation of afferent receptors in the mucosa and airways (irritant receptors and C-fiber afferents) leads to bronchospasm through cholinergic reflexes.

Airway Receptors

Airway receptor stimulation controls airway caliber. Other receptors exist on glands and vessels. Receptors causing constriction of smooth muscle are histamine (H_1), muscarinic (M_3), α_1-adrenergic, adenosine (A_1), SP-P, leukotriene B_4, C_4, D_4, and E_4, prostaglandin D_2 and $F_2\alpha$, platelet activating factor (PAF), thromboxane A_2, and bradykinin (BK). Receptors causing relaxation are beta$_2$-adrenoceptor, adenosine (A_2), prostaglandin E_2 and I_2, histamine (H_2), VIP, and PHM.[15,16]

A β-adrenoceptor is embedded in the cell membrane, and consists of seven folded membrane-spanning segments. It is coupled to adenylate cyclase, also membrane bound, through a stimulatory G_s protein, with production of cyclic-AMP (cAMP) as the final product leading to smooth muscle relaxation. Other receptors, such as alpha$_2$-adrenergic and M_2, are inhibitory to adenylate cyclase through the G_i inhibitory protein.[17]

The action of β-agonists is to cause an immediate drop in the level of calcium, as shown by intracellular calcium indicators.[18] The mechanism whereby this occurs is complex. Cyclic-AMP is involved in multiple actions leading to muscle relaxation, the most recent being stimulation of potassium channels.

BRONCHODILATORS

β-Adrenergic Compounds

The β-agonists are the most potent and versatile of the bronchodilators in the asthmatic and are useful in the COPD patient as well. Epinephrine is the only compound available over-the-counter, marketed as Primatine Mist. With its combined α- and β-adrenergic properties, it has the disadvantage of aggravating hypertension and, with its catecholamine nucleus, a very short duration of bronchodilation. But it undoubtedly serves a useful purpose as an emergency medication for the public. Isoproterenol, the most potent relaxant in this group, was largely superseded in the early 1970s by the β_2-selective compounds, of which isoetharine and metaproterenol (less selective), and albuterol, terbutaline, pirbuterol, and bitolterol are existing Food and Drug Administration (FDA)-approved compounds (Fig. 9–3). β_2-selectivity was achieved by altering the side chain. More prolonged action was achieved by altering the catechol nucleus (present in epinephrine, isoproterenol, isoetharine) to avoid inactivation by tissue catechol-O-methyltransferase. Two new compounds with an ultralong action, designed for twice-daily dosing, are formoterol[19] and salmeterol,[20] presently undergoing FDA evaluation. These bind more tightly to the β_2-receptor site. If approved, they should revolutionize the bronchodilator industry.

Actions of β_2-Selective Compounds
Table 9–1 lists the therapeutic, and deleterious effects of β_2-selective compounds. Their systemic effects depend on the dose and route of administration.[21]

β_1- and β_2-Selectivity
Ahlquist classified adrenergic actions into α- and β-categories, with isoproterenol the prototype of the latter.[22] Lands further distinguished β-actions that increased rate and force of the heart from those relaxing the airways, labeling them β_1 and β_2, respectively.[23] He found that certain alkylated derivatives, such as isoetharine, had β_2-qualities. This distinction became more firmly established with discovery of the β_2-selective compound albuterol (salbutamol), and β_1 and β_2-selective antagonists. Isoproterenol had both β_1- and β_2- actions. Against guinea pig atrium, although isoproterenol and metaproterenol gave a maximum response (E_{max}) that could not be reached by any concentration of albuterol or terbutaline, all gave the same E_{max} with parallel dose–response curves with tracheal relaxation.[24] Among other β_2-actions

β-ADRENERGIC AGONISTS

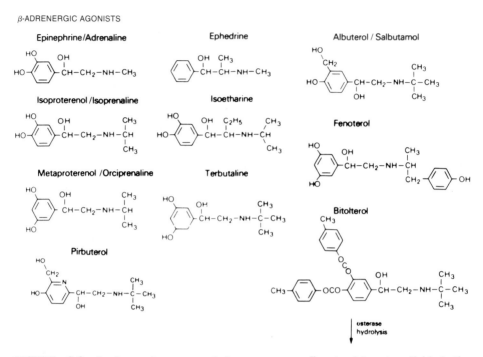

FIGURE   9-3   β-adrenergic compounds in common use. Fenoterol is not available in the United States.

TABLE   9–1.   Actions of β₂-Selective Compounds

Potentially Beneficial	*Potentially Deleterious*
Smooth-muscle relaxation (bronchi, uterus)	Peripheral vasodilation (decreased afterload)
Decreased pulmonary artery pressure (with secondary increased RVEF)	Increased heart rate and LVEF*
Increased mucociliary activity	Increased skeletal muscle tremor
Decreased mediator release	Decreased serum K^+ and increased QT_c interval
Decreased permeability edema	Increased insulin, free fatty acids, glucose
Decreased muscarinic transmission	Decreased PaO_2 (worsened $\dot{V}/\dot{Q}$ ratio)
	Myocardial necrosis (proportional to β₁-component)

* Increased rate and ejection fraction occur secondary to decreased afterload. A minor fraction of cardiac receptors are β₂ and may enhance these responses.

are relaxation of uterine and vascular smooth muscle, skeletal muscle tremor, glycolysis, and a drop in potassium concentration caused by stimulation of the Na–K ATPase of skeletal muscle, causing potassium to enter the cell.

β_2-Selective Compounds and the Heart

β_2-selectivity is not complete, and β_2-actions also affect the heart and circulation. If normal persons inhale four puffs of isoproterenol, metaproterenol, or albuterol by metered-dose inhaler (MDI), isoproterenol produces a sharp increase in pulse, metaproterenol is intermediate, and albuterol produces none.[25] In larger doses, particularly by nebulization or systemically, even albuterol will cause some pulse elevation and increase in cardiac output. For the most part, this is a reflex response to the drop in peripheral resistance. In contrast to isoproterenol, there is little or no increase in contractility (inotropism) and no increase in myocardial oxygen uptake.[26,27] Yet, human hearts contain both β_1- and β_2-receptors, with β_1 being preponderant.[28] β_2-receptors are found in the order SA node > atrium > ventricle. They enhance both rate and force of the atrium.[28] Therefore, β_2-selective compounds do have a direct action on the heart, added to their minor β_1-component.

Kinetics of the Inhalant Route

Relief of bronchospasm in the stable asthmatic by a β_2-agonist delivered by MDI occurs rapidly, half of it within 30 seconds, and the rest peaking at about 60 minutes.[29] Bronchodilation continues for 120 to 150 minutes, and then begins to decline almost to baseline at 4 to 5 hours. Bronchodilation by this route has the advantage of a strong, rapid response, but with the disadvantage of recurring distress between treatments. The specification in some package inserts is two puffs every 4 to 6 hours, not to exceed 12 inhalations per day. In practice, these agents are applied virtually on an as-needed basis.

Only about 10% of the particles expelled by an MDI reach the lung, two-thirds to the larger airways, and one-third to the smaller airways and alveoli.[30] About 80% is deposited in the mouth and pharynx. By contrast, little drug given by wet nebulization is deposited in the mouth. Most of the inefficiency of this latter route is due to drug left behind in the nebulizer chamber, tubing, and atmosphere between breaths.[31] The drug is diluted with normal saline or distilled water to minimize that proportion left behind in the chamber (about 0.7 mL). Efficiency also depends on the particular nebulizer and applicator, pattern of ventilation, and flow rate.[32]

The dose/equivalency ratio between MDI and nebulized drug varies widely in different dose–response studies from 1 : 1 when measured as drug leaving the apparatus and directly inhaled,[33] to 1 : 12.5 in another study measured as drug placed in the chamber.[34] A recent carefully designed study by Mestitz and associates, comparing terbutaline given by MDI and nebulization into a face mask found a twofold difference in efficiency.[35] That is, five puffs from the MDI (1.25 mg) equaled 2.5 mg in the nebulizer, and both were suboptimal on their dose–response curve (Fig. 9–4). Others have shown a tenfold difference in efficiency when albuterol was applied by intermittent positive-pressure breathing (IPPB).[36] Two puffs of MDI (180 μg) were nearly as effective as 2.5 mg by IPPB. The latter's inefficiency was more than made up for by the 12 to 14-fold larger dose placed in the nebulizer. But, if we accept the data of Mestitz and coworkers as representative of a typical setup, 2.5 mg albuterol or 15.0 mg

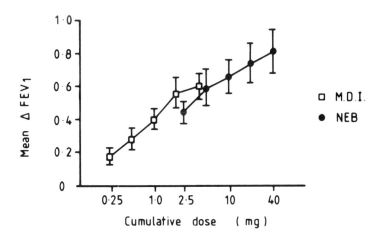

FIGURE 9-4 Cumulative terbutaline response curves comparing metered-dose inhaler (MDI) and liquid nebulization by face mask in stable asthma. Note that two puffs (0.50 mg) by MDI is relatively far down on the dose–response curve in these patients and considerably inferior to nebulization (usually 5.0 mg), but more puffs will equal it. (Mestitz H, et al. Comparison of outpatient nebulized vs metered dose inhaled terbutaline in chronic airflow obstruction. Chest 1989; 96:1237, with permission)

metaproterenol by face mask or mouthpiece is several times as effective as two puffs by MDI.[35] This discrepancy is strikingly illustrated by a comparison by Morely and colleagues of three puffs albuterol by InspirEase to 2.5 mg albuterol and 15.0 mg metaproterenol by nebulization in acute asthma.[37] The MDI was markedly inferior in its FEV_1 response, and albuterol gave a higher peak than metaproterenol (Fig. 9–5).

Cushley and associates conducted cumulative dose–response curve studies from a total of 4.0 mg terbutaline over 90 mintues, measured as dose leaving the apparatus.[33] They compared an MDI, MDI with affixed pear-shaped chamber of 750 mL and a Wright nebulizer delivered directly into the mouth. There was rough equivalence of all three, both in airway response and measured terbutaline in plasma 45 minutes later, 2 to 3 ng/mL. The pear-shaped nebulizer added some efficiency to the MDI. Serum levels were about what one expects from the same dose by mouth.

The peak serum drug levels reached after rapid administration of multiple doses by MDI are clearly significant. Kung and coworkers administered ten puffs of albuterol at 1-minute intervals.[38] Heart rates had already peaked by 5 minutes thereafter (average increase 14 beats per minute), evidently owing to alveolar absorption as experienced by cigarette and crack cocaine addicts. There was no difference with buccal rinsing and gargling. When nebulization takes place over 15 minutes, however, the longer duration must protect against a sharp peak.

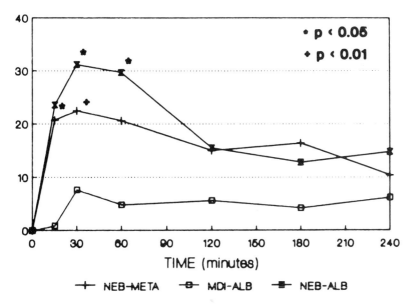

Optimizing Metered-Dose Delivery:
The Physician's Responsibility

One has only to observe patients attempting to use an MDI to realize that any lack of response is usually due to faulty technique. Guidelines for proper use of metered-dose inhalers are listed in Table 9–2. The technique must be suspect in any patient who claims that the inhaler does not help. It is important that patients continue to draw particles slowly in after the actuation of the MDI, rather than only aiming the device into their mouth, a common failing. Physicians must take the time to practice this maneuver with their patients. Probably the most important element in drug therapy of the obstructed patients is correct use of their MDI.

The MDI should be kept clean of particles by keeping the cap on and rinsing frequently. A handy means for gauging the remaining medication is to float the cartridge in water, noting the degree of emersion.

Spacers and Reservoirs

Spacers and reservoirs serve the purpose of removing large droplets that otherwise serve no purpose, but only add toxicity. They also slow down small particles, minimizing their impact on the nasopharynx. Finally, they enable the uncoordinated patient to use an MDI. Spacers are a means to save costs in the hospital during

TABLE 9–2. Steps in Using a Metered-Dose Inhaler

1. Hold inhaler with mouthpiece downward.
2. Shake the container several times.
3. Breathe out normally.
4. Open mouth widely, let mouthpiece touch lip or hold 1/2 to 1 in. from mouth.
5. Start to inhale slowly, then squeeze cartridge to release spray.
6. Continue to inhale as deeply as possible, then hold the breath for approximately 10 seconds, if possible.
7. Wait a minute or so before taking a repeat dose.
8. If there is difficulty following these steps, the addition of a spacer may help.

(Adapted from Ziment I. Pharmacologic therapy of COPD. In: Hodgkin JE, Petty TL, eds. Chronic obstructive pulmonary disease. Philadelphia: WB Saunders, 1987.)

recovery from an acute attack, but the dosing and timing of this are under investigation and in an evolving state.[39]

The Practical Meaning of Functional Antagonism

Functional antagonism refers to the reciprocal relation existing between two agonists with opposing actions. As the concentration of one goes up, the requirement for the counteracting agonist also goes up to maintain stability. This is particularly true for β-agonist protection against muscarinic contraction, both in vitro[40] and in vivo.[41] It is markedly less so for histamine in vitro.[42] Some degree of functional antagonism probably occurs in the asthmatic, although the mixture of contracting and obstructing influences complicates analysis. This was illustrated by the increasing requirement for albuterol by MDI in asthmatics of increasing severity to reach their plateau of response.[43] Such results support the concept that the dose of the β-agonist should be tailored to the severity of bronchospasm, rather than following a fixed schedule.

Tachyphylaxis

Tachyphylaxis means a reduction in drug response with continued exposure. Currently, we believe that tachyphylaxis of airway receptors to β_2-agonists is not a problem for most patients, although we cannot exclude this under some circumstances. It is curious that, whereas the β_2-receptors of the asthmatic's airways are rather resistant to tachyphylaxis, normal airways are not,[44,45] nor are systemic β_2-receptors, such as those modifying peripheral eosinophil count, tremor, and the plasma lactate level.[46] When 1000 μg/day or 4000 μg/day albuterol was given by MDI for 14 days, there was no effect on the FEV_1 dose–response curve to albuterol challenge. However, systemic responses showed a slight reduction after the lower dose, and a considerable reduction after the higher dose.[47] In fact, patients on nebulized albuterol therapy had only a 0.3 mEq drop in serum potassium concentration after a 10-mg challenge.[48] Thus, larger inhaled doses do cause tachyphylaxis of systemic responses.

Although many studies show essentially no drop in FEV_1 response after prolonged exposure, a large multicenter study by Repsher and colleagues showed that after 8 weeks of albuterol at two puffs four times daily, there was a reduction in area under the curve response and a reduction in mean duration of protection.[49] This was also shown in COPD.[50] Asthmatics receiving terbutaline by MDI showed a transient slight increase in nonspecific reactivity for 24 hours after cessation of drug,[51] at least when referred to the placebo. It may be that concomitant use of an inhaled corticosteroid will prevent this modest degree of tachyphylaxis, if it exists. Several studies of the new long-acting β_2-agonists have shown no reduction in effect or dose–response curve after continuous administration, most of them in patients also receiving inhaled corticosteroids.

β-Agonists in Asthma

Dose of Inhaled β-Agonists in Stable Asthma

In stable asthma, the standard FDA-approved dose of an MDI, two puffs four times daily, is suboptimal for many patients, subjecting them to an alternating feast and famine of air. The two-puff dose is relatively far down on the dose–response curve in a moderately severe asthmatic.[35,52] Figure 9–4 brings this out. The response follows a nonlinear logarithmic relation to dose. For example, a nebulized dose of 5.0 mg terbutaline by face mask is more effective than 0.5 mg (two puffs) by MDI, but more puffs will equal it (see Fig. 9–4). Patients often state that they benefit more from liquid nebulization than from their MDI. Although this may be due to faulty technique, it also may be due to a larger effective dose. Many physicians allow their patients to use their MDI as often as needed, with the provision that the need to use it more often than every 3 hours signals a worsening of asthma and the need for either more inhaled corticosteroids or a temporary burst of oral corticosteroids.

Inhaled β-Agonists in the Acute Attack

The conventional treatment of the acute attack, along with other modalities, is administration of nebulized albuterol (2.5 mg) or metaproterenol (15 mg) and to repeat this if the response is not forthcoming. The acute attack, however, requires a larger dose of β-agonist than does stable asthma, and some authorities advocate that the standard dose be repeated at 20-minute intervals for up to six doses until a response occurs.[53] This is essentially continuous nebulization. Patients should be receiving oxygen and be monitored.

An MDI with Aerochamber or a similar space device has been advocated as a substitute for liquid nebulization, since the latter is costly in time and personnel.[54] Newhouse and Dolovich advocate that four puffs of the MDI be given immediately, followed by one puff every minute up to 15 total puffs, or until the patient responds subjectively or develops side effects. This dose may be necessary in the acute situation. As mentioned, when 2.5 mg albuterol or 15 mg metaproterenol by nebulizer were compared with only three puffs of albuterol by MDI into an InspirEase reservoir, the acute MDI response over 4 hours was grossly inferior.[37]

The purpose of bronchodilator therapy is to prevent severe bronchospasm while the acute process is subsiding. This should be possible whether the bronchodilator is delivered by MDI or by nebulizer, provided an adequate dose is used. I favor a nebulizer initially, for at least 24 hours, when a changeover can be made to an MDI–spacer provided the patient is not too fatigued, too dyspneic, or too obstructed, and can master the technique. Four to six puffs every 4 hours over 5 minutes is reasonable for this transitional period, with final return to the usual stable dose. The MDI should be left at the bedside in the event of intercurrent bronchospasm, and the patient's response should be carefully monitored.

Aggressive Nebulization in Poor Responders

More and more studies are appearing using high-intensity nebulization. A comparison of 5.0 mg albuterol at zero and 60 minutes, with the same total dose given continuously over 120 minutes, found no difference.[55] The latter setup may be more convenient in a busy emergency room. Patients should be receiving oxygen and be monitored during such therapy.

The blood levels achieved with high-intensity continuous nebulization are of concern and have been measured in children, giving us some idea of what to expect in the adult. Shuh and associates compared serum albuterol in acute asthmatic children after seven doses of 0.15 mg/kg (5.0 mg maximum per dose), or "high-dose" albuterol, administered over about 1.5 hours (essentially continuously), and one-third this dose ("low dose").[56] The FEV_1 response to the high dose was twice that to the low dose. Serum levels averaged 10 ng/mL in the low-dose group, and 19 ng/mL (maximum 46 ng/mL in the high-dose group). The drop in serum potassium concentration averaged about 20% in both groups. These albuterol levels compare with levels of about 12 ng/mL at steady state when receiving 4 mg albuterol orally every 6 hours.[57] Since the low dose corresponds roughly to dosing 2.5 mg in 2.5 mL saline continuously or every 20 minutes six times, as advocated in severe adult asthma, the levels reached in the latter seem not excessive for the nondiseased heart.

Continuously nebulized terbutaline therapy has been advocated by Moler et al[58] in children with severe asthma using a mean dose of 4 mg/hr by face mask (mean application time of 15.4 hours) and up to 0.4 mg/kg per hour (0.1 to 0.4 mg/kg per hour) and by Kelly and coworkers.[59] The latter found that the response was faster when the dose was equal or greater than 2.0 mg/kg per hour. No arrhythmias or adverse effects were seen. In adults, Nelson advocates 2 mg terbutaline every 20 minutes until a satisfactory response is reached using undiluted drug (1 mg/mL). He may combine this with 0.01 mg/kg up to 0.3 mg subcutaneously every 15 minutes as necessary.[60]

Several intravenous (IV) regimens are published, which are beyond the scope of this chapter, but are summarized elsewhere.[61] Anecdotal experience is often quite impressive, when the regimens have been used after failure of usual treatment. The cardiotoxicity of isoproterenol favors the use of IV terbutaline in the United States.

Subcutaneous Route

The principal need for subcutaneous injection is during an emergency when very rapid bronchodilation is needed, for example, for a patient in the hospital or at home in crisis, and also in the patient with plugged airways who is responding suboptimally to inhaled drug. Appel randomized asthmatics in the emergency room between nebulized metaproterenol given at zero, 30, 60 minutes followed by 0.3 mg epinephrine at 120, 150, and 180 minutes, and the drugs in the reverse order.[62] Although 28 of 46 patients responded briskly to the nebulized drug when given first, 18 did not; however, 13 of these did respond to injected epinephrine. Most of the 54 patients receiving epinephrine first responded, but only 1 of the 6 nonrespondents responded to metaproterenol. Thus, a significant proportion of patients will respond faster to injected, rather than to nebulized, drug in this circumstance. Appel hypothesizes that this is due to airway plugging, since the nonrespondents had twice the duration of buildup of their attack compared with respondents. In our practice, dealing with middle-aged or older veterans, we use subcutaneous terbutaline, rather than epinephrine, and use it liberally along with nebulized drug in the acute attack.

Oral β-Agonists

In the United States we tend to underuse oral β_2-agonists. β_2-agonists undergo first-pass metabolism by mouth, being sulfated by the intestine and liver.[57] Hence, the oral dose is 10 to 20 times the subcutaneous dose. Once oral terbutaline sulfate reaches steady state, it has distributed into tissue reservoirs, presumably fat, and its mean half-life after drug termination averages 17 hours. The practical importance is that a maintenance schedule provides a "floor" of β_2-stimulation, even if a dose is missed. Albuterol sulfate is a little different in its kinetics. Steady-state levels are about twice the levels of a single dose, so accumulation does occur, although the half-life after stopping the drug is about 6.5 hours.[57] Albuterol is available as a slow-release preparation designed for twice-daily dosing. Oral terbutaline is usually administered three times daily. These should provide better control of nocturnal bronchospasm. In our experience, oral β_2-agonists sometimes provide much better control in the occasional patient with erratic response to an MDI, and both can be used together. They can also be combined with theophylline.

We generally begin terbutaline at 2.5 mg every 6 to 8 hours, or albuterol 2 mg (measured as the base) on a similar schedule. Patients will make some adaptation to tremor, and the dose can be doubled if desired. We find oral β-agonists to be well tolerated, even in older patients. Tremor is highly individualized[63] and appears to be less with albuterol than with terbutaline.[64]

β-Agonists in Chronic Obstructive Pulmonary Disease

Inhaled β-Agonists

In the large IPPB Trial Group study, the mean FEV_1 response to isoproterenol was 15%.[65] A useful point was that a single, isolated determination of the bronchodilator response should not be relied on to make therapeutic decisions. Low responses were usually followed by better responses on repeated trial. Patients with the lower FEV_1s (e.g., less than 20% predicted) had higher percentage improvement (averaging 20%) than those with better function.

But even when patients were shown to have fixed obstruction, Berger and Smith found that three puffs of metaproterenol by MDI improved their performance on the 12-minute walk.[66] The reasons are unclear, but there is no reason to withhold inhaled β-agonists on the basis of the bronchodilator response until the patients have tried them empirically.

Unsatisfactory results with an MDI may be due to poor technique, despite much coaching; however the response may be much better to an antimuscarinic agent. We occasionally find a gratifying result. Other approaches are a trial with a spacer, such as an Aerochamber, or a reservoir such as InspirEase. An alternative is the Rotahaler device in which the patient sucks the powdered drug in from a crushed ampule.

All the foregoing approaches have improved our ability to deliver the drug to these patients. A final approach is the use of wet nebulization. The reason most patients obtain relief with these is complex, involving an easier technique, a larger effective dose, and psychologic conditioning. Severely restricted patients, those unable to leave their homes, have usually ended up on such nebulizers. However, larger doses by an MDI in conjunction with a spacer may prove equally effective.

Oral β₂-Agonists

In many clinics, oral β₂-agonists are neglected for COPD patients, perhaps through concern for possible cardiovascular toxicity in the elderly patient, or else through ignorance of their possible benefit. Only recently has there been a suitable study. Mattbaek and colleagues compared oral maintenance terbutaline and placebo in a double-blind, crossover study.[67] Pulmonary function was measured before and 20 minutes after inhalation of 1.0 mg terbutaline from a Nebuhaler, a pear-shaped spacer that improves efficiency of delivery. A thorough attempt was also made to monitor dyspnea during various tasks, and the 6-minute walk distance was obtained. The mean FEV_1 and forced vital capacity (FVC) are listed at the 3-week point in Table 9–3.

Functional analog scales for common patient activities (climbing stairs, carrying shopping bags, walking) showed significant improvement when receiving the oral drug, although the 6-minute walk did not change. No changes occurred in blood pressure, heart rate, or serum potassium levels. Three of 20 patients dropped out because of tremor.

Oral terbutaline and albuterol provide a constant floor of β-agonist stimulation. They probably act more directly on peripheral airways than the inhaled drug. They are valuable in both asthma and COPD when MDI use is not providing consistent benefit.

TABLE 9–3. Effect of Adding Oral Terbutaline, 15 mg/24 h, to Inhaled Terbutaline in COPD

	On Placebo		On Terbutaline	
	Before MDI	After MDI	Before MDI	After MDI
FEV_1	0.86	0.99	0.93	1.02
FVC	1.91	2.24	2.14	2.34

(Adapted from Maltback N, et al. Effects of oral terbutaline in chronic airflow limitation. Chest 1989; 95:1248)

Cardiovascular Toxicity of β-Agonists

Concerns over toxicity have become more important as we have begun to use larger doses of β-agonists in the actue attack, and occasionally during chronic maintenance with usual doses in patients with a diseased heart. The greatest concerns of the FDA have been over myocardial toxicity. The original work on this was done with isoproterenol. The FDA scientists found that a characteristic patchy myocardial necrosis and fatal arrhythmias developed after large systemic doses in the fat rat, dog, and rabbit. These were potentiated by theophylline and corticosteroids, the very drugs used in the severe acute attack.[68,69] Use of β₂-agonists considerably reduced these toxic effects, but did not eliminate them. Hearts from animals that survived these lesions were resistant to further damage. The FDA remains concerned about this potential problem, and continues to evaluate tissue and reports of individual patients for evidence of such lesions. We are left then with balancing the undoubted benefit of vigorous therapy, perhaps with occult lesions, against the occasional and probably rare disaster.

Effect on Pulse Rate

Light and coworkers compared albuterol to isoproterenol by IPPB in stable asthmatics.[70] The ratio of the FEV₁ response to pulse elevation was far superior with albuterol (Fig. 9–6). Five milligrams caused minimal pulse elevation, but 10 and 20 mg produced an increase of 10 to 15 beats per minute. Allon and associates administered nebulized 10 and 20 mg doses of albuterol over only 10 minutes to patients receiving dialysis in an attempt to improve hyperkalemia.[71] The mean pulse rose 5 and 7 beats, respectively, the highest being 22 beats. When ten puffs were given in

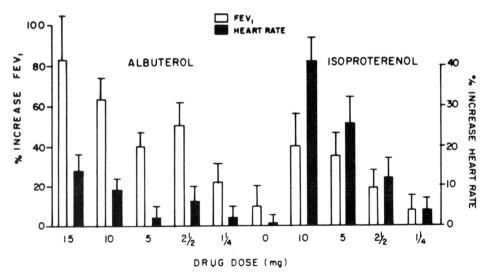

FIGURE   9-6   Comparison of isoproterenol and albuterol dose–response curves by IPPB nebulization in stable asthma. The response of FEV₁ and pulse are time-weighted, mean percentage increases over 6-hour applications. (Light RW, et al. Albuterol and isoproterenol in bronchial asthma. Arch Intern Med 1979;139:639, with permission)

rapid succession from an MDI (1000 μg), the mean pulse elevation was 14 beats, having already peaked by the first measurement at 5 minutes.[38] There was a near doubling of pulse pressure. Current regimens of, for example, 2.5 mg albuterol every 20 minutes times six in the most severe attacks, should produce no more side effects than the quoted studies, since the drug is spaced over 2 hours. Such doses are cumulatively absorbed, and the frequency should be cut back after this. Patients should also be receiving oxygen and be monitored. The ability of 5.0 mg albuterol to product transient asymptomatic arrhythmias in the elderly COPD patient is real[72] and reminds us that this therapy has potentially toxic effects in a patient with a damaged or irritable myocardium.

Effect on Serum Potassium Levels

Subcutaneous injection or nebulization of large doses of β_2-agonists causes a fall in serum K^+ levels by activation of the sodium–potassium (Na–K) ATPase and a rise in plasma insulin concentration, both of which move K^+ into the cells. When two consecutive doses of 0.25 mg terbutaline were injected at 30-minute intervals in asthmatics, the mean drop in serum K^+ value was 0.6 and then 1.1 mEq/L, accompanied by prolongation of the QT_c interval.[73] This could be arrhythmogenic in the irritable heart. Nebulization of 10 and 20 mg albuterol over 10 minutes to patients on dialysis caused a fall of 0.62 and 0.92 mEq/L,[71] respectively, but ten consecutive breaths from an MDI in normal persons dropped K^+ values only 0.2 mEq/L.[74] We have discussed the apparent tachyphylaxis in this response that develops in patients on large maintenance doses.[47,48]

Albuterol versus Fenoterol

The last year has seen serious concern over the use of fenoterol, with reports from New Zealand of an excess of asthma deaths in patients receiving this agonist compared with others, including theophylline. These were collected from the 1981 to 1983 period,[75] and again from 1977 to 1981, using an improved set of controls.[76] Fenoterol is a potent β_2-selective compound, but is reputed to have greater β_1-action than albuterol, as evidenced by similar inotropism to isoproterenol, as judged by shortening of the QS_2 interval.[77] The effect is potentiated with theophylline.[78] One study showed a surprising increase in heart rate with repeated MDI inhalations of fenoterol (two puffs every 10 minutes) that was not seen with albuterol.[79]

Theophylline

As a bronchodilator, theophylline (1,3-dimethylxanthine) offers the advantage of sustained bronchodilation over a 24-hour period and, for some, the ease of taking an oral dose only once or twice daily. It is a popular drug. Combination of theophylline with an inhaled β_2-agonist elevates both peak and trough values of the flow parameters, thereby blunting the discomfort between inhalations. The disadvantages of theophylline mainly center around its variable individual metabolism associated with a narrow therapeutic range.[80,81] Thus, use of theophylline must not be approached casually, but requires a certain minimum knowledge of its complexities for safe administration. Despite the best efforts of the pharmaceutical industry and the FDA to provide guidelines, an unacceptable incidence of toxicity still occurs.

TABLE 9–4. Actions of Theophylline in Humans

Useful Actions	*Adverse Actions*
Bronchodilation	CNS stimulation including seizures (+)
Respiratory stimulation (+) and attenuation of hypoxic respiration depression	Relaxation of lower esophageal sphincter
	Increased gastric volume, acidity (+)
	Vasodilation, increased pulse rate
Increased diaphragm contractility (+) and reduced diaphragm fatigue (+)	Increased myocardial irritability
	Nausea, vomiting
Decreased pulmonary artery pressure	Headache
Increased cardiac output (combination of inotropism, increased rate, decreased peripheral resistance)	Cerebral vasoconstriction
	Decreased red cell mass (+)
Anti-inflammatory effects (including inhibition late phase response, anti-PAF, antipermeability)	Imcreased catecholamines, cAMP, lipolysis, glucose, metabolic acidosis
Relief of syndrome X (angina with negative angiograms) (+)	
Excretion of salt and water (+)	

(+) Denotes adenosine receptor blocking action

Actions of Theophylline

The useful and adverse actions of theophylline are listed in Table 9–4.[81] Many actions are the same as those of a β-agonist, although not by the same mechanism. Because of theophylline's ability to block adenosine receptors (not shared by enprophylline which lacks a 1-methyl group), there are several neuromuscular actions, including the useful ones of stimulation of diaphragmatic function and central respiratory drive, and the potentially dangerous one of general central nervous system (CNS) stimulation and accelerated intracardiac conduction. A recently described effect is inhibition of interferon, resulting in decreased red cell mass.[82] Another interesting effect may be relief of syndrome X (see Table 9–4) by adenosine antagonism.[83] Table 9–4 has to be considered in the context of the serum levels.

Bronchodilation

The mechanisms of bronchodilation by theophylline is still unknown. Its originally proposed action as a cAMP phosphodiesterase inhibitor was later discredited because of discrepancies between relaxing concentrations and changes in whole-muscle cAMP or phosphodiesterase inhibition.[81] However, we now know that only certain isozymes of phosphodiesterase are associated with muscle relaxation, and good correlations can be found between the degree of theophylline inhibition of the low K_m phosphodiesterase and its relaxation of the muscle.[84] Other mechanisms are likely to be involved, which are as yet unknown.

Effect on Respiratory Muscles and Neural Drive

Although theophylline is invaluable in stimulating respiration in neonatal apnea, its stimulatory effect in the adult is thought to be largely due to its effect on the muscles of respiration. In 1981, Aubier and colleagues first published work showing the effect of IV aminophylline (theophylline ethylenediamine) on increasing maximum transdiaphragmatic pressure (Pdi_{max}) elicited by transdermal stimulation of the phrenic nerve.[85] Aminophylline markedly reduced fatigue during resistive loading, and rapidly restored diaphragmatic force if fatigue was first produced. Subsequent papers suggested that the effect was on the muscle and not on respiratory drive,[86] although such an effect had been shown in animals. In the muscle bath, theophylline stimulated calcium influx into the diaphragm through antagonism of adenosine, since verapamil blocked its action and enprophylline had no effect.[87] In severe COPD, long-term theophylline therapy maintains an increased Pdi_{max}, and increased ventilation.[88,89] Theophylline attenuates hypoxic depression of respiration in normal adults,[90] again probably through adenosine antagonism. These actions justify the use of aminophylline in impending respiratory failure, or the patient on a ventilator, but there are no controlled studies to test this.

Effect on the Heart and Circulation

As serum theophylline concentration is increased from 5 to 20 μg/mL, there is a progressively increasing inotropic effect, as indicated by the shortening of the QS_2 interval, representing electromechanical systole.[91] The pulse begins to increase at 15 μg/mL. Theophylline also causes a reduction in both venous and arterial tone, producing a decrease in pulmonary and peripheral vascular resistance. There is an increase in right and left ventricular ejection fraction (RVEF and LVEF), but a decrease in stroke work.[92] In COPD with and without cor pulmonale, the 20% to 30% reduction in mean pulmonary artery pressure persists even with long-term therapy.[93] The combination of 2.5 mg nebulized albuterol and IV aminophylline is synergistic in reduction of the QS_2 interval.[94] For the most part, when levels are in the midtherapeutic range, these should be useful actions in COPD, but with acute theophylline poisoning, serious hypotension and various arrhythmias may develop. Electrophysiologic studies in COPD patients showed acceleration of intracardiac conduction at 15 μg/mL, and this could be instrumental in provoking supraventricular arrhythmias at toxic levels.[95]

Relief of chest pain with theophylline is being observed in syndrome X (effort-induced chest pain or ischemic ECG changes despite normal angiography.) The hypothesis is that theophylline blocks an adenosine-induced hyperemia that is otherwise stealing blood from maximally dilated subendocardial vessels.[83]

Theophylline Kinetics

The half-life of theophylline varies widely in the normal host, and is influenced by disease states and drug interactions. Table 9–5 shows the mean half-lives and their range in several host states. About 90% of theophylline clearance occurs through the mixed function oxidase in the liver, using the cytochrome $P_{448-450}$ system, with the rest by the kidney. This is an inducible system. Table 9–5 lists major and minor drug interactions and their effect on theophylline clearance.[96]

THE ABCs OF THEOPHYLLINE KINETICS. There are a few basic pharmacokinetic principles that a clinician using theophylline, or any drug, should understand. They involve the concept of half-life, clearance, time to steady state, distribution volume,

TABLE 9–5. Effect of Host Factors and Interfering Drugs on Theophylline Clearance and Half-Life (Various Sources)

	$t_{1/2}$ (range) (h)		$t_{1/2}$ (range) (h)
Normal Clearance (Adult nonsmokers 40 mg/kg/hr)		**Clearance Reduced 25–50%**	
Premature infants	30.2 (14.4–57.7)	Cimetidine*	
Newborns	24.0	Ciprofloxacin*	
Children (1–9)	3.7 (2.0–10.0)	Erythromycin course*	
Adults	8.7 (6.1–12.8)	Sustained fever	
	7.7 (5.3–11.3)	Troleandomycin	
Elderly	10.2 (7.1–13.3)	Oral contraceptives	
		Propranolol	
		Allopurinol	
		Clearance reduced 75% or more	
Clearance increased 50–75%		Unstable pt. ICU	
Tobacco, marijuana		Heart failure	
Phenytoin			
Carbamazepine		Pulmonary edema	22.9 (3.1–82)
		Severe liver disease	25.6 (7.1–59)
Clearance increased 25%			
Phenobarbital			
Sulfapyrazone			
High-protein diet			

* Common offenders

and dose-dependent kinetics. They are not difficult in principle, but are terribly important in therapy.

The half-lilfe, $t_{1/2}$, is the time it takes for a compound to fall to half its value when drug is discontinued, or to rise to half its steady-state value when drug is begun. At 1, 2, 3, or 4 half-lives, levels fall to 50%, 25%, 12.5%, and 6.25%, or else rise to 50%, 75%, 87.5%, or 93.75%, respectively.

The half-life is inversely proportional to the clearance, C_1, and directly proportional to the distribution volume, V_D (Eq. 1). The latter varies from 0.3 to 0.7 of ideal body weight for theophylline, averaging 0.45.

$$t_{1/2} = \frac{0.693 \times V_D}{C1} \tag{1}$$

Although we commonly refer to a drug's half-life, the emphasis should be on the individual *clearance* for that drug, and not the half-life. It is the clearance that varies between individuals and that determines the ultimate serum concentration of a drug. Thus, at a constant dose, the mean concentration at steady state, $\bar{C}_{ss}$, is (Eq. 2):

$$\bar{C}_{ss} = \frac{\text{Dose/unit time}}{C1} \tag{2}$$

When loading a drug, however, the distribution volume is also very important and determines the initial serum concentrations until steady state is reached (Eq. 3). For example, a small individual V_D, will result in a higher initial concentration (C), or C_0 (Fig. 9–7).

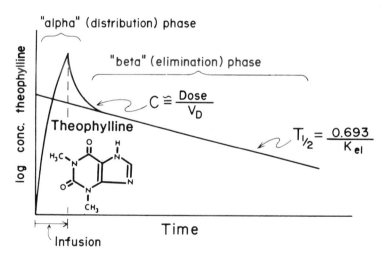

FIGURE 9-7 Behavior of serum theophylline levels following an IV loading dose only. *D*, dose; *C*, serum theophylline; V_D, apparent distribution volume in liters, $T_{1/2}$, half-life, K_{el}, elimination rate constant in min^{-1}. This is a one-compartment model that suffices for clinical purposes, illustrating the dependence of the initial *C* on the *D* and V_D. (Jenne JW. Pulmonary drugs. In: Bone RC ed. Critical care: A comprehensive approach. Park Ridge; American College of Chest Physicians, 1984, with permission)

$$C_0 = \frac{\text{Dose (loading)}}{V_{\text{D}}} \tag{3}$$

Ultimately, however, the $\bar{C}_{ss}$ will return to that level dictated by the clearance (see Eq. 2).

TIME TO STEADY STATE. In medicine we deal with drugs with an enormous range of half-lives. The phenothiazines take days or weeks to reach steady state. Assuming the same V_{D}, a patient in whom the theophylline half-life is 4 hours reaches 87.5% of steady state in 12 hours, whereas one in whom the half-life is 12 hours requires 36 hours, and the level is *three times as high*. This principle is most important when monitoring levels.

CLEARANCE IN THE ELDERLY PATIENT. In my opinion, the dosing recommendations of the package insert for theophylline are excessive for the nonsmoking geriatric adult. The 13 mg/kg per day maximum dose before measurement was based upon kinetic data in a younger population. More recent data, obtained specifically in the elderly, suggests that in persons older than 60 years the clearance falls off (Table 9–6). For example, Vestal and associates found a mean clearance of 30.9 mL/kg per hour (range 19.6 to 48.6) in ten men averaging 70 years in age.[97] This contrasted with a clearance of 45.6 mL/kg per hour in young adults. Assuming 100% drug absorption, we can calculate what the mean theophylline level would be at steady state in the elderly:

$$\bar{C}_{ss} = \frac{0.54 \text{ mg/kg per hr}}{30.9 \text{ mg/kg per hr}} = 17.5 \; \mu g \text{ mL}$$

This figure increases to 27.5 if one uses the lowest clearance in this group of ten patients, and 36.7 with added cimetidine using the lowest clearance value in that portion of the study.

Clearly, the 13 mg/kg dose specified in the package insert as the highest allowable dose before measuring serum levels is too high for the geriatric population. I recommend 10 mg/kg per day instead. In fact, because outliers in even the young adults may have low clearances, it is safer to use this figure for all adult nonsmokers as the first step in dosing (*initial full dose*), preliminary to the final dose adjustment.

DOSE-DEPENDENT KINETICS. In some patients, as one increases the dose of theophylline, levels rise disproportionately owing to near saturation of metabolism. The kinetics are no longer purely first-order, but tend toward zero-order. Dose increases, therefore, should be made with smaller increments than the hoped-for rise

TABLE 9–6. Some Recent Pharmacokinetic Studies in Younger and Older Adults

Ref.	Young Adults		Old Adults	
	Clearance ± SD (mL/kg/hr)	Mean Age	Clearance ± SD (mL/kg/hr)	Mean Age
97	45.5 ± 13.2	26.9	30.9 ± 9.6	70.1
98	57.7	<60.0	32.6	>60.0
99	40.7	25.5	34.7	72

in serum level. For example, if the level is 8 μg/mL on a 300-mg twice-daily regimen, and 15 μg/mL is desired, one should increase the dose to 400 mg twice daily, rather than double it.

DOSE–RESPONSE IN STABLE ASTHMA. Several dose–response studies have been published, the best being those of Mitenko and Ogilvie,[100] as reinterpreted by Rogers and coauthors,[101] and that of Racineux.[102] Both have shown that relaxation by theophylline reaches about 80% of its practical limit (at 20 μg/mL) in the 10 to 15 μg/mL range. Racineux showed that 15 μg/mL of theophylline was the equivalent of two puffs of albuterol when expressed as the percentage of possible improvement in FEV_1, and a little less as specific airway conductance (SG_{aw}). Thus, theophylline, often labeled a "weak bronchodilator" is not so weak (Fig. 9–8).

Theophylline Combined with Inhaled β-Agonists

Most asthmatics today are taking inhaled β_2-agonists as their first choice of bronchodilator. However, more severe asthma, or periodic worsening of asthma, raises the possibility of combined therapy with theophylline. Their worsening of asthma results in a continuing sense of chest discomfort, new exertional limitation, and more frequent use of their inhaler. Addition of theophylline at this time will usually restore their sense of comfort and ease of breathing.

Figure 9–9 shows the effect of adding theophylline, at mean levels of 15.9 μg/mL, to a metaproterenol MDI in 21 asthmatics, receiving beclomethasone diprionate (BDP) by MDI, with a history of recurring severe asthma attacks.[103] They were studied before and after three puffs of metaproterenol followed by two puffs of BDP, given three times during the day. Theophylline significantly raised the peak expiratory flow rate (PEFR) at all three trough periods, and the rise post-MDI was significant after the 7:00 AM treatment. The authors emphasize that the effect of theophylline on PEFR was slight in 18 of 21 patients, but in 3 patients, the effect was

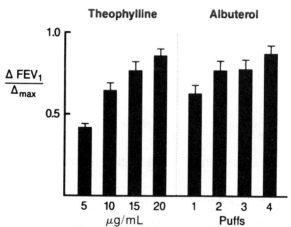

FIGURE   9-8   Dose–response to theophylline and albuterol in stable asthma. Aminophylline was given IV to approximate 5, 10, 15, and 20 μg/mL, and albuterol given as 1, 2, 3, and 4 puffs. The response is calculated in terms of the maximum change in FEV_1 achieved in the study by either means. (Adapted from Racineux JL, et al. Comparison of bronchodilator effects of salbutamol and theophylline. Bull Eur Physiopathol Respir 1981;17:799, with permission)

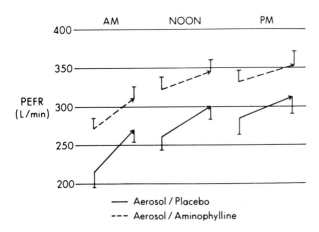

FIGURE 9-9 Mean PEFR before and after three total puffs of metaproterenol by MDI with patients receiving aminophylline or placebo in stable asthma. Theophylline levels average 15.9 $\mu g/mL$. (Appel DW. Effect of aminophylline when added to metaproterenol sulfate and beclomethasone diproprionate aerosol. J Allergy Clin Immunol 1984;73:291, with permission)

marked. Moreover, although theophylline produced some adverse effects, many patients were delighted to be "free of asthma" and thus tolerated the adverse effects.

In this study, the individual variability of response to both the β-agonist and theophylline is emphasized. This carries over into routine patient care. Theophylline is a valuable modality in some patients. Obviously, with increasing asthma severity, one nowadays also increases the dose of inhaled corticosteroid, but the effect of this may not be immediately apparent.

Theophylline in Chronic Obstructive Pulmonary Disease

Use of theophylline is controversial in COPD, in part based on its greater potential for toxicity.[104] Early studies felt that theophylline benefited only a few patients, and some advocated a blinded trial with placebo to make this decision for each patient. Theophylline alone has improved dyspnea[105] and ventilation,[106] and decreased the work of breathing while walking.[107]

Several excellent, recent studies are available. At a mean level of 14.8 $\mu g/mL$, theophylline was compared with placebo in 60 patients preselected by a response of less than 15% (FEV_1) to albuterol (salbutamol) by MDI.[89] After 2 months, the theophylline group showed a mean increase of 13% in FEV_1, 10% in FVC, and an increase in tidal volume from 677 to 766 mL, with no increase in respiratory rate. The mean $PaCO_2$ fell from 48 to 44 mm Hg (these were severe cases) and the mean PaO_2 rose from 62 to 66 mm Hg. The maximum pleural pressure possible (Ppl_{max}) increased with no change in resting swings of Ppl. A reduction in dyspnea occurred as measured by the visual analog scale, from 77 to 58 mm ($p < 0.001$). Table 9–7 gives some figures, when the groups were divided according to $PaCO_2$.

Theophylline produced an increase in tidal volume, but did not increase the resting swings in Ppl. The Ppl_{max} increased by 22%, correlating with the decrease in dyspnea, whereas the improvement in FEV_1 did not. The authors were inclined to believe that the principal effect of theophylline is an increase in diaphragmatic strength. The improved diaphragmatic reserve can be assumed to be beneficial during severe exertion, or impending respiratory failure. This study shows relatively favorable changes despite the fixed obstruction in COPD.

TABLE 9–7. Effect of Maintenance Theophylline on
Ventilation in COPD

	Ppl/Ppl_{max}	Min Vol (L/min)	PaO$_2$ (mm Hg)	PaCO$_2$ (mm Hg)
Normocapnic (n = 24)				
Placebo	0.29	11.6	68	43
Theophylline	0.22	13.6	72	39
Hypercapnic (n = 36)				
Placebo	0.40	10.4	55	54
Theophylline	0.28	12.5	60	49

(Data from Murciano D, et al. A randomized controlled trial of
theophylline in patients with severe chronic obstructive pulmonary
disease. N Engl J Med 1989; 320:1521)

Theophylline–Albuterol Airway Responses in Chronic Obstructive Pulmonary Disease

Richer administered 600 mg theophylline in a rapid-release form to asthmatics
and bronchitics, assessing the effect on PEFR and the serum levels. Flows in the
asthmatics peaked more or less in synchrony with the peak serum levels (19μg/mL),
whereas flows in the bronchitics reached a plateau at about 14 μg/mL theophylline.[108] Barclay and associates gave infusions of theophylline in 5 μg/mL increments
up to the point at which no further increase in FVC occurred, or a maximum of
25 μg/mL.[109] The plateaus in their 12 patients occurred at 9, 9, 12, 12, 14, 17, 17, 17,
20, 23, 23, and 24 μg/mL, but the addition of 400 μg albuterol by MDI produced a
further rise (Fig. 9–10). In a later study, 10 of these subjects were given increasing
albuterol (formerly called salbutamol) doses to a plateau, occurring in 200 μg (2
patients), 1400 μg (4 patients), and 3000 μg (4 patients). Theophylline produced a
further response in only 4 patients (see Fig. 9–10).[110]

Filuk and coworkers gave 800 μg albuterol to 16 bronchitics before and after IV
theophylline administration at a mean level of 24.5 μg/mL.[111] In 8 albuterol responders (the other 8 responded poorly), theophylline still added another 0.13 L
of FEV$_1$ to the 0.16 L with albuterol. When the order was reversed, albuterol added
0.22 L FEV$_1$ after a 0.11-L improvement with theophylline.

Both these studies used very large doses in combination to test the limits of
bronchodilation in a disease supposed to be relatively "irreversible." Large doses of
either an inhaled β_2-agonist or theophylline alone do not exhaust the reversibility in
COPD, and more appears to be achieved with lower doses of the two together.

Combination of Inhaled β-Agonists and Theophylline in Chronic Obstructive Pulmonary Disease

Two recent studies have looked at the separate and combined effects of maintenance theophylline and β-agonists in COPD. Taylor and associates randomized
chronic bronchitics between two puffs of albuterol, theophylline 200 mg four times
daily, their combination, and placebo, making four study groups in all.[112] Spirometry

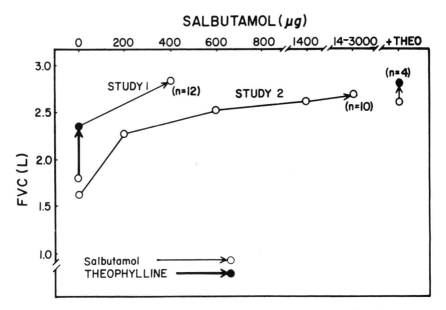

FIGURE 9-10 Mean dose–response curves of FVC response of chronic bronchitics to inhaled albuterol (salbutamol) and theophylline, each being pushed to its limit to illustrate the degree of ultimate reversibility. Theophylline was studied out to its plateau level in 5 μg/mL increments; 6 patients plateaued to albuterol by 1400 μg total, and 4 required 3000 μg. (Combines data from Barclay J, et al. and is taken from Jenne JW. Theophylline as a bronchodilator in COPD and its combination with inhaled beta adrenergic drugs. Chest 1987; 92:7S, with permission)

was conducted 1.5 to 3.0 hours after the MDI. Spirometry showed the greatest improvement in the combined group (Table 9–8), and this group was significantly less likely to relapse (require additional medication).

Guyatt and coworkers studied 19 patients with COPD severe enough to have dyspnea with common tasks, and whose FEV_1 failed to improve more than 25% with an MDI.[113] They compared two puffs of albuterol, theophylline producing mean levels of 12.3 μg/mL, their combination, and placebo. The AM and PM peak flows were done at home, before and after albuterol administration. Functional ability was

TABLE 9–8.   Effect of Theophylline, Albuterol by MDI, and Their Combination in COPD

	Plac	*Theo*	*Alb*	*Theo, Alb*
Mean PEFR	193	205	202	217
Post-FVC	2.36	2.59	2.75	2.88
CRQ-"emotional"	48.3	51.5	54.4	56

(Data from Guyatt GH, et al. Bronchodilators in chronic airflow limitation: effects on airway function, exercise capacity and quality of life. Am Rev Respir Dis 1987; 135:1069)
Plac, placebo; Theo, theophylline; Alb, albuterol.

assessed with a 6-minute walk, a visual analog scale, and the chronic respiratory disease questionnaire (CRQ), which assess dyspnea on five tasks, fatigue, and energy levels. With the exception of the 6-minute walk, the drugs were additive on all scales. Table 9–8 lists some of the values.

Theophylline Toxicity

The extensive literature on toxicity has been reviewed.[114] The range of toxic symptoms is well defined, but large prospective surveys have not been published that provide the true incidence of elevated levels or toxicity. If one starts with emergency room patients, some will be there because of toxicity and the analysis is not random. When 5557 levels were measured in patients presenting to the University of Virginia and VA Medical Center emergency departments, 53% were under 10 μg/mL, 10% were over 20 μg/mL, and 2.8% or 116 of the latter, were over 30 μg/mL. Of these, 12% were due to acute overdose.[115]

The authors developed four grades of toxicity (Table 9–9, Fig. 9–11). Of these, 50% fell in the mild or grade I category, 38% the moderate or grade 2, and 7% severe or life-threatening categories (grades 3 and 4). Serum theophylline concentrations (STC) correlated with severity in the acute, but not the chronic overdoses. Only in the acute cases could one make an accurate prediction of the need for charcoal hemoperfusion from the STC, namely, a level in the 80–100 μg/mL range. Of these, three died of fulminant toxicity with status epilepticus, shock, and ventricular fibrillation or flutter, all with levels over 100 μg/mL. Death occurred in four chronic cases, but three of these had serious underlying disease that could have been responsible without the addition of theophylline. Seven had seizures and one died. Five of these were chronically overmedicated, and all had levels lower than 42 μg/mL. The authors actually conclude that "death directly attributable to toxicity is very uncommon after chronic overmedication."

A much more benign experience has been presented from a large Seattle health maintenance organization which routinely monitors outpatient levels.[116] In a follow-up of 35,909 outpatients who filled 220,000 prescriptions over 9 years, there were 30 hospitalizations for toxicity or 7.8 : 10,000 person-years at risk and no deaths. The authors conclude that serious xanthine toxicity is a relatively rare event.

The distinction between the acute and chronic toxicity presentation was first made by Olson and associates.[117] Patients with acute toxicity present with a picture of hypotension, hypokalemia, and low serum bicarbonate levels. Seizures are rare below 100 μg/mL. In general, patients with chronic toxicity do not have this picture, but seizures or serious arrhythmias usually necessitate levels between 40 and 70 μg/mL (in one case in the Olson series, at only 28 μg/mL). They advised withholding charcoal hemoperfusion in the acute cases unless levels threaten to exceed 100 μg/mL and, rather, apply the conservation measures of oral charcoal, gastric lavage, and saline cathartics. In the chronic case, however, hemoperfusion is advised for levels as low as 40 μg/mL if signs of severe toxicity appear imminent. They urged that every effort be made to determine whether the intake was acute or chronic. Levels are monitored at least every 4 hours to help establish this.

Aitken and Martin also emphasize the inability to predict toxicity from the height of a persistently elevated level.[118] They analyzed 54 consecutive levels over 39.0 μg/mL at the University of Washington Hospitals and the Seattle VA Medical

TABLE 9–9. Manifestations of Toxicity and Grades of Severity*

Grade 1

Vomiting
Abdominal pain
Diarrhea
Nervousness
Tremor
Tachycardia ($>$120 beats per min)
Mild hypokalemia ($>$2.5, $<$3.5 mEq/L)

Grade 2

Hematemesis
Lethargy or disorientation
Supraventricular tachyarrhythmia†
Frequent VPBs
Hypotension (mean blood pressure $<$ 60 mm Hg, improves
  with standard therapy)
Severe hypokalemia ($<$2.5 mEq/L)
Acid–base disturbance (arterial pH $<$ 7.20 or $>$7.60)
Rhabdomyolysis

Grade 3

Seizure, nonrepetitive
Sustained ventricular tachycardia
Shock (mean blood pressure $<$ 60 mm Hg that is refractory to
  standard therapy)

Grade 4

Status epilepticus
Ventricular fibrillation
Cardiac arrest

---

* The grades of toxicity were defined as follows: grade 1, self-limited toxicity that typically has no major impact; grade 2, toxicity that typically requires close observation, electrocardiographic monitoring, or specific medical intervention; grade 3, toxicity that typically requires immediate intervention or often progresses to grade 4 toxicity; and grade 4, toxicity that is often fatal.
† Includes atrial fibrillation or flutter, multifocal atrial tachycardia, and paroxysmal supraventricular tachycardia.
(Sessler CN. Theophylline toxicity: clinical features of 116 consecutive cases. Am J Med 1990; 88:567, with permission)

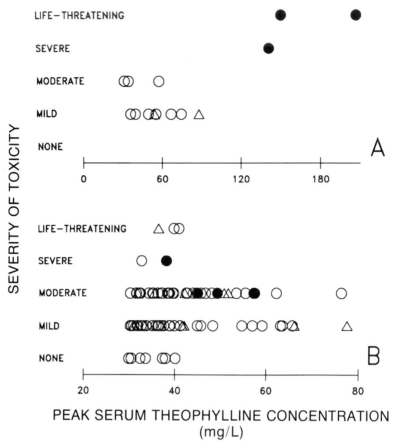

FIGURE   9-11   Correlation of peak serum theophylline concentrations (STC) and severity of toxicity for 14 acute overdose (A) and 102 chronic overmedication (B) cases. Severity of toxicity is displayed as none, mild, moderate, severe, and life-threatening (see text for explanation). Individual cases are depicted as *open circles* (adults) or *triangles* (children). *Solid symbols* denote fatal cases. There was a significant correlation ($X^2 = 7.09$, $p < 0.01$) between STC and the severity of toxicity (maximum toxicity grade) for overdose cases (A) but not for overmedication (B). Multiply by 5.55 to convert mg/L to μmol/L (Sessler CN. Theophylline toxicity; clinical features of 116 consecutive cases. Am J Med 1990; 88:567, with permission)

Center. This series is particularly depressing in the incidence and outcome of seizures, occurring at levels of 43, 43, 45, 45, 52, and 74 μg/mL. Two-thirds of these were receiving intravenous theophylline in the hospital.

In a review of 100 cases of seizures in the literature, Kelly found that the overall mortality was 29%, and mortality or significant neurologic residual 34%.[114] This is lower than the 50% figure usually quoted, perhaps because of the inclusion of children who appear to have a better outcome than adults.

Seizures have been seen with levels in the 20s and 30s. An important predisposing factor is a low serum albumin concentration. The unbound theophylline fraction is also increased with acidosis, hypoxema, and hypocarbia. The existence of previous neurologic damage predisposes to transient seizures at lower levels. Covelli and colleagues observed 17 COPD patients who experienced generalized, witnessed seizures with levels averaging only 26 μg/mL.[119] These had no residual damage; 73% had preexisting neurologic disease.

A much more subtle form of CNS toxicity is the possibility of learning and behavioral problems in children, and an uneasy sense of stimulation, analogous to a "coffee jag" in susceptible patients. Some patients may not feel comfortable receiving the drug. The behavioral issue is very controversial, but has not been adjudged to warrant concern by the FDA on the basis of available data.[96,120] Nevertheless, parents should keep such a possibility in mind if teachers report any problems.

MANAGEMENT OF THEOPHYLLINE TOXICITY. The following scheme for managing chronic overmedication is reasonable. Minor manifestations (nausea, vomiting, headache), with levels under 30 μg/mL can be observed and levels monitored. Levels in the 30s should be under close observation, but this can be done in the clinic. If levels are rising, or associated with minor CNS symptoms (agitation, confusion, disorganization, marked tremors), hospitalization is warranted along with close monitoring and a full press of conservative management. Oral charcoal is given, 20 to 40 g in a slurry every 2 to 4 hours, along with monitoring of levels, vital signs and ECG. Lidocaine suppression is used as indicated for myocardial irritability. I and others[80] advise raising the seizure threshold with prophylactic IV phenobarbital (10 mg/kg over 30 minutes) if the patient shows signs of excessive CNS stimulation, since this induces only drowsiness or light sleep, but could prevent a far worse outcome.

Seizures are treated with diazepam followed by IV phenobarbital (rather than phenytoin), intubation, and oxygenation. Animal studies show a relative ineffectiveness of phenytoin compared with the barbituate in preventing theophylline-induced seizures. Theophylline levels must be lowered rapidly with charcoal hemoperfusion.[121] Kelly has emphasized that those seizures with residuals are cases in whom rapid lowering of theophylline was delayed several hours.[114] Other manifestations of severe toxicity (sustained ventricular tachycardia, shock refractory to therapy, coma) also require hemoperfusion.

APPROACH TO DOSING THAT MINIMIZES TOXICITY. Before beginning a patient on an oral theophylline regimen, the physician should ask himself the following: (1) Is the patient a smoker or nonsmoker? (2) Is he or she elderly (over 60), thin or fat? (3) Does he or she have liver disease, heart failure from time to time, or a history of cardiac arrhythmias? (4) Is he or she receiving interfering drugs (cimetidine, ciprofloxacin or other quinolone, erythromycin, oral contraceptives, propranolol, allopurinol, phenytoin, carbamazepine, or phenobarbital)? The last three increase theophylline elimination.

The patient is instructed about possible side effects. Minor effects, such as gastrointestinal distress are transient, and may be eliminated during an "adaptation" phase at a lower dose. However, I generally start out with a conservative dose, based upon lean body weight, lower in the nonsmoker and elderly (Table 9–10).

Dosing is a two-step process: (1) an initial, conservative dose followed by a serum theophylline level; (2) dose-adjustment to bring levels into the 10–15 μg/mL range. Ideally, levels are measured after 48 hours on no-missed doses, but, if this is inconve-

TABLE 9–10. Theophylline Dosing Recommendations for Adults

IV aminophylline
Off theophylline

Loading	6 mg/kg over 20 min to produce avg level 10 μg/mL (range 7–17)
Maintenance (while critically ill)	
• Nonsmokers, elderly	0.5 mg/kg/hr
• Current smokers	0.8 mg/kg/hr
• Unstable patient	0.2 mg/kg/hr
On theophylline (or not sure)	Draw level, begin maintenance, adjust as needed (1.25 mg/kg = 2.0 μg/mL theophylline)
Monitor	30–60 min after load, adjust up as needed; 18–24 h to detect impending toxic levels

Oral theophylline

Adaptation phase (optional)[109]	1/2 full dose, then full dose
Initial full dose, then adjust	
• Nonsmoker, elderly*	10 mg/kg/hr (range 500–800 mg for 50–80 kg IBW)
• Smoker	13 mg/kg/hr (range 700–1000 mg for 50–80 kg IBW)
Monitor	After 48 h or next appointment, adjust to 10–15 μg/mL using small increments

* In a recent study, 6% of patients (average age 42) on 600 mg/day had peak levels over 20 μg/mL. Therefore, this should probably be the maximum initial full dose.

nient, levels may be done somewhat later. I feel secure in waiting, since I have counseled the patient about side effects, and use a conservative dose. A theophylline level that has been used in dose-adjustment also protects the physician against medicolegal assertions. In a public institution, with multiple doctors prescribing, I prefer a twice-daily preparation, which provides relatively constant levels. However, in a patient with good control, but continued nocturnal bronchospasm, one might switch to a once-daily preparation taken at the evening meal.[122]

Anticholinergics

The introduction of quaternary anticholinergic compounds for COPD patients is a fascinating success story. These compounds block the M_3 receptor on the smooth-muscle membrane, and also the M_1 facilitatory receptor at the parasympathetic ganglion.[123] The M_1 receptor plays a role in reflex bronchoconstriction, such as that induced by SO_2 inhalation, and can be blocked by pirenzepine as well as ipratropium bromide. Some of the current compounds are shown in Figure 9–12 as extensively reviewed.[124] The charged nitrogen of these derivatives prevents systemic absorption and prolongs action. Only atropine sulfate is available for liquid nebulization in the US; ipratropium bromide is available for inhalation from a metered-dose inhaler.

The rank order of efficacy of β-agonists and antimuscarinic compounds differs in asthma and chronic bronchitis, or COPD. This must relate to differences in contrac-

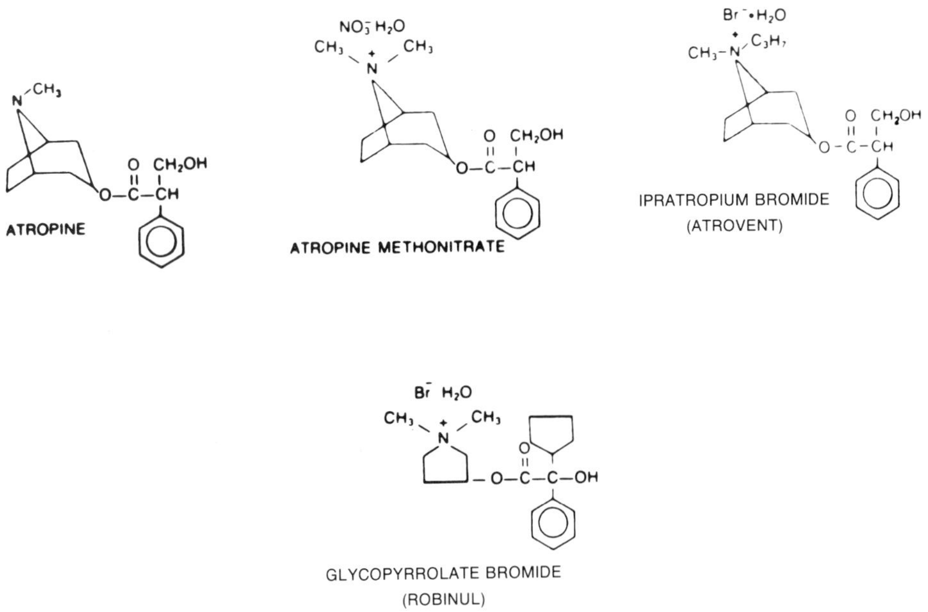

FIGURE   9-12   Structural formulas of atropine and some of the quaternary ammonium cogeners. Note the positive charge on the nitrogen in the quaternary compounds.

tile stimuli in the two diseases.[125] As one increases the dose, β-agonists have a more pronounced effect in the asthmatic over the entire dose range, whereas, in COPD, antimuscarinic compounds are equipotent to begin with, but soon exceed the β-agonist with a higher slope and plateau of effect.[126] However, older asthmatics may respond as well, or even better, to ipratropium.[127] It is questionable whether adding an antimuscarinic adds anything to aggressive β-agonist therapy in treating acute asthma,[128] although the response might be more prolonged.

In COPD, two puffs (40 μg) of ipratropium bromide is a suboptimal dose when measured in terms of the area under the response curves,[129] and yet it is superior overall to two puffs of albuterol.[130] Similar to the β-agonists, these drugs are often underdosed as routinely specified, and it is up to the clinician to tailor them to the needs of the patient. We generally begin the COPD patient on two puffs four times daily of both ipratropium and a β-agonist. The β-agonist gives a more immediate response than the antimuscarinic. Taken together there is an additive and a more sustained effect than large doses of either class alone, as shown with oxitropium bromide (Fig. 9–13).[131,132]

In acute exacerbations of COPD, or in maintenance of some very severe COPD patients, we may resort to nebulized solutions. One may use atropine sulfate, beginning with a dose of 0.0125 mg/kg every 4 to 6 hours and increasing up to as high as 0.075 mg/kg in some patients, as tolerated. Although not approved for this purpose, we have had good experience with glycopyrrolate methylbromide (Robinul), 1.0 mg every 6 hours, which is nearly free of side effects and provides surprisingly prolonged bronchodilation,[133] both in asthma and COPD. When ipratropium becomes avail-

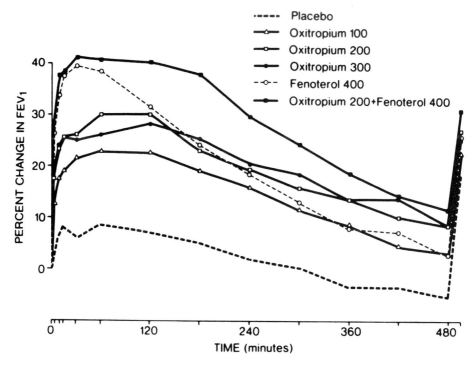

FIGURE 9-13 Dose–response curves (FEV_1) to oxitropium bromide alone and combined with fenoterol by MDI. The subjects were elderly patients with partially reversible obstruction and, thus, may have included some asthmatics. Note that the addition of 200 μg oxitropium adds significantly to what is a very potent bronchodilator in asthmatics. (Frith PA, et al. Oxitropium bromide. Dose–response and time-response study of a new anticholinergic bronchodilator drug. Chest 1986;89:249, with permission)

able in the United States for liquid nebulization, the optimal dose will be at least 0.4 mg.[134]

ANTI-INFLAMMATORY AGENTS

Corticosteroids

Asthmatic inflammation is uniquely sensitive to corticosteroid suppression. However corticosteroids work, they accomplish the following: prevention of the late phase after antigen challenge, increase in FEV_1 and reduction of variability of peak flow rate, and decrease in bronchial hyperreactivity. A correlation has been shown between the FEV_1 response in the individual case given an oral corticosteroid, and the ability of dexamethasone in vitro to suppress certain immunologic events of that patient's cells, such as the generation of monocyte colony-stimulating factor.[135] Asthmatics resistant to steroid improvement of FEV_1 show no suppression. Thus, a major mechanism of steroids is through immunologic means.

Corticosteroids (CS) cause cells to either turn on or turn off synthesis of specific proteins. The known in vivo actions of CS include inhibition of phospholipase A_2

through synthesis of lipocortin; inhibition of production of immune cytokines such as interleukin IL-1, IL-2, IL-3, tumor necrosis factor (TNF)-L, IL-5, granulocyte–macrophage colony-stimulating factor (GMCSF), and receptor activation (IL-2 R) with consequent suppression of the inflammatory response to macrophage stimulation;[136] inhibition of mediator release from alveolar macrophages and eosinophils; inhibition of microvascular permeability with edema suppression; inhibition of mucous secretion, perhaps through suppression of secretagogues.

Changing Roles of Anti-Inflammatory Drugs in Asthma

Traditionally, oral corticosteroids have been reserved for those patients who could not maintain a tolerable existence with the use of bronchodilators alone. Inhaled corticosteroids (ICS) were first restricted to these same patients. This is now changing. Use of ICS or cromolyn is begun in asthma when it becomes clear that the patient needs an inhaled bronchodilator on a routine basis (*i.e.*, several times a day). Not only do these anti-inflammatory agents provide better control of asthma, but they may prevent irreversible damage from developing in the airways over time.

Discovery of Topical Corticosteroids

Probably the single major advance in therapy changing the outlook of the asthmatic has been the discovery that, by adding certain ester groups to the parent corticosteroid molecule, topical activity could be enhanced several hundred-fold, yet with minimal systemic affect (Fig. 9–14). Once absorbed, these compounds are rapidly inactivated. The relative effectiveness of the major compounds, assayed according to their ability to cause vasoconstriction of the abraded skin, is fairly closely reflected in the dose delivered per puff.

With these different potencies, the effective doses expelled from the different products become more comparable. A low dose of beclomethasone dipropionate (BDP), 400 μg/24 hours in eight puffs, is fairly comparable to 800 μg triamcinolone acetonide (TAA) in eight puffs, or 400 μg budesonide (BUD), subject to some variation in efficiency of delivery device. High doses are two or three times these amounts, and can be facilitated by high-potency preparations, as available outside the United States for BDP and BUD. Flunisolide (FLU) is convenient for high dosing.

Spacers are available for these preparations. One can use the valved Aerochamber, and TAA comes with a built-in spacer. Spacers minimize deposition of the drug in the mouth and throat and, along with gargling, reduce the incidence of thrush. The TAA formulation has been shown to avoid the transient bronchospasm and cough sometime seen following BDP, probably owing to the difference in stabilizing ingredients.[137] Hoarseness may also occur secondary to an apparent steroid-induced vocal cord myopathy, with a bowing of vocal cords on phonation.[138] This occurs in a small, but significant, portion of patients and responds to dose reduction.

Inhaled Versus Systemic Corticosteroids

Comparison of ICS in terms of oral CS equivalents is very complex, involving both airway and systemic effects.[139] In terms of flow, however, a recent comparison by Namsirkul and coauthors between 3-week courses of BUD and oral prednisolone is straightforward.[140] In moderate asthmatics, receiving only theophylline and in-

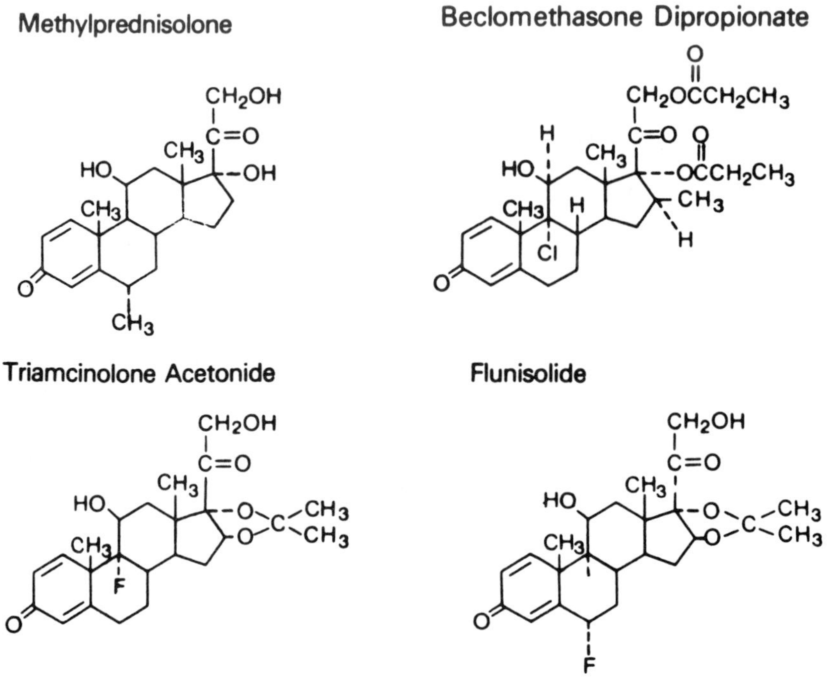

Methylprednisolone

Beclomethasone Dipropionate

Triamcinolone Acetonide

Flunisolide

FIGURE 9-14   Structures of methylprednisolone and three topical corticosteroids used in the United States.

haled β_2-agonists, the improvement in PEFR by 400 μg BUD (in two doses), approximated that by 5 mg prednisolone, and 800 μg BUD that by 10 mg (Fig 9–15). This probably applies to BDP as well.

There are differences in the actions of ICS and oral CS on the airways. For a given effect on flow, topical treatment appears more effective than systemic treatment in reducing bronchial hyperreactivity.[141] This is important from an overall symptomatic viewpoint. Also, a recent study showed the ability of high-dose ICS to further improve that produced by high-dose oral CS.[142] This suggests that systemic steroid is first "blasting out" the small airways so that ICS can reach them. Certainly, this is also true in the acute exacerbation.

Effect on PC$_{20}$

Even though ICS reduces bronchial hyperreactivity, it does not normalize it. What is needed are more long-term studies. Published series have dealt with the effects of only 3 to 8 weeks of ICS in large doses as judged by PC$_{20}$ and diurnal variation in flow. Although a threefold improvement in PC$_{20}$ occurs overall in most studies, many patients, including the most severe, may show no improvement, and PC$_{20}$ may remain well under 1.0.[141] Since the improvement in PC$_{20}$ is a function of both duration and concentration of ICS,[143] perhaps better results can be achieved over a longer period. One would not expect long-standing changes to disappear quickly, nor a healing process to occur adequately in weeks.

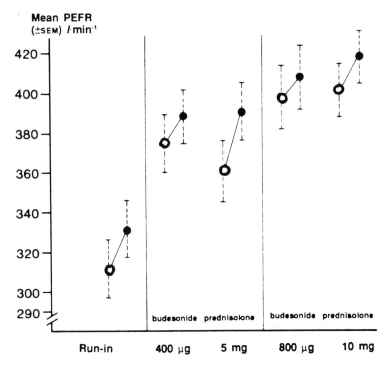

FIGURE   9-15   Comparison of inhaled budesonide (*open circles*) (roughly comparable with beclomethasone dipropionate) and prednisolone (*closed circles*) effects on PEFR in chronic asthma. (Namsirkal D, *et al.* Comparison of inhaled budesonide with oral prednisolone at two dose levels commonly used for the treatment of moderate asthma. Eur Respir J 1989; 2:317, with permission)

Conversion from Oral to Inhaled Corticosteroids

The principal advantage of ICS is the reduction in systemic side effects while preserving or even increasing flow. The effect on the hypothalamic–pituitary (HPA) axis is particularly important. In terms of the morning cortisol level, even 5 mg prednisolone daily causes some reduction, and the reduction is almost complete at 20 mg/day. But suppression by even 1000 μg/24 hour BDP is very slight, and becomes significant at 1600 μg/day. Budesonide has even less effect on the HPA axis.

The withdrawal phase from oral CS during the first 6 months of ICS requires particularly close follow-up. These patients may have acute relapses, and most will require burst oral therapy during exacerbations. Toogood emphasizes that about two-thirds of patients withdrawn from oral CS will ultimately be required to resume *some* regular oral CS.[144]

Some Generalizations for Inhaled Corticosteroids in Asthma

The following points have been made by various authorities, especially Toogood,[144] who has extensive investigational experience:

- Four-times-daily dosing of ICS is superior to twice-daily dosing of the same total dose during periods of asthma instability, but not during stable asthma.
- Many patients who show no response to low doses of ICS do so at a higher dose.
- A higher dose of ICS is required to normalize pulmonary function tests than is required to minimize symptoms.
- More concentrated ICS preparations will increase the success rate.
- Inhaled corticosteroids improve bronchial hyperreactivity more readily than oral CS.
- Asthmatics whose FEV_1 is below 50% of predicted will need some oral corticosteroid, regardless of the dose of ICS.
- Oral CS is essential to clear out the airways during asthma exacerbations; ICS will not reach these airways.
- Both ICS and oral CS will reduce nocturnal bronchospasm. Added bronchodilator will reduce it further.
- Compliance is of overriding importance in the success of ICS.
- The importance of HPA dysfunction from systemic CS is overplayed compared with the importance of reducing the side effects resulting from them. Resistance to stress after withdrawal of oral corticosteroid is generally adequate, although supplemental oral steroid is advised. It is far better to risk this, than the side effects if they are continued.

Side Effects of Oral Corticosteroids

The side effects of oral CS can be divided into effects from brief and those from long-term use, slightly modified from Cochrane.[145] Side effects are not generally a problem in the short-term high-intensity use of corticosteroids in the severe attack, but awareness of their possible occurrence is necessary (Table 9–11). Of more concern are the long-term side effects of corticosteroids (Table 9–12).

Consequently, the extended use of oral corticosteroids should be based on a proved need in that patient, despite the use of inhaled steroids. One should strive to give oral steroids in an alternate-day manner. Short-acting preparations given in the morning on alternate days minimize suppression of the HPA axis, a side effect that is inevitable with daily steroids. Once suppressed, the HPA axis is unable to respond to sudden stressful situations such as surgery, trauma, infection, or even an acute attack

TABLE 9–11. Possible Complications of Acute Use of Corticosteroids

Hypokalemia and alkalosis	Cerebral edema (children)
Fluid and sodium retention	Proximal myopathy
Hyperosmolar–nonketotic coma	Glaucoma
Hypertension	Pancreatitis
Clinical diabetes mellitus	Peptic ulcer and hemorrhage (not proved)
Acute severe psychosis	

TABLE   9–12.   Complications of Long-Term Corticosteroid Use

Common	Uncommon
Suppression of HPA axis	Diabetes mellitus
Change in body shape (centripetal obesity)	Hypertension
Muscle atrophy (negative N_2 balance)	Aseptic necrosis of head of the femur
Skin, capillary fragility (negative N_2 balance)	Impaired wound healing
Osteoporosis–compression fractures of vertebrae, cough fractures of ribs (negative N_2 balance, negative Ca^{++} balance)	Proximal myopathy
	Variations in mood, psychosis
	Impaired response to infections
	Secondary amenorrhea
Growth retardation in young	Cerebral atrophy
Posterior subcapsular contracts	Reactivation of tuberculosis

of asthma, and may continue to remain suppressed up to 12 months after steroids have been stopped. A second advantage of alternate-day therapy is a reduction in other side effects, although children may continue to show growth suppression, and bone losses still occur.

Long-term oral steroid use necessitates periodic check of the blood sugar level, blood pressure, urine calcium level, and eyes. Osteoporosis will be minimized by dietary supplementation of at least 1500 mg calcium every 24 hours, good nutritional status, and as much exercise as possible. Regimens containing vitamin D, etidronate disodium, chlorothiazides, and fluoride are being studied. Results to date with various approaches have been summarized, along with a comprehensive approach employing replacement of gonadal hormones when indicated, and serial measurement of bone density.[146]

Cromolyn Sodium

The potential value of cromolyn for the responsive patient has only gradually become appreciated in the United States. Pediatricians and allergists are aware of its value, particularly in the young atopic asthmatic, but a trial in the older adult asthmatic with an atopic background is also warranted.

Actions of Cromolyn

Cromolyn blocks both the early- and late-phase response after antigen and also blocks exercise-induced bronchospasm. It is protective against toluene diisocyanate (TDI), western red cedar, and metabisulfate. Although the precise mechanisms for cromolyn's action are unknown, a few pertinent observations should be mentioned from among the 6000 papers dealing with this agent as reviewed by Murphy.[147]

Cromolyn is more effective in inhibiting IgE-dependent histamine release from mast cells obtained by brochoalveolar lavage (BAL) than by enzymatic dispersion of human lung, and this reflects differences in the mast cell population of these two sites.[148] It inhibits activation of human neutrophils, eosinophils, and monocytes in vitro.[149] It blocks the appearance of neutrophil chemotactic factor (NCF-A) into serum following antigen challenge,[150] and recruitment of eosinophils into BAL fluid.[151]

Increasing attention is being paid to cromolyn's ability to block neuronal reflexes in the lung. It blocks reflex bronchoconstriction in the dog after capsaicin administration[152] and also response to SO_2 inhalation.[153] Suppression of nervous reflexes may be a much more important aspect of cromolyn's action than realized, since there seems to be a disparity between the considerable symptomatic relief (cough, discomfort) and the relatively small changes in PC_{20} to histamine or methacholine.

Cromolyn's ability to decrease airway reactivity is principally demonstrated during the allergy season. Yet, a decrease in reactivity has also been demonstrated in nonatopic asthmatics of a magnitude equal to that produced by budesonide.[154] Cromolyn's use in the adult chronic asthmatic, undefined as to atopy, was recently shown in a double-blind, placebo-controlled study, to produce both subjective and objective benefit.[155]

Although cromolyn is expensive, it is cost-effective in children owing to the reduced need for hospitalization and emergency room visits.[156] Also, since suppression of the HPA axis may occur in children at a dose of 400 μg/24 hours with beclomethasone dipropionate, cromolyn may be preferable. Furthermore, inhaled corticosteroids do not protect against the immediate response to antigen or exercise.

In the adult, cromolyn's value is in the mild-to-moderate asthmatic. In the severe asthmatic, it does not seem to confer additional benefit to inhaled corticosteroid, and only the latter is generally successful. In the final analysis, when both drugs are effective, cost considerations enter into the choice.

Soon to appear will be nedocromil, a "successor" to cromolyn. Although more potent than cromolyn and thus requiring a lower dose, whether it offers anything beyond cromolyn is not evident from the data and no clinical comparisons are underway to my knowledge. A recent comparison with 400 μg/day BDP in adult asthmatics found BDP to be significantly better.[157]

Methotrexate

For some years, methotrexate has been used for refractory rheumatoid arthritis, since its anti-inflammatory effects occur at a dose below its immunosuppressive effect. It has now been shown in a placebo-controlled study that doses of 15 to 50 mg, given weekly, will allow reduction of oral corticosteroids in most severe asthmatics.[158] In a follow-up of 25 patients completing 18 months or more, the average dose of prednisone was reduced from 26.9 mg/day to 6.9 mg, with loss of cushingnoid features, and no worsening, or improvement in asthma. There was no loss of effectiveness over time. Side effects were minor, consisting of transient nausea on the day of medication (switched to intramuscular thereafter), rash, stomatitis, thinning of hair, and transient transaminase elevation. There was no pulmonary toxicity. More such studies are needed to confirm its usefulness and limitations.

Pulmonary toxicity must be kept in mind, however. Idiosyncratic pulmonary toxicity, consisting of a diffuse infiltrate, shortness of breath, and fever, occurred in 5.5% of 163 patients receiving a mean dose of 10.7 mg/week for rheumatoid arthritis, with a mean period of 80 weeks before onset.[159] These manifestations resolved with discontinuation of drug and corticosteroids. Cumulative dose-related hepatotoxicity may also appear, necessitating repeated liver biopsies in some patients, and the drug may cause malaise, headaches, or leukopenia in some patients at even low doses.

Consequently, although a trial of low-dose methotrexate is justified in the severe steroid-dependent asthmatic receiving sufficient oral steroid to produce long-term side effects, one must become informed about side effects and precautions (e.g., from an experienced rheumatologist) before undertaking such treatment.

Gold

Gold salts have been used for years to treat rheumatoid arthritis, and their injection for treatment of asthma has been advocated by Japanese investigators for years as well. Their effectiveness was shown in the United States in a recent study at a dose of 6 mg/day (auranofin).[160] The role of gold therapy will become clear only as further studies are performed.

Ketotifen

Ketotifen is an interesting oral drug, with both H_1-blocking actions and some experimental anti-inflammatory properties. Its oral capability would make it useful in pediatrics for the mild asthmatic, but studies have not yet been convincing, and further controlled trials are needed to make a case for this drug.[1]

Antihistamines

Older antihistamines have had the side effect of sedation, which has limited their use at an effective dose in the asthmatic. A new generation of H_1 receptor antagonists, lacking sedative properties (inability to cross the blood–brain barrier) and lacking anticholinergic consequences has been introduced. One of these is azelastine, which also has interesting anti-inflammatory properties and can be taken by mouth.[161] These drugs cause some bronchodilation in the stable asthmatics, and reduce wheezing during the allergy season. Their ultimate role remains to be established, but there is certainly potential here.

MUCOLYTIC–EXPECTORANT THERAPY

Many patients with COPD complain bitterly about their inability to bring up mucus lodged in their airways. This problem arises from an inability to mount an adequate expulsive force against increased amounts of mucus, which itself has an increased viscosity and adhesiveness. Furthermore, this mucus is ineffectively propelled by ciliary action which, to make matters worse, is disorganized in the bronchitic.

The pharmacology of drugs that alter mucus behavior is generally unappreciated and underdeveloped in the United States, although well-developed in Europe. But there now exist drugs that modify mucin biochemistry and mucous secretion, with alterations in mucous viscosity. These drugs fall into three categories:[162]

1. *Mucolytics:* drugs that break down the polymeric structure of mucus
2. *Expectorants:* drugs increasing the flow of mucus
3. *Mucoregulating drugs:* drugs that favorably alter the constituents of mucus

What has been lacking are adequate clinical trials. Collection of data is difficult, however. We will describe some of the more prominent agents. More information can be found in the writings of Ziment.[162]

Mucolytic Drugs

The best known are derivatives of L-cysteine. Acetylcysteine is marketed in the United States as Mucomyst in a 10% and 20% solution, which diluted to 5%, is given by inhalation. The free S–S disulfide bonds bind various constituents of mucous glycoproteins, rapidly resulting in a watery constituent, at least in vitro. This drug can produce severe bronchospasm unless accompanied by a β-agonist, but can be useful in certain specific situations, such as mucoid impaction or continued plugging in someone on a ventilator. When given long-term, a few studies have shown benefit. It has not become popular in the United States owing to its taste, odor, and cost.

Expectorant Drugs

Iodides

One can list iodides under this category, although they also have the ability to break up mucus in vitro. They increase the production of mucus in a thinner consistency, an action believed to result from direct stimulation of the glands. A "gastropulmonary mucokinetic vagal" reflex is also believed to play a role in this action, having been demonstrated in animals.

Iodides are administered in two forms. A saturated solution of potassium iodide (SSKI) is the traditional form in the United States, given in water. It contains 1000 mg/mL, so that a dosage of 40 drops per day (10 q.i.d.) delivers about 4.0 g. Disadvantages include a metallic taste and, more importantly, the problem of iodide sensitivity, in the form of an acneiform rash, and hypothyroidism occurring in up to 5% of patients. Therefore, courses of 4 to 6 weeks are preferable, but some patients insist on staying on the drug. If so, thyroid studies are warranted.

More recently, there is interest in iodopropylene glycerol (IPG) marketed as Organidin in the United States. This agent is an isomeric mixture of iodine and glycerol which is absorbed intact and broken down into iodine and glycerol. It is given as 60 mg four times daily by mouth, containing only 120 mg iodine per day. It is not clear why this should be effective in such a low dose when in this form. In one study the overall effect on tracheobronchial clearance could not be shown in 15 bronchitics, but a subgroup of 6 patients with consistent sputum did show a slight increase.[163]

The most extensive study is the National Mucolytic Study, consisting of patients from several centers.[164] It consisted entirely of various subjective gradings, and was controlled by a placebo with about 100 patients in each group. Table 9–13 lists five symptoms with four showing significant improvement, graded on a scale of 1 to 5 (1, none; 2, mild; 3, moderate; 4, marked; 5, severe). Only patients with moderate to severe symptoms are shown here, as these showed the effect of treatment.

The seemingly small differences must be judged with the appreciation that a difference of 1.0 represents the difference between moderate and marked. Curiously, only the patients' and not the physicians' assessments showed significant improvements on these scales and in overall global benefit. Yet, the study is impressive in its scope, and the results sufficiently encouraging to warrant a trial of IPG in those patients particularly bothered by their sputum.

Guaifenesin

Guaifenesin is the most popular expectorant today. Formerly called glyceryl guaiacolate, it consists of a chemical bond between glycerol and the guaicol, a catechol. Its efficacy has been controversial. In large amounts, it is an emetic, and so a stimulant of the gastropulmonary vagal reflex. Thus, it may do so in an adequate dose. It appears to be picked up by the bronchial glands and may stimulate secretion. An early advocate in the United States was Chodosh, who demonstrated a reduced adhesiveness of sputum, but not viscosity, at 2400 mg/day after 20 days.[165] Yet Hirsch and coworkers could not find such an effect at 1600 mg/day, and doubt its existence.[166] The low doses in numerous syrups, up to 800 mg/day, therefore, are not likely to be effective by this mechanism.

Other agents falling in this category are ipecac and terpin hydrate, but hard evidence of their efficacy is lacking.

Mucoregulating Drugs

A number of mucoregulating thiol compounds have been and are being developed containing "blocked"-SH groups (i.e., not free as in N-acetylcysteine).[167] These are taken orally. When studied in humans and animal models, they actually do show the ability to decrease viscosity, increase secretion and thereby fluidity, and increase mucous velocity. Thus, S-carboxymethylcysteine is commonly used in Europe and

TABLE 9–13. Effect of Oral Iodopropylene Glycerol (IPG) on Chest Symptoms in COPD

Symptom	IPG	Placebo	p
Cough frequency	2.90	3.36	(0.007)
Cough severity	3.00	3.18	(NS)
Chest discomfort	2.68	3.05	(0.06)
Dyspnea	3.02	3.44	(0.02)
Ease of bringing up sputum			(0.008)

(Data from Petty TL. The National Mucolytic Study. Results of a randomized, double-blind, placebo-controlled study of iodinated glycerol in chronic obstructive bronchitis. Chest 1990; 97:75)

decreases viscosity of sputum in rheological studies measuring shear stress, as well as increasing secretion of phenol red into tracheobronchial glands in a mouse model.

What is lacking is clinical documentation of the kind used for iodopropylene glycerol (IPG). Nevertheless, the success with IPG in the preliminary results suggest that more such drugs will become available.

CLINICAL MANAGEMENT*

Asthma

Approach to the Asthmatic as an Outpatient

Careful control of airways and a well–thought-out plan for meeting exacerbations will minimize hospitalization or emergency room visits. Two groups have recently published schemes for doing this, using a peak flowmeter to monitor the disease status.[168,169] The elements of these plans are as follows:

1. *Reverse any airway narrowing and record the "best" expiratory flow rate.* This can be done by several means—either a peak bronchodilator response in the mild-to-moderate asthmatic, or a response to large doses of oral corticosteroids plus bronchodilators in the more severely obstructed patients. This can be done during a steroid trial to make the initial diagnosis of asthma.

2. *Provide the patient with a device for monitoring the peak flow rate.* Peak flow is monitored twice daily (morning and night). Some responses to the MDI may be recorded also.

3. *Prescribe drugs to reduce the severity and prevent attacks.* Reduction in airway hyperreactivity through anti-inflammatory drugs is one aspect of this. Another is the use of bronchodilators to prevent and control reduction of airway caliber. A supply of oral corticosteroids is given and their use detailed for self-treatment along with certain prearranged limits of peak flow rate.

4. *The patient is given a "crisis plan"* to institute when peak flow rates drop below certain levels and are sustained over 24 hours. This will involve self-administration of oral steroids, and a call to his or her physician or an emergency room self-referral.

5. *Frequent observations of compliance,* verification of peak flow rates and education are important.

6. *A search for trigger factors is made.* On the basis of history, skin tests, radioallergosorbent test (RAST), a review of possible aggravating factors is made, and should be investigated if clues exist, particularly in refractory cases (Table 9–14).

Airway Reactivity Versus Variability in FEV_1

If a large group of asthmatics is studied, there is a significant correlation between measures of nonspecific reactivity and the severity of asthma, as shown by spirome-

---

* The NHLBI "Guidelines for Asthma," a consensus report of an expert panel, was published and disseminated widely after submission of this manuscript. It bears careful attention and may differ in emphasis and some details.

TABLE 9–14. Possible Trigger Factors
Aggravating Asthma

Gastroesophageal reflux
Chronic sinusitis
Occupational asthma
Food additives (metabisulfites, monosodium glutamate,
   tartrazine)
Aspirin sensitivity, other nonsteroidal anti-inflammatory drugs
Psychological factors
Vocal cord disorders

(Barnes PJ. Difficult asthma. Cause for concern. Br Med J 1989; 299:695)

try, peak flow variability, and response to a bronchodilator.[171] Yet, in longitudinal studies, reactivity measurements in the individual case do not closely reflect severity, as measured by morning peak flow or its diurnal variation.[141,172] Although we need to be cognizant of the dangers of reactivity in the severe asthmatic, it is probably quite adequate to follow their progress through the more conventional means of daily peak flow measurements or spirometry, or both.

Control of Nocturnal Bronchospasm
in the Asthmatic

Nocturnal bronchospasm with early-morning awakening is common in asthmatics, most generally occurring around 4:00 AM. Some 49% of asthmatics have nocturnal symptoms nightly, and 64% have them at least three times a week. About 75% have greater than a 20% drop in peak flow rate.[173] Diurnal variation in peak flow in hospitalized patients can be associated with respiratory arrest, occurring in a more pronounced fashion during the instability of the attack and the immediate period during recovery.[174] These drops, even in stable patients, are associated with significant desaturation and may explain why most deaths in asthma occur at night. There is also an associated increase in bronchial reactivity to methacholine and even to nebulized normal saline during these episodes.[175] The BAL washings show increased numbers of neutrophils and eosinophils at these times.

Treatment of nocturnal bronchospasm by inhaled β_2-agonists taken at 10:00 PM using the longer-acting bitolterol is inferior to twice-daily dosing of a slow-release theophylline preparation, producing mean levels of 12 to 14 $\mu g/mL$. Theophylline markedly reduces the number of desaturation episodes (fall greater than 4%) without interference with the sleep architecture.[176] Those patients who find that a twice-daily theophylline preparation still does not control nocturnal bronchospasm may do better with a once-daily preparation (e.g., Uniphyl) taken at 6:00 to 7:00 PM with the evening meal, since theophylline levels will peak at about 14 $\mu g/mL$ 10 hours later, while their trough levels the next day are still adequate.[122]

Inhaled corticosteroids will reduce the frequency of nocturnal bronchospasms, the effect usually becoming obvious in 3 weeks.[177] This may be due to suppression of airway hyperreactivity. A sustained-release oral β_2-agonist can also be used alone or combined. It will be advantageous when longer-acting β_2-agonist inhaled preparations become available in the US. Thus, the physician has strong tools to combat nocturnal bronchospasm. Attention to this symptom in the asthmatic is an important part of proper management.

Escalation of Therapy for Outpatient Asthma

Table 9–15 is a suggested approach in controlling asthma, according to symptoms or PEFR, as judged by twice-daily measurements. This plan is similar to published schemes.[168,169]

As conditions improve, one attempts to return to the previous dose until it becomes clear that more is needed. The patients should be given a plan, as specified by Beasley.[169] This plan should state what PEFR measurements warrant a change in steroid therapy (see Table 9–15).

TABLE 9–15. Suggested Self-Management Plan for Escalating Therapy According to Severity

Stable Asthma	
If	*Then commence as needed*
Mild or intermittent symptoms	1. PRN use of beta MDI and 2. Cromolyn if seasonal
More or less constant symptoms requiring multiple use MDI/day	1. Begin inhaled CS (low dose) or cromolyn
Constant symptoms despite above	1. Increase inhaled CS (up to 3× usual dose) 2. Add theophylline and/or oral β-agonists
Constant symptoms despite above that cause discomfort during normal activities (or PEFR < 60%)	1. Begin daily oral CS (as needed) and cut back to q.o.d. when possible

Deteriorating Asthma	
If	*Then*
Progressive discomfort over several days, or PEFR < 50% over 24 h or need for MDI < 3 h	Begin "burst" therapy of oral CS until PEFR returns to 80%. Contact physician.

Asthma in Crisis	
If	*Then*
PEFR < 150–200 L/min	Self administer 60 mg oral prednisone, take 4–6 puffs MDI, go to emergency room If attacks characteristically come on abruptly, self administer 0.25–0.5 mg epinephrine or terbutaline sc.

The Acute Attack Requiring Emergency Room Treatment

The asthmatic or COPD patient's life will probably be punctuated by one or more trips to the emergency room. If properly managed in the use of burst therapy of corticosteroids, most asthma visits can be avoided. But if this is necessary, the final episode usually comes on a background of poor control. One study of 44 adults found a mean period of 5 weeks of poorly controlled wheezing before a rapid deterioration over 24 hours.[178] The severity of the acute attack was not related to the duration of acute wheezing. Recovery was slow, most reaching 70% of predicted values after 7 days in the hospital. Sudden deterioration from a background of good control is uncommon in adults.

In children and some adults, however, sudden deterioration may occur, based on excessive airway reactivity.[179] When 15 steroid-dependent patients aged 9 to 15 were divided into those deteriorating over 8 hours after onset of wheezing, and those more gradually, the rapid patients exhibited markedly enhanced nonspecific airway reactivity during the interim phase and had a history of respiratory arrests and hypoxic seizures. Yet, their stable baseline function was better than the slower group. These patients warrant the use of self-medication with a subcutaneous injection of epinephrine or terbutaline.[180]

In 55 adult asthmatics requiring hospitalization, the initial PEFR was not predictive of the recovery time.[181] Host factors associated with prolonged recovery were age, intrinsic asthma, duration of attack, poor long-term control, and use of maintenance oral corticosteroids. Fanta and coworkers did find that patients with an FEV_1 below 30% predicted, averaging 20%, required a longer time in the emergency room, and were often finally hospitalized.[182] Although such severely depressed function may rapidly bounce back with intensive bronchodilator treatment, it allows little further deterioration and should be treated vigorously with steroids at the outset.

Turner-Warwick has identified asthmatics with greatly fluctuating PEFRs as *brittle* asthmatics, who are responsive to bronchodilators, but not to corticosteroids.[183] Such patients require enormous doses of β-agonists to be comfortable, and this need must be acknowledged. This may be related to the phenomenon of steroid resistance, which is believed to be quite rare. However, studies in unselected asthmatics suggest that they have a range of corticosteroid responsiveness that is highly correlated with the ability of steroids to suppress lymphokine function,[184] and this provides a good reason to use large doses of corticosteroids in the acute attack.

Severity Assessment in the Emergency Room

The majority of asthma attacks in the emergency room will respond sufficiently to aggressive therapy to be discharged home after several hours' observation, often on an oral or intramuscular repository corticosteroid regimen, and with close follow-up. But there are certain features and serious abnormalities of objective measurements in the emergency room that indicate a potential life-threatening attack and the need for hospitalization. These have been discussed by various authors (Table 9–16).[185–187]

Patients with an FEV_1 of 0.75 to 1.0 L may or may not respond sufficiently to emergency room treatment to avoid hospitalization, but those with values under

TABLE 9–16. Features Suggestive of a Life-Threatening Attack

Central cyanosis	Tachypnea over 30/min
Profuse diaphoresis	Pulsus paradoxus over
Severe respiratory distress	15–18 mm Hg
and inability to lie flat	Tachycardia over 120
Exhaustion	PEFR under 100 L/min
Sternocleidomastoid	FEV_1 under 1.0 L
retraction	PaO_2 under 60; $PaCO_2$ over
Inspiratory wheezing	40
Silent chest	ECG abnormalities
Disturbance of	Pneumonia; pneumothorax
consciousness	

0.75 L are usually admitted, particularly since there is little room for further deterioration in this unstable state. A patient unable to perform an FEV_1 or PEFR determination will often require intubation, although others may respond sufficiently to aggressive management.

Principles of Drug Management in the Severe Acute Asthma Attack

1. Consecutive or continuous nebulization of β-agonists over 120 minutes are the mainstay of therapy in the most severe cases, providing supplemental O_2 and ECG monitoring are used.
2. Subcutaneous administration of a β-agonist is warranted if the patient has not responded to the initial nebulization (e.g., after two cycles of albuterol). This can be epinephrine or terbutaline (the latter preferred in older adults). This may be repeated once with close ECG monitoring.
3. Intravenous corticosteroids are indicated in

   • Patients with a history of steroid use
   • Patients with a prolonged buildup (e.g., more than 24 hours)
   • Patients with an FEV_1 below 1.0 L
   • Older asthmatics
   • Asthmatics with a history of intubation

   The optimum IV dose of methylprednisolone has been determined in a random comparison of 15, 40, and 100 mg every 6 hours.[188] The 15-mg dose was inferior to the others, whereas nothing more was gained by the 100-mg dose over 40 mg. Alternatively, IV hydrocortisone is used, 4 mg/kg or 200 mg, every 6 hours.

4. Aminophylline or theophylline should be maintained only while a stat level is obtained. Some physicians would not use theophylline unless the acute attack is responding poorly, but I believe that there are ample reasons to use it in the most severe cases.

5. Although inhaled anticholinergics are not now standard therapy, they may be valuable in the resistant case.
6. In some quarters, IV terbutaline[61] is a final alternative to intubation, although intubation may be more prudent when little experience exists with this approach. The IV terbutaline may also be useful in the refractory case on a ventilator.

Treatment Phases

1. *Initial phase: the first 4 hours.* The patient is receiving O_2 and monitored, with an IV line, and receives one or more cycles of nebulized β-agonist, with additional drug subcutaneously if the response is poor. Corticosteroids IV are bolused. Theophylline is adjusted or may be loaded.
2. *Stabilization phase: the next 24 hours.* A nebulized β-agonist is given every 4 hours and IV corticosteroids continued. Theophylline is maintained with a check of level particularly after 18 to 24 hours. Systemic β-agonist may be added in the more severe cases. Close surveillance of blood gas levels continues and spirometry or PEFR is measured at the bedside to document improvement.
3. *Resolution phase: the next several days.* Continued daily flow measurements document the return to near-normal levels, which may be rapid (1 to 2 days), or prolonged (7 to 10 days). Nebulization can be replaced by a MDI-spacer at increased doses (4 to 6 puffs every 4 hours) with the aid and assessment by respiratory therapist and nursing staff. Corticosteroids are given orally in large, divided doses (e.g., 60 mg prenisolone every 24 hours), with theophylline continued orally at the same dose. Upon discharge, oral corticosteroids are tapered on an every-morning schedule and inhaled steroids maintained, with early follow-up and further dose adjustment.

Chronic Obstructive Pulmonary Disease

Approach to the Outpatient with Chronic Obstructive Pulmonary Disease

- Onset of dyspnea in early or midadulthood?
- Episodic dyspnea, exercise-induced attacks?
- Childhood asthma, childhood respiratory problems?
- History of allergic rhinitis, nasal polyps, strong family allergies?
- Peripheral or sputum eosinophilia, elevated IgE?
- Brisk bronchodilator response (over 20%); fluctuating FEV_1s, normal D_LCO despite severe obstruction of flow?
- Marked wheezing on physical exam?

Patients with any of the foregoing deserve a steroid trial to rule out asthma, or an asthmatic component to their COPD, using 40 mg prednisone or prednisolone each morning for 14 days; obtain spirometry before and after. A significant increase in FEV_1 over that on optimal bronchodilator therapy (over 20%) suggests an asthmatic component to COPD, or simple asthma and no COPD. Patients with COPD with steroid-responsive component will benefit from inhaled or oral corticosteroids.

Bronchodilator Therapy

One of the more β_2-selective agents (albuterol, terbutaline, pirbuterol) is given every 4 to 6 hours by MDI, more during exacerbations (Table 9–17). Oral β_2-agonists may be begun if patients are unable to master the MDI, have erratic control, or prefer an oral route. The MDI technique should be checked regularly by the physician. When there is suboptimal technique, a spacer may be used (Aerochamber, InspirEase, Nebuhaler, Breathancers), or a breath-actuated device (Rotahaler, Autohaler-pending).

In general, COPD patients respond strongly to antimuscarinic compounds, but patients will note that the response is not as immediate as to a β_2-agonist (Table 9–18). Antimuscarinics by MDI should be given together with a β-agonist. Together, they provide additive and prolonged response.[131] Ipratropium can be used in larger doses than two puffs, as the 40-μg dose is suboptimal. Liquid nebulization of β-agonists and antimuscarinics is another option, providing even more drug deposition than the MDI, some say equivalent to eight to ten puffs. These are prescribed for those with the most severe COPD and asthma. This method should also be tried in patients with poor inhaler technique.

Slow-release theophylline compounds (Table 9–19) are part of our standard therapy for COPD, usually in a dose of 300 mg twice daily (nonsmoker) or 400 twice daily (smoker) as the initial dose, adjusted later to bring levels close to 15 μg/mL for maximum effect. Theophylline levels are checked yearly after this, when the patient's status changes, or when interfering drugs are added (see Table 9–10).

Antibiotics, Antivirals

The use of prophylactic antibiotics is a standard approach for acute exacerbations of bronchitis in the COPD patient, but has been difficult to justify in placebo-controlled comparisons. Nevertheless, their use makes considerable sense in the hope to accomplish two things: (1) suppression of bacterial complications of acute bronchitis; and (2) prevention of bronchopneumonia or bronchiolitis as sequelae.

Acute bronchitis usually begins and continues as a viral infection, and only the occasional case is likely to develop serious bacterial complications. Yet, it is worth treating many cases with prophylactic antibiotics to prevent or suppress one instance of pneumonia or a life-threatening bacterial bronchitis. Such a useful purpose will not be easy to document statistically and, recognizing this, most physicians continue to advise self-administered antibiotics for signs and symptoms of acute bronchitis.

The antibiotics used must cover the pneumococcus, and preferably also *Haemophilus influenzae*, since both bronchitis and pneumonia can also be seen with the latter organism or in combination with *Streptococcus pneumoniae*. A course of ampicillin (2.0 g/day for 10 days) or trimethoprim–sulfamethoxazole (Bactrim, Septra) is the most economical, although a number of alternatives exist.[189] The latter is more effective against *Moraxella* (*Branhamella*) *catarrhalis*, now recognized as a common pathogen.

In the patient with COPD or asthma who has probably been exposed to influenza A, amantadine is given as soon as possible in a dose of 100 mg twice daily for ten days.[6] If repeated exposures are likely, the drug can be given for as long as 90 days. The dose should be reduced in patients with renal insufficiency or a history of seizures. Amantadine is also used in the early treatment of influenza A, if begun within 48 hours of the onset of symptoms, to be continued for 5 days.

Immunization

In the United States, there are about 200,000 cases of pneumococcal pneumonia yearly, and the mortality from the 50,000 cases with bacteremia is as high as 50%, despite antibiotics, usually in patients older than 60 years. The pneumococcal vaccine contains antigens to 23 serotypes, or about 80% of the pneumococcal strains. Once given, revaccination may be considered after 6 years in the older, very high risk individual,[190] although, owing to the severity of reaction to the vaccine, the package insert does not advise this.

Influenzal vaccination against current strains should be given yearly, usually in the fall, in time to build antibodies against the winter epidemic.

α_1-Antitrypsin Deficiency

The incidence of the PiZZ phenotype in North America is estimated to be between 1 : 3,500 and 1 : 1,670 and, therefore, it is one of the most common serious genetic conditions.[191] This phenotype has true levels of α_1-antitrypsin (AAT) of 2.5 to 7 μM, compared with the normal range (MM phenotype) of 20 to 48 μM. These levels are commonly quoted as 20 to 45 and 150 to 350 mg/dL, respectively, in commercial laboratories, but are 35% to 40% too high.

At the present time, patients with the ZZ phenotype, and the rarer phenotype combinations that give a threshold level under 11 μM, are treated with bronchodilators and augmentation of their AAT levels with its very costly human serum concentrate (Prolastin) given IV. This is given to those persons older than 18 years whose pulmonary function is abnormal, regardless of the degree, in hope of preventing further deterioration. The dose is generally administered weekly, but trials are underway with monthly infusions. Although Prolastin has been heat-treated, patients should be immunized against hepatitis B, and screened for the human immunodeficiency virus (HIV). An NIH registry for patients older than 18 with severe deficiency has been established.

Adjunctive Drugs

Although we do not wish to add further pharmacopeial burden to our patients, there are sometimes situations that call for relief of more than shortness of breath, for example, suppression of a disturbing cough, or relief of a patient who is anxious, depressed, or sleepless. A more complete discussion of these drugs is found in reviews by Ziment[189] and by Altose and Hudgel.[192]

COUGH SUPPRESSANTS. As a nonnarcotic, dextromethorphan, 15 to 60 mg three to four times daily, is the most suitable in the COPD patient with constant, irritating nonproductive cough. It can also be given in a slow-release form. Small doses of narcotic drugs may be necessary, but the workup for cough should be carried out insofar as possible.

PSYCHOACTIVE DRUGS. Psychoactive drugs fall into the categories of anxiolytics, hypnotics, and antidepressants. For relief of anxiety, the older benzodiazepines and

(*Text continues on p. 186*)

TABLE 9–17. β-Adrenergic Preparations

Product/ Manufacturer	Oral Form	Subcutaneous	MDI	Nebulized Dose (Adult)
Epinephrine				
Aqueous epinephrine		0.3–0.5 mg q20' up to 3x 1:1000,1 mg/mL		200 μg
Primatine Mist, Whitehall Bronkaid Mist, Winthrop Medihaler-Epi, Riker			(not recommended) 270 μg 160 μg	
Isoproterenol				
Various Manufacturers			45–131 μg/puff (1–2 puffs q2–4h)	0.25–10% (1–2 inhal 0.25%) by hand bulb; 2.5 mL 0.05% by compressor)
Isoetharine				
Isoetharine HCl Inhal, Roxane Bronkometer, Winthrop			0.34 mg/puff, 200 puffs (2–3 puffs q4h)	0.1%, 0.125%, 0.2% (3–5 mL undil)

Drug / Manufacturer	Oral	Inhalation (MDI)	Nebulizer/Solution
Ephedrine sulfate Various manufacturers	Various (15–60 mg) 25–50 mg syrup q4–6h		
Metaproterenol Alupent, Boehringer Metaprel, Dorsey	10, 20 mg tablets 10 mg/mL syrup (20 mg q4–6h)	0.65 mg/puff, 200 puffs (2–3 puffs q4–6h)	0.6% unit dose of vial of 2.5 mL (15 mg); 0.3 mL of 5% (15 mg) with 2.5 mL saline q2–4h
Terbutaline Brethine, Geigy Bricanyl, Merill Dow	2.5–5 mg tablets (2.5–5 mg q6–8h)	0.2 mg/puff, 300 puffs (1–2 puffs q4–6h)	0.1% (1 mg/mL) (0.25–0.5 mg q6–8h)
Albuterol/ **Salbutamol** Ventolin, Glaxo Proventil, Schering	2,4 mg tablets 2 mg/mL 5 mL syrup (2–4 mg q6–8h)	90 μg/puff, 200 puffs (1–2 puffs q4–6h)	0.5 mL of 0.5% (2.5 mg) with 2.5 mL saline q2–6h
Pirbuterol Maxair, 3M Riker		0.2 mg/puff, 300 puffs (1–2 puffs q4–6h)	
Bitolterol mesylate Tornalate, Breon		0.37 mg/puff, 300 puffs (1–3 puffs q4–6h)	

TABLE 9–18. Other Categories

Category	Strength	Dosing
Anticholinergics		
Atropine sulfate, Dey	0.2% (1 mg), 0.5% (2.5 mg) in 0.5 mL unit dose	0.025–0.075 mg/kg q6h by neb.
Ipratropium bromide (Atrovent, Boehringer)	20 μg/puff, 300 puffs	2–3 puffs q4–6h
Cromolyn Sodium		
(Intal, Fisons)	20 mg/capsule by Spinhaler	1–2 capsules q.i.d.
(Intal solution, Fisons)	800 μg/puff, 200 puffs	2 puffs q.i.d.
(Intal solution, Fisons)	20 μg/2 mL ampoule by nebulizer	1 amp q.i.d.
Corticosteroids		
Tablets		
Prednisone, prednisolone	1-50 mg	10-20 mg/day, q.o.d.
Parenteral		
Cortisol, hydrocortisone (Solu-Cortef, Upjohn)	100, 250, 500, 1000 mg Na succinate powder	4 mg/kg q4–6h until response, then daily
Methylprednisolone (Solu-Medrol, Upjohn)	40, 125, 500, 1000 mg Na succinate powder	1–2 mg/kg q4–6h until response, then daily
Aerosol		
Beclomethasone dipropionate (Beclovent, Glaxo; Vanceril, Schering)	42 μg/puff, 200 puffs	2 puffs q.i.d.
Triamcinolone acetonide (Azmacort, Rorer)	100 μg/puff, 240 puffs	2 puffs q.i.d.
Flunisolide (Aerobid, Key)	250 μg/puff, 100 puffs	2 puffs b.i.d.

the barbituates are contraindicated in COPD because of respiratory depression. However, a number of newer agents exist with short half-lives and minimal depression and can be given in low doses. Buspirone (Buspar) is a recent drug that must be given for several weeks to become effective, rather than occasional use.

For sleeplessness, COPD patients with CO_2 depression will tolerate single doses of flurazepam (Dalmane), 15 to 30 mg or triazolam (Halcion), 0.0625 to 0.125 mg). In the patient that warrants an antidepressant, Dudley and Sitzman consider doxepin[193] to be the drug of choice in COPD, and nortriptyline (Aventyl, Pamelor) to be an alternative.[194]

RESPIRATORY STIMULANTS. In the patient with COPD with increasing CO_2 retention, one can consider the use of medroxyprogesterone (Provera). In a dose of 20 mg three times daily, this hormone produced a mean drop of 7 mm Hg in PCO_2 while awake and 8 mm Hg while asleep, with corresponding rises in PO_2.[195] Individual results were quite variable. This agent will cause a loss of libido and potency in about

TABLE 9-19. Theophylline Preparations (Incomplete Listing)

Dosage Form	Theophylline Content	Dosing Interval	
Liquids			
		Pediatric	Adult
Elixophyllin (20% alcohol)	5.3 mg/mL	q4–6h	q6–8h
Choledyl pediatric syrup, Parke Davis	6.4 mg/mL	q4–6h	q6–8h
Somophyllin, Fisons	18 mg/mL	q4–6h	q6–8h
Rapid-release tablets			
Theophylline, various mfrs.	100, 200 mg	q4–6h	q6–8h
Aminophylline, various mfrs.	78.9, 157.8 mg	q4–6h	q6–8h
Theolair, Riker	225 mg		
Sustained-release tablets			
Aminodur Duratabs, Berlex	240 mg (scored)	q8h	q12h
Constant-T, Geigy	200, 300 mg (scored)	q8h	q12h
Choledyl SA, Warner Lambert	256, 364 mg	q8h	q12h
Theolair SR, Riker	250, 500 mg (scored)	q8h	q12h
Theochron, Forest	300 mg	q8h	q12h
Theo-Dur, Key	100, 200, 300 mg (scored)	q8h	q12h
Uniphyl, Purdue-Frederick	200, 400 mg (scored)	q8h	q12–24h
Sustained-released capsules			
Somphyllin-CRT, Fisons	65, 130, 260 mg	q8h	q12h
Theobid, Glaxo	130, 260 mg		
Slo-Phyllin Gyrocaps, Rorer	60, 125, 250 mg	q6–8h	q8–12h
Theo-Dur Sprinkle, Key	50, 75, 125, 200 mg	q8–12h	q12h
Slo-bid Gyrocaps, Rorer	50, 100, 200, 300 mg	q12h	q12h
Theo-24, Searle	100, 200, 300 mg	q12h	q24h
Rectal			
Somophyllin, Fisons	51.4 mg/mL	q6h	q6–8h
Aminophylline suppositories (various)	125, 250 mg	q6h	q6–8h
Parenteral			
Aminophylline, various mfgs.	25 mg/mL = 20 mg/mL theo		
Theophylline in 5% dextrose, Travenol	200 mg/50 mL and 100 mL	Constant infusion	
	400 mg/100, 250, 500 mL	or q6–8h	
	800 mg/500, 1000 mL		

10% of men. Other respiratory stimulants have been used in COPD, such as almitrine bimesylate (used in Europe), acting apparently both as a central stimulant and possibly through an effect on ventilation–perfusion matching,[196] and methylphenidate (Ritalin).[189]

In the sleep apnea syndrome, medroxyprogesterone offers some improvement in fewer than one-half of the patients. Protriptyline enhances respiratory activation of upper airway muscles and may be helpful in mild to moderate sleep apnea, but has the potentially serious side effects of constipation, urinary retention, ataxia, and confusion.[192]

CORTICOSTEROIDS. If a course of daily oral corticosteroid (e.g., 40 mg prednisone each morning) is given for 10 to 14 days to a population of COPD patients, carefully screened to exclude asthmatics and stabilized on bronchodilators, a few will show a significant further increase in FEV_1. These steroid responders can be maintained on the lowest alternate day dose that maintains their improvement. Many will not respond to inhaled corticosteroids, although they should be given a trial.

The literature on steroid responsive COPD to 1978 has been critically reviewed by Sahn and associates,[197] and to 1986 by Eliasson and associates.[198] A peripheral eosinophilia is more common in responders. Indeed, some of these may be asthmatics who have escaped detection because of an uncharacteristic presentation. My own practice is to pay particular attention to any history of childhood respiratory disease, a personal or family history of atopic disease, or a history of wheezing or shortness of breath in earlier adulthood. A serum IgE level higher than 200 IU suggests allergy.

I also carefully analyze all previous spirometry. Fluctuations beyond 25% or so in prebronchodilator values of FEV_1, or a response to bronchodilator over 20%, suggest the possibility of an asthmatic component. Any of these features warrant a steroid trial and, indeed, some would give a steroid trial irrespective of any such features. The trial must be controlled and deliberate, with pre- and poststeroid spirometry. A response of 20% or more, which is maintained, is convincing. There may also be patients who claim considerable improvement, despite the absence of objective documentation. This poses a dilemma, and such patients are usually left on a steroid dose that is low enough to avoid long-term side effects.

Long-term daily corticosteroids may in some manner slow the progression of severe chronic obstructive disease. In an uncontrolled study, Postma and colleagues followed serial spirometry of 65 patients who began prednisone at a dose of 15 mg/day (men) and 10 mg/day (women).[199] While receiving the steroid, the FEV_1 did not decline, or it actually improved. When the steroid was stopped or reduced to 7.5 mg or less (because of concern over side effects), the FEV_1 declined. It appeared that this initial dose was strongly associated with both survival and maintenance of FEV_1, but with a prohibitive incidence of side effects. However, given these studies, substitution of inhaled corticosteroids, with or without a lower oral dose, may be beneficial and deserves study.

Drug Management of the Acute Exacerbation of Chronic Obstructive Pulmonary Disease

The acute exacerbation may come on gradually or very abruptly, even within a matter of 1 or 2 hours. The PCO_2 may increase precipitously, since these patients are often CO_2 retainers, or close to it. Exacerbations of COPD are not well understood and usually entail an extended crisis for the patient, often lasting several weeks, which must run its course. There is increased dyspnea, usually increased cough and sputum, further elevation of their mean pulmonary artery pressure (only slightly improved by supplemental O_2), a deterioration of blood gas values and spirometry, and sometimes a leukocytosis. Intensification of bronchodilator therapy seems helpful, but often patients receive little more than they would at home, except for close observation. Presumably, most episodes begin with a viral infection, but often there is no indication of an infectious process.

These patients are older and may have heart disease. They must be monitored during the initial stages of treatment, and their PO_2 maintained in the 60s. It seems prudent to treat them less aggressively with β-agonists than a patient with a severe asthmatic attack, and to limit their β-agonist nebulization to two cycles, followed initially by an every-4-hour schedule. An antimuscarinic agent may be nebulized simultaneously. Injection of 0.25 mg terbutaline subcutaneously may improve the patient if he or she fails to respond to nebulization.

Substitution of an MDI-spacer for nebulization can be made after initial stabilization, at the same doses and the same indications as discussed under treatment of acute asthma. Both β-agonists and an antimuscarinic can be delivered by MDI. Such an approach requires frequent evaluation of the patient, however, and should not be done on an automatic basis.[200]

In our institution, most of these patients are already receiving theophylline, and levels are just optimized to 10 to 15 $\mu g/mL$. Although a recent controlled study comparing nebulized metaproterenol, with and without theophylline, failed to show a significant advantage to theophylline in the overall rate of FEV_1 recovery, examination of the premetaproterenol values is suggestive of theophylline benefit over the first 48 hours.[201] In such a comparison, the hoped-for advantage of the drug may not be revealed by group comparisons. Particularly with theophylline, in this situation, one hopes that at least some patients out of the group would experience an improvement in diaphragmatic function or fatigue that would justify its use.

Large doses of corticosteroid in the first 72 hours have been advocated, based on the controlled study of Albert and coworkers, showing a more vigorous FEV_1 response in patients on 0.5 mg/kg methyprednisolone IV every 6 hours for 72 hours.[202] This study was recently criticized, based on a calculated noncomparability of pre-bronchodilator baseline spirometry that allowed more room for improvement in the steroid group,[203] but the criticism itself is quite speculative. In fact, a recent study suggests that corticosteroids are indeed beneficial.[204] From those COPD patients with a history of multiple relapses, 45 well-matched pairs of emergency room visits in 30 patients were found in whom one visit was treated with corticosteroids and one was not. Steroid treatment consisted of an IV dose (mean of 365 mg hydrocortisone equivalents) followed by either a tapering oral dose of prednisone or a temporary increase. The 48-hour relapse rate was much lower in the steroid-treated visit (8.9% vs. 33.3%, $p = 0.005$).

This study should settle the question. Although some patients might be steroid-responders, there is likely to be a nonspecific anti-inflammatory effect of the steroid as well. Finally, antibiotics are also usually begun for possible prevention of bacterial complications.

REFERENCES

1. Barnes PJ. A new approach to the treatment of asthma. N Engl J Med 1989; 321:1517.

2. James AL, Pare PD, Hogg JC. The mechanics of airway narrowing in asthma. Am Rev Respir Dis 1989;139:242.

3. Samter M. Asthma bronchiale and histeminempfindlichkeit. Z. Gesamte Exp Med 1933;89:24.

4. Cockcroft DW, Killian DN, Mellon JJA, Hargreave FE. Bronchial reactivity to inhaled histamine: a method and clinical survey. Clin Allergy 1977;7:235.

5. Hargreave FE, Ryan G, Thomson NC, et al. Bronchial responsiveness to histamine and methacholine in asthma: measurement and clinical significance. J Allergy Clin Immunol 1981;68:347.

6. Greenspon LW, Parrish B. Inhibition of methacholine-induced bronchoconstriction in patients with chronic obstructive pulmonary disease. Am Rev Respir Dis 1988;137:281.

7. Cockcroft DW, Murdock KY. Comparative effects of inhaled salbutamol, sodium cromoglycate, and beclomethasone diproprionate on allergy-induced early asthmatic responses, late asthmatic responses and increased bronchial responsiveness to histamine. J Allergy Clin Immunol 1987;79:734.

8. Cartier A, Thomson NC, Frith PA, Roberts RS, Hargreave FE. Allergen-induced increase in bronchial responsiveness to histamine: relationship to the late asthmatic response and change in airway caliber. J Allergy Clin Immunol 1982;70:170.

9. Metzger WJ, Zavala D, Richerson HB, et al. Local allergen challenge and bronchoalveolar lavage of allergic asthmatic lungs. Am Rev Respir Dis 1987;135:433.

10. Cockcroft DW, Killian DN, Mellon JJ, et al. Bronchial reactivity to inhaled histamine: a method and clinical survey. Clin Allergy 1977;7:235.

11. Laitinen LA, Heino M, Laitenen A, Kava T, Haahtela T. Damage of the airway epithelium and bronchial reactivity in patients with asthma. Am Rev Respir Dis 1985;131:599.

12. Beasley R, Roche WR, Roberts JA, Holgate ST. Cellular events in the bronchi in mild asthma and after bronchial provocation. Am Rev Respir Dis 1989;139:806.

13. Brown PJ, Greville HW, Finucane K. Asthma and irreversible airflow obstruction. Thorax 1984;39:131.

14. Barnes PJ. The third nervous system in the lung. Thorax 1984;39:561.

15. Goldie RC. Receptors in asthmatic airways. Am Rev Respir Dis 1990;141:S151.

16. Barnes PJ. Airway receptors. In: Jenne JW, Murphy S, eds. Drugs therapy for asthma. Research and clinical practice. New York: Marcell Dekker, 1987:67.

17. Lefkowitz R. Adrenergic receptors. Models for the study of receptors coupled to guanine nucleotide regulatory proteins. J Biol Chem 1988;283:4993.

18. Takuwa Y, Takuwa N, Rasmussen H. The effect of isoproterenol on intracellular calcium concentration. J Biol Chem 1988;263:762.

19. Becker AB, Simons FER, McMillan JL, Faridy T. Formoterol, a new long-acting selective β_2 adrenergic receptor agonist. Double-blind comparisons with salbutamol and placebo in children with asthma. J Allergy Clin Immunol 1989;84:891.

20. Ullman A, Svedmyr N. Salmeterol, a long acting inhaled β_2 adrenoceptor agonist: a comparison with salbutamol in adult asthmatic patients. Thorax 1988;43:674.

21. Larsson S, Svedmyr N. Bronchodilating effect and side effects of β_2-adrenoceptor stimulants by different modes of administration (tablets, metered aerosol and combinations thereof). A study with salbutamol in asthmatics. Am Rev Respir Dis 1977;116:861.

22. Ahlquist RP. A study of adrenotropic receptors. Am J Physiol 1948;153:586.

23. Lands AM, Arnold A, McAuliff JP, et al. Differentiation of receptor systems activated by sympathomimetic amines. Nature 1967;214:597.

24. Brittain RT. A comparison of the pharmacology profile of salbutamol with that of isoproterenol, orciprenaline (metaproterenol) and trimetoquinol. Postgrad Med J 1971;47:11.

25. Kennedy MCS, Simpson WT. Human pharmacological and clinical studies on salbutamol: a specific beta-adrenergic bronchodilator. Br J Dis Chest 1969;65:163.

26. Gibson DG, Coltart DJ. Hemodynamic effects of intravenous salbutamol in patients with mitral valve disease: comparison with isoproterenol and atropine. Medicine 1971;47:40.

27. Naylor WG, McInnes I. Salbutamol and orciprenaline-induced changes in myocardial function. Cardiovasc Res 1972;6:725.

28. Lemoine H, Schonell H, Kaumann A. Human cardiac beta-adrenergic receptors: subtype heterogeneity delineated by direct radioligand binding. Br J Pharmacol 1988; 95:55.

29. Roth MJ, Wilson AF, Novey HS. A comparative study of the aerosolized bronchodilators isoproterenol, metaproterenol and terbutaline in asthma. Ann Allergy 1977;38:16.

30. Newman SP, Pavia D. Aerosol deposition in man. In: Moren F, Newhouse MT, Dolovich MB, eds. Aerosols in medicine. Amsterdam: Elsevier Publishing, 1985:193.

31. Wilson A. Aerosol dynamics and delivery systems. In: Jenne JW, Murphy S, eds. Drug therapy for asthma. Research and clinical practice. New York: Marcel Dekker, 1987:389.

32. Hess DR, Horney D, Snyder T. Medication-delivery performance of either eight small-volume, hand held nebulizers: effects of diluent, volume, gas flowrate, and nebulizer model. Respir Care 1989;34:712.

33. Cushley MJ, Lewis RA, Tattersfield AE. Comparison of three techniques of inhalation on the airway response to terbutaline. Thorax 1983;38:90.

34. Harrison BA, Pierce RJ. Comparison of wet and dry aerosol salbutamol. Aust N Z J Med 1983;13:29.

35. Mestitz H, Copeland JM, McDonald CF. Comparison of outpatient nebulized vs. metered dose inhaled terbutaline in chronic air flow obstruction. Chest 1989;96:1237.

36. Nelson HS, Spector SL, Whitsett TL, George RB, Dwek JH. The bronchodilator response to inhalation of increasing doses of aerosolized albuterol. J Allergy CLin Immunol 1983;72:371.

37. Morely TF, Marozan E, Zappasodi SJ, Gordon R, Griesback R, Giudice JL. Comparison of beta adrenergic agents delivered by nebulizer versus metered dose inhaler with hospitalized patients. Chest 1988;94:1205.

38. Kung M, Croley SW, Phillips BA. Systemic cardiovascular and metabolic effects associated with the inhalation of an increased dose of albuterol. Influence of mouth rinsing and gargling. Chest 1977;91:382.

39. Summer W, Elston R, Tharpe L, Nelson S, Haponik E. Aerosol bronchodilation delivery methods. Relative impact on pulmonary function and cost of respiratory care. Arch Intern Med 1989;149:618.

40. Karlsson J-A, Persson CGA. Influence of tracheal contraction on relaxant effects in vitro of theophylline and isoproterenol. Br J Pharmacol 1981;74:73.

41. Jenne JW, Shaughnessy TK, Druz WS, Manfredi CJ, Vestal RE. In vivo functional antagonism between isoproterenol and bronchoconstrictants in the dog. J Appl Physiol 1987;63:812.

42. Russell JA. Differential inhibitory effect of isoproterenol on contractions of canine airways. J Appl Physiol 1984;57:801.

43. Barnes PJ, Pride NB. Dose-response curves to inhaled beta-adrenoceptor agonists in normal and asthmatic subjects. Br J Pharmacol 1983;15:677.

44. Holgate ST, Baldwin CJ, Tattersfield AE. Beta-adrenergic resistance in normal human airways. Lancet 1977;2:375.

45. Jenne JW. Whither beta adrenergic tachyphylaxis? J Allergy Clin Immunol 1982; 70:413.

46. Jenne JW, Chick W, Strickland RD, Wall FJ. Subsensitivity of beta responses during therapy with long-acting beta-2 preparation. J Allergy Clin Immunol 1977;59:383.

47. Lipworth BJ, Struthers AD, McDevitt DG. Tachyphylaxis to systemic but not to airway responses during prolonged therapy with high dose inhaled salbutamol in asthmatics. Am Rev Respir Dis 1989;140:586.

48. Ebden P, Farrow PR, Shaw D, Cookson JB. 75 deaths in asthmatics prescribed home nebulizers. Br Med J 1987; 294:972.

49. Repsher LH, Anderson JA, Bush RK, et al. Assessment of tachyphylaxis following prolonged therapy of asthma with inhaled albuterol aerosol. Chest 1984;85:34.

50. Georgopoulos D, Wong D, Anthonien NR. Tolerance to beta$_2$ agonists in patients with chronic obstructive pulmonary disease. Chest 1990;97:280.

51. Vathenen AS, Knox AJ, Higgens BG, Britton JR, Tattersfield AE. Rebound increase in bronchial responsiveness after treatment with inhaled terbutaline. Lancet 1988;1:554.

52. Spector SL, Gomez MG. Dose-response curves to inhaled beta-adrenoreceptor agonists in normal and asthmatic subjects. J Allergy Clin Immunol 1977;59:280.

53. Drugs for asthma. Med Lett 1987;29:11.

54. Newhouse M, Dolovich M. Aerosol therapy: nebulizer versus metered dose inhaler. Chest 1987;91:799.

55. Colacone A, Wolkove N, Stern E, Afilalo M, Rosenthal TM, Kreisman H. Continuous nebulization of albuterol (salbutamol) in acute asthma. Chest 1990;97:693.

56. Shuh S. High dose continuous nebulization of albuterol for severe asthma is more effective than low dose. Pediatrics 1989;83:513.

57. Jenne JW, Ahrens RC. Pharmacokinetics of beta-adrenergic compounds. Part II. Inhaled route. In: Jenne JW, Murphy S, eds. Drug therapy for asthma. Research and clinical practice. New York: Marcel Dekker, 1987:213.

58. Moler FW, Hurwitz ME, Custer JR. Improvement in clinical asthma score and Paco$_2$ in children with severe asthma treated with continuously nebulized terbutaline. J Allergy Clin Immunol 1988;81:1101.

59. Kelly HW, McWilliams BC, Katz R, Murphy S. Safety of frequent high dose nebulized terbutaline in children with acute asthma. Ann Allergy 1990;64:229.

60. Nelson HS. Adrenergics in asthma. J Respir Dis 1986;7:43.

61. Murphy S, Kelly HW. Appendix. In: Jenne JW, Murphy S, eds. Drug therapy for asthma. Research and clinical practice. New York: Marcel Dekker, 1987:1044.

62. Appel DW, Karpel JP, Sherman M. Epinephrine improves expiratory flow rates in patients with asthma who do not respond to inhaled metaproterenol sulfate. J Allergy Clin Immunol 1989;84:90.

63. Jenne JW, Ridley DF, Marcucci R, Druz WS, Rook JC. Objective and subjective tremor responses to oral beta-2 agents on first exposure. Am Rev Respir Dis 1982;126:607.

64. Jenne JW, Valcarenghi G, Druz WS, Starkey PW, Yu C, Shaughnessy TK. Comparison of tremor responses to orally administered albuterol and terbutaline. Am Rev Respir Dis 1986;134:708.

65. Antonisen NR, Wright EC, IPPB Trial Group. Bronchial response in COPD. Am Rev Respir Dis 1986;133:1171.

66. Berger H, Smith D. Effect of inhaled metaproterenol on exercise performance in patients with stable "fixed" airway obstruction. Am Rev Respir Dis 1988;138:624.

67. Mattbaek N, Garsdal P, Christensen H, Bro H, Rasmussed FV. Effects of oral terbutaline in chronic airflow limitation. Chest 1989;95:1248.

68. Joseph X, Whitehurst VE, Bloom S, Balazs T. Enhancement of cardiotoxic effects of beta-adrenergic bronchodilators by aminophylline in experimental animals. Fundam Appl Toxicol 1981;1:443.

69. Sly RM, Jenne JW, Cohn J. Toxicity of beta-adrenergic drugs. In: Jenne JW, Murphy S, eds. Drug therapy for asthma. Research and clinical practice. New York: Marcel Dekker, 1987:953.

70. Light RW, Taylor RW, George RB. Albuterol and isoproterenol in bronchial asthma. Arch Intern Med 1979;139:639.

71. Allon M, Dunlay R, Copkney C. Nebulized albuterol for acute hyperkalemia in patients on dialysis. Ann Intern Med 1989;110:426.

72. Higgins RM, Cookson WOCM, Lane DJ, John SM, McCarthy GL, McCarthy ST. Cardiac arrhythmias caused by nebulized beta-agonist therapy. Lancet 1987;2:863.

73. Clifton GD, Hunt BA, Patel R, Burki NK. Effects of sequential doses of parenteral terbutaline on plasma levels of potassium and related cardiopulmonary responses. Am Rev Respir Dis 1990;141:575.

74. Lipworth BJ, McDevitt DG, Struthers AD. Electrocardiographic changes induced by inhaled salbutamol after treatment with bendrofluazide: effects of replacement therapy with potassium, magnesium, and triamterene. Clin Sci 1990;78:255.

75. Crane J, Pearce N, Flatt A, et al. Prescribed fenoterol and death from asthma in New Zealand, 1981–83: case–control study. Lancet 1989;1:917.

76. Pierce N, Grainger J, Atkinson M, et al. Case–control study of prescribed fenoterol and death from asthma in New Zealand. 1977–1981. Thorax 1990;42:14.

77. Crane J, Burgess C, Beasley R. Cardiovascular and hypokalemic effects of inhaled salbutamol, fenoterol and isoprenaline. Thorax 1989;44:136.

78. Flatt A, Burgess C, Windom H, Beasley R. The cardiovascular effects of inhaled fenoterol alone and during treatment with oral theophylline. Chest 1989;96:1317.

79. Tandon MK. Cardiopulmonary effects of fenoterol and salbutamol aerosols. Chest 1980;77:429.

80. Hendeles L, Weinberger M. Theophylline. A "state of the art" review. Pharmacotherapy 1983;3:2.

81. Jenne JW. Physiology and pharmacodynamics of theophylline. In: Jenne JW, Murphy S, eds. Drug therapy for asthma. Research and clinical practice. New York: Marcel Dekker, 1987:297.

82. Bakris GL, Sauter ER, Hussey JL, Fisher JW, Gaber AO, Winsett R. Effect of theophylline on erythropoetin in patients with erythrocytosis after renal transplant. N Engl J Med 1990;323:8690.

83. Enndin M, Picano E, Lattanzi F, L'Abbat CA. Improved exercise capacity with acute aminophylline administration in patients with syndrome X. J Am Coll Cardiol 1989;14:1450.

84. Polson JB, Krzanowski JJ, Szentivanyi A. Inhibition of a high affinity cyclic AMP phosphodiesterase and relaxation of canine tracheal smooth muscle. Biochem Pharmacol 1982;31:3403.

85. Aubier MA, DeTroyer A, Sampson M, Macklem PT, Roussos C. Aminophylline improves diaphragmatic contractility. N Engl J Med 1981;305:249.

86. Aubier MA, Murciano D, Viires N, Lecocquic Y, Palacios S, Pariente YR. Increased ventilation caused by improved diaphragmatic efficiency during aminophylline infusion. Am Rev Respir Dis 1983;27:148.

87. Aubier MA, Murciano D, Viires N, Lecocquic Y, Pariente R. Diaphragm contractility enhanced by aminophylline: role of extracellular Ca^+. Appl Physiol 1983;54:460.

88. Murciano D, Aubier MA, Lecocquic Y, Pariente R. Effect of theophylline on diaphragmatic strength and fatigue in patients with chronic obstructive pulmonary disease. N Engl J Med 1984;311:349.

89. Murciano D, Auclair M-H, Pariente R, Aubier M. A randomized controlled trial of theophylline in patients with severe chronic obstructive pulmonary disease. N Engl J Med 1989;320:1521.

90. Georgopoulos D, Holtby SG, Perezanski D, Anthonisen NR. Aminophylline effects on ventilatory response to hypoxia and hyperoxia in normal adults. J Appl Physiol 1989;67:1150.

91. Vestal RE, Erickson CE Jr, Musser B, Ozaki L, Halter JB. Effect of intravenous aminophylline on plasma levels of catecholamines and related cardiovascular and metabolic responses. Circulation 1983;67:162.

92. Parker JO, Ashekian PB, DiGeorgi S, et al. Hemodynamic effects of aminophylline in chronic obstructive pulmonary disease. Circulation 1967;35:365.

93. Matthay RA, Berger SA, Davies R, et al. Improvement in cardiac performance by oral long-term theophylline in chronic obstructive pulmonary disease. Am Heart J 1982;104:1022.

94. Burgess CD, Crane J, Graham AN, Maling TJB. The hemodynamic effects of aminophylline and salbutamol alone and in combination. Clin Pharmacol Ther 1986;40:550.

95. Erickson CE Jr, Writer SL, Vestal RE. Theophylline-induced alterations in cardiac electrophysiology in patients with chronic obstructive pulmonary disease. Am Rev Respir Dis 1987;135:322.

96. Weinberger M. Managing asthma. Baltimore: Williams & Wilkins, 1990.

97. Vestal RE, Cusack BJ, Mercer GD. Aging and drug reactions. I. Effects of cimetidine and smoking on the oxidation of theophylline and cortisol in healthy men. J Pharmacol Exp Ther 1987;241:488.

98. Au WYW, Dutt AK, DeSoyza N. Theophylline kinetics in chronic obstructive lung disease in the elderly. Clin Pharmacol Ther 1985;37:472.

99. Shin S-G, Juan D, Rammohan M. Theophylline pharmacokinetics in normal elderly subjects. Clin Pharmacol Ther 1988;44:522.

100. Mitenko PA, Ogilvie RI. Rational intravenous doses of theophylline. N Engl J Med 1973;289:600.

101. Rogers RM, Owens GR, Penock BE. The pendulum swings again: towards a rational use of theophylline [editorial]. Chest 1985;87:280.

102. Racineux JL, Troussier J, Tureant A. Comparison of bronchodilator effects of salbutamol and theophylline. Bull Eur Physiopathol Respir 1981;17:799.

103. Appel DW. Effect of aminophylline when added to metaproterenol sulfate and beclomethasone diproprionate aerosol. J Allergy Clin Immunol 1984;73:291.

104. Hill NS. The use of theophylline in "irreversible" chronic obstructive pulmonary disease. An update. Arch Intern Med 1988;148:2579.

105. Mahler DA, Matthay RA, Snyder PE, Wells CK, Loke J. Sustained release theophylline reduces dyspnea in non-reversible obstructive airway disease. Am Rev Respir Dis 1985;131:22.

106. Lakshminarayan S, Sahn SA, Weil JV. The effect of theophylline on ventilatory responses in normal men. Am Rev Respir Dis 1978;117:33.

107. Jenne JW, Siever JR, Druz WS, Solano JW, Cohen SM, Sharp JT. The effect of maintenance theophylline therapy on lung work in severe COPD while standing and walking. Am Rev Respir Dis 1984;130:600.

108. Richer C, Mathiew M, Bah H, Thurley C, Duroux P, Gludicelli J-F. Theophylline kinetics and ventilatory flow in chronic asthma and chronic airflow obstruction: influence of erythromycin. Clin Pharmacol Ther 1982;31:579.

109. Barclay J, Whiting B, Merideth PA, Addis CW. Theophylline–salbutamol interaction. Bronchodilator responses to salbutamol at maximally effective plasma theophylline concentrations. Br J Clin Pharmacol 1981;11:203.

110. Barclay J, Whiting B, Addis CJ. The influence of theophylline on maximal response to salbutamol in severe chronic obstructive pulmonary disease. Eur J Clin Pharmacol 1982;22:389.

111. Filuk RB, Easton PA, Anthonisen NR. Response to large doses of salbutamol and theophylline in patients with chronic obstructive pulmonary disease. Am Rev Respir Dis 1985;132:871.

112. Taylor DR, Buick B, Kinly C, Lowry RC, McDevitt DG. The efficacy of orally administered theophylline, inhaled salbutamol, and a combination of the two as chronic therapy in the management of chronic bronchitis with a reversible air flow obstruction. Am Rev Respir Dis 1985;131:747.

113. Guyatt GH, Townsend M, Pugsley SO, et al. Bronchodilators in chronic airflow limitation: effects on airway function, exercise capacity and quality of life. Am Rev Respir Dis 1987;135:1069.

114. Kelly HW. Theophylline toxicity. In: Jenne JW, Murphy S, eds. Drug therapy for asthma. Research and clinical practice. New York: Marcel Dekker, 1987:925.

115. Sessler CN. Theophylline toxicity: clinical features of 116 consecutive cases. Am J Med 1990;88:567.

116. Derby LE, Jick SS, Langbis JC, Johnson LE, Jick H. Hospital admission for xanthine toxicity. Pharmacotherapy 1990;10:112.

117. Olson KR, Benowitz NL, Woo OF, Pond SM. Theophylline overdose: acute single ingestion versus chronic repeated overmedication. Am J Emerg Med 1985;3:386.

118. Aitken ML, Martin TR. Life-threatening theophylline toxicity is not predictable by serum levels. Chest 1987;91:10.

119. Covelli HD, Knodel AR, Keppner BT. Predisposing factors to apparent theophylline-induced seizures. Ann Allergy 1985;54:411.

120. Creer TL, McLoughlin JA. The effects of theophylline on cognitive and behavioral performance [editorial]. J Allergy Clin Immunol 1989;83:1027.

121. Park GD, Spector R, Roberts RJ, et al. Use of hemoperfusion for treatment of theophylline intoxication. Am J Med 1983;74:961.

122. Martin RJ, Cicutto LC, Ballard RD, Goldenheim PD, Cherniack RM. Circadian variation in theophylline concentrations and the treatment of nocturnal bronchospasm. Am Rev Respir Dis 1989;139:475.

123. Lammers J-WJ, Minette P, McCusker M, Barnes PJ. The role of pirenzepine-sensitive (M_1) muscarinic receptors in vagally mediated bronchoconstriction in humans. Am Rev Respir Dis 1989;139:446.

124. Gross NJ, Skorodin MS. Anticholinergic agents. In: Jenne JW, Murphy S, eds. Drug therapy in asthma. Research and clinical practice. New York: Marcel Dekker, 1987:615.

125. Gross NJ, Skorodin MS. Anticholinergic antimuscarinic bronchodilator. Am Rev Respir Dis 1984;139:856.

126. Marlin GE, Bush DE, Berend N. Comparison of ipratropium bromide and fenoterol in asthma and chronic bronchitis. Br J Clin Pharmacol 1976;6:647.

127. Ullah MI, Newman GB, Saunders KB. Influence of age on response to ipratropium and salbutamol in asthma. Thorax 1981;36:523.

128. Summers QA, Tarala RA. Nebulized ipratropium in the treatment of acute asthma. Chest 1990;97:430.

129. Allen J, Campbell AH. Dose response of ipratropium bromide assessed by two methods. Thorax 1979;34:137.

130. Braun SR, McKenzie WN, Copeland C, et al. A comparison of the effect of ipratropium and albuterol in the treatment of chronic obstructive airway disease. Arch Intern Med 1989;149:544.

131. Bryant DH, Rogers P. Oxitropium bromide: an acute dose response study of a new anticholinergic drug in combination with fenoterol in asthma and chronic bronchitis. Pulmon Pharmacol 1990;3:55.

132. Frith PA, Jenner B, Dangerfield R, Atkinson J, Drennan E. Oxitropium bromide. Dose-response and time-response study of a new anticholinergic bronchodilator drug. Chest 1986;89:249.

133. Walker FB, Kaiser DL, Kowal MB, Suratt PM. Prolonged effect of inhaled glycopyrrolate in asthma. Chest 1987;91:49.

134. Gross NJ, Petty TL, Friedman M, Skorodin MS, Silvers GW, Donohue JF. Dose response to ipratropium as a nebulized solution in patients with chronic obstructive pulmonary disease. Am Rev Respir Dis 1989;139:1188.

135. Wyllie AH, Poznansky MC, Gordon ACH. Glucocorticoid-resistant asthma: evidence for a defect in mononuclear cells. In: Kay AB, ed. Asthma. Clinical pharmacology and therapeutic progress. Oxford: Blackwell Scientific Publications, 1986.

136. Guyre PM, Girard MT, Morganelli PM, Mangeniello PD. Glucocorticoid effects on the production and actions of immune cytokines. J Steroid Biochem 1988;30:89.

137. Shim CS, Williams MH. Cough and wheezing from beclomethasone diproprionate aerosol is absent after triamcinolone acetonide. Arch Intern Med 1987;106:700.

138. Williams AJ, Baghat MS, Stableforth DE, Cayton RM, Shenoi PM, Skinner C. Dysphonia caused by inhaled steroids: recognition of a characteristic laryngeal abnormality. Thorax 1983;38:813.

139. Toogood JA, Baskerville J, Jenning B, Lefcoe NM, Johansson SA. Bioequivalent doses of budesonide and prednisone in moderate and severe asthma. J Allergy Clin Immunol 1989;84:688.

140. Namsirkal D, Chaisupemongkollarp S, Chantadisai N, Bamberg P. Comparison of inhaled budesonide with oral prednisolone at two dose levels commonly used for the treatment of moderate asthma. Eur Respir J 1989;2:317.

141. Jenkins CR, Woolcock AJ. Effect of prednisone and beclomethasone diproprionate on airway responsiveness in asthma: a comparative study. Thorax 1988;43:378.

142. Salmeron S, Guerin J-C, Goard P, et al. High doses of inhaled corticosteroids in unstable chronic asthma. Am Rev Respir Dis 1989;140:167.

143. Kraan J, Koeter GH, Van Der Mark TW, et al. Dosage and time effects of inhaled budesonide on bronchial hyperreactivity. Am Rev Respir Dis 1988;137:44.

144. Toogood JA. Corticosteroids. In: Jenne JW, Murphy S, eds. Drug therapy for asthma. Research and clinical practice. New York: Marcel Dekker, 1987:719.

145. Cochrane GM. Systemic steroids in asthma. In: Clark TJH, ed. Steroids in asthma. Auckland: ADIS Press, 1983:103.

146. Luckert BP, Raisz LG. Glucocorticoid-induced osteoporosis: pathogenesis and management. Ann Intern Med 1990;112:352.

147. Murphy S. Cromolyn sodium: basic mechanisms and clinical usage. In: Pediatric asthma, allergy and immunology. New York: Mary Ann Liebert, 1988:237.

148. Flint KC, Leung KBP, Pierce FL, Hudspith BN, Brostoff J, Johnson NMCI. Human mast cells recovered from bronchoalveolar lavage: their morphology, histamine release, and effects of sodim cromoglycte. Clin Sci 1985;68:427.

149. Kay AB, Walsh GM, Moqbel R, et al. Disodium cromoglycate inhibits activation of human inflammatory cells in vitro. J Allergy Clin Immunol 1987;80:1.

150. Atkins PC, Norman ME, Zweiman B. Antigen-induced neutrophil chemotactic activity in man. Correlation with bronchospasm and inhibition by disodium cromoglycate. J Allergy Clin Immunol 1978;62:149.

151. Diaz P, Galleguillos FR, Gonzalez MC, Pantin CFA, Kay AB. Bronchoalveolar lavage in asthma: the effect of disodium cromoglycate (cromolyn) on leukocyte counts, immunoglobulins, and complement. J Allergy Clin Immunol 1984;286:722.

152. Harris MG. Bronchial irritant receptors and a possible new mode of action for cromolyn sodium. Ann Allergy 1981;46:156.

153. Myers DJ, Bigby BG, Boushey HA. The inhibition of sulfur dioxide bronchoconstriction in asthmatic subjects by cromolyn is dose-dependent. Am Rev Respir Dis 1986;133:1150.

154. Lowhagen O, Rak I. Effect of sodium cromoglycate and budesonide on bronchial hypereactivity in non-atopic asthmatics. Respiration 1984;46:105.

155. Petty TL, Rollins DR, Christopher K, Good JT, Oakley R. Cromolyn sodium is effective in adult chronic asthmatics. Am Rev Respir Dis 1989;139:694.

156. Ross RN, Morris M, Sakowitz SR, Berman BA. Cost-effectiveness of including

cromlyn sodium in the treatment program for asthma: a retrospective, record-based study. Clin Ther 1988;10:187.

157. Svendsen UG, Frolund L, Madsen F, Nielsen NH. A comparison of the effects of nedocromil sodium and beclomethasone diproprionate on pulmonary function, symptoms, and bronchial responsiveness in patients with asthma. J Allergy Clin Immunol 1989; 84:224.

158. Mullarkey MF, Lammert JK, Blumenstein BA. Long-term methotrexate treatment in corticosteroid-dependent asthma. Ann Intern Med 1990;112:577.

159. Carson CW, Cannon GW, Egger MJ, Eard JR, Clegg DO. Pulmonary disease during the treatment of rheumatoid arthritis with low dose pulse methotrexate. Semin Arthritis Rheum 1987;16:186.

160. Bernstein DI, Bernstein IL, Bodenheimer SS, Pietrusko RG. An open study of auranofin in the treatment of steroid-dependent asthma. J Allergy Clin Immunol 1988;81:6.

161. Tinkelman DG, Bucholtz GA, Kemp JP, et al. Evaluation of the safety and efficacy of multiple doses of azelastine to adult patients with bronchial asthma. Am Rev Respir Dis 1990;141:569.

162. Ziment I. Hydration, humidification, and mucokinetic therapy. In: Weiss EB, Segal MS, Stein M, eds. Bronchial asthma mechanisms and therapeutics. Boston: Little, Brown & Co, 1985:758.

163. Pavia D, Agnew JE, Glassman JM, et al. Effects of iodopropylidene glycerol on tracheobronchial clearance in stable, chronic bronchitic patients. J Respir Dis 1985;67:177.

164. Petty TL. The National Mucolytic Study. Results of a randomized, double-blind, placebo-controlled study of iodinated glycerol in chronic obstructive bronchitis. Chest 1990;97:75.

165. Chodosh S, Medici TC. The expectorant effect of glyceryl guiacolate [letter]. Chest 1973;64:543.

166. Hirsch SR, Zastrow JE, Kory RC. The expectorant effect of glyceryl guiacolate in patients with chronic bronchitis. A controlled in vitro and in vivo study. Chest 1973;63:9.

167. Brage PC, Ziment I, Allegra L. Classification of agents that act on bronchial mucus. In: Braga PC, Allegra L, eds. Drugs in bronchial mucology. New York: Raven Press, 1989:59.

168. Woolcock AJ. Use of corticosteroids in treatment of patients with asthma. J Allergy Clin Immunol 1989;84:975.

169. Beasley R, Cushley M, Holgate ST. A self management plan in the treatment of adult asthma. Thorax 1989;44:200.

170. Barnes PJ. Difficult asthma. Cause for concern. Br Med J 1989;299:695.

171. Ryan G, Latimer KM, Dolovich J, Hargrave FE. Bronchial responsiveness to histamine: relationship to diurnal variation of leak flow rate, improvement after bronchodilator and airway caliber. Thorax 1982;37:423.

172. Josephs LK, Gregg I, Mullee MA, Holgate ST. Non-specific bronchial reactivity and its relationship to the clinical expression of asthma. A longitudinal study. Am Rev Respir Dis 1989;190:350.

173. Turner-Warwick M. Epidemiology of nocturnal asthma. Am J Med 1988;85(1B):6.

174. Hetzel MR, Clark TJH. Adult asthma. In: Clark TJH, Godfrey S, eds. Asthma. London: Chapman & Hall, 1983:457.

175. Martin RJ, Cicutto LC, Ballard RD. Factors related to the nocturnal worsening of asthma. Am Rev Respir Dis 1990;141:33.

176. Zwillich CW, Neagley SR, Cicutto L, White DP, Martin RJ. Nocturnal asthma therapy. Inhaled bitolterol versus sustained-release theophylline. Am Rev Respir Dis 1989;139:470.

177. Dahl R, Pedersen B, Hagglof B. Nocturnal asthma: effect of treatment with oral

sustained-release terbutaline, inhaled budesonide, and the two in combination. J Allergy Clin Immunol 1989;83:811.

178. Bellamy D, Collins JV. "Acute" asthma in adults. Thorax 1979;34:36.

179. Bhagat RG, Grunstein MM. Comparison of responsiveness to methacholine and exercise in subgroups of asthmatic children. Am Rev Respir Dis 1984;129:221.

180. Bateman JRM, Clarke SW. Sudden death in asthma. Thorax 1979;34:40.

181. Jenkins PF, Benfield GFA, Smith AP. Predicting recovery from acute asthma. Thorax 1981;36:835.

182. Fanta CH, Rossing TH, McFadden ER. Emergency room treatment of asthma: relationship among therapeutic combinations, severity of obstruction and time course of response. Am J Med 1981;72:416.

183. Turner-Warwick M. On observing patterns of airflow obstruction in chronic asthma. Br J Dis Chest 1977;71:72.

184. Poznanski MC, Gordon ACH, Douglas JG, Krajewski AS, Wyllie AH, Grant IWB. Resistance to methylprednisolone in cultures of blood mononuclear cells from glucocorticoid-resistant asthmatic patients. Clin Sci 1984;67:639.

185. Rebuck AS, Read J. Assessment and management of severe asthma. Am J Med 1971;51:788.

186. Snider GL. Staging therapy to severity of asthma. In: Weiss EB, Segal MS, Stein M, eds. Bronchial asthma. Mechanisms and therapeutics. 2nd ed. Boston: Little, Brown & Co, 1985:

187. Fischl MA, Pitchenik A, Gardner LB. An index predicting relapse and need for hospitalization in patients with acute asthma. N Engl J Med 1981;305:783.

188. Haskell RJ, Wong BM, Hansen JE. A double-blind randomized clinical trial of methylprednisolone in status asthmaticus. Arch Intern Med 1983;143:1324.

189. Ziment I. Pharmacological therapy of obstructive airway disease. In: Hodgkin JE, ed. Chronic obstructive pulmonary disease. Clin Chest Med 1990;11:461.

190. American Thoracic Society official statement. Prevention of infleunze and pneumonia. Am Rev Respir Dis 1990;142:487.

191. American Thoracic Society. Guidelines for the approach to the patient with severe hereditary alpha-1-antitrypsin deficiency. Am Rev Respir Dis 1989;140:1494.

192. Altose MD, Hudgel DW. The pharmacology of respiratory depressants and stimulants. Clin Chest Med 1986;7:481.

193. Dudley DL, Sitzman J. Psychological evaluation and treatment of chronic obstructive pulmonary disease. In: Sweenay AJ, Grant I, eds. Chronic obstructive pulmonary disease: a behavioral prespective. New York: Marcel Dekker, 1988:183.

194. McDonald G, Borson S, Gayle T, et al. Nortriptyline effectively treats depression in COPD. Am Rev Respir Dis 1989;139(4 part 2).

195. Skatrud JB, Dempsey JA, Iber C, et al. Correction of CO_2 retention during sleep in patients with chronic obstructive pulmonary disease. Am Rev Respir Dis 1981;124:260.

196. Watanabe S, Kanner RE, Cotillo AG, et al. Long-term effects of almitrine bimesylate in patients with hypoxemic chronic obstructive pulmonary disease. Am Rev Respir Dis 1989;140:1269.

197. Sahn JA. Corticosteroids in chronic bronchitis and pulmonary emphysema. Chest 1978;73:389.

198. Eliason O, Hoffman J, Trueb D, et al. Corticosteroids in COPD. A clinical trial and reassessment of the literature. Chest 1986;89:484.

199. Postma DS, Steenhuis EJ, Van derWeele LT, Sluiter HJ. Severe chronic airflow obstruction: can corticosteroids slow down progression? Eur J Respir Dis 1985;65:56.

200. Berry RB, Shinto RA, Wong FH, Despars JA, Light RW. Nebulizer vs spacer for bronchodilator delivery in patients hospitalized for acute exacerbations of COPD. Chest 1989;96:1241.

201. Rice KI, Leatherman JW, Duane PG, et al. Aminophylline for acute exacerbations of chronic pulmonary disease—a controlled trial. Ann Intern Med 1987;107:305.

202. Albert RK, Martin TR, Lewis SW. Controlled clinical trial of methylprednisolone in patients with chronic bronchitis and acute respiratory insufficiency. Ann Intern Med 1980;92:753.

203. Glenny RW. Steroids in COPD. The scriptures according to Albert. Chest 1987;91:289.

204. Murata GH, Gorby MS, Chick TW, Halpern AK. Intravenous and oral corticosteroids for the prevention of relapse after treatment of decompensated COPD. Chest 1990;98:845.

205. Jenne JW. Pulmonary drugs. In: Bone RC, ed. Critical care. A comprehensive approach. Park Ridge, IL: Am College Chest Physicians, 1984:223.

206. Jenne JW. Theophylline as a bronchodilator in COPD and its combination with inhaled beta adrenergic drugs. Chest 1987;92:7S.

ROBERT M. KACMAREK

CARLOS A. VazFRAGOSO

10

Aerosol Therapy

The rationale behind the medications used in obstructive pulmonary disease comes from an understanding of its pathophysiology. It is currently accepted that the disease process involves an imbalance between proteases and protease inhibitors, acute and chronic inflammation, and altered cell proliferation.[1] The end result is tissue destruction, with disruption of the respiratory air spaces, replacement of ciliated columnar cells by squamous and goblet cell metaplasia, submucosal gland and smooth-muscle hypertrophy, infiltration by inflammatory cells, scarring, and various degrees of bronchial hyperreactivity.[2] These morphologic changes then contribute to increasing obstruction, sputum production, respiratory infections, or hyperinflation, leading to various levels of respiratory disability.[3] Therapy is aimed at slowing the decrement in the 1-second forced expiratory volume (FEV_1) and maximizing respiratory function. The first line of therapy often involves aerosolized medications. These are convenient for the patient and have the benefit of providing treatment locally where it is most needed, while minimizing systemic toxicities. This chapter focuses on the therapeutic role of aerosolized medications and their different modes of delivery in patients with chronic pulmonary disease.

BRONCHODILATORS

Bronchodilators are usually included as a first-line treatment in asthma and chronic obstructive pulmonary disease (COPD) in acute and chronic settings. The therapeutic goals are a reduction in the level of obstruction, primarily by inducing smooth-muscle relaxation, and an improvement in bronchopulmonary hygiene by increasing the rate of mucociliary clearance.[4] There are three major classes of bronchodilators currently in clinical use: sympathomimetics, anticholinergics, and methyl xanthines.

Sympathomimetics

The sympathomimetics refer to the β-agonists. Their mechanism of action involves the activation of β_2-receptors on the smooth muscle of the airway, leading to activation of the enzyme adenylate cyclase and an increase in cyclic-AMP (cAMP).[5] This results in a decrease in intracellular calcium concentration and eventual smooth-muscle relaxation. The various β-agonists differ, depending on the degree of their

β_2-selectivity. In general, the more β_2-selective the agent, the less the cardiovascular side effects for a given level of bronchodilation. This advantage, however, may be lost as the dose is increased. Additionally, the more β_2-selective agents have a greater delay in their peak effects, but a greater duration of action. Dosage of all β_2-agents is individualized, as some patients require larger than standard doses, but still exhibit minimal toxicity.[6] Examples of the various β_2-agonists and their respective characteristics are listed in Table 10–1. Another potential benefit of the sympathomimetics includes improvements in the rate of mucociliary clearance.[7,8] The evidence for this is sketchy, but has been shown to occur with both epinephrine and albuterol.[7,8]

The modes of delivery that are available for sympathomimetics include oral, aerosol, and parenteral. For the newer β_2-selective agonists, aerosolized preparations are the mode of choice, since their onset and duration of action is appropriate for short- and long-term therapy and the level of toxicity is low for the doses considered. The aerosol may be delivered by a metered-dose inhaler (MDI), with or without a spacing device, or by nebulizer. In certain clinical situations, the oral tablet form, with sustained release, may be of complementary value to the aerosol therapy, especially for overnight treatment. Whatever the ultimate route of administration or the delivery system, it is critical to consider the patient's ability to carry out the prescription. Modes of delivery are discussed later in the chapter.

The side effects of the sympathomimetics, especially in the case of the β_2-selective agonists, are usually minimal and well tolerated, but may include various degrees of tachycardia, palpitations, hypertension, nervousness, tremor, nausea, and vomiting. Additionally, patients may develop hypokalemia,[9] reduced arterial oxygen tensions,[10] arrhythmias (primarily supraventricular extrasystoles and tachycardias),[11] and ECG abnormalities (prolongation of the QT_c interval and depression of T-wave amplitude).[9,12] These changes could be accentuated when other classes of bronchodilators are being used concomitantly or during exacerbations of asthma or COPD when there can be coexisting hypoxia, acidosis, and cardiovascular disease.[9,11,12]

Anticholinergics

The anticholinergics are becoming more and more accepted as a first line of treatment in COPD. Their mechanism of action is most likely related to their ability to block muscarinic receptors in smooth muscle and to inhibit the cholinergically mediated reflex bronchoconstriction.[13,14] Atropine has long been known to be an effective bronchodilator, but its undesirable anticholinergic side effects have limited its use. Ipratropium bromide, a congener of methylatropine, is an even better bronchodilator, but without many of the problems associated with atropine.[13,14] At doses that provide bronchodilation there are minimal effects on bronchopulmonary secretions, cardiovascular parameters, glaucoma, or urinary retention.[13,14] They appear to be as effective, if not better, than the β-agonists in chronic bronchitis, but less so in asthma.[15,16] They may also enhance the effectiveness of the β_2-agonists, theophylline and steroids.[16,17] Another anticholinergic that is not currently available in the United States is oxitropium bromide,[18] which may be even more selective, more potent, and have a longer duration of action. Glycopyrrolate[19,20] is a quaternary anticholinergic

TABLE 10-1. Aerosolized Sympathomimetics

Drug	Brand Name(s)	Agonist Effect	Peak Effect (min)	Duration of Action (h)	Method of Administration	Strength	Standard* Dosage
Epinephrine	Adrenalin	$\beta_1 > \beta_2$	3–5	1–1.5	Nebulizer	1:100(1.0%)	0.25–0.5 mL
Racemic epinephrine	MicroNefrin VapoNefrin Asthma Nefrin	$\beta_1 = \beta_2$	3–5	1–1.5	Nebulizer	2.25%	0.25–0.5 mL
Isoproterenol sulfate	Isuprel	$\beta_1 = \beta_2$	5–15	1–1.5	Nebulizer MDI	1:200(0.5%) 131 μg/puff	0.25–0.5 mL 1–2 puffs
Isoetharine mesylate	Bronkosol	$\beta_1 < \beta_2$	15–60	2–4	Nebulizer MDI	1% 340 μg/puff	0.25–0.5 mL 1–2 puffs
Metaproterenol sulfate	Alupent Metaprel	$\beta_1 < \beta_2$	30–60	3–4	Nebulizer MDI	5% 0.65 mg/puff	0.3 mL 2–3 puffs
Terbutaline sulfate	Brethaire Brethine Bricanyl	$\beta_1 << \beta_2$	10–30	4–6	MDI	0.2 mg/puff	2 puffs
Albuterol	Proventil Ventolin	$\beta_1 << \beta_2$	30–60	4–6	Nebulizer MDI	0.5% 90 μg/puff	0.5 mL 2 puffs
Bitolterol mesylate	Tornalate	$\beta_1 <<< \beta_2$	60	3–6	MDI	0.37 mg/puff	2 puffs
Fenoterol	N/A	$\beta_1 <<< \beta_2$	30–60	6–8	MDI	0.2 mg/puff	1–2 puffs
Pirbuterol acetate	Maxair	$\beta_1 <<< \beta_2$	30–60	5	MDI	0.2 mg/puff	2 puffs
Salmeterol	N/A	$\beta_1 <<< \beta_2$	60	12	MDI	Not determined	Not determined

* Doses should be individualized to the patient's needs and level of toxicity.
β_1, inotropic and chronotropic effects; β_2, bronchodilation, vasodilation, and tremors.
N/A, not yet available in the United States.

that has also been shown to be an effective bronchodilator, with minimal side effects. Table 10–2 summarizes the various anticholinergics currently available.

The mode of delivery for the anticholinergics has been limited to aerosolized preparations, whether it be by MDI or by nebulizer. Currently, ipratropium bromide is available only in the MDI form in the United States. Alternatively, glycopyrrolate may be given by nebulizer.

Methyl Xanthines

The aerosolized preparations of the methyl xanthines are highly irritating and much less effective than the β-agonists, and thus are not in clinical use.[21] Therefore, they are administered by either the intravenous route or by the enteral route. The role of these agents in the treatment of obstructive airways disease is discussed in Chapter 9.

STEROIDS

In the introduction, a brief description of the pathophysiology of obstructive airways disease was presented. On the basis of that discussion, it can be seen that steroids, by virtue of their anti-inflammatory properties (Table 10–3), could have a significant therapeutic effect. In particular, the inflammatory reaction and the bronchial hyperreactivity that is observed could be minimized. In addition, steroids may enhance the effectiveness of bronchodilators, especially the β-agonists. All of this could lead to reduced obstruction, decreased sputum production and, ultimately, improvements in respiratory function. This is an ideal scenario, but the potential toxicity of steroids (Table 10–4) requires one to be highly selective and to consider other alternatives.

The patient with the best risk to benefit ratio for steroids is one who has demonstrated some degree of "reversibility." *Reversibility* is not easily defined, in view of the large component of fixed airway obstruction that is present in COPD, but it may be suggested by (1) a history of bronchial hyperreactivity, or previous significant responses to an inhaled bronchodilator during pulmonary function testing (PFTs); (2) a clinical course that is remarkable for periods of documented improvements in obstruction; (3) elevated IgE levels, with or without systemic or sputum eosinophilia; (4) sputum production as a major feature of the presentation; or (5) a therapeutic response by PFTs to a 2- to 3-week course of a moderate dose of prednisone (0.5 mg/kg per day). Once reversibility has been demonstrated and bronchodilator therapy has been maximized, the next step is to establish the lowest dose of steroid that is required to obtain the desired therapeutic endpoint. The endpoint must be individualized, as it may differ, depending on whether it is an acute or chronic setting. Steroids may be administered orally, by aerosol, or parenterally (intramuscular or intravenous), with the route of delivery being largely determined by the amount one wishes to prescribe. Inhaled steroids should be considered when the prednisone dose requirements fall to approximately 10 mg or less and, consequently, are rarely ever used acutely. When the oral prednisone dose is above 10 to 20 mg/day, inhaled steroids may be used as adjuncts, but not as substitutes, in an attempt to achieve as low a systemic dose as possible, thereby minimizing toxicity. They are usually administered by an MDI, with or without a spacing device, and to ensure

TABLE   10-2.   **Aerosolized Anticholinergics**

Drug	Brand Name(s)	Anticholinergic Effect	Peak Effect (min)
Atropine sulfate	Dry-Dose atropine	+++	30–60
Ipratropium bromide	Atrovent	+	60–120
Glycopyrrolate	Robinul	+	30–60
Oxitropium bromide	Experimental agent	+	120

maximal benefit should be given after a bronchodilator treatment. Table 10–5 summarizes the various aerosolized forms of steroids currently available.

The side effects of inhaled steroids are minimal when used judiciously.[22] They include those related to oropharyngeal deposition, such as a sore throat, hoarseness, and oral candidiasis. These are minimized by a proper technique when administering the MDI, rinsing the mouth after use, or use of a spacing device. Suppression of the hypothalamic–pituitary–adrenal axis is a potential complication when large doses of the drug are administered. The level of suppression can vary from patient to patient, but is unusual at doses below 1500 μg/day.[23]

ANTIBIOTICS

When antibiotics are given systemically in the treatment of COPD exacerbations, there is a significant benefit, especially when the presentation is associated with changes in the baseline sputum production (i.e., due to increasing bronchitis).[24] The need for aerosolized forms of antibiotics has not been a major issue in COPD owing to the availability of effective systemic antibiotics with minimal toxicity and relatively good lung tissue penetration, and because of the respiratory pathogens involved and the episodic nature of the attacks. The same is not true when considering cystic fibrosis (CF).[25] Here, the disease is more persistent and the respiratory pathogens are such (*Pseudomonas* species) that there is significant drug resistance, requiring antibiotics with relatively poor tissue penetration and high toxicities (aminoglycosides). As a result, the experience with aerosolized antibiotics has largely been limited to CF in the United States. It should be emphasized that this discussion on aerosolized antibiotics is limited to bronchitic episodes. In the setting of pneumonia, systemic therapy is the primary mode of delivery, as sepsis and other related complications may occur.

TABLE   10-3.   **Anti-Inflammatory Properties of Steroids**

Reduce microvascular permeability
Reduce the inflammatory response (cellular and cytokines)
Reduce the down-regulation of β_2-receptors
Reduce bronchial hyperreactivity

TABLE 10-2. (*continued*)

Duration of Action (h)	Method of Administration	Strength	Standard Dosage
3–4	Nebulizer	0.29% or 0.5%	0.025 mg/kg
4–6	MDI	18 μg/puff	2–3 puffs
6	Nebulizer	0.2 mg/mL	5 mL
6–8	MDI	100 μg/puff	2 puffs

MUCOLYTICS

Numerous mucolytic agents (mercaptoethanol sulfate, bromhexine hydrochloride, deoxyribonuclease, trypsin, chymotrypsin, streptokinase, and L-arginine) have been available over the years; however, only one, acetylcysteine (Mucomyst) is currently recommended for use.[26,27] Acetylcysteine is the N-acetyl derivative of the amino acid L-cysteine. It disrupts the structure of mucus molecules by substituting its own sulfhydril groups for the disulfide bonds in the mucus.[27] In acute increases in secretion volume and viscosity, acetylcysteine does reduce the viscosity of secretions and enhance removal. However, provided appropriate systemic hydration is maintained, there appears to be no indication for the routine use of this agent in the long-term management of patients with COPD. Major side effects of this agent are bronchospasm and bronchorrhea.[26] As a result, it should always be administered after, or in conjunction with, a bronchodilator (see Table 10–6). In addition to being nebulized, acetylcysteine may be directly instilled through an artificial airway. Periodic instillations of 5 mL of the 10% solution in tracheostomized patients, followed by suctioning, does help prevent crusting of secretions and airway obstruction. Instillation does not normally produce the level of bronchospasm noted with nebulization, but coordination with bronchodilator therapy is still recommended.

TABLE 10-4. **Toxic Effects of steroids**

Osteoporosis
Hypertension
Diabetes mellitus
Aseptic necrosis
Myopathy
Peptic ulcer disease
Susceptibility to infections
Skin fragility
Metabolic alkalosis
Psychosis
Cataracts
Adrenal suppression

TABLE 10-5. Inhaled Steroids

Drug	Brand Name(s)	Method of Administration	Strength	Standard Dosage
Dexamethasone sodium phosphate	Decadron Respihaler	MDI	84 μg/puff	3 puffs
Beclomethasone dipropionate	Beclovent, Vanceril	MDI	42 μg/puff	2 puffs
Triamcinolone acetonide	Azmacort	MDI	100 μg/puff	2 puffs
Flunisolide	Aerobid	MDI	250 μg/puff	2 puffs

COMBINATION THERAPY

There is reasonable evidence to suggest that the efficacy of a drug is enhanced when used in combination with other drugs, and toxicity may be minimized by the resultant ability to use lower doses. This has been seen with the β-agonists and anticholinergics, methyl xanthines, and steroids.[28–30] In general, the physiologic abnormality of COPD is such that, depending upon the severity of symptoms, combination therapy becomes the rule, rather than the exception.

BLAND AEROSOLS

Historically, the use of intermittent or continuous bland aerosols (water, normal saline solution) has been recommended in the management of the patient with chronic pulmonary disease.[31,32] However, contrary to popular belief, the short-term intermittent use of bland aerosols does not deposit sufficient fluid on the airway to liquify secretions. A typical 10- to 20-minute bland aerosol treatment delivers only 1 to 2 mL of fluid to the airway surface,[33] and the mucous gel layer is relatively impervious to absorption of water.[34,35] It is theorized that these aerosols enhance sputum production by irritation of subepithelial cough receptors in the trachea and bronchi, initiating a vagally mediated reflex production of mucus, cough, and increased airways resistance.[35,36] There is, however, a small group of patients with cystic fibrosis who may benefit from the periodic administration of bland aerosol therapy by ultrasonic nebulizer. This group of patients presents with thick, tenacious

TABLE 10-6. Mucolytics

Drug	Brand Name	Method of Administration	Strength	Standard
Acetylcysteine	Mucomyst	Nebulizer*	20%	3–5 mL
			10%	6–10 mL
		Instillation	10%	5 mL

* Administer after, or in conjunction with, a bronchodilator.

secretions, despite maintenance of systemic hydration. The output of ultrasonic nebulizers (3 to 6 mL/minute) greatly exceeds that of mechanical nebulizers (0.5 to 1.0 mL/minute), as a result the volume of fluid deposited on the airway may be sufficient to enhance bronchial hygiene, in spite of the short-term application (20 to 30 minutes).

The routine use of bland aerosols is rarely indicated, except as a diluent during the delivery of other nebulized pharmacologic agents. Appropriate systemic hydration combined with other bronchial hygiene techniques (proper breathing techniques, cough, and postural drainage) appear more appropriate than bland aerosols in maintaining airway clearance. In the patient with a tracheostomy, nocturnal continuous bland aerosol therapy or humidity therapy is frequently indicated because the upper airway is permanently bypassed. However, many patients do acclimate to tracheostomy without the need for bland aerosol therapy. In general, the factor determining need is the patient's ability to handle his or her secretions. If systemic hydration and other bronchial hygiene techniques are able to ensure secretion clearance, continuous bland aerosol or humidity therapy is unnecessary.

When continuous aerosol or humidity therapy is used, the question of heating the system always arises. When a humidifier is used, the system should be heated to 32° to 35°C, or insufficient water vapor will be delivered to the airway to prevent insensible water loss. However, if an aerosol is used, heating is dependent on patient comfort. Whether the aerosol is heated or not, sufficient water is normally delivered to the airway to correct a water deficit. In the case of the unheated aerosol, the water carried in particulate form is converted to water vapor as the gas temperature increases upon entering the patient.

MODE OF AEROSOL DELIVERY

Aerosolized pharmacologic agents can be delivered by a variety of devices; however, the most common and efficient methods are the gas-powered nebulizer and the MDI. Either of these two approaches may be used during spontaneous breathing or during intermittent positive-pressure breathing (IPPB). Aerosols deposit on surfaces of the respiratory tract by sedimentation and inertial impaction, the larger (more than 5-μm mass median diameter; MMD) aerosol particles settle in the upper respiratory tract, whereas particles of 2- to 5-μm MMD settle in the airways and smaller particles (1- to 2-μm MMD) deposit at the alveolar level.[37,38]

Regardless of the method used to administer an aerosolized pharmacologic agent, an appropriate-breathing pattern is necessary to ensure maximum penetration and deposition of the drug within the lung (see Table 10–7). Factors affecting penetration and deposition include the route (oral or nasal breathing): generally a larger volume of the drug deposits in the nose and nasal pharynx than in the mouth and oral pharynx; inspiratory flow rate: a peak inspiratory flow rate of less than 30 L/minute ensures greater peripheral deposition[39] than higher flows; and lung volume at which the drug is inhaled. Lung volume is primarily a concern with MDIs. Contrasting data[40,41] exist concerning the most appropriate lung volume to begin inhalation of a drug from an MDI. Some believe the drug should be inhaled during the last 20% of an inspiratory capacity maneuver, whereas others believe the MDI should

TABLE 10-7.   Breathing Pattern with MDIs and Nebulizers

Inspire through a wide-open mouth
Inspire slowly over a 2- to 3-second period, or longer
Inspire to total lung capacity
Position MDIs at lips to about 4 cm from the mouth
With MDIs, activate shortly after inspiration has begun
Hold maximum inspiration for 5–10 seconds.

be activated after the first 20% of the inspiratory capacity is inspired. Most do agree inhalation of the drug should occur during a near inspiratory capacity maneuver. Finally, a breath hold of 5 to 10 seconds enhances peripheral deposition by ensuring sufficient time for settling and inertial impaction.[39] Also, to avoid deposition in the mouth, the mouth should be opened wide during inspiration and, if an MDI is used, it should be held at lips to about 4 cm from the mouth when activated.[42,43]

Jet Nebulizers

The most common method of delivering an aerosolized drug is through a jet nebulizer. These units produce an aerosol on a continuous basis and must be powered by a compressed gas source. With all jet nebulizers, a relatively large volume of drug (see Table 10–1) must be used, since almost all of the drug nebulized is lost to environment. The efficiency of jet nebulizers is dependent on several factors, including

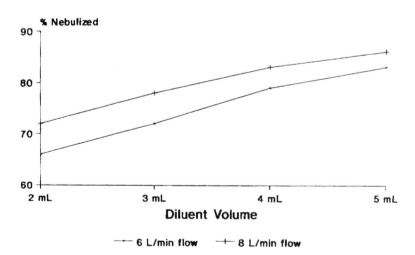

— 6 L/min flow   — 8 L/min flow

FIGURE 10-1   Relation between gas flow and diluent volume on percentage of total drug volume nebulized. A diluent volume of 4 to 5 mL with a nebulizer flow of 8 L/min results in the largest drug volume delivered. (Hess D, et al. Medication–delivery performance of eight small-volume, hand-held nebulizers: effects of diluent volume, gas flow rate and nebulizer model. Respir Care 1988;34:717, with permission)

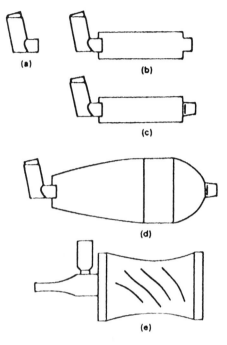

FIGURE 10-2 Schematic of common MDI delivery systems currently available: (*a*) actuator alone; (*b*) open-end straight tube; (*c*) Aerochamber (Monaghan Medical Corp., Plattsburg, NY; (*d*) Nebuhaler (Astra Pharmaceutical Products, Worcester, MA; (*e*) InspirEase (Key Pharmaceuticals). (Kim CS, et al. Oropharyngeal deposition and delivery aspects of metered dose inhaler aerosols. Am Rev Respir Dis 1987;135:157, with permission)

volume of fluid to be nebulized, flow of gas into the nebulizer, and nebulizer design (Fig. 10–1). Regardless of design, jet nebulizers all have a *dead volume*,[44,45] that is, a volume of fluid that cannot be nebulized because of the design and operation of the unit (Fig. 10–2). In addition, as the nebulization of the fluid continues, the solution cools because of evaporate heat loss,[46] and the solution becomes more concentrated.[47] Cooling of the solution has also been associated with a decrease in aerosol particle size,[47] believed to result from a greater amount of water evaporating from the aerosol particles as the gas is warmed to room rather than to body temperature.[48]

As a result, the following guidelines should be followed when prescribing aerosol therapy with a jet nebulizer: (1) The total volume of solution should be about 4 mL.[49,50] This appears to be the optimal volume ensuring maximal drug delivery in spite of the dead volume. (2) The gas flow to the nebulizer should be set between 6 and 8 L/minute.[49,50,51] (3) Ideally, a compressor delivering room air is used to power the jet nebulizer. The higher the relative humidity of the gas driving the nebulizer, the more stable the particle size.[48] (4) Although impractical to achieve, the temperature of the nebulizer should be kept constant (room temperature or higher) throughout the treatment.

Metered-Dose Inhalers

The MDI devices deliver a single squirt or puff of a pharmacologic solution with each actuation. The puff lasts only a fraction of a second and must be inhaled promptly. Proper use of an MDI requires appropriate instruction and the capability of coordinating hand and breathing movements.[52,55] Instruction is a key factor, without which results of therapy vary considerably.[56,57] It is essential that a skilled health care worker instruct and supervise the initial use of these devices to maximize effect.[58,59]

In patients with difficulty coordinating hand–breathing movements, the use of spacers (see Fig. 10–2) greatly improves the efficiency of lung penetration and deposition.[53,54] When an MDI is used with a spacer, the patient actuates the MDI, aerosolizing the solution into the spacer, then inspires the aerosol from the spacer by use of a mouthpiece. The spacer serves two functions: to contain the aerosol to eliminate the need for hand–breath coordination, and to allow for impaction and fall out of large aerosol particles that would otherwise deposit in the mouth and pharynx and cause adverse effects.[48,55] The development of spacers has greatly increased the number of patients capable of benefiting from properly using MDIs.

Jet Nebulizers Versus Metered-Dose Inhalers

Which is preferable for a given patient, a jet nebulizer or MDI? Given the available data, it appears that MDIs, without[60–64] or with spacers,[65–68] produce the same physiologic response as a jet nebulizer, provided equivalent quantities of the drug are deposited on the airway and the patient is able to properly use the MDI. As a result, in the setting of acute airways obstruction (status asthmaticus), a jet nebulizer is preferred. With both devices, only about 10% of the aerosol produced actually deposits in the lower respiratory tract (Figs. 10–3 and 10–4).[69,70] With MDI, the remainder is deposited in the mouth and pharynx, in the spacer, or is exhaled, whereas during continuous jet nebulization, a large volume of aerosol is lost to the environment, left in the nebulizer as dead volume, deposited in the mouth and pharynx, or exhaled.

Cost, complexity, and patient ability to use the device properly essentially determine which of these should be used. Since the MDI, even with spacer, is much less costly than the jet nebulizer,[48,60,61] and the MDI is much easier to maintain, in *patients capable of properly using* an MDI, the MDI is the method of choice. However, the efficiency of the MDI falls rapidly if used improperly. Patient ability to appropriately use the MDI is the single factor determining the method of aerosol

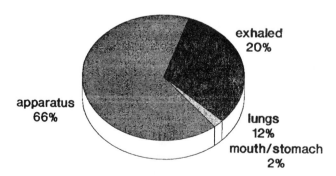

FIGURE   10-3   Distribution of nebulizer volume deposition from jet nebulizers. (Adapted from Lewis RA, Fleming JS. Fractional deposition from a jet nebulizer: How it differs from a metered-dose inhaler. Br J Dis Chest 1985;79:361)

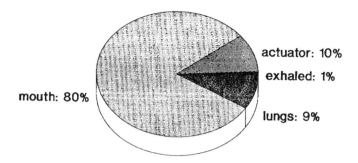

FIGURE   10-4   Distribution of nebulizer volume deposition from MDIs. (Adapted from Newman SP, et al. Deposition of pressurized aerosols in the human respiratory tract. Thorax 1981;36:52)

administration. Given the available information, the MDI is always the first choice for mode of delivery.

Intermittent Positive-Pressure Breathing

An alternate approach to the delivery of aerosolized drugs is the use of intermittent positive-pressure breathing (IPPB). Historically, this mode of delivery was frequently employed; however, no data indicating enhanced physiologic response with IPPB has ever been established. In the NIH-sponsored study comparing IPPB therapy with compressor nebulizer therapy in patients with COPD, no difference was noted in any of the outcome measurements between these two techniques for aerosolizing bronchodilators.[71] As a result, there is no indication for the use of IPPB as a means of delivering aerosolized medication in outpatients with obstructive airways disease.

REFERENCES

1. Nadel JA. General principles and diagnostic approach to obstructive lung disease. In: Murray JF, Nadel JA, eds. Textbook of respiratory medicine. Philadelphia: WB Saunders, 1988.

2. Mitchell RS, Silvers GW, Dart GA, et al. Morphologic correlations in chronic airway obstruction. Am Rev Respir Dis 1968;97:54.

3. Snider GL. Chronic bronchitis and emphysema. In: Murray JF, Nadel JA, eds. Textbook of respiratory medicine. Philadelphia: WB Saunders, 1988.

4. Schwartzstein RM, Weiss ST. Sympathomimetic bronchodilators, anticholinergics, and cromolym sodium. In: Kacmarek RM, Stoller JK, eds. Current respiratory care. Toronto: BC Decker, 1988.

5. Stiles GL, Caron MG, Lefkowitz RJ. β-Adrenergic receptors: biochemical mechanisms of physiological regulation. Physiol Rev 1984;64:661.

6. Jenkins S, Moxham J. High-dose salbutamol in chronic bronchitis: comparison of 400 μg, 1 mg, 1.6 mg, 2 mg and placebo delivered by Rotahaler. Br J Dis Chest 1987;81:242.

7. Foster WM, Bergofsky EH, Bohning DE, Lippmann M, Albert RE. Effect of adrenergic agents and their mode of action on mucociliary clearance in man. J Appl Physiol 1976;41:146.

8. Fazio F, Lafortuna D. Effects of inhaled salbutamol on mucociliary clearance in patients with chronic bronchitis. Chest 1981;80:S827.

9. Crane J, Burgess CD, Graham AN, Maling TJB. Hypokalaemic and electrocardiographic effects of aminophylline and salbutamol in obstructive airways disease. NZ Med J 1987;100:309.

10. Tai E, Read J. Response of blood gas tensions to aminophylline and isporenaline in patients with asthma. Thorax 1967;22:543.

11. Eidelman DH, Sami MH, McGregor M, Cosio MG. Combination of theophylline and salbutamol for arrhythmias in severe COPD. Chest 1987;91:808.

12. Flatt A, Burgess C, Windom H, Beasley R, Purdie G, Crane J. The cardiovascular effects of inhaled fenoterol alone and during treatment with oral theophylline. Chest 1989;96:1317.

13. Cugell D. Clinical pharmacology and toxicology of ipratropium bromide. Am J Med 1986;81(S5A):18.

14. Gross NJ. Ipratropium bromide. N Engl J Med 1988;319:486.

15. Comparison of the anticholinergic bronchodilator ipratropium bromide with metaproterenol in chronic obstructive pulmonary disease: a 90-day multicenter study. Am J Med 1986;81(S5A):81.

16. Easton PA, Jadue C, Dhingra S, Anthonisen NR. A comparison of the bronchodilating effects of a beta-2-adrenergic agent (albuterol) and an anticholinergic agent (ipratropium bromide) given by aerosol alone, or in sequence. N Engl J Med 1986;315:735.

17. Lightbody IM, Ingram CC, Legge JS, Johnston RN. Ipratropium bromide, salbutamol, and prednisolone in bronchial asthma and chronic bronchitis. Br J Dis Chest 1978;72:181.

18. Frith PA, Jenner B, Atkinson J. Effects of inhaled oxitropium and fenoterol, alone and in combination, in chronic airflow obstruction. Respiration 1986;50(suppl2):294.

19. Walker FB, Kaiser DL, Kowal MB, Suratt PM. Prolonged effect of inhaled glycopyrrolate in asthma. Chest 1987;91:49.

20. Gal TJ, Suratt PM, Lu JY. Glycopyrrolate and atropine inhalation: comparative effects on normal airway function. Am Rev Respir Dis 1984;129:871.

21. Bohadana AB, Peslin R, Teculescu D, Polu JM, Belleville F, Massin N. The bronchodilator action of theophylline aerosol in subjects with chronic airflow obstruction. Bull Eur Physiopathol Respir 1980;16:13.

22. Clark TJH. Safety of inhaled corticosteroids. Eur J Respir Dis 1982;63(suppl122):235.

23. Smith MJ, Hodson ME. Effects of long-term inhaled high-dose beclomethasone dipropionate on adrenal function. Thorax 1983;38:676.

24. Anthonisen NR, Manfreda J, Warren CPW, Hershfield ES, Harding GKM, Nelson NA. Antibiotic therapy in exacerbations of chronic obstructive pulmonary disease. Ann Intern Med 1987;106:196.

25. Hodson ME. Antibiotic treatment aerosol therapy. Chest 1988;94:156S.

26. Seligman M. Mucolytics. In: Kacmarek RM, Stoller J, ed. Current respiratory care. Toronto: BC Decker, 1988.

27. Rau JL. Respiratory Care Pharmacology. 3rd ed. Chicago: Mosby—Year Book Medical Publishers, 1989.

28. Barnabe R, Pirrelli M, Rossi M. Combined inhalation of fenoterol and ipratropium bromide in long-term therapy of chronic reversible airway obstruction. Respiration 1986;50(suppl2):232.

29. Dullinger D, Kronenberg R, Niewoehner DE. Efficacy of inhaled metaproterenol and orally administered theophylline in patients with chronic airflow obstruction. Chest 1986;89:171.

30. Ajewski Z, Popiak B. The relation between permanent administration of Atrovent and the dose of steroid in chronic bronchitis [Abstract]. Scand J Respir Dis [Suppl] 1979;103:205.

31. Cushing IE, Miller WF. Nebulization therapy. In: Safar P, ed. Respiratory therapy. Philadelphia: FA Davis, 1965.

32. Miller WF. Aerosol therapy in acute and chronic respiratory disease. Arch Intern Med 1973;131:148.

33. Rau JL. Humidity and aerosol therapy. In: Barnes TA, ed. Respiratory care practice. Chicago: Mosby–Year Book Medical Publishers, 1988.

34. Dulfano JJ, Adler KB. Physical properties of sputum: VII Rheologic properties and mucociliary transport. Am Rev Respir Dis 1973;107:140.

35. Pavia D, Thomson ML, Clarke SW. Enhanced clearance of secretions from the human lung after the administration of hypertonic saline aerosol. Am Rev Respir Dis 1978;117:199.

36. Gold WM. Vagally-mediated reflex bronchoconstriction in allergic asthma. Chest 1973(suppl);63:11.

37. Morrow PE. Aerosol characterization and deposition. Am Rev Respir Dis 1974;110:88.

38. Swift DL. Aerosols and humidity therapy: generations and respiratory deposition of therapeutic aerosols. Am Rev Respir Dis 1980(suppl);122:71.

39. Newhouse MT, Ruffin RE. Deposition and path of aerosolized drugs. Chest 1978(suppl);73:936.

40. Riley DJ, Liu RT, Edelman NH. Enhanced responses to aerosolized bronchodilator therapy in asthma using respiratory maneuvers. Chest 1978;76:501.

41. Newmen SP. Effects of various inhalation modes on the deposition of radioactive pressurized aerosols. Eur J Respir Dis 1982(suppl);119:57.

42. Eriksson NE, Haglind K, Hidinger KG. A new inhalation technique from Freon aerosols: terbutaline aerosol with a tube extension in a two-day crossover comparison with salbutamol aerosol. Allergy 1980;35:617.

43. Pedersen S. Aerosol treatment of bronchoconstriction in children, with or without a tube spacer. N Engl J Med 1983;308:1328.

44. Massey DG, Miyauchi D, Fournier-Massey G. Nebulizer function. Bull Eur Physiopathol Respir 1982;18:655.

45. Arossa W, Quagliotti F, Sola M, Spinaci S, DeCandussio G. Different performance of two commercial nebulizers. Respiration 1984;46:128.

46. Wood JA, Wilson RSE, Bray C. Changes in salbutamol concentration in the reservoir solution of a jet nebulizer. Br J Dis Chest 1986;80:164.

47. Phipps PR, Gonda I. Droplets produced by medical nebulizers: some factors affecting their size and solute concentration. Chest 1990;97:1327.

48. Hess D. How should bronchodilators be administered to patients on ventilators? Respir Care (editorial) 1990;35:399–404.

49. Clay MM, Pavia D, Newman SP, Lennard-Jones T, Clarke SW. Assessment of jet nebulizers for lung aerosol therapy. Lancet 1983;2:592.

50. Hess D, Horney D, Snyder T. Medication-delivery performance of eight small-volume, hand-held nebulizers: effect of diluent volume, gas flow rate, and nebulizer model. Respir Care 1989;34:717.

51. Kradjan WA, Lakshminarayan S. Efficiency of air compressor-driven nebulizers. Chest 1985;87:512.

52. Konig P. Spacer devices used with metered-dose inhalers: breakthrough or gimmick? Chest 1985;88:276.

53. Tobin MJ, Jenouri G, Danta I, Kim C, Watson H, Sackner MA. Response to bronchodilator drug administration by a new reservoir aerosol delivery system and a review of other auxiliary delivery systems. Am Rev Respir Dis 1982;126:670.

54. Kim CS, Eldridge MA, Sackner MA. Oropharynx deposition and delivery aspects of metered-dose inhaler aerosols. Am Rev Respir Dis 1987;135:157.

55. Newmen SP, Moren F, Pavia D, Little F, Clarke SW. Deposition of pressurized suspension aerosols inhaled through extension devices. Am Rev Respir Dis 1981;124:317.

56. Self TH, Brooks JB, Lieberman P, Ryan MR. The value of demonstration and role of the pharmacist in teaching the correct use of pressurized bronchodilators. Can Med Assoc J 1983;128:129.

57. DeTullio PL, Corson ME. Effect of pharmacist counseling on ambulatory patients' use of aerosolized bronchodilators. Am J Hosp Pharm 1987;44:1802.

58. Armitage JM, Williams SJ. Inhaler technique in the elderly. Age Aging 1988;17:275.

59. Allen SC, Prior A. What determines whether an elderly patient can use a metered dose inhaler correctly? Br J Dis Chest 1986;80:45.

60. Jasper AC, Mohsenifar Z, Kahan S, Goldberg H, Koerner SK. Cost–benefit comparison of aerosol bronchodilator delivery methods in hospitalized patients. Chest 1987;91:614.

61. Summer W, Elston R, Tharpe L, Nelson S, Haponik EF. Aerosol bronchodilator delivery methods: relative impact on pulmonary function and cost of respiratory care. Arch Intern Med 1989;149:618.

62. Mestitz H, Copland JM, McDonald CF. Comparison of outpatient nebulized vs metered dose inhaler terbutaline in chronic airflow obstruction. Chest 1989;96:1237.

63. Jenkins SC, Heaton RW, Fulton IJ, Moxham J. Comparison of domiciliary nebulized salbutamol and salbutamol from a metered-dose inhaler in stable chronic airflow limitation. Chest 1987;91:804.

64. Gunawardena KA, Smith AP, Shankleman J. A comparison of metered-dose inhalers with nebulizers for the delivery of ipratropium bromide in domiciliary practice. Br J Dis Chest 1986;80:170.

65. Turner JR, Corkery KJ, Eckman D, Gelb AM, Lipavsky A, Sheppard D. Equivalence of continuous flow nebulizer and metered-dose inhaler with the reservoir bag for treatment of acute airflow obstruction. Chest 1988;93:476.

66. Stauder J, Hidinger KG. Terbutaline aerosol from a metered-dose inhaler with a 750 mL spacer or as a nebulized solution. Respiration 1983;44:237.

67. Gervais A, Begin P. Bronchodilatation with a metered-dose inhaler plus an extension, using tidal breathing vs jet nebulization. Chest 1987;92:822.

68. Berry RB, Shinto RA, Wong FH, Despars JA, Light RW. Nebulizer vs spacer for bronchodilator delivery in patients hospitalized for acute exacerbations of COPD. Chest 1989;96:1241.

69. Lewis RA, Fleming JS. Fractional deposition from a jet nebulizer: how it differs from a metered dose inhaler. Br J Dis Chest 1985;79:361.

70. Newman SP, Pavia D, Moren F, Sheahan NF, Clarke SW. Deposition of pressurized aerosols in the human respiratory tract. Thorax 1981;36:52.

71. The IPPB Trial Group. Intermittent positive pressure breathing therapy of chronic obstructive pulmonary disease: a clinical trial. Ann Intern Med 1983;99:612.

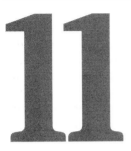

WALTER J. O'DONOHUE, JR.

Oxygen Therapy in Pulmonary Rehabilitation

No modality of therapy available today is more effective than continuous or near-continuous oxygen to increase survival and improve quality of life for patients with chronic obstructive pulmonary disease (COPD) and hypoxemia. Multicenter clinical trials conducted in North America and the United Kingdom[1,2] have demonstrated the value of long-term oxygen therapy (LTOT) to prolong survival in patients with COPD. Furthermore, these studies found that near-continuous oxygen (18 h/day) was superior to oxygen provided only for 12 to 15 hours daily, including the nocturnal hours. In the North American Nocturnal Oxygen Therapy Trial (NOTT) neuropsychological function was improved to a significantly greater degree in those patients receiving near-continuous oxygen.[3]

Analysis of data from the National Institutes of Health (NIH) multicenter intermittent positive-pressure breathing (IPPB) study,[4] when correlated with the NOTT study,[5,6] indicates that correction of hypoxemia in patients with COPD improves survival to levels expected for patients with similar degrees of obstructive lung disease without hypoxemia. Hypercapnia was present in about 50% of the NOTT study patients, but did not appear to alter this improved survival when hypoxemia was corrected. The factors that therefore appear to have the greatest relevance to survival in COPD patients are (1) hypoxemia, (2) pulmonary hypertension,[7] and (3) the severity of the fixed obstructive dysfunction. Hypoxemia and pulmonary hypertension are physiologically related, and treatment with oxygen can correct hypoxemia and reduce, but not totally eliminate, pulmonary hypertension.[8-10] In addition to the increased survival and improved neuropsychological function, oxygen can increase exercise tolerance and reduce dyspnea.[11-13] Recent studies suggest that the mode of oxygen delivery (e.g., nasal cannula versus transtracheal catheter or high flow versus low flow) may alter exercise tolerance substantially.[14-16] Oxygen therapy also can reduce the hematocrit in patients with hypoxemia and erythrocytosis.[8,12] These are all very important physiologic effects that are essential to optimize pulmonary rehabilitation.

When used in conjunction with a program for pulmonary rehabilitation, oxygen therapy allows patients with hypoxemia to exercise more safely, to increase exercise tolerance, and to experience a better quality of life. An exercise prescription can be developed, while monitoring cardiac and metabolic function, with the oxygen flow adjusted to avoid arterial oxygen desaturation. Patients can then continue this program either at a rehabilitation center or at home, with periodic modifications in the prescription based on appropriate reassessment. Thus, many patients with chronic pulmonary disease not only have been able to live longer, but also have enjoyed more active lives and, in some cases, have been able to maintain gainful employment.

ECONOMICS OF OXYGEN THERAPY

Although the total cost of home oxygen therapy is unknown, it has been estimated that approximately 800,000 patients are receiving outpatient oxygen therapy at a cost of nearly 1 billion dollars each year. Medicare pays about 60% of the cost, with a total reimbursement of over 500 million dollars yearly. Each physician and respiratory health care provider has a responsibility to be sure that oxygen is used appropriately and only when medically indicated. The Health Care Financing Administration (HCFA) has established precise guidelines for oxygen reimbursement based on the consideration that oxygen is "durable medical equipment" (DME). Medically, oxygen is considered to be a drug, but Medicare coverage does not include outpatient medications for other medical conditions. Fortunately, for patients with hypoxemia, HCFA pays for home oxygen as DME, but one of the prices we pay for this coverage is a very complex Certification of Medical Necessity form that must be completed by a physician or a member of the physician's staff and must be renewed on a yearly basis. It is considerably easier to prescribe severely addicting narcotics than it is to order home oxygen therapy.

In 1988, Congress legislated a new system for reimbursement of DME known as the "6-Point Plan." This plan provided for prospective reimbursement of all DME, with oxygen and oxygen equipment constituting approximately 45% of the total cost. The 6-Point Plan for oxygen was based on the primary assumption that all oxygen delivery systems are clinically equal and cost neutral. There were no built-in safeguards to assure that patients would receive the type of equipment ordered by the physician and judged to be medically most appropriate. The 6-Point Plan created a financial disincentive for some DME providers to supply liquid oxygen systems, since HCFA recognizes no clinical or cost difference between liquid oxygen and oxygen from a concentrator. As a result, in some rural areas and areas where there is no competition among oxygen suppliers, it has become difficult to obtain liquid oxygen

TABLE 11-1. Cost Components of Home Oxygen Therapy

Equipment and equipment inventory
Setup and educational costs
Administration and overhead
Delivery, supply, and maintenance
Oxygen: liquid and compressed
Profit

TABLE 11-2. Problems Resulting from the 6-Point Plan for Reimbursement of Oxygen and Oxygen Equipment

Inadequate historical data base to determine appropriate reimbursement

Assumption that all oxygen systems are clinically equal and cost neutral:
  Inadequate reimbursement for liquid ambulatory systems
  Reluctance of oxygen suppliers to provide liquid oxygen to rural patients

Disincentive for the use of oxygen conserving devices that deliver less than 1 L/min (50% reduction in reimbursement)

Absence of safeguards to assure that patients receive the most appropriate oxygen delivery system for their management and rehabilitation

for patients who need ambulatory equipment. Since most patients with COPD and hypoxemia are able to live active and longer lives with oxygen therapy, liquid oxygen systems with ambulatory units that can be transfilled at home by the patient are necessary to allow full activity and to facilitate pulmonary rehabilitation. High-pressure cylinders on wheels (strollers) are portable, but not ambulatory, and are suitable only for patients who occasionally leave the home for visits to their physician or who take infrequent trips away from their stationary unit. The "standard of care" for most patients receiving home oxygen therapy is liquid oxygen for ambulation.[17,18]

The 6-Point Plan also discourages the use of oxygen-conserving devices that can reduce the oxygen flow to less than 1 L/minute since reimbursement is reduced by 50% when flow rates of less than 1 L/minute are utilized. The total cost of supplying oxygen is almost never reduced by 50% simply because a lower flow rate is being used. The factors that are important in determining the true cost of home oxygen are presented in Table 11–1. The least important of these costs is the cost of oxygen itself (about 10 cents/lb for liquid oxygen). Reducing the amount of oxygen being used can reduce cost by allowing fewer home deliveries of liquid or cylinder oxygen, but not to the magnitude of 50%. The problems introduced by the 6-Point Plan are summarized in Table 11–2.[19]

REGULATIONS FOR REIMBURSEMENT OF HOME OXYGEN

The current HCFA requirement for documentation of hypoxemia with an arterial PO_2 of 55 mm Hg or less or an arterial PO_2 of 56 to 59 mm Hg, along with evidence of cor pulmonale or erythrocytosis, is derived directly from the requirements for entry into the NOTT study.[1] The HCFA also added arterial oxygen saturations of 88% or less or 89% with cor pulmonale or erythrocytosis as a means of documenting hypoxemia by a less invasive approach and also because it is difficult to obtain an arterial blood gas sample during sleep or exercise. In addition to these oxygen tension and saturation limits, HCFA now recognizes that patients should be clinically stable and receiving optimum therapy before LTOT is prescribed. (This was originally stated by HCFA as "other means of therapy should have been tried before oxygen is prescribed.") The actual measurement of arterial oxygen tension or saturation must be done by a Medicare "qualified" laboratory with the intent being that the oxygen provider will not also perform the test that certifies the need for therapy. Finally, a Certificate of Medical Necessity (Form HCFA-484) must be submitted by the physician. Yearly renewal is required for all patients who qualify for LTOT, but repeat blood gas analysis is not necessary. Currently, HCFA requires that the physician reevaluate the patient within 90 days before renewal. This is now resulting in unnecessary office visits, since many of these patients can be seen on a yearly basis or sometimes less frequently if they are clinically stable, and these visits are not usually in synchrony with the request for renewal of oxygen therapy.

In the past, HCFA has stated a preference for the arterial blood gas analysis that certifies the need for home oxygen therapy to be done in the hospital. In a five-state survey of patients using oxygen concentrators, the Office of the Inspector General[20] found that more than 30% of patients who received oxygen concentrators because of abnormal arterial blood gas measurements obtained during hospitalization were no longer using oxygen at all or to the extent being billed. This study also found that the physician often played a minor role in the entire process, commonly functioning only as the "signer of the Certificate of Medical Necessity." In many cases, the Certificate of Medical Necessity was being completed by the oxygen supplier with the physician having no documentation of the certification. As a result of this study, HCFA issued a new Certification of Medical Necessity form (Form HCFA-484) that was initially designed to require 25 minutes for the physician or a member of the physician's office staff to complete. The form has recently been reduced in length by approximately 50% to a single page that uses a checklist format for many of the options, reducing time for completion considerably. The form still has major shortcomings when used universally for initial certification, recertification, and renewal, or if the patient requires different oxygen flow rates at rest, during exercise, and with sleep. Completion can be very time-consuming if the necessary information and dates are not readily available to the physician. The HCFA requiremens for reimbursement of oxygen are summarized in Table 11–3.

TABLE   11-3.   Medicare Requirements for Home Oxygen Therapy

1. $PaO_2 \leq 55$ mm Hg or saturated $O_2 \leq 88\%$ breathing ambient air
2. PaO_2 56–59 mm Hg or saturated O_2 89% with:
   Evidence of cor pulmonale
   Erythrocytosis (Hct > 56%)
3. Optimum medical management before certification for long-term oxygen therapy
4. Recertification in 60–90 days after hospital discharge, if the patient was not previously receiving home oxygen
5. Measurement of PaO_2 or saturated O_2 by a Medicare qualified laboratory (preference for a hospital laboratory)
6. Physician submission of Form HCFA-484
7. Recertification yearly with physician evaluation within 90 days

APPROPRIATE OXYGEN THERAPY

The Report of the Office of the Inspector General[20] made both HCFA and the medical community more aware that oxygen may be necessary for patients to be discharged from the hospital, but often this is not justification for lifetime oxygen therapy. With increasing pressure for early hospital discharge brought about by the Prospective Payment System, many patients are still recovering from an acute respiratory illness when they leave the hospital, and they may need supplemental oxygen until full recovery has occurred. The Third National Oxygen Consensus Conference[17] recommended that when home oxygen is prescribed at the time of hospital discharge, arterial blood gases should be repeated in 1 to 3 months when the patient is clinically stable and receiving optimum therapy. At this point, the decision for long-term oxygen therapy can be made; and if the patient qualifies for LTOT, this is usually a lifetime commitment. Recent studies indicate that oxygen can have a reparative effect on the lungs within 6 months that can result in a reducton in alveolar–arterial oxygen gradient and an increase in the arterial PO_2 that is attributable to the beneficial effects of oxygen therapy itself and not to changes in clinical stability.[21] On the basis of the best knowledge available today, when LTOT is prescribed for a clinically stable patient who meets the current criteria for supplemental oxygen, it should not be discontinued later, even if the patient no longer meets *initial* blood gas requirements for therapy. Repeat blood analyses should be used to follow the course of the disease and to guide overall management of the patient and not to determine continuing need for oxygen therapy.

By allowing arterial oxygen saturation measurements to be used to document the need for oxygen therapy, some potential problems are presented. Arterial oxygen saturation measurements of 88% do not always correlate with an arterial PO_2 of 55 mm Hg or less owing to multiple physiologic and technical factors that can affect the determination. Nocturnal desaturation has also been noted to occur in clinically normal and healthy individuals.[22] Therefore, the medical standard for *continuous* LTOT should be based on a resting arterial blood gas measurement with the patient breathing ambient air.[23] Measurement of arterial oxygen saturation is useful to document hypoxemia during sleep when there is evidence of *clinical disease*, such as cor pulmonale, in the absence of hypoxemia during the waking hours. In many patients, other sleep disturbances may be present, such as obstructive or central sleep apnea, that may require treatment other than oxygen therapy. In some patients with chronic lung disease, the only abnormality associated with cor pulmonale may be nocturnal desaturation that is correctable by use of supplemental oxygen. Other patients with COPD and nocturnal desaturation may have mild elevations in pulmonary vascular resistance without cor pulmonale, and there is no conclusive evidence of benefit from oxygen therapy in these individuals.[24]

Some patients with chronic lung disease may not have resting hypoxemia, but may have desaturation during exercise. If dyspnea or exercise tolerance are improved with oxygen therapy, then oxygen should be prescribed during exercise and may be very important for pulmonary rehabilitation. If desaturation occurs only with exercise, this should not be used as a means to justify continuous oxygen therapy. Often oxygen is used as a "tonic" for dyspnea, without documentation of benefit. Most often severe dyspnea is due to mechanical dysfunction of the lungs and chest wall, and if hypoxemia is not present, oxygen therapy is not justified. In those patients who have qualified for LTOT, measurements of arterial oxygen saturation is useful to titrate the oxygen flow at rest, during various levels of exertion, and during sleep. In this context, oxygen saturation measurements may be used to write a more complete oxygen prescription. Arterial oxygen saturation measurements are also useful to monitor acute changes in respiratory status.

For a discussion of the various modes of oxygen therapy as well as oxygen-conserving devices, see Chapter 19.

SUMMARY

Given well-conducted clinical trials, it is quite evident that oxygen is beneficial for patients with COPD who have resting hypoxemia. From these data we assume that oxygen benefits patients with similar levels of hypoxemia resulting from other forms of cardiopulmonary disease; however, definitive studies have not been done. We have also been able to observe beneficial effects from correction of nocturnal hypoxemia in patients with cor pulmonale, even in the absence of hypoxemia during the waking hours. Oxygen is beneficial in reducing dyspnea and increasing exercise tolerance when exercise-induced hypoxemia is present. Once oxygen has been started in a clinically stable patient with COPD and hypoxemia, repeat arterial blood gas or saturation measurements are not necessary for recertification. The PaO_2 may rise as a result of the beneficial effects of the therapy. Until future studies are performed to verify that stopping the therapy does not result in more rapid progression of pulmonary hypertension and reversal of the benefits that have been achieved, continuous oxygen therapy should be provided for the lifetime of each patient once he or she has qualified for LTOT.

REFERENCES

1. Nocturnal Oxygen Therapy Trial Group. Continuous and nocturnal oxygen therapy in hypoxemic chronic obstructive lung disease: a clinical trial. Ann Intern Med 1980;93:391.

2. Report of the Medical Research Council Working Party. Long term domiciliary oxygen therapy in chronic cor pulmonale complicating chronic bronchitis and emphysema. Lancet 1981;1:681.

3. Heaton RK, Grant I, McSweeney AJ, Adams KM, Petty TL. Psychologic effects of continuous and nocturnal oxygen therapy in hypoxemic chronic obstructive pulmonary disease. Arch Intern Med 1983;143:1941.

4. The Intermittent Positive Pressure Breathing Trial Group. Intermittent positive pressure breathing therapy of chronic obstructive lung disease: a clinical trial. Ann Intern Med 1983;99:612.

5. Anthonisen NR, Wright EC, Hodgkin JE, IPPB Trial Group. Prognosis in chronic obstructive pulmonary disease. Am Rev Respir Dis 1986;133:14.

6. O'Donohue WJ Jr. The future of home oxygen therapy. Respir Care 1988;33:1125.

7. Neff TA, Petty TL. Long-term continuous oxygen therapy in chronic airway obstruction: mortality in relationship to cor pulmonale, hypoxia and hypercapnia. Ann Intern Med 1970;72:621.

8. Levine BE, Bigelow DB, Hamstra RD, et al. The role of long-term continuous oxygen administration in patients with chronic airway obstruction with hypoxemia. Ann Intern Med 1967;66:639.

9. Abraham AS, Cole RB, Bishop JM. Reversal of pulmonary hypertension by prolonged oxygen administration to patients with chronic bronchitis. Circ Res 1968;23:147.

10. Weitzemblum E, Sautegeau A, Ehrhart M, Mammosser M, Pelletier A. Long-term oxygen therapy can reverse the progression of pulmonary hypertension in patients with chronic obstructive pulmonary disease. Am Rev Respir Dis 1985;131:493.

11. Cotes JE, Gilson JC. Effect of oxygen on exercise ability in chronic respiratory insufficiency: use of portable apparatus. Lancet 1956;1:872.

12. Petty TL, Finigan MM. Clinical evaluation of prolonged ambulatory oxygen therapy in chronic airway obstruction. Am J Med 1968;45:242.

13. Woodcock AA, Gross ER, Geddes DM. Oxygen relieves breathlessness in "pink puffers." Lancet 1981;1:907.

14. Wesmiller SW, Hoffman LA, Sciurba FC, Ferson PF, Johnson JT, Dauber JH. Exercise tolerance during nasal cannula and transtracheal oxygen delivery. Am Rev Respir Dis 1990;141:789.

15. Couser JI, Make BJ. Transtracheal oxygen decreases inspired minute ventilation. Am Rev Respir Dis 1989;139:627.

16. Dewan NA, Bell CW. Effect of high-flow and low-flow oxygen delivery via transtracheal catheter and nasal cannula on exercise tolerance and sensation of dyspnea. Chest 1991;100:52S.

17. Conference Report. New problems in supply, reimbursement and certification of medical necessity for long-term oxygen therapy. Am Rev Respir Dis 1990;142:721.

18. Petty TL, O'Donohue WJ Jr. Ambulatory oxygen: the standard of care. Chest 1990;98:791.

19. O'Donohue WJ Jr. New problems in home oxygen therapy. Am Rev Respir Dis 1989;140:1813.

20. US Department of Health and Human Services, Office of Inspector General, Office of Audit. National review of medical necessity for oxygen concentrators, 1990. Audit Control No. A-04-88-02058.

21. O'Donohue WJ Jr. Effect of oxygen therapy on increasing arterial oxygen tension in hypoxemic patients with stable chronic obstructive pulmonary disease while breathing ambient air. Chest 1991;100:968.

22. Block AJ, Boysen PG, Wynne JW, Hunt LA. Sleep apnea, hypopnea, and oxygen desaturation during sleep in normal subjects. N Engl J Med 1979;300:513.

23. Conference Report. Problems in prescribing and supplying oxygen for Medicare patients. Am Rev Respir Dis 1986;134:340.

24. Fletcher EC, Luckett RA, Miller T, Fletcher JG. Exercise hemodynamics and gas exchange in patients with chronic obstructive pulmonary disease, sleep desaturation, and a daytime PaO_2 above 60 mm Hg. Am Rev Respir dis 1989;140:1237.

CATHERINE CERTO

12

Chest Physical Therapy

Chest physical therapy is widely used as an adjunct for management of patients with acute and chronic pulmonary disease. It may also be used prophylactically in those patients who may be at risk of developing pulmonary complications secondary to diagnostic procedures or surgical interventions such as abdominal surgery. In the last 20 years modern advances in cardiopulmonary medicine, technology, research, and pharmacology have improved the long-term outlook of patients with chronic pulmonary disease. Chest physical therapy is an important component of pulmonary rehabilitation.

Pulmonary care is shared by numerous health care professionals, including nurses, physical therapists, occupational therapists, respiratory therapists, and exercise physiologists. It is not uncommon to find these health care providers treating patients at various stages in the health care spectrum. This includes, but is not limited to, intensive care units (ICU), respiratory intensive care units (RICU), neonatal intensive care units (NICU), and inpatient or outpatient rehabilitation centers.

The type of patient in need of these services may have medical or surgical diagnoses, complications, a need for ventilatory support, neurologic or spinal cord injury, and includes children with a myriad of cardiopulmonary disorders.

The responsibilities of each of these health care professionals will vary depending on the needs and goals of the patient population. These responsibilities run the spectrum of functional and physical assessment of upper and lower extremities, including strength, coordination, endurance, sitting, standing, walking, balance, and mobility needs (wheelchair, walker, and such). Cardiopulmonary treatments, commonly referred to as *chest physiotherapy* (or *chest physical therapy*), include bronchopulmonary hygiene procedures, such as postural drainage and manual techniques, breathing exercises, muscle reeducation, chest mobilization, and therapeutic exercises designed to improve functional capacity. Inherent in each of these treatments is a component of patient education and psychosocial support.

There is a feeling by many that even though chest physical therapy has been used extensively as a treatment intervention for years, little objective data supports its value in the management of individuals with pulmonary problems in either the inpatient or outpatient setting. However, newer investigational approaches help provide a physiologic understanding of how chest physical therapy modalities work, which methods are most beneficial, and which disease entities may benefit from specific techniques.[1]

The purpose of this chapter is to discuss the various chest physical therapy techniques that should be considered for the evaluation and treatment of patients at various stages of pulmonary dysfunction.

RATIONALE AND GOALS

To provide a rationale for therapeutic intervention and to understand the possible outcomes of that intervention, the provider of pulmonary care must have a clear understanding and working knowledge of the following: normal anatomy and physiology of the pulmonary system, pathophysiology of the disease process, and the characteristics of each of the numerous lung diseases. These health care providers must also comprehend the needs of pulmonary patients during an acute crisis or exacerbation as well as during long-term maintenance therapy so that appropriate assessment and treatment protocols can be initiated.

The overall goals for the pulmonary patient are to maintain a patent airway, improve gas exchange, enhance cough effectiveness, reduce pain, increase chest mobilization, and maintain or improve functional capacity. The physical therapy techniques that should be considered in an attempt to achieve these goals will be considered in the remainder of this chapter. These chest physical therapy techniques are performed in combination with general exercise to maintain or improve functional capacity.

PULMONARY ASSESSMENT

Any treatment should be performed subsequent to a thorough assessment of the patient. This assessment of patients with pulmonary dysfunction is one of the most critical aspects of rehabilitative medicine. A chest examination is coupled with objective information obtained from arterial blood gases, pulmonary function tests, chest radiography, graded exercise tests, and microbiologic studies of sputum.

A chest examination should be performed by all health care professionals involved in the treatment of patients with pulmonary dysfunction. The basic elements of the assessment are the same for both acute and chronic pulmonary patients; what differs is the emphasis and intervention.

Multiple objectives are considered when performing a chest examination. First is the identification of the patient's problem. Next is the recognition of any coexisting signs and symptoms of pulmonary or cardiac disease. Third, the therapist establishes if there is a need for further evaluative procedures to verify findings or to rule out other problems. Fourth is the identification of treatment goals for both the pulmonary aspect of care and, frequently, musculoskeletal problems and, then, the formulation of a treatment plan to achieve these multiple goals.

Components of the chest examination include inspection, auscultation, palpation, and percussion. In addition, the examination should evaluate pulmonary musculature. An understanding of the muscles of ventilation and their adaptation to pulmonary disease is an essential prerequisite for accurate evaluation and successful program planning.

The next section reviews the pulmonary treatments commonly performed by pulmonary health care providers and the effectiveness of these treatments relative to therapeutic goals.

TREATMENTS DESIGNED TO ENHANCE VENTILATION AND AERATION

Since alveolar ventilation depends on the magnitude of tidal volume and dead space,[2] the intervention administered is designed to increase alveolar ventilation by increasing the tidal volume or by decreasing dead space ventilation, or both, ultimately improving oxygenation. These strategies include controlled-breathing techniques and positioning techniques.

CONTROLLED-BREATHING TECHNIQUES

Breathing exercises are used for patients throughout the spectrum of care, acute to chronic. *Breathing exercises* is a term that encompasses techniques such as pursed-lips breathing, diaphragmatic breathing, and segmental breathing. Studies such as those of Barach and Miller observed the improvement of dyspnea in patients with chronic obstructive pulmonary disease (COPD) when they prescribed breathing-training techniques, such as pursed-lips breathing, the bending-forward posture, and abdominal breathing.[3,4]

It is well established that long-term physiologic adaptations of COPD cause an increase in the work of breathing and a significant reduction in the efficiency of the respiratory musculature. Diseases such as emphysema, obstructive bronchitis, bronchiectasis, and cystic fibrosis cause a myriad of alterations, such as loss of pulmonary recoil, obstruction of small airways, and increased airways resistance, that ultimately can lead to hyperinflation of the lungs. This hyperinflation eventually has a significant adverse effect on the diaphragm. The diaphragm becomes increasingly flattened, its muscle fibers shorten, and its radius of curvature increases, causing it to function on a less advantageous length–tension curve. The resultant phenomenon, according to Celli, is a reduction in the diaphragm's ability to generate useful inspiratory pressure.[5] Further alterations caused by hyperinflation, such as changes in the surface and angles of the ribs, cause greater demands on the respiratory muscles. The results of these changes clinically manifest themselves by increases in respiratory rate. These increases in rate promote further air-trapping, inspiratory muscle dysfunction, weakness, and fatigue.[1]

The goals of breathing exercises are to (1) improve abdominal breathing and thereby improve function of the diaphragm; (2) control respiratory rate and decrease the work of breathing; (3) assist the patient in relaxation and thereby allay dyspnea; (4) increase the strength, coordination, and efficiency of breathing patterns; (5) prevent or reverse atelectasis; and (6) mobilize and maintain mobility of the chest wall.

Pursed-Lips Breathing

Pursed-lips breathing is effective in reducing the respiratory rate and relieving dyspnea. It has been suggested that this method of breathing may improve ventilation and

TABLE   12-1.   The Objectives and Potential Outcomes of Pursed-Lips Breathing Exercises

Therapeutic objectives	Alleviate dyspnea
	Increase tolerance
Physiologic objectives	Increase alveolar ventilation
	Increase oxygenation
	Reduce the work of breathing
Potential outcomes	Elimination of accessory muscle activity
	Reduced respiratory rate
	Increased arterial oxygen tension
	Decreased carbon dioxide tension
	Increased exercise tolerance

(Humberstone N. Respiratory assessment and treatment. In: Irvin S, Tecklin J, eds. Cardiopulmonary physical therapy. St. Louis: CV Mosby, 1990, with permission)

oxygenation. Table 12–1 lists the objectives and potential outcomes of pursed-lips–breathing exercises. Pursed-lips breathing is frequently used spontaneously by COPD patients. Two methods of pursed-lips breathing have been reported. The preferred method advocates passive expiration,[4] and the other suggests abdominal muscle contraction through expiration.[6] In the latter, the patient must be taught not to exhale forcefully, since this method increases bronchiolar collapse.

Research in this area gives no clear mechanism for the physiologic responses for pursed-lips breathing. Thoman and colleagues investigated the effect of this type of breathing on ventilation in subjects with COPD.[7] They discovered that this breathing pattern decreased respiratory rate and increased tidal volume. Furthermore, they demonstrated improved alveolar ventilation as measured by $PaCO_2$ and suggested that the decrease in respiratory rate was the mechanism for such improvement.

Ingram and Schilder, investigated the effects of pursed-lips breathing and found that this type of breathing reduced both the peak and mean expiratory flow rates.[8] In addition, patients who claim to benefit from this technique obtained a greater reduction in "nonelastic" resistance across the lung than those who denied such improvement.

Mueller and colleagues reevaluated the influence of pursed-lips breathing on ventilation and oxygenation.[9] Their results support previous findings of decreased respiratory rate and increased tidal volume. In addition, they suggest that these effects are sustained during exercise. Later research by Casiari and coworkers evaluated the effect of pursed-lips breathing on exercise tolerance in patients with severe COPD.[10] They reported that pursed-lips breathing improved exercise tolerance without increasing the respiratory rate or decreasing the PO_2.

Although research has not given clear explanations of the benefits of pursed-lips breathing, it appears to be an effective treatment tool. Health care professionals should continue to teach this type of breathing to patients who complain of dyspnea both at rest and during exercise.

Positioning Techniques

Positioning is the basis of every chest physical therapy treatment, regardless of the goal of the treatment. Potential goals of positioning may include draining secretions, improving the ventilation/perfusion ($\dot{V}/\dot{Q}$) ratio, or maximizing the mechanical advantage of musculature. Two commonly used positions, the head-down (Trendelenburg) and the leaning-forward position often relieve dyspnea in COPD patients. Table 12–2 lists objectives and potential outcomes. These positions are also effective for ambulatory COPD patients and may improve ventilation and oxygenation. In contrast, acutely ill patients may not tolerate these positional changes, and a combination of side-to-side positioning may be more effective.

One of the results of emphysema is a depressed flat diaphragm, a diaphragm that is a poorly functioning muscle. Therefore, for effective treatment, patients should be placed in positions that assist the diaphragm. Barach noted that proper positions appear to alleviate dyspnea by reducing the respiratory effort and this is accompanied by a decline in accessory breathing musculature use.[3] He also speculated that the elevation of the diaphragm by the upward shift in weight of the abdominal content influenced these improvements.

It is well known that the head-down position is a difficult position for COPD patients to assume and to maintain. This position often increases venous return, intracranial pressure, and abdominal pressure on the diaphragm. Any of these changes may alter the patient's physiologic state, vital signs, and breathing patterns. Therefore, patients seem most comfortable when a maximum of 20° head-down is assumed.[1] The bending-forward posture is more widely used for COPD patients and can be assumed during sitting or walking, or when using a walker or a cane (Fig. 12–1A,B). When considering the effects of various positions on respiratory muscle function, careful thought should also be given to the mechanics of breathing and gas distribution.

Studies have reported the hydrostatic force exerted on the diaphragm by the abdominal contents, and a greater force exerted on the dorsal aspect of the dia-

TABLE 12-2. Objectives and Potential Outcomes of Position Changes

Therapeutic objective	Alleviate dyspnea
Physiologic objective	Increase oxygenation
	Improve ventilation
Potential outcome	
Prone	Increased arterial oxygen tension in bilateral lung disease
Supine	Decreased arterial oxygen tension in bilateral lung disease
Lateral	Decreased arterial oxygen tension lying on the affected lung in unilateral lung disease
	Decreased arterial oxygen tension lying on the left side in bilateral lung disease
	Improved arterial oxygen tension lying on the unoperated side after thoracotomy (relative to supine)

(Humberstone N. Respiratory assessment and treatment. In: Irvin S, Tecklin J, eds. Cardiopulmonary physical therapy. St Louis: CV Mosby, 1990, with permission)

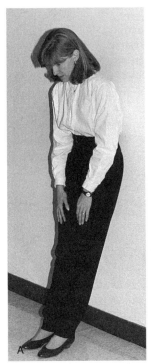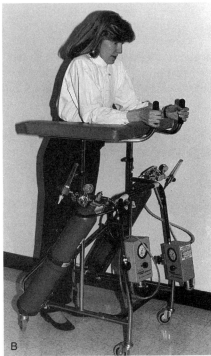

FIGURE   12-1   (**A**) The forward-leaning position. (**B**) A high-wheeled walker that allows assumption of the forward-leaning posture.

phragm has been observed in the supine position.[11-13] Also noted was that for COPD subjects in the supine position, the excursion of the curvature of the diaphragm is smaller at the dorsal aspect. The fibers appear lengthened, thereby placing the muscle at a mechanically advantageous length and ultimately improving diaphragmatic strength. These changes, along with previously recognized declines in accessory breathing musculature, probably account for the improved dyspnea these patients experience when placed in the supine or bent-forward position.

Positioning for the breathless patient is also effective in promoting comfort and relaxation. This is especially effective when the leaning-forward posture is used during exercise. Delgado and associates observed a decrease in dyspnea and an improved exercise tolerance in patients with COPD who exercised in the leaning-forward posture.[13] These patients usually developed paradoxical diaphragmatic motion with upright exercise, and with this posture change, there was a return of normal chest wall–abdominal motion in some cases and a shift to only partial inspiratory paradox in others.

Breathing Exercises

Breathing exercises are used throughout cardiopulmonary management and form the basis of every treatment. Normal persons who regularly perform aerobic exercise use breathing exercises as an adjunct to their routine. The relation between oxygen consumption and minute ventilation varies during increasing levels of exercise, up to maximal oxygen consumption. During light to moderate exercise, ventilation increases linearly with oxygen uptake. With more intense exercise, the minute ventilation takes a sharp upswing from increases in oxygen consumption.

On the other hand, consider the plight of the patient with COPD who has a low vital capacity, copious secretions, bronchospasm, pain, and other symptoms that increase energy expenditure, even at rest. These patients often breathe shallowly and rapidly. This compromised pattern of breathing becomes progressive until they develop respiratory failure. For these individuals, a program of breathing exercises may have some physiologic benefit. Breathing exercises should promote slow, deep inspiration through the nose to take advantage of upper airway function. A prolonged holding of the breath at maximal inspiration and a relaxed expiration with or without pursed-lips breathing should be performed. These breathing exercises should be performed by those patients with COPD who have dyspnea and bronchospasms.

Frequently, the therapist's hand(s) placed over the surface of the chest or lung area being emphasized during these exercises can assist the patient with recognition of breathing patterns and control over respiration rate and muscle function.

Although these exercises may have a favorable effect on respiration rate and muscle function, they may not improve alveolar ventilation and oxygenation.[14] Grassino and coworkers developed a plausible explanation for the inability of COPD patients to spontaneously breathe slowly and deeply.[15] Several indices of muscle fatigue were monitored in a small group of COPD patients, during normal resting breathing and during an imposed breathing pattern with an increase in tidal volume, a slow-breathing rate, a long inspiratory phase, and a brisk exhalation. After only 6 to 10 minutes, the slow, deep-breathing pattern caused diaphragmatic fatigue. Deep breathing, however, in patients with asthma produces bronchoconstriction.[16] Therefore, caution is used when teaching breathing exercises to these patients.

Diaphragmatic-Breathing Exercises

Encouraging the use of diaphragmatic breathing in the management of COPD is one of the best methods employed to improve the mechanics of breathing. Although any patient with chronic lung disease may use diaphragmatic-breathing exercises, it appears to be most advantageous to patients with hyperinflated lungs and depressed, flattened diaphragms.

If performed properly diaphragmatic-breathing exercises purport to enhance diaphragmatic descent during inspiration and diaphragmatic ascent during expiration.[17] Observation of the patient's breathing pattern along with palpation will identify whether respiratory muscles are used correctly and effectively. Close observation of accessory muscle use, inward movement of the lower ribs, and lack of abdominal distention on inspiration will identify COPD patients with diaphragmatic dysfunction.

Although the techniques for teaching diaphragmatic-breathing exercises vary, in principle they are similar. That is, they all use a sequential approach and begin with patients assuming a comfortable position, usually sitting. One method for teaching

TABLE   12-3.   Steps for Teaching Diaphragmatic Breathing Exercises

1. Place the patient's dominant hand over the midrectus abdominis area.
2. Place the patient's nondominant hand on the midsternal area.
3. Direct the patient to inhale slowly through the nose.
4. Instruct patient to watch the dominant hand as inspiration continues.
5. Encourage the patient to direct the air so that the dominant hand gradually rises as inspiration continues.
6. Caution the patient to avoid excessive movement under the nondominant hand.
7. Apply firm counterpressure over the patient's dominant hand just before directing the patient to inhale.
8. Instruct the patient to inhale as you lessen your counterpressure as inspiration continues.
9. Practice the exercise until the patient no longer requires the manual assistance of the therapist to perform the exercise correctly.
10. Progress the level of difficulty by sequentially removing auditory, visual, and tactile cues. Thereafter, progress the exercise by practicing seated, standing, and walking.

(Humberstone N. Respiratory assessment treatment. In: Irvin S, Tecklin J, eds. Cardiopulmonary physical therapy. St Louis: CV Mosby, 1990, with permission)

diaphragmatic-breathing exercises is described in Table 12–3. Once learned, diaphragmatic-breathing exercises should be practiced several times a day. The sequence is most effective if taught with the patient in different positions that increase the difficulty of the procedure, as well as in combination with pursed-lips exhalation and a leaning-forward position to attain maximum benefit.

The actual results or alterations attributed to the use of diaphragmatic-breathing exercises as a treatment modality are still controversial and the subject of significant research. For instance, many therapists use diaphragmatic-breathing exercises with COPD patients in an effort to minimize the use of accessory musculature as well as to strengthen the diaphragm. However, the inference that strong diaphragms increase ventilation has not been validated. The ability of diaphragmatic-breathing exercises to alter the distribution of ventilation in chronically obstructed patients has not been observed,[18,19] and its effect in normal subjects is still unclear.

The effect of diaphragmatic breathing on oxygenation is not yet clear. Earlier reports demonstrated a significant improvement in arterial oxygen saturation in selected patients with diaphragmatic breathing.[4] Later studies failed to substantiate such results. More recent findings, however, suggest that diaphragmatic breathing may affect oxygenation indirectly by altering regional pulmonary perfusion.[20]

Early research evaluated the effect of diaphragmatic breathing on the mobility of the diaphragm. Studies give little credence to an increase in diaphragmatic motion in either normal subjects or patients with chronic obstructive lung disease.[21] However, more recent studies report improved diaphragmatic excursion in selected patients.[22,23]

The most positive support of diaphragmatic-breathing exercises is associated with the reduced rate of postoperative pulmonary complications in patients with any thoracic or abdominal surgery.[24]

Segmental-Breathing Exercises

Chest wall compliance alterations can account for localized ventilation abnormalities. These instances require a more specialized technique (segmental-breathing exercises or lateral costal breathing) to emphasize specific lung problems. Some of these problems are atelectasis, pneumonia, muscle splinting from pain, especially postoperative pain, and thus hypoventilation, scoliosis, or kyphosis. Each technique uses manual counterpressure to encourage the expansion of a specific part of the lung. Table 12–4 lists the steps for one method of administering segmental breathing exercises. Table 12–5 lists objectives and potential outcomes of segmental breathing.

Advanced therapeutic approaches to physical therapy treatment often include neurophysiologic patterns of movement of the upper extremities. These techniques are often used as an adjunct to segmental breathing (Fig. 12–2), and have additional influence on thoracic cage mobility. Repeated contractions can be especially helpful. The patient is asked to take a deep breath and hold it. He or she is then asked to breath more, more, and more, while repeated stretch is given. This is especially effective if administered over the sternum or in the lateral costal area.

Research validating the effectiveness of segmental breathing is limited. Most studies that have taken place have attempted to validate the premise that ventilation can be directed to a predetermined area.[17]

Campbell and Friend attempted to study the effects of lateral basal expansion on ventilation.[25] Their conclusion failed to demonstrate improvements in ventilation of patients with emphysema when using segmental breathing as a treatment. However, a study by Vraciu and Vraciu did find less postoperative pulmonary complications in patients who had been treated with segmental breathing exercises as a prophylactic treatment.[24] Since more than one type of breathing exercises were performed as part

TABLE 12-4.   Steps for One Method of Administering Segmental Breathing Exercises

1. Identify the surface landmarks demarcating the affected area.
2. Place the therapist's hand or hands on the chest wall overlying the bronchopulmonary segment or segments requiring treatment.
3. Apply firm pressure to that area at the end of the patient's expiratory maneuver. (Pressure should be equal and bilateral across a median sternotomy incision.)
4. Instruct the patient to inspire deeply through his or her mouth, attempting to direct the inspired air toward your hand, saying "Breathe into my hand."
5. Reduce hand pressure as patient inspires. (At end inspiration, the instructor's hand should be applying no pressure on the chest.)
6. Instruct the patient to hold his or her breath for 2 to 3 sec at the completion of inspiration.
7. Instruct the patient to exhale.
8. Repeat sequence until patient can execute breathing maneuver correctly.
9. Progress the exercises by instructing the patient to use his or her own hands or a belt to execute the program independently.

(Humberstone N. Respiratory assessment and treatment. In: Irvin S, Tecklin J, eds. Cardiopulmonary physical therapy. St. Louis: CV Mosby, 1990, with permission)

TABLE 12-5. Objectives and Potential Outcomes of Segmental Breathing Exercises

Therapeutic objective	Alleviate dyspnea
Physiologic objectives	Increase alveolar ventilation
	Increase oxygenation
Potential outcomes	Prevent accumulation of pleural fluid
	Prevent accumulation of secretions
	Decrease paradoxical breathing
	Decrease "panic"
	Improve chest mobility

(Humberstone N. Respiratory assessment and treatment. In: Irvin S, Tecklin J, eds. Cardiopulmonary physical therapy. St Louis: CV Mosby, 1990, with permission)

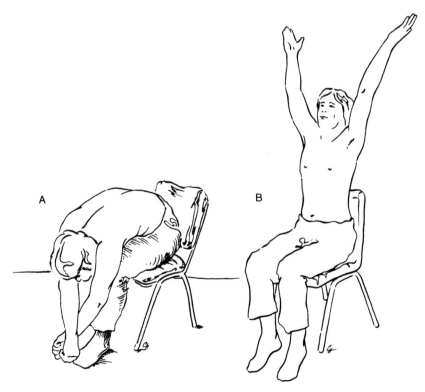

FIGURE 12-2 (**A**) Total pattern exercise. Patient exhales during flexion. (**B**) Patient stretches and breathes in during the extension phase. (Frownfelter D. Chest physical therapy and pulmonary rehabilitation, an interdisciplinary approach. 2nd ed. Chicago: Year Book Medical Publishers, 1987, with permission)

of the protocol, it was difficult to identify the exact contribution of segmental breathing.

TREATMENTS TO ENHANCE SECRETION CLEARANCE

Effective mucociliary transport and effective cough are required for normal secretion clearance. This dual system protects the airways by trapping and eliminating inhaled materials. When either of these mechanisms functions improperly, secretions increase and set off a cycle of physiologic alterations, causing mucous accumulation in the airways and impaired gas exchange. Inflammation, infection, airway obstruction, atelectasis, and pneumonia are a few conditions that result in an accumulation of secretions. When the amount of mucous secretions overwhelms the function of the mucociliary transport system, the secretions can no longer be cleared efficiently.

Table 12–6 lists some of the causes of impaired mucociliary transport. If these secretions can be cleared from the pulmonary system by an effective cough, then proper gas exchange can occur. Conversely, many patients have impaired cough. Patients with muscle weakness are generally unable to give an effective cough because they are unable to generate enough intrapleural pressure. Patients with pain as a result of surgery, trauma, or pulmonary dysfunction are often unwilling to cough. After abdominal surgery, patients are often unable to cough owing to a period of diaphragmatic dysfunction.[26] Finally, patients with airflow limitations have ineffective coughs because expiratory flow rates are greatly reduced.

Goals of treatment include improvement of airway clearance, ventilation, and exercise tolerance; reduction in work of breathing and, ultimately, restoration of the patient to fullest potential in the inpatient, outpatient, pulmonary rehabilitation, and home care setting.[27] Techniques used in chest physical therapy include postural drainage, chest percussion and vibration, cough, and forced expiratory technique (FET). Treatment setting for inpatients may vary from the intensive care unit to the

---

TABLE   12-6.   Some of the Causes of Impaired Mucociliary Transport

- Hypoxia or hyperoxia
- Cuffed endotracheal tube
- Dehydration
- Electrolyte imbalance
- Infection
- Loss of ciliated respiratory epithelium
- Inhaled dry gases
- Cigarette smoke
- Anesthetics and analgesics
- Pollutants

(Humberstone N. Respiratory assessment and treatment. In: Irvin S, Tecklin J, eds. Cardiopulmonary physical therapy. St Louis: CV Mosby, 1990, with permission)

chronic care area for the surgical (pre- and postoperative) and the medical patient, ranging from the neonate to the very elderly.

Optimal pulmonary rehabilitation includes home program planning which helps the patient and family understand and participate in self-care. A follow-up program should include restructuring of the treatment plan and identification of interdisciplinary resources for information and assistance.[27]

Postural Drainage

Postural drainage, along with percussion, shaking, and vibration are used to enhance secretion clearance. In some cases, hydration, humidity, aerosol, and drug therapy performed before beginning postural drainage is effective in enhancing secretion clearance.

By positioning a patient such that the segmental bronchi from a particular lung segment are perpendicular to the ground, secretions that have accumulated in that segment will move to a more central segment, from which they can more easily be removed by coughing. Figure 12–3A,B, and C show postural drainage positions for each bronchopulmonary segment of the lungs. The head-down position (Trendelenburg) is generally used with drainage angles between 10° and 45°,[1] except for the upper lobes, which are drained with the patient flat.

On the other hand, large angles are often poorly tolerated by many patients with severe airway obstruction. Patients with COPD were shown to have little changes in lung volume and no decline in arterial oxygen saturation when assessed with small

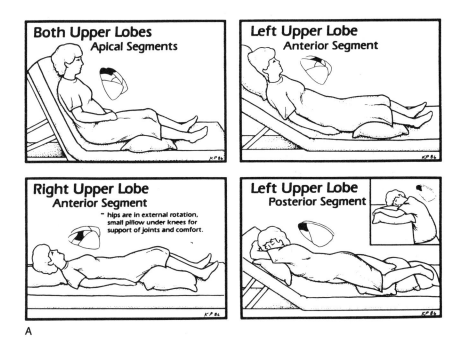

A

FIGURE   12-3   (A) Suggested positions for postural drainage of the upper lobes. (*continued*)

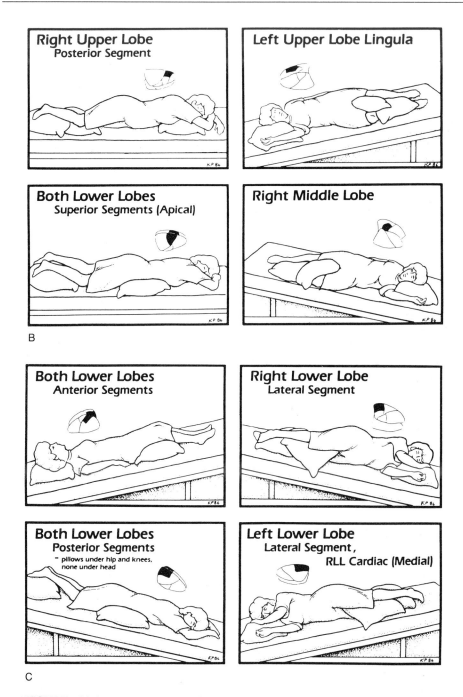

FIGURE 12-3 (*continued*)   (**B**) Suggested positions for postural drainage of the upper, middle, and lower lobes. (**C**) Suggested positions for postural drainage of the lower lobes. (Frownfelter D. Chest physical therapy and pulmonary rehabilitation, an interdisciplinary approach. 2nd ed. Chicago: Year Book Medical Publishers, 1987, with permission)

increment angles of the head-down tilt.[28] Significant decreases in PaO_2 commonly occur in patients with unilateral lung disease when positioned with the diseased lung down. Increases in PaO_2 were reported when patients were positioned with the affected side up.[12,29]

It is common for patients to maintain each posture for a 20-minute period. When percussion, shaking, or vibration is used as an adjunct, the time period for each posture position can be decreased. Although these are the optimal positions for effective treatment, they may have adverse physiologic consequences for some patients (Table 12–7). An inhaled bronchodilator can be administered 10 to 20 minutes before treatment. There are known adverse effects of dehydration, however, the beneficial effects of hydration on the viscoelastic properties of bronchial mucus, as well as on the ease of expectoration, are still unclear.[30] For patients with large amounts of sputum and difficulty expectorating, postural drainage can be performed two to three times daily, depending on the amount of accumulated secretions, and should last for approximately 30 to 40 minutes per session. Controlled cough or the forced expiratory technique (FET) after a session of postural drainage is essential to clearing bronchial secretions.

Postural drainage is frequently used in patients with chronic dysfunction. Ambulatory patients quickly learn to use selected drainage positions that benefit them the most. However, no studies have shown postural drainage to be helpful for patients with COPD in the chronic setting if these individuals are producing less than 1 oz or 30 mL of sputum per day.[31]

Percussion

Percussion (or clapping) is applied with the therapist's cupped hands over the surface of the lung segment being drained. The percussion technique releases the secretions from the wall of the tracheobronchial tree into the lumen of the airway. The cupping of the hands provides a cushion of air between the hands and the chest wall, in an effort to eliminate irritation and discomfort. The technique need not be extremely forceful to be effective. The force of the percussion must be determined for each patient, taking into account such factors as condition of the chest, pain, secretion

TABLE   12-7.   Some of the More Common Contraindications to Positions

Contraindications to the Trendelenberg position
Neurologic problems: recent neurosurgery, increased intracranial pressure, headaches, aneurysm precautions
Circulatory problems: pulmonary edema, congestive heart failure, recent myocardial infarction, unstable arrhythmias, unstable blood pressure
Abdominal problems: obesity, large abdominal masses, distention (ascites, pregnancy), hiatus hernia, nausea and vomiting, recent food consumption

Contraindications of side-lying
Vascular problems: axillofemoral bypass graft
Musculoskeletal injuries: fractures with fixation of the humerus, flail chest

(Starr J. Management of the individual with pulmonary dysfunction. Alexandria, VA: In Touch Prof Dev Ser, Am Phys Ther Assoc, 1990, with permission)

density, secretion volume, and tolerance. Surface areas over bony prominences should be avoided. Percussion should not be performed over ribs 11 and 12 because they are not stabilized by an attachment to the sternum by cartilage. Special consideration should be taken over the anterior and lateral chest wall areas. If necessary, the therapist may choose to percuss with one hand and still have an effective treatment. When percussion is coupled with the appropriate postural drainage position, the probability of secretion removal is enhanced.

For postoperative patients, shorter and more frequent treatments appear to be more effective. No percussion should be done over the area of the incision. A pillow held over the incision will accomplish a splinting effect and enhance tolerance of the treatment. If percussion is not tolerated well by the patient, shaking or vibration alone will be generally satisfactory.

Table 12–8 lists special considerations when administering percussion to patients with cardiovascular, pulmonary, oncologic, and other medical conditions.

Shaking or Rib Springing

There are clinical conditions that seem to necessitate a more aggressive approach by the therapist. If the patient has a mobile chest wall, which should be evaluated by the therapist before commencement of this treatment, shaking may be indicated. Shaking, either vigorous or moderate, is a bouncing rib cage maneuver applied to the chest wall throughout the expiratory phase of breathing, which is designated to produce a more rapid and efficient mobilization of secretions. It is commonly used following percussion in the appropriate postural drainage position. It can also be effective if performed in conjunction with breathing exercises.

Vibration

Vibration is the isometric contraction of the therapist's upper extremities producing vibration that is transmitted from the therapist's hands to the patient's thorax during the expiratory phase of respiration. Vibration with compression should follow the normal chest movement and is most effective when administered during exhalation. Care should be taken if the patient exhibits a stiff, inelastic chest wall, as pathologic fractures may occur. Vibration is generally administered following percussion or can be performed in lieu of percussion. Vibration may be preferred for an acutely ill patient, for a patient in acute respiratory distress, or for a patient who is still ventilator-dependent postoperatively and not hemodynamically stable enough to tolerate percussion. Vibration may also be effective in patients with chronic COPD. In some instances, the therapist may choose to alternate between percussion and vibration techniques. Table 12–9 lists the potential objectives and outcomes of these combined treatment modalities.

TREATMENTS ADMINISTERED TO ENHANCE COUGH

Once secretions have been mobilized and moved to the central airways, clearance techniques are employed. A properly performed cough or huff (cough against an open glottis) should bring secretions to the back of the throat ready for expectoration.

TABLE 12-8. Conditions for Which Caution in Application of Therapeutic Percussion Has Been Recommended

Cardiovascular Conditions
Chest wall pain
Unstable angina
Hemodynamic lability
Low platelet count
Anticoagulation therapy
Unstable or potentially lethal dysrhythmias

Orthopedic Conditions
Osteoporosis
Prolonged steroid therapy
Costal chondritis
Osteomyelitis
Osteogenesis imperfecta
Spinal fusion
Rib fracture or flail chest

Pulmonary Conditions
Bronchospasm
Hemoptysis
Severe dyspnea
Untreated lung abscess
Pneumothorax
Immediately after chest tube removal
Pneumonia or other infectious process
Pulmonary embolus

Oncologic Conditions
Cancer metastatic to ribs or spine
Carcinoma in the bronchus
Resectable tumor

Miscellaneous Conditions
Recent skin grafts
Burns
Open thoracic wounds
Skin infection thorax
Subcutaneous emphysema head and back
Immediately after cataract surgery

(Adapted from Humberstone N. Respiratory assessment and treatment. In: Irvin S, Tecklin J, eds. Cardiopulmonary physical therapy. St. Louis: CV Mosby, 1990, with permission)

TABLE 12-9. Objectives and Potential Outcomes of Postural Drainage and Adjunctive Techniques such as Percussion and Vibration

Therapeutic objective	Eliminate retained secretions
Physiologic objective	Improve mucociliary transport
Potential outcomes	Increase volume expectorated
	Improve clearance of thick secretions
	Reduce airway resistance
	Improve compliance
	Reduce the work of breathing
	Improve oxygenation and ventilation
	Reduce the rate of postoperative pulmonary complications
	Shorten hospitalization

(Humberstone N. Respiratory assessment and treatment. In: Irvin S, Tecklin J, eds. Cardiopulmonary physical therapy. St Louis: CV Mosby, 1990, with permission)

Cough

Cough, either voluntary or reflex, is the simplest method to clear secretions from the larger airways. The therapist improves cough effectiveness by evaluating a patient's cough and determining if improvement is needed by increasing the volume inspired, by augmenting the compression force generated, or by eliciting a cough reflex.[17] Proper cough requires the patient to inhale deeply, close the glottis, create an increase in intrathoracic pressure by contracting the abdominals (bearing down), then release the glottis and expel the air while continually contracting the abdominals.

Most therapists attempt to find a few reliable tricks to assist patients who have difficulty coughing. One of these is to find a comfortable position for the patient. In most instances, patients cough best when sitting up straight or leaning forward.[32] The position of the diaphragm in either of these positions puts the patient in a position that facilitates exhalation. Each patient, as well as each medical condition, should be considered when attempting to facilitate coughing. This is especially true when one considers that a critical depth of airway mucus is required before cough becomes beneficial.[33,34]

In some patients, uncontrolled coughing may induce fatigue, chest wall pain, and dyspnea or even bronchospasm. Controlled cough or forced expiratory technique (huffing or FET) have been used as alternatives to the usual cough techniques.

Huffing is the alternative used to facilitate removal of secretions in patients who have a truly ineffective cough owing to weakness, pain, or a low vital capacity. The patient is asked to take a deep inhalation and rapidly contract the abdominal muscles for a forced expiration through an open airway. A huff is a good alternative because it does not cause a great deal of increased intrathoracic pressure.[35] Because of this, more airways remain patent and make expiration and secretion removal more effective. For many weaker pulmonary patients, huffing is a good way to build up pressure for a cough and not allow the patient to fatigue as quickly. All too often these patients try too hard to cough, with obvious signs of fatigue and strain.

The FET consists of one or two huffs performed from mid- to-low lung volumes, followed by a period of relaxed, controlled diaphragmatic breathing and a cough. The sequence is repeated until secretions are mobilized. The huffs are enhanced by the patient briskly adducting their arms to compress the chest wall. In addition to causing less fatigue, FET appears to decrease cough-induced damage with focal ciliary impairment in flow-limited airway segments.[36] Use of FET has been effective with patients who have cystic fibrosis and bronchiectasis, and should be useful in any patient with excessive secretions or ciliary impairment.[37]

TREATMENTS ADMINISTERED TO REDUCE PAIN AND ENHANCE CHEST MOBILIZATION

In addition to the use of breathing exercises and pulmonary hygiene to maintain optimal function in chronic pulmonary patients, upper extremity and trunk exercises are crucial for long-term joint mobility and trunk flexibility. Long-term pulmonary disease causes muscular adaptations that may alter posture and cause chronic pain. On the other end of the spectrum, patients with abdominal or thoracic surgery frequently remain immobile because of pain, fear, or immediate postoperative weakness. Strong emphasis is placed on mobilization of these patients in addition to pulmonary hygiene. Upper extremity and trunk exercises are incorporated into the treatment to prevent loss of motion and muscle atrophy in both inpatient and outpatient rehabilitation programs. Figure 12–4A through F demonstrates mobilization exercises commonly used in the treatment of acute and chronic pulmonary patients.

Pain and pain tolerance vary from individual to individual and are generally indicative of tissue damage. Therapists use many strategies in the management of pain. For instance, just the tone of voice or gentle approach to patient treatment can relieve anxiety in a patient and reduce pain. Merely changing position can also relieve pain. Recently, the treatment of pain for pulmonary hygiene has included transcutaneous electrical nerve stimulation (TENS). This is a noninvasive, nonpharmacologic and low-cost method of managing pain in any setting.

Research in the area of TENS has reported a lower incidence of atelectasis and reduced number of intensive care days,[38] reduced pain perception and, therefore, reduced pharmacologic intervention,[39] and a positive effect on pulmonary function.[40]

TREATMENTS ADMINISTERED TO ENHANCE FUNCTIONAL CAPACITY

The hazards of both bed rest and sedentary life-style have been well documented and, therefore, progressive exercise programs have been implemented in both the inpatient and outpatient setting as soon as most patients are hemodynamically stable. As the

(*Text continues on p. 242*)

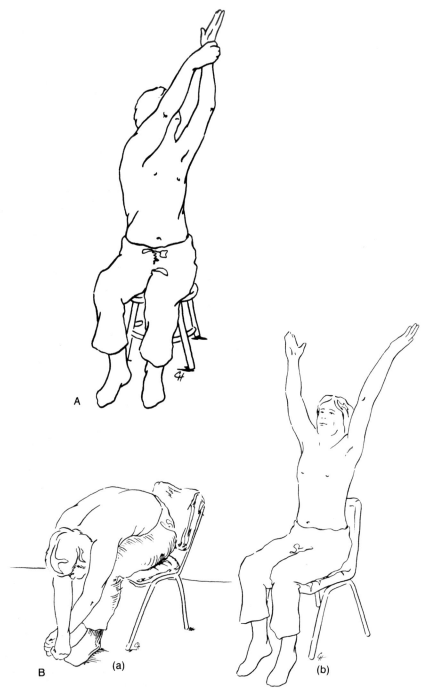

FIGURE 12-4 (**A**) Chest mobilization using trunk rotation and PNF (proprioceptive neuromuscular facilitation [chopping and lifting]) patterns. (**B**) (**a**) Total pattern exercise. Patient exhales during flexion. (**b**) Patient stretches and breathes in during the extension phase. (*continued*)

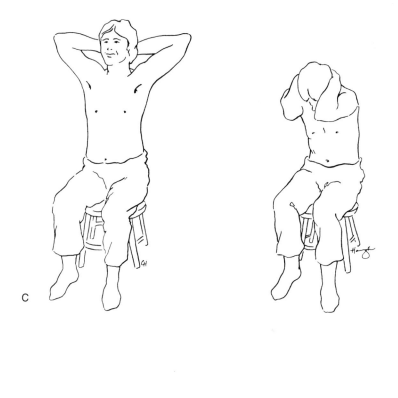

C

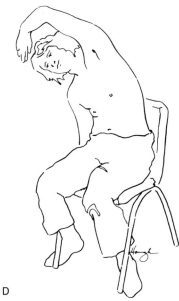

D

FIGURE   12-4 (*continued*)   (**C**) Chest mobilization exercise: breathe in during extension, breathe out during flexion. (**D**) Chest mobilization, lateral flexion; patient exhales during lateral bending. (*continued*)

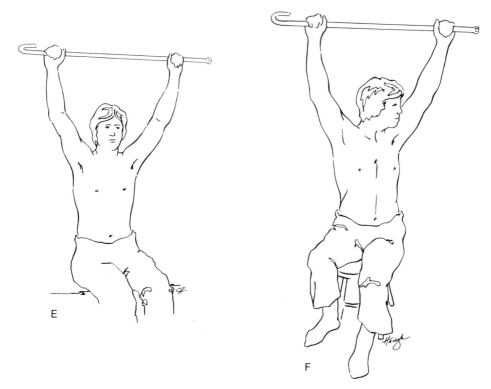

FIGURE   12-4 (*continued*)   (**E**) Cane exercise. Patient may do flexion–extension or rotation exercise (all coordinated with proper breathing patterns). (**F**) Cane exercises for chest mobilization. Patient exhales as he rotates his trunk. (Frownfelter D. Chest physical therapy and pulmonary rehabilitation, an interdisciplinary approach. 2nd ed. Chicago: Year Book Medical Publishers, 1987, with permission)

patient's condition improves, activities that are more aerobic are introduced as a means of enhancing functional capacity.

The effects of physical training on cardiopulmonary performance in patients with COPD have been the subject of many investigations. Aerobic activities, such as bicycling, treadmill walking, and upper extremity activities, have increased the patient's ability to exercise with reduced oxygen consumption. Exercise training to improve exercise endurance, and exercises designed to improve the strength and endurance of the respiratory muscles are discussed elsewhere in the text.

SUMMARY

Pulmonary rehabilitation programs acknowledge the concept that pulmonary disease requires comprehensive medical management. This includes the treatment of acute exacerbations or complications, followed by an attempt to improve and maintain optimal functional levels. If pulmonary rehabilitation is to continue to be a successful mode of treatment, the goals of the program should include, but are not limited to, achieving optimal levels of functional capacity, preventing deterioration, and decreasing morbidity and mortality.[41] Given these goals and given the difficulty in management of the patient with chronic pulmonary disease, individual, allied health professionals have included the techniques of postural drainage, percussion, vibration, cough facilitation, breathing exercises, and the use of humidity and bronchodilators as an adjunct to the exercise components of pulmonary rehabilitation.

A regular program that includes chest physical therapy may help mobilize secretions and clear the airways for effective ventilation during exercise. Symptoms of fatigue may not affect patients to the point of discontinuance of their walking or cycling program. Zadai suggests that patients who usually complain of excess secretions appear to be able to exercise without undue difficulty when chest physical therapy is a part of their regular program.[41] Additionally, in some patients, the use of an effective cough at regular intervals is all that is needed to clear airways, since the increased amounts of secretions owing to exercise appear to mobilize secretions centrally.[41]

Many questions remain unanswered in the area of therapeutic interventions as an adjunct to pulmonary rehabilitation. Ongoing research validating the effects of all chest physical therapy elements is critical. It is imperative that all health care professionals involved in this area of care strive for the highest quality of care, in light of the need for cost-efficient management, with treatment interventions that have sound theoretical foundations.

REFERENCES

1. Faling J. Chest physical therapy. In: Burton G, Hodgkin J, Ward J, eds. Respiratory care: a guide to clinical practice. 3rd ed. Philadelphia: JB Lippincott, 1991.
2. Comroe JH. Physiology of respiration. 2nd ed. Chicago: Year Book Medical Publishers, 1974.
3. Barach AL, Beck GJ. The ventilatory effects of the head-down position in pulmonary emphysema. Am J Med 1954;16:55.
4. Miller WF. A physiologic evaluation of the effects of diaphragmatic breathing training in patients with chronic pulmonary emphysema. Am J Med 1954;17:471.
5. Celli BR. Respiratory muscle function. Clin Chest Med 1986;7:567.
6. Westreich N. Breathing retraining. Minn Med 1970;53:621.
7. Thoman RL, Stoker GL, Ross JC. The efficacy of pursed-lips breathing in patients with chronic obstructive pulmonary disease. Am Rev Respir Dis 1966;93:100.
8. Ingram RH, Schilder DP. Effect of pursed-lip expiration on the pulmonary pressure–flow relationship in obstructive lung disease. Am Rev Respir Dis 1967;96:381.
9. Mueller RE, Petty TL, Filley GF. Ventilation and arterial blood gas changes induced by pursed lips breathing. J Appl Physiol 1970;28:784.
10. Casiari RJ, Fairsbter RD, Harrison A, et al. Effects of breathing retraining in patients with chronic obstructive pulmonary disease. Chest 1981;79:393.
11. Piehl MA, Brown RS. Use of extreme position changes in acute respiratory failure. Crit Care Med 1976;4:13.
12. Zack MB, Pontoppidan H, Kazemi H. The effects of lateral positions on gas exchange in pulmonary disease. A prospective evaluation. Am Rev Respir Dis 1974;110:49.
13. Delgado HR, Braun SR, Skatrud JB, et al. Chest wall and abdominal motion during exercise in patients with chronic obstructive pulmonary disease. Am Rev Respir Dis 1982;126:200.
14. Milic-Emili J, Aubier M. Some recent advances in the study of the control of breathing in patients with chronic obstructive lung disease. Anesth Analg 1980;59:865.

15. Grassino A, Bellemare F, Laporta D. Diaphragm fatigue and the strategy of breathing in COPD. Chest 1984;85(suppl):51S.

16. Gayrard P. Bronchoconstrictor effects of a deep inspiration in patients with asthma. Am Rev Respir Dis 1975;111:433.

17. Humberstone N. Respiratory assessment and treatment. In: Irvin S, Tecklin J, eds. Cardiopulmonary physical therapy. St. Louis: CV Mosby, 1990.

18. Brach BB, et al. Xenon washout patterns during diaphragmatic breathing: studies in normal subjects and patients with chronic obstructive pulmonary disease. Chest 1977;71: 735.

19. Grimby G, et al. Effects of abdominal breathing on the distribution of ventilation in lung disease. Clin Sci Mol Med 1975;148:193.

20. Hughes RC. Does abdominal breathing affect regional gas exchange. Chest 1979;76:258.

21. Innocenti DM. Breathing exercises in the treatment of emphysema. Physiotherapy 1966;52:437.

22. Willeput R, Vachaudez JP, Lenders D, et al. Thoracoabdominal motion during chest physiotherapy in patients affected by chronic obstructive lung disease. Respiration 1983;44:204.

23. Sackner MA, Gonzalez HF, Jenouri G, et al. Effects of abdominal and thoracic breathing on breathing pattern components in normal subjects and in patients with chronic obstructive pulmonary disease. Am Rev Respir Dis 1984;130:584.

24. Vraciu JK, Vraciu RA. Effectiveness of breathing exercises in preventing pulmonary complications following open heart surgery. Phys Ther 1977;57:1367.

25. Campbell E, Friend J. Action of breathing exercise in pulmonary emphysema. Lancet 1955;1:325.

26. Dureuil B, Vires N, Cantineau JP, et al. Diaphragmatic contractility after upper abdominal surgery. J Appl Physiol 1986;61:1775.

27. A definition of chest physical therapy. Cardiopulmonary section. Am Phys Ther Assoc Q 1983(Spring); 4(1) Issue I.

28. Marini JJ, Tyler ML, Hudson LD, et al. Influence of head-dependent positions on lung volume and oxygen saturation in chronic air-flow obstruction. Am Rev Respir Dis 1984;129:101.

29. Huseby J, Hudson L, Stark K, et al. Oxygenation during chest physiotherapy [Abstract]. Chest 1976;70:430.

30. Shim C, King M, Williams MH Jr. Lack of effect of hydration on sputum production in chronic bronchitis. Chest 1987;92:679.

31. Murray JF. The ketchup-bottle method. N Engl J Med 1979;300:1155.

32. Burford JG, George RB. Respiratory physical therapy in the treatment of chronic bronchitis. Semin Respir Infect 1988;3:55.

33. King M, Phillips DM, Gross D, et al. Enhanced tracheal mucus clearance with high frequency chest wall compression. Am Rev Respir Dis 1983;128:511.

34. Evans JN, Jaeger MJ. Mechanical aspects of coughing. Pneumonologie 1975;152: 253.

35. Hietpas BG, Roth RD, Jensen WM. Huff coughing and airway patency. Respir Care 1979;24:710.

36. Smaldone GC, Itoh H, Swift DL, Wagner HN Jr. Effect of flow-limiting segments and cough on particle deposition and mucociliary clearance in the lung. Am Rev Respir Dis 1979;120:747.

37. Pavia D, Agnew JE, Clarke SW. Cough and mucociliary clearance. Bull Eur Physiopathol Respir 1987;23(suppl 10):41S.

38. Rosenberg M. Transcutaneous electrical nerve stimulation for the relief of post-operative pain. Pain 1978;5:129.

39. Stratton S, Smith M. Postoperative thoracotomy: effect of transcutaneous electrical nerve stimulation on forced vital capacity. Phys Ther 1980;60:45.

40. Sahn SA, Nett LM, Pelty TL. Ten year follow-up of a comprehensive COPD. Chest 1980;77(suppl 2):31.

41. Zadai CC. Rehabilitation of patients with chronic obstructive pulmonary disease. In: Irwin S, Tecklin J, eds. Cardiopulmonary physical therapy. St. Louis: CV Mosby, 1990:491.

MIRIAM SCANLAN

LUCY KISHBAUGH

DEBORAH HORNE

Life Management Skill in Pulmonary Rehabilitation

Evaluation and treatment of basic life management skills, including activities of daily living and leisure function are an important step in assisting patients with chronic pulmonary disease to maximize their quality of life. Assisting the patient with environmental adaptations will enhance self-esteem, improve social role performance, and promote a higher level of function. This increased functional level will result in an improvement in quality of life.[1,2] The interrelations among quality of life, neuropsychological functioning, physiologic variables, age, and social position (Fig. 13–1) was considered in the Nocturnal Oxygen Therapy Trial (NOTT) study.[3] This study was a multisite collaborative study designed to compare the effectiveness of nocturnal and continuous oxygen therapy for patients who have chronic obstructive pulmonary disease (COPD) with notable hypoxemia. Findings in this study indicate that the quality of life for patients with COPD was impaired in almost all aspects of functioning, including basic self-care, home management activities, and social, recreational, and leisure activities.

WORKING WITH THE REHABILITATION TEAM

The information in this chapter will provide an overview of the evaluation and treatment of functional deficits, including activities of daily living (ADL) and leisure. This information is based on the multidisciplinary treatment approach, which is used in our pulmonary rehabilitation program at the National Jewish Center for Immunology and Respiratory Medicine, Denver, Colorado. This program is primarily an outpatient rehabilitation program. However, the services that will be described in this chapter can be provided in various settings, by an assortment of health care professionals trained in the management of patients with chronic pulmonary disease. In the Denver program, an occupational therapist is responsible for assessment and treatment of functional deficits related to activities of daily living and vocational needs, and a recreational therapist is responsible for identification and treatment of problems related to leisure well-being. These services enable the patient to lead a full and satisfying life through the recognition, evaluation, and treatment of physical limitations, especially those limitations that are the result of chronic pulmonary disease. To

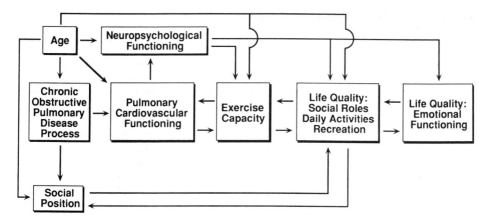

FIGURE   13-1   Hueristic model for interrelating chronic obstructive pulmonary disease and other variables that affect quality of life. (McSweeney J, et al. Life quality of patients with chronic obstructive pulmonary disease. Arch Intern Med 1982; 142:473, with permission)

maximize the effectiveness in achieving the program goals, the staff must have a thorough understanding of all evaluations and treatment that are completed by other members of the multidisciplinary team.

REVIEW OF THE MEDICAL RECORD

Basic medical information should be available for the occupational or recreational therapist responsible for evaluation of the problems associated with ADL and leisure function through review of the medical record and consultation with other members of the multidisciplinary team. Information that should be considered as part of the chart review has been outlined in Table 13–1. A thorough review of this data is essential before proceeding with the patient evaluation, which is then followed by identification of the patient problems, goals, and the development of a treatment plan.

EVALUATION OF ACTIVITIES OF DAILY LIVING

Evaluation of ADL provides the foundation from which the treatment objectives are formed and a plan for therapy is initiated. As part of the evaluation process, the occupational therapist will examine a patient's ability to manage the basic activities of daily living in such a way that personal satisfaction and comfort is attained.[4]

The Interview Process

An interview with the patient and family begins the assessment process. Important components of a good interview include observation, listening, and the ability to ask the right question.[5] It is important to observe the patient for comprehension, breathing pattern during conversation, posture, ability to ambulate, and interaction with family members. When listening during an interview, the therapist should be

TABLE 13-1. **Medical Record Review**

Report	*Information*	*Application to Treatment*
Social support	Family support; community resources	Home program planning; equipment needs
Medical history	Diagnosis, severity; medical management; associated conditions	Previous, current functional level; establish precautions; evaluate associated problems
Pulmonary function	FEV_1; VC; arterial blood gases	Plan realistic goals for completion of ADL and leisure; use of O_2 with ADL and leisure activities
Exercise test	Workload, HR, BP, cardiac precautions, limiting factors, METs	Correlate MET levels with ability to complete ADL and leisure; consider for activity modification
Medication	Bronchodilator, cardiac, blood pressure, psychotropic, and steroid medications	Affect fine/gross motor performance, cognitive ability, strength, and endurance
Physical therapy	Evaluation of strength, endurance, orthopedic dysfunction, posture, gait	Influence on ability to perform functional tasks, including ambulation
Psychosocial	Emotional response—coping style; family interrelations; level of stress	Ability/desire to learn and make life-style modification; need for stress management
Dietary	Underweight, overweight, special dietary requirements	Consider need for energy management techniques, food preparation techniques, and intake changes

aware of the patients' perceptions of their self-concept, motivation, attitude about their illness, and their personal goals for rehabilitation. Follow-up questions might include the following:

- What is your current living situation? Support system?
- With what self-care or other daily tasks and responsibilities are you having more shortness of breath or fatigue than is comfortable or tolerable?
- Do you use oxygen? Please describe when you use your oxygen. Is it at rest, with activity, during sleep, or continuous? What liter flow do you use?
- Do you require any adaptive equipment at home or for the car?
- What tasks do you want to continue doing independently? What tasks would you be comfortable having someone else do for you?
- Could you describe a typical day?
- What activities cause you to have shortness of breath?

- How does your lung problem interfere with your life and the things you enjoy doing?
- Are you employed? If so, has your breathing problem interfered with your employment and how?

The interview should provide an initial impression of the problems that the patient is currently experiencing with activities of daily living[6] along with the patient's and family's expectations. This information, including the patient's stated goals, is essential for successfully implementing an effective treatment program.

Functional Assessment Questionnaire

The next step in the evaluation process includes administration of a self-report questionnaire to the patient. The answers from this questionnaire will permit the evaluation of the patient's individual status, prediction of future problems, and the development of a plan for treatment.[7,8] There are questionnaires available for the measurement of activities of daily living; however, we have found that most of these measure the patient's physical capacity to perform a task, rather than address the symptoms of shortness of breath and generalized fatigue. Currently, we are using the Functional Status Questionnaire[9] which works well for the COPD population with questions based on an "in the past month" time frame.

Other questionnaires that also have good application for the COPD population are the Satisfaction with Performance Scaled Questionnaire[10] and the Subjective ADL Rating Scale for the Pulmonary Rehabilitation Patient.[11] The Satisfaction with Performance Scaled Questionnaire measures the degree of satisfaction that an individual experiences while performing an array of basic and instrumental activities of daily living. This questionnaire considers the relations among satisfaction with life, performance of daily responsibilities, quality of life, and treatment planning. The Subjective ADL Rating Scale for the Pulmonary Rehabilitation Patient measures changes in the performance of ADL before and after participation in an outpatient pulmonary rehabilitation program. This subjective rating scale will facilitate discussion with patients concerning treatment goals and may also be used for measurement of patient outcomes. These are just a few of the questionnaires we have found useful in this patient population.

Upper Extremity Evaluation and the Functional Task

The final phase in the evaluation of functional deficits associated with activities of daily living includes an upper extremity evaluation and the performance of a functional task. Objective parameters monitored routinely as part of the functional task evaluation include measurement of the rate of perceived exertion (RPE) and rate of perceived dyspnea (RPD) (Table 13–2),[12,13] heart rate response, respiratory rate, and oxygen saturation. Attention should also be given to the patterns of breathing used during the initial evaluation and, subsequently, during the treatment process. Some of the inefficient breathing patterns seen in patients with pulmonary disease are as follows:[14,15]

TABLE   13-2.   Instruction for Evaluation of Perceived Exertion and Dyspnea

1. The patient is shown a 10-point rating scale of perceived exertion and dyspnea. They are asked to use the associated descriptions to rate their perception of exertion and dyspnea.

Perceived Exertion Scale		*Perceived Dyspnea Scale*	
0	No effort	0	No shortness of breath (SOB)
0.5	Just noticeable effort	0.5	Slight SOB or breathing
1		1	
2	Light effort	2	Mild SOB or breathing
3	Moderate effort	3	Moderate SOB
4		4	
5	Strong effort	5	Strong or hard breathing
6		6	
7	Very strong effort	7	Severe breathing or SOB
8		8	
9	Very, very strong effort	9	
10	Maximum effort	10	SOB so severe you need to stop and rest

2. The patient is queried about how much effort or shortness of breath he or she is experiencing at the time, depending on the symptoms.
3. Explain the RPE and RPD scale in the following manner:
   a. *Perceived Exertion:* "Try to estimate how hard you feel the work is; that is, we want you to rate the degree of perceived exertion you feel. By perceived exertion, we mean the total amount of exertion and physical fatigue. Do not concern yourself with any one fact, such as leg pain, shortness of breath, or work grade, but try to concentrate on your total inner feeling of exertion. Try to estimate as honestly and objectively as possible."[16]
   b. *Perceived Dyspnea:* "I will be asking you to quantify the amount of your shortness of breath. The scale is from zero to 10. Zero represents no shortness of breath and 10 is so much SOB that you have to stop the activity and rest."

(Adapted from Borg G: Psychophysical bases of perceived exertion. Med Sci Sports Exercise 1982;14:377)

Breath holding or interrupting the regular breathing rhythm during activities

A very short or slight gasp, using the upper chest or accessory muscles, giving little time for air exchange in the lungs and producing a shallow breathing pattern

Forced exhalation, more than normal, causing small airway collapse; not to be confused with pursed-lips breathing

Failure to lengthen exhalation to compensate for airway collapse in patients with air trapping

Irregular, jerky pattern, rather than smooth-flowing, even, and rhythmic breathing

Unnecessary raising of shoulders in an attempt to take in air, or throwing the head back slightly

Paradoxical diaphragmatic movement, with the diaphragm ascending during
inspiration

Asychronous breathing, with minimal abdominal movement, but with
outward rib cage motion during inspiration

The upper extremity evaluation consists of a standard occupational therapy
screening of upper extremity range of motion, strength, endurance, sensation, and
coordination.[17] Attention should be focused on evaluation of strength and endurance
for muscle groups of the hips, shoulders, and trunk, which appear to be the most
affected by steroids.[18] Generalized weakness and deconditioning are associated with
inactivity in the patient with COPD. Often these individuals must rely heavily on
accessory muscle use to do the work of breathing and, at the same time, call upon
these same muscles to stabilize the rib cage and assist with unsupported upper
extremity work.[19–21] Consequently, these muscles often suffer from the overuse
syndrome.

The 12-Minute Walk Evaluation

The 12-minute walk evaluation has been used extensively as part of the basic functional evaluation of patients with chronic pulmonary disease. Cooper originally
described the 12-minute run test as a means of evaluating the level of physical fitness
in young subjects.[22] This test was useful because of the close correlation with the
oxygen uptake measured on the treadmill. McGravin and coworkers found that a
modified version of this test, the 12-minute walk, had good application for evaluating
function in patients with chronic pulmonary disease.[23,24]

The test provides patients with practical knowledge about their endurance with
walking and their ability to pace themselves. Patient awareness of their physiologic
response to exercise and their walking ability is increased. Additional benefits of this
test include the ease of administration, limited equipment and space requirements,
consistent and reproducible results, and that it is a functional activity with universal
importance to patients. The steps in administration and interpretation of this test are
as follows:[25]

PROCEDURE
1. Perform test on a flat, premeasured track.
2. Monitor COPD patients using portable oximetry.
3. Titrate patient with oxygen if desaturation occurs (below 89%).
4. Monitor heart rate at rest, and at 6 and 12 minutes.
5. Complete the test a second time to eliminate learning effect as suggested
   by McGavin.[23]
6. Record results of second test (parameters recorded include distance
   covered, total number of rests, rate of perceived exertion, rate of
   perceived dyspnea, heart rate, oxygen saturation, oxygen liter flow).

PATIENT INSTRUCTIONS
1. Explain purpose of test and basic procedure.
2. Discourage talking during the test, as it interferes with breathing.
3. Explain perceived exertion and dyspnea scale (see Table 13–2).

4. Perform standing stretches with the therapist.
5. Instruct patient to rest as needed.
6. Start test.
7. Cover as much distance as possible for the duration of test.

TEST INTERPRETATION
1. Evaluate individual pacing skills (i.e., rests, rate of perceived exertion, rate of perceived dyspnea).
2. Note breathing patterns during test.
3. Correlate RPE with heart rate.
4. Correlate RPD with SaO_2.
5. Evaluate endurance for functional ambulation by noting distance walked, number of rests, and abnormal gait deviations.
6. Calculation of miles per hour:

$$\frac{\text{distance walked (in ft)}}{5280} = \text{miles walked}$$

$$\frac{\text{miles walked in 12 min.}}{0.2} = \text{miles/hour}$$

7. Approximate energy requirement in metabolic equivalents (METs) for horizontal walking[24]

Miles/hour	Estimated METS (0% grade)
1.7	2.3
2.0	2.5
2.5	2.9
3.0	3.3
3.4	3.9

(Adapted from Guidelines for Exercise Testing, 3rd ed. American College of Sports Medicine, Lea & Febiger, 1986)

Functional Task Performance

Selection of a functional task for performance should be done after reviewing information collected from the initial interview, self-care questionnaire, and performance on the 12-minute walk and exercise test. It is important to consider activities that the patient must be able to manage as part of their basic self-care or to consider specific activities the patient has a strong desire to successfully perform. We have standardized three functional tasks for evaluation. Performance of the functional task is used to establish a baseline for planning treatment and measuring outcomes. The three functional tasks used for testing may include:

- washing hands and face, brushing teeth, combing hair while seated at the sink (1.5 METs)
- changing bed linens (3.5 METs)
- work simulation (5 METs).

TABLE   13-3.   Energy Expenditure in METs

Physical Conditioning Activities	METS	Recreation Activities	METS
Walking (1.7–2 mph)	2.3–2.5	Painting (sitting)	1.5
Walking (2.5–3 mph)	2.9–3.3	Playing cards	1.5–2.0
Stationary cycling (slowly)	3.5	Playing piano	2.0
Walking (3.4–3.75 mph)	3.6–3.9	Driving a car	2.0
Calisthenics	4.5	Canoeing (2.5 mph)	2.5
Cycling (outdoors) (6 mph)	4–5	Horseback riding (walk)	2.5
Swimming (crawl, 1 ft/sec)	5.0	Golf (power cart)	2–3
Stationary Cycling (vigorous)	6–7	Volleyball (6-man team)	3.0
Jogging (5 mph)	7–8	Golf (pulling clubs)	3–4
Housework and Occupational Activities			
Sitting at a desk or eating	1.5	Horseshoes	3.5
Typing	2.0	Sailing (small boat)	3–4
Dusting furniture	2.0	Ballroom dancing (foxtrot)	4–5
Preparing a meal	2–2.5	Tennis (doubles)	4–5
Auto repair	2–3	Ice or roller skating (9 mph)	5–6
Riding lawn mower	2–3	Stream fishing (wading)	5–6
Sweeping	3.0	Horseback riding (trot)	6.5
Making beds	3.0	Square dancing	6–7
Vacuuming	3.5	Tennis (singles)	6–7
Ironing (standing)	3.5	Water skiing	6–7
Cleaning windows	3.5	Downhill skiing (light)	6–7
Mopping	3.5	**Self-Care Activities**	
Hanging wash	3.5	Sitting/eating	1–2
Raking leaves	3.5	Wheelchair propulsion	2.0
Pushing light power mower	3–4	Meal preparation	2.5
Hoeing	4.5	Tub bath/dressing	2–3
Carpentry	5.5	Shower (seated or standing)	3–4
Digging a garden	5–6	Walking downstairs	5.0
Washing car	6.0	Ambulation with crutches	6.5
Mowing with hand mower	6.5		

A MET equals 3.5 mL/kg/min of oxygen consumption. These values are based on a person weighing 150 lb (70 kg).
(Adapted from Blair SN, et al. Guidelines for graded exercise testing and prescription. 3rd ed. Philadelphia: Lea & Febiger, 1986; and McArdle WD, et al. Exercise physiology: energy, nutrition, and human performance. Philadelphia: Lea & Febiger, 1986)

These three tasks represent progressions in physical exertion and the use of the upper extremities. Correlation of these tasks with MET levels (Table 13–3) can provide patients with information about physical activities, household and occupational tasks, and recreation that they may be able to accomplish independently or with slight modification (Fig. 13–2). A MET is the amount of energy required while the body is at rest (1 MET = 3.5 mL/kg/min. of oxygen consumption). In other words, it is the amount of energy needed to maintain basic bodily functions. Other activities are expressed as requiring a multiple of this resting requirement. Emotional stress, extremes of temperature, skill and coordination, self-confidence, physical fitness, body position, and posture are some factors that can alter energy requirements in any individual. It is important to remember these factors when reviewing the results of the functional task evaluation and when making recommendations to patients about their ability to perform certain activities. Remember that the numbers are only approximations, and there are many variables that may affect the performance of a given activity. The form used for scoring the performance of the functional task is shown in Table 13–4. The use and scoring of this form provides a more objective way to measure improved performance of a specific functional task. Individual section scores, as well as a cumulative score, provide objective information to assist the therapist in identifying problems, planning follow-up treatment, and evaluating outcomes.

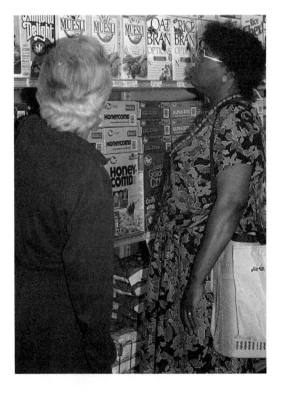

FIGURE 13-2 Household–occupational task modification. (Courtesy of National Jewish Center for Immunology and Respiratory Medicine, Denver, CO)

TABLE 13-4. Functional Task Performance Test Form

Name: _____ Diagnosis: _____

MET Level: _____ FEV$_1$: _____ % Predicted _____ **Weight (kg):** _____ **Age:** _____
(Achieved on Stress Testing)

Functional task selected: _____ **12-min walk** _____

Task MET Level _____   (Does regularly) _____   (Does not do regularly) _____

1. **Independence:**   Activity Completed: Yes or No _____

2. **Physiologic Parameters**   Liters of O$_2$ _____

	Heart Rate	SaO$_2$	Respirations	
Before	_____	_____	_____	
Post (IPA)*	_____	_____	_____	
5 min Post	_____	_____	_____	
Change from baseline	_____	_____	_____	Score _____

3. **Time:** _____   4. **Number of rests:** _____

5. **Subjective rating:**   Perceived Dyspnea Pre-Task: _____
   Perceived Exertion (IPA*) _____ Perceived Dyspnea (IPA*) _____ Score _____

6. **Breathing pattern characteristics:**
   (Recorded during the test—not part of total score)

   _____ Deep   _____ Shallow
   _____ Slow   _____ Rapid
   _____ Smooth/rhythmical   _____ Irregular
   _____ Uncontrolled/poor pacing   _____ Inappropriate use of O$_2$

7. **Energy management techniques: Present/Absent**   Score _____

8. **Comments:** _____

9. **Cumulative score for functional task:** _____
   Rating: Good _____   Fair _____   Poor _____

* IPA; Immediate post-activity.
(Adapted from Cromwell F, ed. Occupational therapy for the energy deficient patient: Monitored dressing evaluation–physiologic assessment of cardiac work tolerance. New York: Haworth Press, 1986)

ASSESSMENT AND TREATMENT TO MAXIMIZE ACTIVITIES OF DAILY LIVING

Objective information collected from the patient evaluation will be used to make an overall assessment of problems, establish treatment goals, and proceed with implementation of a treatment plan. Table 13–5 outlines the steps used in processing the data collected during the functional evaluation. The general goal of occupational therapy is to restore and maximize independence to perform basic and instrumental ADL. Specific treatment goals include the following:

1. Minimize shortness of breath with basic and instrumental ADL
2. Achieve the most effective breathing pattern possible through instruction in specific breathing techniques
3. Increase functional endurance for ADL
4. Apply principles of energy and time management

TABLE 13-5. Assessment and Treatment of Functional Deficits

Evaluation	Problems Identified	Treatment (group or individual)
Functional task	Shortness of Breath/fatigue with ADLs	Individual ADL Rx
	Inefficient breathing pattern	Breathing retraining
	Increased use of accessory muscles of respiration	Maximize use of diaphragmatic breathing
	Poor pacing or energy management techniques	Instruction and practice of energy management, relaxation, stress management techniques
12-min walking	Gait abnormalities	Gait training Lower extremity strengthening
	Decrease in functional endurance for ambulation	Endurance training
Upper extremity evaluation	Decreased upper extremity strength	Progressive resistive exercise
	Decreased upper extremity endurance	Upper extremity endurance training
	Postural abnormalities	Posture exercise
Vocational issues	Difficulty maintaining employment	Identify specific issues
	Lack knowledge of job modifications	Explore possible strategies
	Lack knowledge of vocational options	Vocational interest testing Resume preparation Referral to vocational rehabilitation

5. Provide relaxation and stress management techniques
6. Increase awareness of the use of adaptive equipment
7. Assist the patient's family with understanding options for managing ADL after discharge
8. Explore issues related to employment

Individual Versus Group Treatment of Functional Activities of Daily Living Deficits

Treatment goals are met through a variety of methods. Patients can benefit from a combination of individual and group treatment sessions. The severity of a patient's problems usually determines to what extent a patient will be treated individually or in a group session. Family members are encouraged to attend either or both sessions. This facilitates the patient's comprehension of treatment and promotes compliance. Individual treatment allows the therapist to focus on specific needs, and it is most frequently used for those who are experiencing marked problems with basic ADL. Sessions are also important for patient instruction on specific breathing techniques, such as pursed-lips and diaphragmatic breathing. This allows patients to practice performance until they can incorporate the concepts of energy management and effective-breathing techniques into routine performance.

Group treatment is often preferred because of the positive effect of group interactions, including an opportunity to share common problems and resolutions. The size of the group should remain small to facilitate discussion. Lower-functioning patients may be seen in group treatment after receiving individualized instruction in specific deficit areas. Sessions on energy management in the home, stress management,[28] physical relaxation training,[29] and employment issues are appropriate topics for group sessions (Table 13–6).

Breathing Training and Energy Management

Management of breathlessness should be an integral part of the treatment program for patients with chronic pulmonary disease.[30] Breathing is taken for granted, and normal variations in regularity are not noticed by most persons, except during strenuous work, exercise, or emotional upsets. Little attention is required to bring breathing back into control for normal persons. However, for those with pulmonary disease, becoming aware of when to expect disruptions in breathing patterns enables them to control "normal" breathlessness to some extent. Appropriate breathing patterns and the use of energy management techniques should be incorporated into

TABLE   13-6.   Functional ADL Group Program Session

Group Session	Process Objective	Teaching Strategy
Energy management	Present information to increase knowledge of energy management	Instruct in components of energy management Group problem-solving of difficult task to apply above
Physical relaxation training	Acquire knowledge of benefits of relaxation techniques for pulmonary patients Demonstrate appropriate relaxation techniques	Instruct and schedule practice in various relaxation techniques
Stress management	Increase knowledge of normal life-style stresses, and interaction of stress and chronic disease Identify individual stresses	Stress awareness exercises Instruction in psychophysiologic responses to stress and stress reduction techniques
Employment issues	Identify employment issues for pulmonary patients Acquire knowledge of possible work modifications, job options, and retraining	Group discussion from general outline of employment issues Group problem-solving of several specific employment issues

all aspects of treatment. This includes group and individual treatment sessions for ADL and leisure function.

For patients with severe pulmonary disease, it is the unsupported upper extremity activities that cause the most shortness of breath.[19–21] Often, these patients must rely heavily on accessory muscles to do the work of breathing, and when these muscles are used for supporting the arms, they are unavailable to assist with breathing. In addition, trunk muscles are being used to stabilize the rib cage, and breathing becomes more difficult. Patients experience the most difficulty with basic self-care tasks that involve working over their shoulders, such as shaving, hair care, and other personal-grooming tasks. Instructions should be provided in ways to modify the use of the upper extremities for all activities. They can learn to apply "breathing awareness principles" during those activities that cause severe shortness of breath.

BREATHING AWARENESS PRINCIPLES

1. Minimize arm movement against gravity or overhead. If you must work at this level, do a few movements, relax the arms down, breathe properly (no breath holding), and resume the activity.
2. Emphasize the use of O_2 with ADL and leisure activities when prescribed.
3. Complete tasks after inhaled medication treatments when possible.
4. Coordinate breathing with all activities (e.g., exhale when pushing a vacuum and inhale with pulling).
5. Recognize that talking, laughing, eating, and coughing, all are exhaling patterns that interrupt the regular rhythm of breathing and accommodate accordingly.
6. Realize that activities requiring great concentration or steadiness may place additional demands on breathing.
7. Consider body position and posture when completing activities (e.g., minimize bending when possible).

Individual treatment sessions may be required to allow work on breathing and energy management with specific home management tasks. Coordinated breathing with body movements is practiced to give the patient a basis for future problem solving with any activity that may be undertaken. Patients are taught to think through a task and then visualize the movements and steps involved in completion of that task. When breathlessness is ensuing, it is important for the patient to pause and breathe through pursed lips while it is still possible to get breathing under control.

Oximetry is used as an adjunct to these individual treatment sessions if patients are receiving oxygen. This allows the therapist to interpret and document whether a patient maintains adequate O_2 saturations during ADLs. The guideline at this institution is to maintain saturation at 90% or above. Oximetry provides useful feedback to the patient. The patient can be taught that:

- Body motions or positions (especially unsupported upper extremity) cause decreased O_2 saturation.
- Sensation of shortness of breath does not necessarily mean the O_2 saturation is too low.
- Shortness of breath correlates most closely with the work of breathing.

- Adequate saturation can be maintained if efficient breathing techniques are employed, such as pursed-lips breathing.
- Incorporating pacing in performance of activities can decrease dyspnea, maintain saturation, and ultimately reduce fatigue.

Since shortness of breath and fatigue are the most prominent symptoms treated by the occupational therapist, attaining the best application of energy management techniques is essential. It is suggested that energy management be used as a generic concept encompassing various components of traditional occupational therapy treatment. The following general principles on energy management should be considered:[6,15,30,31]

1. Energy conservation techniques
2. Work efficiency
3. Proper body mechanics
4. Time management
5. Pacing skills

Ultimately, if patients are able to apply some of these important principles of breathing and energy management, they will have increased confidence in performance of functional and leisure activities.

Treatment of Vocational Issues

The patient's occupational status is easily determined during the initial interview process. Information should be gathered on employment status, including specific questions concerning full-time or part-time employment, retirement, and disability. It is important to consider factors that contribute to the patients' ability to maintain employment while managing their chronic pulmonary disease. Patients with COPD who are employed must deal with issues related to increased absenteeism, unreasonable physical demands, environmental irritants, and the need for oxygen or medications while working.

Educational sessions that explore job issues related to chronic pulmonary disease can help patients develop coping skills for independent problem solving. This might include possible job modifications, such as a change in working hours, altered responsibilities, changing work station to avoid irritants, or wearing a mask. Appropriate management of medication and potential side effects pose another challenge to patients wishing to maintain employment; difficulty with memory, concentration, or shakiness are some of the side effects that interfere with employment. Medication schedules should be organized into a patient's work schedule.

Frequently, vocational changes must be considered for patients who have employment and health issues that cannot be successfully managed together (see Chapter 18 for more detailed information on this topic).

EVALUATION OF LEISURE FUNCTION

A satisfying leisure life-style has been determined to be an integral element in attaining a more satisfying quality of life. Ragheb and Griffin confirmed that the higher the frequency of participation in leisure activity, the better the life satisfaction of the older adult.[32] One of the changes that a person experiences with chronic disease is a change in life-style. The need to make life-style adjustments because of chronic illness and aging can directly affect a person's satisfaction and participation in meaningful leisure activities.[33,34] Often, new recreational resources need to be tapped, and patients must learn to cope with their illness by learning new recreational pursuits (Fig. 13–3) or ways to adapt to previous interests.

A process of leisure education can assist patients with developing personally fulfilling leisure life-styles. Through guided activities, the patients have an opportunity to explore feelings, values, and beliefs related to the leisure experience. Through this exploration, a person's leisure repertoire will be improved. Improved leisure function will positively affect the person's entire well-being.

Leisure Diagnostic Battery

The leisure functioning of patients with chronic lung disease should be considered in the overall evaluation and treatment of functional deficiency. A practical plan for improvement of leisure function is developed by referencing information gathered from the ADL and leisure diagnostic battery evaluation (LDB).[35]

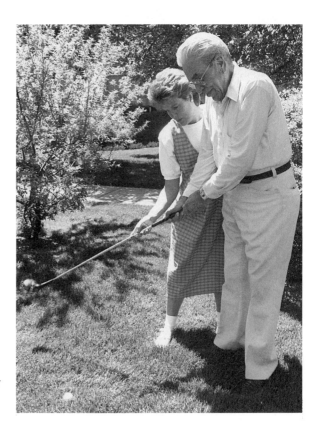

FIGURE 13-3 Active life-styles delay functional consequences of chronic disease. (Courtesy of National Jewish Center for Immunology and Respiratory Medicine, Denver, CO)

TABLE 13-7. Guidelines for Use of the Leisure Diagnostic Battery (LDB) with Adult Pulmonary Patients

Leisure Evaluation	Test Form Used	Score/ Interpretation	Recommendations Leisure Education Enrichment Program (LEEP); see Table 13-8)
1. Initial screening	LDB short form	Above 3.4	LEEP unit 1 and 2 "recommended" Leisure and society Leisure and Well-Being
		3.4 or below	Complete evaluation
2. Complete evaluation	LDB long form		
	a. Scale F (Barriers)	10 or above in subscale	Unit 3 (breaking down barriers)
	b. Scale G (Leisure preferences)	Less than 5 on each subscale	Unit 4 (Leisure in my life)
	c. Scale H (Knowledge of leisure opportunities and resources)	60% or below	LEEP; unit 4 and unit 5 (Implementing my leisure plan)

The LDB was designed to identify an individual's perception of freedom in leisure, and for those individuals identified with deficiencies, to further identify the factors limiting perceived freedom. The purpose of the LDB evaluation is to:

1. assess the patient's leisure functioning
2. determine areas in which improvement of current leisure functioning are needed
3. determine the effect of the leisure education and enrichment program on leisure functioning
4. facilitate research on the value, purpose, and outcome of leisure experience for pulmonary patients

The LDB is a collection of instruments used to evaluate leisure function and make treatment recommendations (Table 13–7). This instrument was originally developed for use with adolescents (version A), but has since been modified for use in the adult population (version B, short form; and C, long form). The LDB short form is administered to all of the patients in our pulmonary rehabilitation program. This questionnaire consists of 25 items and requires approximately 10 minutes to complete. It serves as a quick screening tool for identification of potential problems with leisure function.

The LDB long form is used if more detailed evaluation is indicated by the scoring of the short form. The long form consists of the folllowing three scales:

Scale F: Barriers to leisure experience. Used to determine problems that an individual encounters when trying to select, or participate in leisure experiences.

Scale G: Leisure preference. Used to determine an individual's pattern of selecting activities. In addition, this scale measures preference for mode or style of involvement.

Scale H: Knowledge of leisure opportunities and resources. Used to determine the individual's knowledge of specific information concerning leisure opportunities and community resources (this scale was adapted from the long form—adolescent version by National Jewish Center staff).

Interpretation of the long form is based on the cumulative score for all three scales, as well as the individual score for each scale. Detailed information on use of the leisure diagnostic battery can be found in the *The Leisure Diagnostic Battery—Users Manual.*[35]

TREATMENT OF LEISURE DYSFUNCTION

Information gathered from the patient's medical record, interview, and results of the LDB are used to identify problems associated with leisure functioning. The general goal for treatment of the patients is to assist in development of a greater awareness of their values, beliefs, and attitudes toward leisure. Through this increased awareness, patients can begin to explore their needs for satisfying participation in recreation activities (Fig. 13–4). Upon discharge the patient will be able to successfully implement a personally fulfilling leisure component to their life. Our leisure education enrichment program (LEEP) was designed to meet the needs of patients with chronic lung disease (Table 13–8). The goals of LEEP are to:

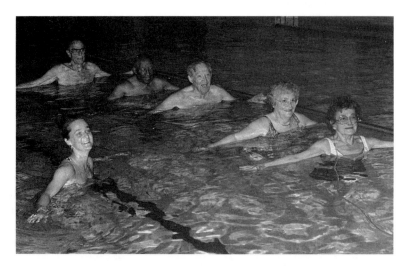

FIGURE   13-4   Fitness-related leisure activities promote wellness and increase quality of life. (Courtesy of National Jewish Center for Immunology and Respiratory Medicine, Denver, CO)

TABLE 13-8. Leisure Education Enrichment Program (LEEP)

Group Session	Objective	Teaching Strategies
Leisure and society (Unit 1)	Introduce information to increase awareness of the role leisure plays in society	Group instructional activities: "Benefits of leisure" "Time use diary" "Working for leisure"
Leisure and well-being (Unit 2)	Present information that demonstrates the relation between leisure and health	Group instructional activities: "How's your sense of self responsibility?" "How long will you live?" "Stress quiz"
Leisure in my life (Unit 3)	Exploration of personal beliefs, values, attitudes, styles, and resources related to leisure	Individual/group instructional activities: "Twenty things I love to do" "12-foot room" "Leisure inventory" "The leisure balance"
Breaking down barriers (Unit 4)	Facilitate recognition and management of barriers affecting leisure participation	Individual instructional sessions: "Barriers to your enjoyment" "Leisure barriers" "Boxed in" "Leisure alternatives"
Implementing my leisure plan (Unit 5)	Instruct patient in development of a leisure plan for use after discharge	Individual instructional sessions: "Get ready" "Leisure contact" "Leisure gothic goals" "Leisure activity self-contract"

(LEEP developed in consultation with Dr. Jane Kaufman, PhD, Director of Therapeutic Recreation, University of Northern Colorado and the Recreation Therapy Staff at National Jewish Center. Teaching strategies adapted from Stumbo NJ, Thompson SR. Leisure education: a manual of activities and resources. Peoria, IL, Center for Independent Living and Easter Seals 1986; and McDowell, CF. Leisure wellness: concepts and helping strategies, vol 1–10. OR: Sunmoon Press, 1983)

- provide an awareness of the importance of a healthy leisure life-style to overall quality of life
- assist the individual in exploring personal values, attitudes, and beliefs toward leisure
- assist the individual in recognizing barriers to leisure participation
- encourage independence or utilization of support persons and organizations for leisure participation
- expand awareness of leisure opportunities that are personally applicable
- encourage the patient to develop a leisure plan for discharge
- provide the patient with opportunities for recreation upon discharge
- provide general information on how to access leisure information and activities in the community
- explore methods of activity modification

Treatment can be provided in group education sessions or through individual leisure counseling sessions for patients with more significant problems.[36,37] The first three basic units of the LEEP program may be implemented in a group setting. Most patients seen for a pulmonary rehabilitation program could benefit from the basic units (Units 1 and 2), regardless of their score on the LDB or their present life-style. Persons who are seen for rehabilitation are often close to retirement and have given little thought to how they will spend their unstructured time. In addition, many patients who are not currently having difficulty with leisure function are likely to experience problems as their disease progresses. Through educational sessions, patients have the opportunity to learn the importance of leisure and planning for social and recreational activities.

Units 3, 4, and 5 of the LEEP program should be completed by patients who are having significant problems in leisure function, as identified on the LDB scales F, G, and H. These units can be provided in small group or individual sessions. Individual leisure counseling is recommended for patients with low total scores on the LDB long form. Leisure counseling facilitates and promotes self-awareness of leisure attitudes and values. It also encourages the development of problem-solving and decision-making related to participation in personally rewarding leisure activities.

LIFE MANAGEMENT HOME PROGRAM RECOMMENDATIONS

Home program recommendations should be developed following completion of the discharge evaluation. The therapist evaluates the patient's readiness for discharge, including improvement in ability to complete ADL and leisure interests and understanding of information provided during the course of treatment. This can be done most effectively through patient and family discussion and demonstration of specific techniques. The interdisciplinary team should make every effort to coordinate home recommendations. Written recommendations provided to the patient will assist in the implementation of a home program. Home program information should include specific application of breathing techniques, use of energy conservation techniques, recommendations for adaptive equipment, and a review of community resources that may be helpful. A plan for follow-up visits and involvement in an ongoing com-

TABLE 13-9. Sample Home Activity Plan

SAMPLE HOME ACTIVITY PLAN
(65-year-old married female COPD, MET level 3.0, living in 3-bedroom house with retired husband)

Time	Monday	Tuesday	Wednesday	Thursday	Friday	Saturday	Sunday
6:00 AM	Treatment Medications	Same as Monday	Same as Monday	Same as Monday	Same as Monday	Same as Monday	Same as Monday
7:00	Breakfast	*	*	*	*	*	*
8:00	ADL/dress	*	*	*	*	*	*
9:00	Light housework (husband vacuums)			Husband cleans bathroom		Patient light housework	
10:00		Grocery shop alone-light		Heavy grocery shop with husband		Husband cleans kitchen floor	
11:00	Food preparation		Beauty shop		Food preparation	Food preparation	Church
NOON	Med Tx/lunch	*	*	*	*	*	Treatment
1:00		Errands					Meal out
2:00		Volunteer 2 h		Crafts at Sr. Center 2 h	Shopping at mall 2 h	Visit friends relatives	
3:00	Relaxation	*	*	*	*	*	*
4:00	Walking/exercise	*	*	*	*	*	*
5:00	Supper home	Supper out	Supper home	Supper out	Supper home	Supper home	Supper home
6:00-7:00	Handwork, read, TV, and etc.		Movie	Handwork			
8:00-10:00	Treatment/news	*	*	*	*	*	*

* Same as previous day.
Appropriate Tasks: Light housekeeping (dusting, laundry, changing bed), grocery shopping, and food preparation.
Options: with increased endurance and activity tolerance: Pool exercise class, additional volunteer hours, day trips with Senior Center, vacation away.
This schedule should be kept flexible; use it as a guide and experiment with the balance of task.

265

munity-based group program will facilitate compliance with home recommendations.

Completion of a home activity plan (Table 13–9) will assist the patient and family with organization of information provided during treatment.

SUMMARY

It is not clear if the issues we covered in this chapter can influence physiologic function of the pulmonary patients that come to us for rehabilitation. However, we do feel that patients can experience a satisfying, purposeful life, regardless of the effects of their physiologic function. We believe that rehabilitation is all about showing the patient there is a reason to live and providing methods for adaptation to a life with chronic disease. Patients must be given the confidence to try new methods of performing tasks and be provided with the option of experiencing activities that they may not have previously considered possible.

Acknowledgments

Sylvia Talkington, R. N., Case Manager PRIDE Program
National Jewish Center for Immunology and Respiratory Medicine

REFERENCES

1. Stewart AL, et al. Functional status and well-being of patients with chronic conditions. JAMA 1989;263:907.

2. Packa DR, Branyon ME, Kinney MR, Khan SH, Kelley R, Miers LJ. Quality of life of elderly patients enrolled in cardiac rehabilitation. J Cardiovasc Nurs 1989;3(2):33.

3. McSweeney J, Grant I, Heaton R, Adams K, Timms R. Life quality of patients with chronic obstructive pulmonary disease. Arch Intern Med 1982;143:473.

4. Rogers JC. The spirit of independence: the evolution of a philosophy. AOTA 1982;36:709.

5. Willard H, Spackman C. Occupational therapy. 5th ed. Philadelphia. JB Lippincott, 1978:151.

6. Ogden LD, de Renne C. Chronic obstructive pulmonary disease: program guidelines for health professionals. Laurel, MD: Ramsco, 1985.

7. Kane A, Kane R. Uses and abuses of measurements. Assessing the elderly, a practical guide to measurement. 11th ed. Lexington, MA: Lexington Books, 1981.

8. Spiegel JS, Madlyn HS, Spiegel TM. Evaluation self-care activities: comparison of a self-reported questionnaire with an occupational therapist interview. Br J of Rheumatol 1985;24:357.

9. Jett A, Davies A, Clearly P, et al. The functional status questionnaire. J Gen Intern Med 1986;1:143.

10. Yerxa E, Burnett-Beaulieu S, Stocking S, Azen S. Development of the satisfaction with performance scaled questionnaire. Am J Occup Ther 1988;42:215.

11. Phillips M. A subjective ADL rating scale for the pulmonary rehabilitation patient. In: Occupational therapy for energy deficit patient. New York: Haworth Press, 1986:1.

12. Borg G. Psychological bases of perceived exertion. Med Sci Sports Exercise 1982;14:377.

13. Mahler D. Dyspnea: diagnosis and management. Clin Chest Med 1987;8:215.

14. Lareau S, Larson JL. Ineffective breathing pattern related to airflow limitation. Nurs Clin North Am 1987;22:179.

15. Tangri S, Woolf CR. The breathing pattern in chronic obstructive pulmonary disease during the performance of some common daily activities. Chest 1973;63:126.

16. Pollock M, Wilmore J, Fox F. Evaluation and prescription for prevention and rehabilitation. In: Exercise in health and disease. Philadelphia: WB Saunders, 1984:191.

17. Trombly C, Scott AD. Evaluation and assessment. In: Occupational therapy for physical dysfunction. Baltimore: Williams & Wilkins, 1977:125.

18. Bowyer SL, LaMothe MP, Hollister JR. Steroid myopathy: incidence and detection in an asthmatic population. J Allergy Clin Immunol 1985;76:234.

19. Celli BR, Rassulo J, Make BJ. Dyssynchronous breathing during arm but not leg exercise in patients with chronic airflow obstruction. N Engl J Med 1982;307:485.

20. Criner GJ, Celli BR. Effect of unsupported arm exercise on ventilatory muscle recruitment in patients with severe chronic airflow obstruction. Am Rev Respir Dis 1988;138:856.

21. Make BJ. Pulmonary rehabilitation: myth or reality? Clin Chest Med 1986;7:519.

22. Cooper KH. A means of assessing maximal oxygen intake. JAMA 1968;203:201.

23. McGavin CR, Gusta SP, McHardy GJR. Twelve-minute walking test for assessing disability in chronic bronchitis. Br Med J 1976;1:822.

24. McGavin CR, Artvinli M, Naoe H, McHardy GJR. Dyspnea, disability and distance walked: comparison of estimates of exercise performance in respiratory disease. Br Med J 1978;2:241.

25. Blair SN, Gibbons LW, Painter P, Pate RP, Taylor CB, Will J. Guidelines for exercise testing and prescription. 3rd ed. Philadelphia: Lea & Febiger, 1986.

26. McArdle WD, Katch FI, Katch VL. Exercise physiology: energy, nutrition and human performance. Philadelphia: Lea & Febiger, 1986.

27. Cromwell, FS. Occupational therapy for the energy deficient patient. New York: Haworth Press, 1986.

28. Frain M, Valiga T. The multiple dimensions of stress. Aspen, CO: Aspen Systems Corporation, 1979.

29. Renfroe K. Effect of progressive relaxation on dyspnea and state of anxiety in patients with COPD. Heart Lung 1988;17:408.

30. Moser K, Archibald C, Hansen P, Ellis B, Whelan D. Shortness of breath: a guide to better living and breathing. St Louis: CV Mosby, 1983.

31. O'Ryan J, Burns, D. Pulmonary rehabilitation: from hospital to home. Chicago: Yearbook Medical Publishers, 1984.

32. Ragbeh M, Griffith H. The contribution of leisure participation and leisure satisfaction to life satisfaction of older persons. Leisure Satisfaction Res 1982;14:295.

33. Wade MG. Constraints on leisure. Springfield:1987;22:335.

34. McDowell CF, Clark P. Assessing the leisure needs of older persons. Meas Eval Guidance 1982;15:228.

35. Witt P, Ellis G. The leisure diagnostic battery—users manual. State College, PA: Venture Publishing, 1987.

36. Gunn S, Peterson C. Therapeutic recreation program design: principles and procedures. Englewood Cliffs, NJ: Prentice-Hall, 1978.

37. Edwards PB. Leisure counseling techniques: individual and group counseling step-by-step. 3rd ed. Los Angeles: Constructive Leisure, 1980.

38. Stumbo NJ, Thompson SR. Leisure education: a manual of activities and resources. Peoria, IL: Center for Independent Living and Easter Seals, 1986.

39. Mc Dowell CF. Leisure wellness: concepts and helping strategies, vol. 1–10. Eugene, OR: Sun Moon Press, 1983.

BARTOLOME R. CELLI

14

Arm and Leg
Exercise Training in
Pulmonary Rehabilitation

The short- and long-term effects of systematic exercise conditioning has been the subject of extensive investigation. In normal persons, it is known that participation in a well-designed exercise training program results in several objective changes:

1. There is increased maximal oxygen uptake, primarily owing to increases in blood volume, hemoglobin level, and heart stroke volume, although changes in the peripheral utilization of oxygen have not totally been ruled out.
2. With specific training, there is increase in muscular strength and endurance, primarily resulting from enlargement of muscle fibers and improved blood and energy supply.
3. There is better muscle coordination.
4. There is a change in body composition with increased muscle mass and loss of adipose tissue.
5. There is an improved sensation of well-being.

In patients with obstruction to airflow, participation in a similar program will result in different outcomes, depending on the severity of the obstruction. Patients with mild-to-moderate disease will, as a rule, manifest the same findings as normal subjects, whereas, as we shall discuss later, patients with the severe form will be able to increase exercise endurance and improve their sensation of well-being with little if any increase in the maximum oxygen uptake.

In patients with COPD, tolerance to exercise is decreased. The most important factors thought to contribute to this limitation of exercise in patients with COPD are alterations in pulmonary mechanics, abnormal gas exchange, dysfunction of the respiratory muscles, alterations in cardiac performance, malnutrition, and development of dyspnea. Other factors deserve to be mentioned, but are less well characterized. They include active smoking, abnormal peripheral muscle function, and polycythemia. The most severely affected patients cannot exercise to the levels at which the training effect is thought to occur (above anaerobic threshold). Fortunately, a large body of evidence supports exercise training as a beneficial therapeutic tool that is useful in helping these patients achieve their full potential.

PHYSIOLOGIC ADAPTATION TO TRAINING

There are several principles that apply to exercise training, and we must understand them in the context of prescribing exercise to patients with severe pulmonary problems. They are the specificity of training, the intensity and duration of the exercise load, and the detraining effect.

Specificity of Training

The principle of training specificity is based on the observations that programs can be tailored to achieve specific goals and that the training of muscles or muscle groups is beneficial only to the trained muscle.

The use of high-resistance, low-repetition stimulus increases muscle strength (weight lifting), whereas a low-resistance, high-repetition program increases muscle endurance. This specificity of training is achieved by increasing the number of myofibrils in certain muscle fibers (white) to promote strength or by increasing the number of capillaries and mitochondria to promote endurance.

The training is specific to the trained muscle. Clausen and associates trained subjects' arms and legs and found that the decreased heart rate observed with arm muscle training could not be transferred to the leg group and vice versa.[1] Davies and Sargeant showed that if training was completed for one leg, the beneficial effect could not be transferred to exercise involving the untrained leg.[2] More recently, Belman and Kendregan confirmed these findings in patients with chronic obstructive pulmonary disease (COPD).[3] They examined the effect of 6-weeks training in eight patients who trained only their arms and seven patients who trained only their legs. They observed improved exercise for only the extremity that the patients trained. Interestingly, they failed to see any changes in muscle enzyme content of biopsies taken before and after the exercise training program.[3]

Intensity and Duration of the Exercise Load

Both factors profoundly affect the degree of the training effect. Athletes will usually train at maximal or near-maximal levels to rapidly achieve the desired effects. On the other hand, middle-aged nonathletes may require less intensive exercise. Siegel and coworkers showed that training sessions of 30 minutes about three times a week for 15 weeks significantly improved maximal oxygen uptake if the heart rate was raised over 80% of predicted maximal rate.[4] In patients with chronic lung disease, the issue of exercise intensity and duration has been studied by different investigators, as we shall review later, but it would appear that the more sessions there are and the more intense these are (as a function of maximal performance), the better the results.

In their work, Belman and Kendregan exercised patients at 30% of maximal, and after 6 weeks of four-times weekly training during which the load was increased as tolerated, they observed significant improvement in endurance time for 9 of the 15 patients. It is possible that the relatively low training level (30% of maximal) may help explain why 6 of their patients failed to increase their endurance time. In contrast, Niederman and associates started the exercise at a 50% maximal cycle ergometer level, increased its intensity on a weekly basis, and observed endurance improvement in most patients.[5] Other authors have used higher starting exercise levels and have achieved higher endurance.[6-9]

The best study is that of Casaburi and colleagues, who studied 19 patients with COPD who could achieve anaerobic threshold [moderate COPD with a mean ± SD 1-second forced expiratory volume (FEV_1) of 1.8 ± 0.53 L] before and after randomly assigned, low-intensity (50% of maximal) or high-intensity (80% of maximal) exercise.[10] They showed that the high-intensity training program was more effective than the low-intensity one. They also observed a drop in ventilatory requirement for exercise, after training, that was proportional to the drop in lactate at a given work rate. Therefore, it seems that training is achieved if the intensity of exercise is at least 50% of maximal and that it can be increased as tolerated.

The number of exercise sessions is also a matter of debate.[3,11,12] As shown in Table 14–1, in general, as the number of sessions are increased, so is the change in observed endurance time. Since stopping the exercise results in a loss of the training effect, the optimal plan should involve an intense-training phase and a maintenance phase. This latter part is very difficult to implement and results in the frequently observed failure to maintain and preserve the beneficial effects achieved through the training.

Detraining Effect

The detraining principle is based on observations that the effect achieved by training is lost after the exercise is stopped. Sattin and associates showed that bed rest in normal subjects resulted in a significant decrease in maximal oxygen uptake within 21 days of resting. It took between 10 and 50 days for the values to return to those seen before resting.[12] Keens and coworkers examined ventilatory muscle endurance after training in normal subjects who had undergone ventilatory muscle training. Within 1 month of having stopped training, the subjects had lost the training effect that they had achieved.[13]

Our exercise program is based on the data and concepts developed in the foregoing. Patients are exercised at 60% of the maximal work achieved in a test day. This work is increased on a weekly basis, as tolerated by the patient. We aim to complete 24 sessions. This is achieved more quickly if the patient is in the hospital because the sessions are completed on a daily basis, whereas they require longer with outpatients,

TABLE 14-1. Number of Sessions of Exercise in Those Studies that Summarized the Improvement in Exercise Endurance

Author (Ref)	Sessions	Endurance Change (%)
Belman[3]	45	50
Epstein[40]	19	30
Make[11]	12	12

for sessions are held on a three-times-a-week basis. Each session lasts 30 minutes if tolerated by the patient, otherwise it is begun as tolerated and no further load is provided until the patient can complete the 30 minutes of the session. A close communication exists between the person in charge of the training and the rehabilitation-planning team.

LEG EXERCISE

Many studies have shown that the inclusion of leg exercise in the training of patients with lung disease is beneficial.[14–18] Cockcroft and associates randomized 39 dyspneic patients, younger than 70 years and not receiving oxygen, to a treatment group that spent 6 weeks in a rehabilitation center where they underwent graduated exercise training, and a control group that received medical care but no advice to exercise.[19] The control group served as such for 4 months and was then admitted to the rehabilitation center for 6 weeks. Just as the treated patients, they were instructed to exercise at home afterward. Both groups were similar at baseline. After rehabilitation, only 2 of the 16 control subjects manifested improvement in dyspnea and cough, whereas 16 of the 18 patients included in the treatment group manifested improvement in these symptoms. More importantly, the treated patients showed significant improvement in the 12-minute walk and in the peak oxygen uptake when compared with the controls.[19] In a different setting, Sinclair and Ingram randomized 33 patients with chronic bronchitis and dyspnea to two groups. The 17 patients in the treatment group exercised by climbing up and down on two 24-cm steps twice daily. The exercise time was increased to tolerance. The patients exercised at home and were evaluated by the treatment team weekly. The control group did not exercise, but were all reassessed after 6 months. There were no changes in the degree of airflow obstruction in either group. Similarly, there was no improvement in strength of the quadriceps, the minute ventilation, or heart rate. In contrast, the 12-minute walk distance significantly increased in the patients who were trained.[20] These two studies are particularly important in that they were well designed and used randomization in the assignment of patients to the specific treatment groups (Table 14–2).

Numerous studies that have used patients as their own controls have shown similar results, with significantly increased exercise endurance. The mechanism by which this improvement occurs remains a matter of debate. Several studies, including those of Paez and coworkers[18] and Mohsenifar and associates[6] have demonstrated a

TABLE 14-2. Controlled Trial of Exercise and Rehabilitation in Patients with Chronic Airflow Obstruction

Author (Ref)	No. Patients	Duration	Course	Results
Cockcroft[19]	18 treated	Daily	16 wks	↑ 12-min walk
				↑ $\dot{V}o_2$
	16 controls			No change
Sinclair[20]	17 treated	Daily	40 wks	↑ 12-min walk
	16 control			No change

drop in heart rate at a similar work level, a hallmark of a training effect for the specific exercise. This is perhaps related to a decrease in the exercise lactate level, as suggested by Woolf and Suero.[21] More recent evidence in support of a training effect is provided by the study of Casaburi and colleagues.[10] In their group of trained patients with COPD they showed a reduction in exercise lactic acidosis and ventilation after patients were trained. Furthermore, the reduction was proportional to the intensity of the training. There was a 12% decrease in the rise of lactic acidosis in patients trained with the low-work rate (50% of maximum) and 32% decrease in those trained with the high-work rate (80% of maximum). In both groups there were significant decreases in heart rate after training.[10] Other studies have failed to document either an increase in maximum O_2 uptake, or a decrease in heart rate or lactate level at similar work levels. The most important study in this group is the one by Belman and Kendregan that failed to show a decrease in heart rate at the same workload as represented by the oxygen consumption per unit time ($\dot{V}O_2$). These authors went further and analyzed the enzyme content of muscle biopsies before and after training. They observed no change in this parameter. Interestingly, nine of the treated patients improved their exercise endurance. As stated previously, it is possible that this study used too low a training effort, since training was started at 30% of the maximum achieved during their testing.[3]

Two recent studies addressed the issue of whether patients with the most severe COPD can undergo exercise training. The reason for this question is because patients with severe COPD do not exericse to the intensity required to reach an anaerobic threshold or to train the cardiovascular system. Niederman and colleagues exercised 33 patients with different degrees of COPD (FEV_1 ranging from 0.33 to 3.82 L).[5] When they evaluated the response to training, there was no correlation between the degree of obstruction and the observed improvement. In other words, the patients with very low FEV_1 were as likely to improve as the patients with a high FEV_1. Similarly, ZuWallack and associates evaluated 50 patients with COPD (FEV_1 ranged from 0.38 to 3.24 L) before and after exercise training. They observed an inverse relation between the baseline 12-minute walk distance and $\dot{V}O_2$ and the improvement. They concluded that patients with poor performance, on either the 12-minute walking distance or maximal exercise test, are not necessarily poor candidates for a pulmonary rehabilitation program. From this data it seems prudent to conclude that any patient capable of undergoing leg exercise training will benefit from a program that includes leg exercises.

When one considers the type of exercise training to be prescribed, again different studies have used different training techniques. Most studies include walking, both as a measure of exercise tolerance[22] and of the training program. The classic 12-minute walk, for which the distance walked over 12 minutes is recorded, is particularly good for patients with moderate to severe COPD, but it may not be taxing enough for patients with a smaller degree of airflow obstruction. We have evaluated stair climbing and have shown that the peak oxygen uptake can be estimated from the number of steps climbed during a symptom-limited test.[23] Several studies have used treadmill testing or step testing, even though the training has been done with the patient walking. Oxygen uptake is higher for stair climbing or treadmill testing than for the more commonly used leg ergometry,[23] presumably because the former uses more

TABLE   14-3.   Training Method for Leg Exercise

1. Train at 60% of maximal work capacity*
2. Increase work every 5th session as tolerated
3. Monitor: dyspnea, heart rate
4. Increase work after 20–30 min of submaximal targeted work
    is achieved
5. Aim for 24 sessions

* Work capacity as determined by an exercise test, not necessarily by
evaluating heart rate (see text for discussion).

body muscles than leg cycling. Leg ergometry has become very popular in its use as a testing device and has been the training apparatus for most recent studies. It is certainly smaller than the treadmill and, with relatively inexpensive units in the market, it is possible to place several together and train groups of patients simultaneously. In our pulmonary rehabilitation program, we complete testing on an electrically braked ergometer, whereas the training is done in mechanically controlled ergometers. Table 14–3 practically describes how we train our patients. The program may be tailored to each individual and to the available training equipment.

ARM EXERCISE

Most of our knowledge about exercise conditioning in patients undergoing rehabilitation is derived from programs emphasizing leg training. This is unfortunate, because the performance of many everyday tasks requires not only the hands, but also the concerted action of other muscle groups that partake in upper torso and arm positioning. Some of the muscles of the upper torso and shoulder girdle serve a dual function (respiratory and postural). Muscles such as the upper and lower trapezius, latissimus dorsi, serratus anterior, subclavius, and pectoralis minor and major possess a thoracic and an extrathoracic anchoring point. Depending on the anchoring point, they may help position the arms or shoulder or, if given an extrathoracic fulcrum (such as fixing the arms in a supported position), they may exert a pulling force on the rib cage. In patients with chronic airflow obstruction, as severity worsens, the diaphragm loses its force-generating capacity, and the muscles of the rib cage become more important in the generation of inspiratory pressures.[24] When patients perform unsupported arm exercise, some of the shoulder girdle muscles have to decrease their participation in ventilation and, if the task involves complex purposeful arm movements, the pattern of ventilation may be affected. Tangri and Wolf used a pneumobelt to study breathing patterns in seven patients with COPD while they performed simple activities of daily living, such as tying their shoes and brushing their teeth.[25] The patients developed an irregular and rapid pattern of breathing with the arm exercise. After the exercise, the patients breathed faster and deeper, which according to the authors was done to restore the blood gas levels to normal.

We have explored the ventilatory response to unsupported arm exercise and compared it with the response to leg exercise in patients with severe chronic lung disease.[26] Arm exercise resulted in dyssynchronous thoracoabdominal excursion that was not solely due to diaphragmatic fatigue. The dyspnea that was reported by the patients was associated with a dyssynchronous breathing pattern. We concluded that unsupported arm exercise could shift work to the diaphragm and, in some way, lead to dyssynchrony. To test this hypothesis, we have used pleural–gastric pressure (Ppl–Pg) plots (determined with gastric and endoesophageal balloons) and evaluated the changes as well as the ventilatory response to unsupported arm exercise and compared it to leg cycle ergometry in normal subjects and patients with airflow obstruction.[27,28] We documented increased diaphragmatic pressure excursion with arm exercise and alterations in the pattern of pressure generation, with more contribution by the diaphragm and abdominal muscles of respiration and less contribution by the inspiratory muscles of the rib cage. Our knowledge of ventilatory response to arm exercise was based on arm cycle ergometry. It is known that, at a given work load in normal subjects, arm cranking is more demanding than leg cycling, as shown by higher $\dot{V}o_2$, expired volume per unit time ($\dot{V}E$), heart rate, blood pressure, and lactate production.[29-31] At maximal effort, however, $\dot{V}o_2$, $\dot{V}E$, cardiac output and lactate levels are lower during arm than leg cycle ergometry.[32,33]

Very little is known about the metabolic and ventilatory cost of simple arm elevation. Two recent reports underscore the importance of arm position in ventilation. Banzett and coworkers showed that arms bracing increases the capacity to sustain maximal ventilation when compared with lifting the elbows from the braced position.[34] Maestro and associates observed a decrease in the maximum attainable workload and increases in oxygen uptake and ventilation at any given workload when normal subjects exercised with their arms elevated.[35] We have recently evaluated the metabolic and respiratory consequence of simple arm elevation in patients with COPD.[36] Elevation of the arms to 90° in front of them results in a significant increase in $\dot{V}o_2$ and $\dot{V}co_2$. There were concomitant increases in heart rate and $\dot{V}E$. When ventilatory muscle recruitment patterns were evaluated with the use of continuous recording of Pg and Ppl, there was a shift in the contribution to ventilation, by the different muscle groups, toward increased diaphragmatic and abdominal muscle use. The observations suggest that if we trained the arms to perform more work, or if we decreased the ventilatory requirement for the same work, we should improve the patient's capacity to perform activities of daily living.

There are several studies that have used both arm and leg training and have shown that the addition of arm training results in improved performance, and that the improved performance is, for the most part, task-specific. In their study, Belman and Kendregan showed a significant increase in arm exercise after exercise training.[3] Lake and coworkers randomized patients to arm exercise, leg exercise, and arms and legs exercise. There were increases for arm ergometry in the arm group, for leg ergometry in the leg group, and increased improvement in sensation of well being when both exercises were combined.[37] Ries and coworkers studied the effect of two forms of arm exercise—gravity-resistance and modified proprioceptive neuromuscular facilitation—and compared them with no arm exercise in a group of 45 patients with COPD who were involved in a comprehensive, multidisciplinary pulmonary rehabilitation program. Even though only 20 patients completed the program, they showed improved performance on tests that were specific for the training. The patients reported a decrease in fatigue in all tests performed.[38] It is noteworthy that in

TABLE 14-4. Training Methods for Supported (Ergometry) Arm Exercise Training

1. Train at 60% of maximal work capacity*
2. Increase work every 5th session as tolerated
3. Monitor: dyspnea, heart rate
4. Train for as long as tolerated up to 30 min
5. Aim for 24 sessions

---

* Work capacity as determined by an exercise test, not necessarily by evaluating heart rate (see text for discussion).

the study of Keens and coworkers, a group of patients with cystic fibrosis underwent upper extremity training consisting of swimming and canoeing for 1.5 hours daily. At the end of 6 weeks, there was increased upper extremity endurance, but most importantly, there was an increase in maximal sustainable ventilatory capacity that was similar to that obtained with ventilatory muscle training.[13] This suggests that ventilatory muscles could be trained by using an arm exercise training program.

Because simple arm elevation results in a significant increase in $\dot{V}E$, $\dot{V}O_2$, and $\dot{V}CO_2$, we studied 14 patients with COPD before and after 8 weeks of three-times weekly, 20-minute sessions of unsupported arm and leg exercise as part of a comprehensive rehabilitation program to test whether arm training decreases ventilatory requirement for arm activity. There was a 35% decrease in the rise of $\dot{V}O_2$ and $\dot{V}CO_2$ brought about by arm elevation. This was associated with a significant decrease in $\dot{V}E$.[39] Because the patients also trained their legs, we could not conclude that the improvement was due to only the arm exercise. To answer this question, we have recently completed a study of 26 patients with COPD who were randomized to either unsupported arm training (11 patients) or resistance-breathing training (14 patients). After 24 sessions, arm endurance increased for only the patients in unsupported arm-training group, but not for those in the resistance-breathing group. Interestingly, maximal inspiratory pressure increased significantly for both groups, indicating that by training the arms, we could be inducing ventilatory muscle training for those muscles of the rib cage that hinge on the shoulder girdle.[40]

On the basis of the information available, we include arm exercise in our rehabilitation program. As seen in Tables 14–4 and 14–5, the methods for supported and unsupported arm exercise vary in their implementation. Arm ergometry is performed

TABLE 14-5. Method for Unsupported Arm Training

1. Dowl (weight = 750 g)
2. Lift to shoulder level for 2 min. Rate equal to breathing rate
3. Rest for 2 min
4. Repeat sequence as tolerated for up to 32 min
5. Monitor: dyspnea, heart rate
6. Increase weight (250 g) every 5th session, as tolerated
7. Aim for 24 sessions

for 20 minutes per session. We start at 60% of the maximal work achieved in the test run. The work is increased weekly, as tolerated. Dyspnea and heart rate are monitored. *Maximal work capacity* is defined as the watts that the patient is capable of achieving. If the patient's limiting symptom is dyspnea at minimal work, we have him or her exercise at 60% of the work that makes him or her stop. In the most severely affected patients, the heart rate is unreliable, since they may be tachycardic even at rest and may not show any significant increase with exercise. In these patients, dyspnea may be a more reliable index to follow. In contrast, unsupported arm exercise training is achieved by having the patient lift a dowel (750 g) to shoulder level at the same rhythm as the patient's breathing rate. The sequence is repeated for 2 minutes, with a 2-minute resting period. The exercises are repeated for 30 minutes. Dyspnea and heart rate are monitored. The load is increased by 250 g weekly, as tolerated. We aim to complete 24 sessions.

In conclusion, an increasing body of evidence has indicated that arm exercise training results in improved performance for arm activities. There also is a drop in the ventilatory requirements for similar upper extremity activities. All this should result in an improvement in the capacity of the patients to perform activities of daily living.

SUMMARY

This chapter has reviewed the physiologic correlates of exercise training and addressed the specific training of legs and arms. A critical review of the literature indicates that exercise conditioning that includes leg and arm training improves exercise performance and seems to have physiologic explanations different from simple dyspnea desensitization. The practical aspects of implementation of an exercise program within the context of pulmonary rehabilitation are reviewed. They are attainable by anyone interested in them and result in a rewarding component of any program.

REFERENCES

1. Clausen JP, Clausen K, Rasmussen B, Trap-Jensen J. Central and peripheral circulatory changes after training of the arms or legs. Am J Physiol 1973;225:675.

2. Davis CT, Sargeant AJ. Effects of training on the physiological responses to one and two legged work. J Appl Physiol 1975;38:377.

3. Belman MJ, Kendregan BA. Exercise training fails to increase skeletal muscle enzymes in patients with chronic obstructive pulmonary disease. Am Rev Respir Dis 1981;123:256.

4. Siegel W, Blonquist G, Mitchell JH. Effects of a quantitated physical training program on middle-aged sedentary men. Circulation 1970;41:19.

5. Niederman MS, Clemente PH, Fein A, et al. Benefits of a multidisciplinary pulmonary rehabilitation program. Improvements are independent of lung function. Chest 1991;99:798.

6. Mohsenifar Z, Horak D, Brown H, Koerner SK. Sensitive indices of improvement in a pulmonary rehabilitation program. Chest 1983;83:189.

7. Holle RH, Williams DB, Vandree JC, Starks GL, Schoene RB. Increased muscle efficiency and sustained benefits in an outpatient community hospital-based pulmonary rehabilitation program. Chest 1988;94:1161.

8. Zack M, Palange A. Oxygen supplemented exercise of ventilatory and nonventilatory muscles in pulmonary rehabilitation. Chest 1985;88:669.

9. ZuWallack RL, Patel K, Reardon JZ, Clark BA, Normandin EA. Predictors of improvement in the 12-minute walking distance following a six-week outpatient pulmonary rehabilitation program. Chest 1991;99:805.

10. Casaburi R, Patessio A, Ioli F, Zanabouri S, Donner S, Wasserman K. Reductions in exercise lactic acidosis and ventilation as a result of exercise training in patients with obstructive lung disease. Am Rev Respir Dis 1991;143:9.

11. Make BJ, Buckolz J. Exercise training in COPD patients improves cardiac function. Am Rev Respir Dis 1991;143:80A.

12. Sattin B, Blonquist G, Mitchell JH, et al. Response to exercise after bed rest and training. Circulation 1968;38:1.

13. Keens TG, Krastins IR, Wannamaker EM, Levinson H, Crozier DN, Bryan AC. Ventilatory muscle endurance training in normal subjects and patients with cystic fibrosis. Am Rev Respir Dis 1977;116:853.

14. Moser KM, Bokinsky GC, Savage RT, et al. Results of comprehensive rehabilitation programs. Arch Intern Med 1980;140:1596.

15. Beaumont A, Cockcroft A, Guz A. A self-paced treadmill walking test for breathless patients. Thorax 1985;40:459.

16. Christie D. Physical training in chronic obstructive lung disease. Br Med J 1968;2:150.

17. Hughes RL, Davidson R. Limitations of exercise reconditioning in COPD. Chest 1983;83:241.

18. Paez PN, Phillipson EA, Mosangkay M, et al. The physiologic basis of training patients with emphysema. Am Rev Respir Dis 1967;95:944.

19. Cockcroft AE, Saunders MJ, Berry G. Randomized controlled trial of rehabilitation in chronic respiratory disability. Thorax 1981;36:200.

20. Sinclair DJ, Ingram CG. Controlled trial of supervised exercise training in chronic bronchitis. Br Med J 1980;1:519.

21. Woolf CR, Suero JT. Alterations in lung mechanics and gas exchange following training in chronic obstructive lung disease. Chest 1969;55:37.

22. McGavin CR, Gupta SP, McHardy GJ. Twelve minute walking test for assessing disability in chronic bronchitis. Br Med J 1976;1:822.

23. Pollock M, Roa J, Benditt J, Celli BR. Stair climbing (SC) predicts maximal oxygen uptake in patients with chronic airflow obstruction. Chest 1990;98:585A.

24. Martinez FJ, Couser J, Celli BR. Factors that determine ventilatory muscle recruitment in patients with chronic airflow obstruction. Am Rev Respir Dis 1990;142:276.

25. Tangri S, Woolf CR. The breathing pattern in chronic obstructive lung disease, during the performance of some common daily activities. Chest 1973;63:126.

26. Celli BR, Rassulo J, Make B. Dyssynchronous breathing associated with arm but not leg exercise in patients with COPD. N Engl J Med 1968;314:1485.

27. Criner GJ, Celli BR. Effect of unsupported arm exercise on ventilatory muscle recruitment in patients with severe chronic airflow obstruction. Am Rev Respir Dis 1988;138:856.

28. Celli BR, Criner GJ, Rassulo J. Ventilatory muscle recruitment during unsupported arm exercise in normal subjects. J Appl Physiol 1988;64:1936.

29. Bobbert AC. Physiological comparison of three types of ergometry. J Appl Physiol 1960;15:1007.

30. Davis JA, Vodak P, Wilmore JH, Vodak J, Kwitz P. Anaerobic threshold and maximal power for three modes of exercise. J Appl Physiol 1976;41:549.

31. Steinberg J, Astrand PO, Ekblom B, Royce J, Sattin P. Hemodynamic response to work with different muscle groups, sitting and supine. J Appl Physiol 1967;22:61.

32. Reybrouck T, Heigenhouser GF, Faulkner JA. Limitations to maximum oxygen uptake in arm, leg and combined arm–leg ergometry. J Appl Physiol 1975;38:774.

33. Martin TW, Zeballos RJ, Weisman IM. Gas exchange during maximal upper extremity exercise. Chest 1991;99:420.

34. Banzett R, Topulus G, Leith D, Natios C. Bracing arms increases the capacity for sustained hyperpnea. Am Rev Respir Dis 1988;138:106.

35. Maestro L, Dolinage T, Avendano MA, Goldstein R. Influence of arm position in ventilation during incremental exercise in healthy individuals. Chest 1990;98:113(S).

36. Martinez FJ, Couser J, Celli BR. Factors influencing ventilatory muscle recruitment in patients with chronic airflow obstruction. Am Rev Respir Dis 1990;142:276.

37. Lake FR, Hendersen K, Briffa T, et al. Upper limb and lower limb exercise training in patients with chronic airflow obstruction. Chest 1990;97:1077.

38. Ries AL, Ellis B, Hawkins RW. Upper extremity exercise training in chronic obstructive pulmonary disease. Chest 1988;93:688.

39. Couser J, Martinez F, Celli B. Effect of pulmonary rehabilitation (PR) including arm exercise on ventilatory muscle function during arm elevation (AE) in patients with chronic airflow obstruction (CAO). Am Rev Respir Dis 1989;139:232A.

40. Epstein S, Breslin E, Roa J, Celli B. Impact of unsupported arm training (AT) and ventilatory muscle training (VMT) on the metabolic and ventilatory consequences of unsupported arm elevation (UAE) and exercise (UAEx) in patients with chronic airflow obstruction. Am Rev Respir Dis 1991;143:81A.

CHARLES F. EMERY

Psychosocial Considerations Among Pulmonary Patients

Although medical advances over the past 20 years have contributed to increased survival rates among patients with chronic obstructive pulmonary disease (COPD), they have not led directly to commensurate improvements in quality of life. Patients living with COPD often must endure many years of progressive and debilitating physical illness, leading to profound psychosocial ramifications of surviving with this disorder. Psychosocial functioning among COPD patients can be defined in terms of three general categories: first, indicators of both psychological distress and psychological well-being (e.g., depression, anxiety, life satisfaction); second, behavioral adaptations, as defined by the person's capacity for functional, social, and recreational activity; and third, neuropsychological or cognitive functioning (e.g., memory, problem-solving ability). These three broadly defined areas of psychosocial functioning overlap and interact, contributing to a wide range of psychosocial phenomena among patients with COPD. Experimental and clinical studies of COPD patients have reported on numerous areas of psychosocial distress and dysfunction, ranging from mild depression and cognitive dysfunction to acute episodes of severe psychological distress and chronic social withdrawal. The clinical psychosocial presentation of the COPD patient, therefore, may be quite complicated, and requires thorough assessment and treatment of psychosocial factors. This chapter will address the psychosocial issues involved in COPD, including (1) the psychological, behavioral and cognitive changes observed among COPD patients; (2) the common techniques employed for psychological, behavioral, and cognitive assessment among COPD patients; and (3) considerations for treatment of psychosocial factors in pulmonary rehabilitation.

PSYCHOLOGICAL AND EMOTIONAL ADJUSTMENT

Much of the past literature pertaining to psychological functioning of COPD patients is descriptive.[1,2] The descriptive accounts of psychological complications associated with COPD have paralleled the relatively few empirical studies that have been conducted in this area. Taken together, the descriptive, clinical, and empirical data provide a vivid picture of the psychological distress that afflicts many patients with COPD. One of the most commonly reported emotional consequences of COPD is depression,[1,3] and the prevalence of depression among COPD patients has been reported to range from 51% to 74%.[1,4] Depression among COPD patients is usually characterized by sleep disturbance, reduced appetite, decreased energy, reduced libido, and feelings of hopelessness and pessimism,[3] as well as social withdrawal, sense of failure, poor concentration, and sometimes suicidal ideation.[5] In most patients there are multiple sources of depression, ranging from negative self-assessment to restrictions in a number of areas of behavioral functioning, including occupational restrictions, reduced recreational activities, and decreased social contacts. The resulting clinical syndrome of depression may further reinforce the patient's social isolation and physical inactivity.[5]

Another commonly described emotional consequence of COPD is anxiety, with one study reporting disabling anxiety in as many as 96% of patients.[1] Anxiety is often manifested in various ways, including exaggerated body movements, rapid speech, and physiologic changes, such as palpitations, tachycardia, dyspnea, or sweating. The anxious patient's thought content is frequently characterized by exaggerated fear of death and obsessive rumination. The patient may also experience episodes of faintness or difficulty concentrating.[6] One of the most fearful symptoms of anxiety is dyspnea, and anxiety has been associated closely with symptoms of dyspnea,[7] especially among COPD patients.[8] In COPD patients, anxiety may be triggered by dyspnea; subsequently, the anxiety may contribute to further dyspneic episodes. Thus, COPD patients are more likely to experience physical symptoms of anxiety that exacerbate the physical symptoms of the illness.

In addition to depression and anxiety, several other emotional consequences of COPD have been described, including irritability, somatic preoccupation, dependency, and frustration,[3] as well as a sense of embarrassment.[9] Prigatano and colleagues found significantly greater impairment in psychological well-being among 985 COPD patients, compared with a matched control group of 25 subjects, on five out of six scales from the Profile of Mood States (POMS).[10] The COPD patients, in comparison with controls, experienced greater tension, depression, anger, and fatigue, as well as less vigor. Results of personality testing indicated that COPD patients were extremely concerned with bodily functions and were notably depressed and anxious.[10] These results are consistent with results of another study suggesting that COPD patients tend to suffer from reactive depression.[4] However, results from psychological testing must be interpreted cautiously because symptoms of psychological distress may be confounded with symptoms of physical illness.

Indeed, past studies have demonstrated psychophysiologic effects of pulmonary disease, suggesting that the psychological state or mood of the COPD patient may be directly related to physical functioning. For example, psychological arousal, as in significant levels of anxiety, anger, or even euphoria, is associated with increased energy expenditure, elevated respiratory ventilation, higher oxygen consumption, and skeletal muscle tension. On the other hand, reductions in psychological arousal, as in feelings of apathy or depression and deep relaxation, are associated with reduced energy expenditure, decreased respiratory ventilation, lower oxygen consumption, and relaxation of skeletal muscles.[11] The extreme manifestation of either emotional state may contribute to increased symptoms among patients with COPD.[5]

Thus, a cyclic pattern of emotional changes and physical changes may readily evolve. For example, the patient's illness may contribute initially to mild depression and symptoms of depression (i.e., fatigue, appetite change, and reduced energy). The depression, in turn, may reinforce behavior consistent with the patient's illness (e.g., reduced energy expenditure, decreased respiratory ventilation). Because the emotional and physical changes of the patient become so closely interrelated, it is often difficult for the patient with COPD to break the pattern.

Researchers have also suggested that patients with COPD avoid expressing strong emotions, such as anger, to prevent the physiologic arousal (e.g., increased heart rate, shortness of breath) that may accompany those emotions.[12] As a consequence, COPD patients may be inclined to avoid expressing their feelings or emotions in general. The reluctance of COPD patients toward expressing their emotions is consistent with clinical descriptions of alexithymia among COPD patients, which has been observed, especially among patients with chronic asthma. *Alexithymia* is defined as a patient's inability to label affective states verbally.[13] Kleiger and Dirks described two groups of alexithymic asthmatics:[14] one group, scoring high on an indicator of panic–fear, manifested diffuse, poorly articulated distress; whereas the second group, which scored low on the panic–fear dimension, demonstrated an unusual absence of distress at times when it might have been expected. This latter group would be consistent with descriptions of patients high in denial. Denial early in the progression of COPD may be adaptive (as it is for other chronic health problems such as coronary artery disease)[15] in that it may help the patient to accept decreases in physical capacity. However, denial may also keep the patient from seeking or following necessary medical advice and, thereby, contribute to increased morbidity and mortality. Thus, denial is one of the most significant psychological factors to be addressed in the treatment of the patient with COPD.

BEHAVIORAL ADJUSTMENT

The patient with COPD is frequently confronted with changes in physical capabilities that affect overall activity level and behavior. Numerous areas of life functioning are often directly affected, including work performance as well as other activities of daily living (ADL). Barstow has described significant life-style impairments among COPD patients, including difficulty in bathing, grooming, dressing, eating, sleeping, and mobility.[16] Patients with COPD are less likely to be employed than their peers,[10] and they may be more likely to experience sexual dysfunction.[17–19] McSweeny and colleagues[4] examined four dimensions of life quality (emotional functioning, social role functioning, activities of daily living, and recreational pastimes) among 233 hypoxemic COPD patients compared with 73 healthy controls matched by age, gender, race, and neighborhood. They found significant decrements in all four areas among the COPD patients, who experienced greater difficulty with home management, as well as reductions in social interaction, mobility, sleep, and recreational activities.[4]

The COPD patient's psychosocial assets include not only individual characteristics and psychological resources, but also social supports that are available to the patient in the community. All of the patient's psychosocial assets, taken together, may play a critical role in the patient's ability to cope adaptively. Increased morbidity and mortality have been associated with low psychosocial assets.[2] On the other hand, greater psychosocial assets have been associated with improved response to rehabilitation.[20] Many times, the patient's difficulty in coping with social and behavioral changes will have a severely detrimental effect on both rehabilitation and psychological well-being.[21] In fact, it has been suggested that the emotional distress, especially depression and anxiety, observed among COPD patients may be a direct result of physical restrictions that are placed on their life-style by the illness.[4] Thus, the COPD patient may initially experience the loss of social and recreational opportunities, as well as reduced functional ability, followed by emotional upheaval and reluctance to pursue or initiate an active course of rehabilitation.

Assessment of Psychological and Behavioral Functioning

Numerous psychological test instruments have been employed to assess psychological and behavioral functioning among COPD patients.

One of the most frequently used measures of psychological functioning is the Minnesota Multiphasic Personality Inventory (MMPI).[22] The MMPI is a 566-item measure providing ten dimensions of personality functioning (hysteria, depression, hypochondriasis, psychopathic deviance, gender identification, paranoia, psychasthenia, schizophrenia, mania, and social introversion), with three validity scales. In addition, numerous other indicators of psychological functioning can be scored from the MMPI, including hostility, alcoholism, alexithymia, and ego strength. Because of the number of studies of COPD patients that have made use of MMPI data, it has great clinical and research use. It is especially useful in diagnosing psychiatric illness that is overlaid on COPD, such as instances of characterologic disturbances or borderline psychosis. However, its length may preclude its use in many settings. The MMPI has recently undergone a revision, MMPI-2, which is now available for clinical use and research studies.

Another measure that has come into widespread use in recent years is the Sickness Impact Profile (SIP),[23] which comprises 136 questions covering 12 categories of health-related dysfunction. It has proved to be a reliable measure of the influence of disease states on a wide range of daily activities. The questionnaire may be administered to the patient or may be self-administered, and for each statement the patient is asked to agree or disagree. Scales of the SIP reflect limitations in physical functioning (ambulation, mobility, body care, movement), as well as in social functioning (social interaction, communication, alertness, and emotional behavior). The inventory also assesses more complex behaviors related to health (e.g., sleep, appetite). For each scale of the SIP, the respondent's score is the percentage of impairment in that area.

The Hopkins Symptom Check-List (SCL-90-R)[24] is a 90-item multidimensional symptom inventory measuring various aspects of emotional disturbance. Respondents rate on a five-point scale the incidence of symptoms such as headache, nausea, and nervousness during the previous 2 weeks. The questionnaire provides a global symptom measure (GSI) as well as nine clinical subscales, including depression, anxiety, and hostility.

The Profile of Mood States (POMS)[25] consists of a 65-item list of adjectives. The respondent is asked to rate, on a five-point scale, the degree to which each adjective describes his or her functioning during the preceding week. The questionnaire provides an overall mood score, as well as six mood subscores (tension–anxiety, depression–dejection, anger–hostility, fatigue, vigor, confusion–bewilderment).

The Katz Activity Scale (KAS)[26] includes separate forms for the patient and the patient's relative to complete. The questionnaire encompasses a range of emotional, social, and leisure-time activities and the respondent rates, on a four-point scale, the degree to which each statement is true of the patient.

The Multiple Affect Adjective Check-List (MAACL)[27] consists of a list of 132 adjectives. The respondent is instructed to mark any adjective that describes how he or she has been feeling during the previous several months.

Other indicators of psychological distress and well-being that are frequently used in research studies include (1) the Center for Epidemiological Studies—Depression Inventory (CES-D),[28] a 20-item scale assessing symptoms associated with depression during the preceding week; (2) the State Trait Anxiety Inventory (STAI),[29] a 40-item measure of tension and worry; (3) the Psychological General Well-Being Scale (PGWB),[30] a 22-item scale providing a summary measure of psychologic functioning as well as six subscores (anxiety, depression, positive well-being, self-control, general health, vitality); (4) the Life Satisfaction Index (LSI),[31] a 20-item scale, developed especially for use with older adults, assessing satisfaction with life; and (5) the Multidimensional Health Locus of Control Scale (MHLOC),[32] an 18-item scale assessing perceptions of control in various aspects of health behavior.

NEUROPSYCHOLOGICAL ADJUSTMENT

In addition to emotional changes associated with COPD, cognitive or neuropsychological changes also have been observed in numerous studies of COPD patients, especially those who are hypoxemic.[33,34] In one study of a small group of hypoxic COPD patients ($N = 11$), Huppert found that reduced partial pressure of oxygen (PaO_2) was correlated with impaired memory, but not impaired mental speed.[33] Prigatano and his colleagues found that mildly hypoxemic COPD patients manifested neuropsychological impairments in memory, abstract reasoning, and perceptual motor speed, even when age and education were partialled out.[34] The COPD patients in their study demonstrated a subtle, but significant, impairment in higher cerebral problem-solving skills, with no indication of greater fatigue effects, depression, or reduced motivation contributing to the impairments. The authors suggest that lower levels of blood oxygenation may contribute to inefficiencies in neural functioning, consistent with the observation that chronic reduction of PaO_2 may contribute significantly to cognitive deficits.[35] Likewise, Fix and colleagues found impairments among COPD patients on tests of nonverbal and higher-cognitive skills.[36] They also found a significant correlation between performance on the cognitive indices and PaO_2, and they concluded that PaO_2 may be the most important contributor to neuropsychological deficits in COPD patients.[36]

Grant and associates examined the relation of neuropsychological impairment to several physical markers of COPD severity, including PaO_2, oxygen saturation (SaO_2), carbon dioxide retention ($PaCO_2$), lung function indicators, and blood pressure.[37] Their sample comprised 302 COPD patients with hypoxemia, ranging from mild to severe, from two intervention trials. They found that hypoxemia was the only medical variable consistently predictive of neuropsychological performance and, although there were deficits in simple motor skills and concentration, language and verbal memory appeared relatively unaffected. They also found neuropsychological impairment to be associated with low levels of blood oxygen (PaO_2) and SaO_2, even though there was no evidence of carbon dioxide retention, which itself has been related to deficits in cognitive performance. The researchers conclude that cognitive decrements may result from reduced central cholinergic activity, which can best be improved with greater oxygenation of the brain.[37]

These changes in cognitive functioning observed among COPD patients are critically important from both a practical and a medical viewpoint. First, memory problems may be associated with forgetting to take prescribed medications or missing important appointments; abstract reasoning skills are vital to the patient's capacity to devise solutions to daily problems; and sequencing of information and activities is also crucial for activities such as driving a car, or for patients in a pulmonary rehabilitation program who may be expected to follow an exercise routine independently.

In view of the decrements in neuropsychological functioning observed among patients with COPD and the suggestion that oxygenation of the brain may contribute to enhanced functioning, studies have been conducted exploring the ameliorative effects of oxygen therapy among this group. Early studies, examining the effect of continuous oxygen therapy among COPD patients, found that impairments in visual–spatial function and simple motor movement could be partially reversed.[38,39] Subjects in one study also indicated reduced depression and somatic preoccupation following oxygen treatment.[38] A later study[39] included electroencephalographic (EEG) evaluations and found a correlation between EEG abnormalities and neuropsychological impairment. However, both of these early studies involved pretesting of subjects on room air and posttesting on supplemental oxygen. One logical question raised by the methodology of these studies is the extent to which brief administration of O_2 at posttest might have enhanced neuropsychological performance. Although there have been reports among healthy older subjects of enhanced neuropsychological performance following brief administration of O_2,[40] Wilson and colleagues conducted a study of ten hypoxemic COPD patients who were administered O_2 treatment during testing and found no evidence of enhanced functioning as a result of brief O_2 treatment.[41]

The question of optimal administration of O_2 has been addressed in subsequent research endeavors. Because COPD patients experience hemoglobin oxygen desaturation, especially during sleep, it was of interest to examine the extent to which nocturnal oxygen therapy could be as effective as continuous oxygen in reducing cognitive deficits. The Nocturnal Oxygen Therapy Trial (NOTT), a large, multicenter clinical study, was designed to evaluate the performance of patients prescribed continuous oxygen treatment (COT) versus those prescribed only nocturnal oxygen treatment (NOT) after 6 months and 12 months of treatment.[42] After 6 months, both groups performed significantly better than an age-matched control group on three neuropsychological measures. Results at 12 months, assessing a subset of COT and NOT patients, indicated that the COT patients demonstrated mild neuropsychological improvement over NOT patients during the second 6 months of oxygen therapy. Thus, prolonged and continuous oxygen treatment contributed more substantially to improved neuropsychological functioning than nocturnal oxygen treatment. Heaton and colleagues suggest that there may be, in fact, two different mechanisms contributing to the beneficial effects of oxygen on the brain.[42] The short-term administration of oxygen is thought to affect hypoxic neurons by stimulating enzyme systems responsible for producing neurotransmitters. Long-term oxygen is thought to affect brain metabolism and, possibly, the formation of neurotransmitters.[42]

Assessment of Neuropsychological Functioning

A number of measures have been used in clinical research studies of COPD patients to determine neuropsychological functioning.

The Wechsler Adult Intelligence Scale—Revised (WAIS-R)[43] is one of the most widely used cognitive assessment batteries, providing a measure of overall intellectual functioning as well as indicators of functioning on six verbal subtests and five performance subtests. One of the most common WAIS-R performance subtests used in neuropsychological assessment is the Digit Symbol subtest.

The Wechsler Memory Scale[44] is a brief test with seven subscales assessing temporal orientation, logical memory, and figural memory. The revised WMS has higher reliability[45] than the original scale and is frequently used for cognitive assessment and as a screening measure to determine whether additional testing may be indicated.

The Aphasia Screening Test[46] is the most widely used test for aphasia, and it is included in many neuropsychological test batteries including the Halstead–Reitan battery. The screening test comprises 51 items assessing aphasic disability as well as other associated communication problems.

The Trail Making Test[47] is an easily administered test of visual conceptual and visual motor tracking, and is highly vulnerable to the effects of brain injury. The test is divided into two parts, A and B, with part B representing a more complex task than part A.

The Halstead–Reitan Neuropsychologic Test Battery for Adults[48,49] is an extensive, commonly used neuropsychological assessment instrument. The entire battery generally requires a full day to complete, and it is often administered in two sittings. The battery comprises five subtests yielding seven scores, from which are derived three impairment measures: (1) the Halstead Impairment Index (HII), based on the seven scores; (2) the Average Impairment Rating (AIR), based on the seven scores of the HII plus five subtests from the WAIS-R, the Trail Making Test (B), and the Aphasia Screening Test; and (3) the Brain Age Quotient (BAQ), based on three of the seven scores of the HII, the Trail Making Test (B), as well as the Digit Symbol and Block Design subtests from the WAIS-R. The BAQ is useful with older samples because it is age-corrected.

The Lafayette Clinic Repeatable Neuropsychological Test Battery[50] includes a number of tests from the Halstead–Reitan battery as well as a variety of other timed tests measuring neuropsychological functions such as verbal fluency, visual scanning, and fine hand coordination. It is useful in studies involving repeated measurements of neuropsychological functioning because alternative forms are available for all of the subtests in the battery that are susceptible to practice effects.

The Stroop Test[51] provides a measure of the subject's ability to shift perceptual sets to meet changing demands of the test. It has been used in several studies examining neuropsychological performance of healthy older adults[52,53] and in at least one study of COPD patients.[36]

RELATION BETWEEN AREAS OF PSYCHOSOCIAL FUNCTIONING

McSweeny and coauthors have suggested that there are significant interrelations between neuropsychological functioning, physiologic functioning, and the quality of life among COPD patients.[4] In one study, significant correlations were found between overall scores on the SIP and neuropsychological impairment.[4] Prigatano and associates also found that cognitive impairment on the Average Impairment Rating was significantly correlated with SIP scores, and that cognitive impairment was somewhat more highly correlated with physical limitation than with social limitation on the SIP.[10]

In addition, Grant and coworkers demonstrated a relation between pulmonary function and neuropsychological performance;[37] and the psychophysiologic studies of COPD patients suggest a significant relation between emotional factors and pulmonary function.[5] Because most patients with COPD are older adults, age also is an important factor, affecting both psychosocial functioning and physiologic functioning through several pathways.

Thus, data from studies of COPD patients demonstrate interrelations among various aspects of psychosocial functioning, in addition to relations between physiologic functioning and overall psychosocial functioning. Figure 15–1 depicts the hypothesized multidimensional and multidetermined nature of psychosocial functioning in COPD patients.

EXERCISE REHABILITATION

Intervention studies exploring the effects of exercise rehabilitation on psychosocial factors have helped further explain the relation between psychosocial functioning and physiologic functioning. Several controlled studies have been conducted on the effects of exercise on psychological well-being among COPD patients. During a study of 39 COPD patients participating in a 6-week exercise program, exercisers experienced significantly greater subjective benefits than controls, and they significantly increased the distance covered during a 12-minute walk.[54] McGavin and colleagues studied the effects of a 3-month unsupervised home stair-climbing program on 12 COPD patients compared with 12 randomized control subjects.[55] Subjects in the exercise group indicated subjective gains in sense of well-being as well as decreased breathlessness, increased distance during a 12-minute walk, and improved performance on the bicycle ergometer. The nonexercise control subjects did not change. Although a randomized study of COPD patients assigned to aerobic exercise ($n = 9$) or to a waiting group ($n = 6$) found no significant effect on depression or anxiety,[56] a

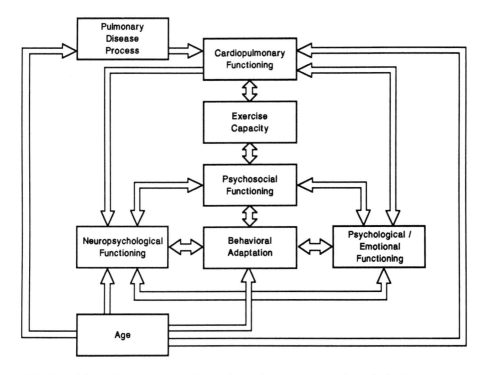

FIGURE   15-1   Model for describing relation between areas of psychologic dysfunction in patients with chronic obstructive pulmonary disease. (Adapted from McSweeny AJ, et al. Life quality of patients with chronic obstructive pulmonary disease. Arch Intern Med 1982; 142:473)

more recent study of 64 patients participating in a comprehensive pulmonary rehabilitation exercise program found significant improvements in psychological well-being, especially depression and anxiety, as assessed with the SCL-90 and the PGWB.[57] In addition, significant improvement was found on measures of neuropsychological functioning, including the Trail Making test and the Digit Symbol subtest from the WAIS-R. However, the latter study did not include a control group. Agle and colleagues studied 21 patients participating in a 4-week comprehensive exercise rehabilitation program and found that improved functional capacity was correlated with enhanced psychological well-being, but not with improved physiologic functioning.[21] Furthermore, subjects who improved significantly in the exercise program began the program with fewer psychological symptoms of depression, anxiety, and somatic preoccupation. Fishman and Petty also found improvement among COPD patients in a study with a 1-year follow-up.[35] Subjects in their study demonstrated reductions in affective distress, which was thought to be related to improvement in physical functioning.

    Thus, the data indicate that exercise rehabilitation itself may serve to enhance psychological functioning among COPD patients. After participation in an exercise program, COPD patients endorse fewer symptoms of depression and anxiety, as well as reduced somatic symptoms. Another important treatment outcome of rehabilitation for COPD patients is confidence or self-efficacy in symptomatic control and exercise performance. Kaplan and associates found specific efficacy expectations for exercise enhanced exercise compliance and general activity level among COPD patients participating in exercise rehabilitation. The studies in this area are few, and most suffer from methodologic problems, such as lack of randomized control groups, small numbers of subjects, and wide variability in the frequency and intensity of the exercise programs. Because pulmonary rehabilitation programs often involve several components in addition to exercise, including education and social support, further research, with randomized control groups, is necessary to understand the mechanisms by which the various components of pulmonary rehabilitation may be responsible for the observed changes.

TREATMENT CONSIDERATIONS

Given the apparent benefits of exercise for psychological well-being among patients with COPD, exercise is clearly a useful psychosocial intervention for these patients. However, given the multidetermined nature of psychosocial functioning in this group, exercise should not be viewed as a panacea. Indeed, successful treatment of COPD patients must be multimodal. Several studies have examined other treatment options for addressing the various symptoms of psychosocial distress among COPD patients.

Renfroe studied 20 COPD patients randomly assigned either to 4 weekly sessions of progressive muscle relaxation (PMR) ($n = 12$) or to a no-treatment control group ($n = 8$).[59] Dyspnea and anxiety were measured before beginning each session of the treatment program, as well as at the conclusion of each session. In addition, heart rate (HR), respiratory rate (RR), forced vital capacity (FVC), and forced expiratory volume in 1 second (FEV_1) were also measured. Patients in the PMR condition were better able to control anxiety, dyspnea, and HR than were patients assigned to the control condition. Kabat-Zinn and associates also found that COPD patients were better able to control episodes of dyspnea following a 10-week program of meditation.[60] Patients in their study were able to reduce the frequency and severity of dyspnea, and they indicated greater confidence in their ability to cope with dyspnea. Biofeedback-assisted relaxation has also been thought to help relieve dyspnea through generalized reduction of muscle tension. However, only a few studies of biofeedback have been conducted among COPD patients, and no studies have examined the effectiveness of biofeedback separately from a pulmonary rehabilitation program.[61]

Past studies of COPD patients participating in traditional group psychotherapeutic interventions, have indicated largely disappointing results.[2,21] These reports suggested that COPD patients became defensive and hostile in traditional psychotherapy. However, other research indicates that psychotherapy may contribute to improved psychological functioning of patients with COPD and should be incorporated into the rehabilitation program.[62,63] The data presented in this chapter further confirms that COPD patients will benefit from psychosocial interventions that allow them to view their emotional responses to the illness in the context of normal behavioral adaptation. Patients with COPD may benefit from both cognitive approaches toward modifying their patterns of thinking, as well as behavioral approaches toward altering the psychophysiologic response to stress, through relaxation. For COPD patients to cope with their condition, they may need help in accepting both their physical limitations and physical strengths, to minimize their psychological distress and maximize their functional capabilities. If denial persists as a primary defense mechanism, the COPD patient may be prevented from appreciating the progress that is made in a rehabilitation program.

Neuropsychological functioning of COPD patients is also important to assess and adequately address in a rehabilitation program. If deficits are observed, the treatment program may need to be modified to accommodate the patient, with all instructions given the patient made as clear and simple as possible. In addition, it may be necessary to enlist the support of the patient's family or friends to encourage compliance with medical or exercise regimens, and the patient may need external environmental cues for following prescribed treatment regimens.

From a developmental perspective, it is known that interindividual differences tend to become greater with age.[64] Thus, all 60-year-olds are not functioning at comparable levels either physically or psychosocially and, among patients with COPD, individual differences may be substantially more pronounced. In addition to the effects of aging per se on individual performance levels, the effects of COPD contribute even more variability, with COPD affecting individual performance in a variety of ways. Thus, it is crucial that COPD patients be given individualized treatment plans, and that health care providers working with COPD patients not make faulty assumptions about patients, based on experiences with other similar-appearing patients.

SUMMARY

Psychosocial functioning of COPD patients may be assessed in several ways, including psychological or emotional functioning, behavioral and social adaptations, and neuropsychological or cognitive functioning. In all of these areas, COPD patients exhibit impairments that may have a direct influence on their physical condition. Adequate assessment of the patient's level of psychosocial functioning is an important first step. Treatment of psychosocial deficits may include exercise rehabilitation in addition to specific behavioral approaches to stress reduction and modification of stress-related behaviors, such as smoking and sexual dysfunction. In addition, cognitive and cognitive–behavioral approaches may be useful in individual and group counseling of COPD patients. Future research may help to better explain the relation between psychosocial functioning and physiologic functioning, and especially to explore the mechanisms by which exercise and exercise capacity may effect both neuropsychological functioning and psychological well-being.

REFERENCES

1. Agle DP, Baum GL. Psychological aspects of chronic obstructive pulmonary disease. Med Clin North Am 1977;61:749.

2. Dudley DL, Verhey JW, Masuda M, Martin CJ, Holmes TH. Long-term adjustment, prognosis, and death in irreversible diffuse obstructive pulmonary syndromes. Psychosom Med 1969;31:310.

3. Sandhu HS. Psychosocial issues in chronic obstructive pulmonary disease. Clin Chest Med 1986;7:629.

4. McSweeny AJ, Grant I, Heaton RK, Adams KM, Timms RM. Life quality of patients with chronic obstructive pulmonary disease. Arch Intern Med 1982;142:473.

5. Dudley DL, Glaser EM, Jorgenson BN, Logan DL. Psychosocial concomitants to rehabilitation in chronic obstructive pulmonary disease—part 1: psychosocial and psychological considerations. Chest 1980;77:413.

6. Dudley DL, Glaser EM, Jorgenson BN, Logan DL. Psychosocial concomitants to rehabilitation in chronic obstructive pulmonary disease—part 2: psychosocial treatment. Chest 1980;77:544.

7. Heim E, Blaser A, Waidelich E. Dyspnea: psychophysiologic relationships. Psychosom Med 1972;34:405.

8. Kinsman RA, Yarousch RA, Fernandez E, Dirks JF, Schocket M, Fukuhara J. Symptoms and experiences in chronic bronchitis and emphysema. Chest 1983;83:755.

9. Guyatt GH, Townsend M, Berman LB, Pugsley SO. Quality of life in patients with chronic airflow limitation. Br J Dis Chest 1987;81:45.

10. Prigatano GP, Wright FC, Levin D. Quality of life and its predictors in patients with mild hypoxemia and chronic obstructive pulmonary disease. Arch Intern Med 1984;144:1613.

11. Dudley DL, Martin CJ, Holmes TH. Psychophysiologic studies of pulmonary ventilation. Psychosom Med 1964;26:645.

12. Dudley DL, Wermuth C, Hague W. Psychosocial aspects of care in the chronic obstructive pulmonary disease patient. Heart Lung 1973;2:289.

13. Sifneos P. The prevalence of "alexithymic" characteristics in psychosomatic patients. In: Freyberger H, ed. Topics of psychosomatic research. Basel: S Karger, 1973.

14. Kleiger JH, Dirks JF. Psychomaintenance aspects of alexithymia: relationship to medical outcome variables in a chronic respiratory illness population. Psychother Psychosom 1980;34:25.

15. Blumenthal JA. Assessment of patients with coronary heart disease. In: Keefe FJ, Blumenthal JA, eds. Assessment strategies in behavioral medicine. New York: Grune & Stratton, 1982.

16. Barstow RE. Coping with emphysema. Nurs Clin North Am 1974;9:137.

17. Conine TA, Evans JH. Sexual adjustment in chronic obstructive pulmonary disease. Respir Care 1982;26:871.

18. Kass I, Updegraff K, Muffly RB. Sex in chronic obstructive pulmonary disease. Med Aspects Hum Sex 1972;6:33.

19. Petty TL. Health, sex, and better quality of life for your COPD patient. Med Aspects Hum Sex 1986;20:70.

20. Rowlett DB, Dudley DL. COPD: psychosocial and psychophysiological issues. Psychosomatics 1978;19:273.

21. Agle DF, Baum GL, Chester EH, Wendt M. Multidiscipline treatment of chronic pulmonary insufficiency: psychologic aspects of rehabilitation. Psychosom Med 1973;35:41.

22. Dahlstrom WG, Welsh GS, Dahlstrom LE. An MMPI handbook. rev ed. Minneapolis: University of Minnesota Press, 1972.

23. Bergner M, Bobbitt RA, Carter WB, Gilson BS. The sickness impact profile: development and final revision of a health status measure. Med Care 1981;19:787.

24. Derogatis LR. SCL-90-R: administration, scoring and procedures manual II. Towson, MD: Clinical Psychometrics Research, 1983.

25. McNair DM, Lorr M, Droppleman LF. Manual for the profile of mood states. San Diego: Educational and Industrial Testing Service, 1971.

26. Katz MM, Lyerly SB. Methods of measuring adjustment and social behavior in the

community: I. Rationale, description, discriminative validity and scale development. Psychol Rep 1963;13:503.

27. Zuckerman M, Lubin B. Manual for the multiple affect adjective checklist. San Diego: Educational and Industrial Testing Service, 1965.

28. Radloff L. The CES-D scale: a self-report depression scale for research in the general population. Appl Psychol Measure 1977;1:385.

29. Spielberger CE, Gorsuch RL, Luschene RE. Manual for the state trait anxiety inventory. Palo Alto, CA: Consulting Psychologist Press, 1970.

30. Dupuy HJ. Utility of the National Center for Health Statistics' general well-being schedule in the assessment of self-representations of subjective well-being and distress. In The National Conference on evaluation in alcohol, drug abuse and mental health programs. Washington, DC: ADAMHA, 1974.

31. Neugarten BL, Havighurst RJ, Tobin SS. The measurement of life satisfaction. J Gerontol 1961;16:141.

32. Wallston KA, Wallston BS, DeVellis R. Development of the multidimensional health locus of control (MHLC) scales. Health Educ Monogr 1978;6:160.

33. Huppert FA. Memory impairment associated with chronic hypoxia. Thorax 1982;37:858.

34. Prigatano GP, Parsons O, Wright E, Levin DC, Hawryluk G. Neuropsychological test performance in mildly hypoxemic patients with chronic obstructive pulmonary disease. J Consult Clin Psychol 1983;51:108.

35. Fishman DB, Petty TL. Physical, symptomatic and psychological improvement in patients receiving comprehensive care for chronic airway obstruction. J Chron Dis 1971;24:775.

36. Fix AJ, Golden CJ, Daughton D, Kass I, Bell CW. Neuropsychological deficits among patients with chronic obstructive pulmonary disease. Int J Neurosci 1982;16:99.

37. Grant I, Prigatano GP, Heaton RK, McSweeny AJ, Wright EC, Adams KM. Progressive neuropsychological impairment and hypoxemia: relationship in chronic obstructive pulmonary disease. Arch Gen Psychiatry 1987;44:999.

38. Krop H, Block AJ, Cohen E. Neuropsychologic effects of continuous oxygen therapy in chronic obstructive pulmonary disease. Chest 1973;64:317.

39. Block AJ, Castle JR, Keitt AS. Chronic oxygen therapy treatment of chronic obstructive pulmonary disease at sea level. Chest 1974;65:279.

40. Jacobs EA, Winter PM, Alvis HJ, Small SM. Hyperoxygenation effect on cognitive functioning in the aged. N Engl J Med 1969;281:753.

41. Wilson DK, Kaplan RM, Timms RM, Dawson A. Acute effects of oxygen treatment upon information processing in hypoxemic COPD patients. Chest 1985;88:239.

42. Heaton RK, Grant I, McSweeny AJ, Adams KM, Petty TL. Psychologic effects of continuous and nocturnal oxygen therapy in hypoxemic chronic obstructive pulmonary disease. Arch Intern Med 1983;143:1941.

43. Wechsler D. The Wechsler adult intelligence scale—revised (manual). New York: Psychological Corporation, 1981.

44. Wechsler D, Stone C. Wechsler memory scale. New York: The Psychological Corporation, 1973.

45. Russell EW. A multiple scoring method for the assessment of complex memory functions. J Consult Clin Psychol 1975;43:800.

46. Halstead WC, Wepman JM. The Halstead–Wepman aphasia screening test. J Speech Hearing Disord 1959;14:9.

47. Reitan RM. Validity of the trail making test as an indicator of organic brain damage. Percept Motor Skills 1958;8:271.

48. Halstead WC. Brain and Intelligence. Chicago: University of Chicago Press, 1947.

49. Reitan RM, Davison LA. Clinical neuropsychology: current status and applications. New York: Hemisphere, 1974.

50. Lewis R, Kupke T. The Lafayette Clinic repeatable neuropsychological test battery: its development and research applications. Paper presented at the annual meeting of the Southeastern Psychological Association, Hollywood, Florida, 1977.

51. Stroop JR. Studies of interference in serial verbal reactions. J Exp Psychol 1935;18:643.

52. Blumenthal JA, Emery CF, Madden DJ, et al. Cardiovascular and behavioral effects of aerobic exercise training in healthy older men and women. J Gerontol Med Sci 1989;44:M147.

53. Dustman RE, Ruhling RO, Russell EM. Aerobic exercise training and improved neuropsychological function of older individuals. Neurobiol Aging 1984;5:35.

54. Cockcroft AE, Saunders MJ, Berry G. Randomised controlled trial of rehabilitation in chronic respiratory disability. Thorax 1981;36:200.

55. McGavin CR, Gupta SP, Lloyd EL, McHardy JR. Physical rehabilitation of chronic bronchitis: results of a controlled trial of exercises in the home. Thorax 1977;32:307.

56. Gayle RC, Spitler DL, Karper WB, Jaeger RM, Rice SN. Psychological changes in exercising COPD patients. Int J Rehabil Res 1988;11:335.

57. Emery CF, Leatherman NE, Burker EJ, MacIntyre NR. Psychological outcomes of a pulmonary rehabilitation program. Chest 1991;100:613.

58. Kaplan RM, Atkins CJ, Reinsch S. Specific efficacy expectations mediate exercise compliance in patients with COPD. Health Psychol 1984;3:223.

59. Renfroe KL. Effect of progressive relaxation on dyspnea and state anxiety in patients with chronic obstructive pulmonary disease. Heart Lung 1988;17:408.

60. Kabat-Zinn J, Tarbell S, French C. Functional status of patients with COPD following a behavioral pulmonary rehabilitations program. Presentation at the annual meeting of the Society of Behavioral Medicine, Boston, Massachusetts, 1988.

61. Parker SR. Behavioral science aspects of COPD: current status and future directions. In: McSweeny AJ, Grant I, eds. Chronic obstructive pulmonary disease: a behavioral perspective. New York: Marcel Dekker, 1988.

62. Greenberg GD, Ryan JJ, Bourlier PE. Psychological and neuropsychological aspects of COPD. Psychosomatics 1985;26:29.

63. Lustig FM, Haas A, Castillo R. Clinical and rehabilitation regime in patients with chronic obstructive pulmonary disease. Arch Phys Med Rehabil 1972;53:315.

64. Baltes PB, Willis SL. Toward psychological theories of aging and development. In: Birren JE, Schaie KW, eds. Handbook of the psychology of aging. New York: Van Nostrand Reinhold, 1977.

HOWARD M. KRAVETZ

NAN PHEATT

16

Sexuality in the Pulmonary Patient

"Until death do us part." Filled with the heady expectation of lifelong love, our patients and their marriage partners vowed, probably decades ago, to knit together their spirits, bodies, and futures. In many cases the fabric of their love, though worn and occasionally stretched, held firmly together through the years like a child's trusty blanket. But now, tensed by day-in, day-out lung disease, it is quite likely that those threads are unraveling. The couples now face a kind of parting before death they could not have anticipated and have few tools to deal with.

Intimacy is especially important to patients with chronic obstructive pulmonary disease (COPD) because it is a powerful antidote to the depression and isolation that most patients feel so keenly. Yet, ironically, intimacy is especially hard for many patients with lung disease to achieve. Barrel-chested and stooped, they feel physically unattractive. Forced to retire from work and even household chores, they feel socially nonproductive. Robbed of their self-esteem, our patients feel permanently and desperately unlovable.

As health care providers, committed to restoring our patients to their fullest possible experience of life, we must not overlook the critical importance of love and intimacy in making our patients' lives worth living. But few of us are prepared by medical school or experience to ask our patients about their intimate relations or to offer them help in bracing those relations. Less than two dozen studies on specific aspects of sexual adjustment to COPD have been published. Even the *Textbook of Sexual Medicine*[1] by Kolodny and colleagues assigns only three pages to the topic.

Meanwhile our patients, many of whom are seniors, are unlikely to raise questions about lovemaking because they sense our reticence, and they do not wish to be considered brash.

Therefore, the first step in helping our patients become reconnected with their capacity for intimacy and love is a personal one. We must reexamine our own feelings about sexuality and intimacy; we must recognize how our own moral and religious upbringing has shaped those feelings, and we must be willing to see if those feelings, probably a vestige from adolescence, are still appropriate.

For many years, I [Howard M. Kravetz] did not feel comfortable discussing sexuality with my patients. I was born an Orthodox Jew, attended a Jesuit college, and was initiated into medicine in the heart of Protestant Boston. These exposures gave me a broad view of religion, but also a narrow view of sexuality.

When I later joined a group practice in Arizona, I noticed my colleagues also felt uncomfortable about discussing sexuality with their patients. None of us was especially eager to follow up on the few questions about sexual adjustment we had perfunctorily included on our long medical history intake form. This consensus of silence served to reinforce our separate decisions to let someone else address our patients' concerns about intimacy.

Then one day, one of my patients—a widower—appeared at the office in an obvious state of depression. His clothes and demeanor showed his self-respect was flagging, and he was losing interest in fighting his rather debilitating case of emphysema. Realizing his mental state was more critical than his physical state, I suggested that he find someone with whom to share dinner and conversation. At his next office visit, he was a new man—neat, smiling, ready again to fight for his life. I later learned the explanation for his metamorphosis was a friendship with a woman that had deepened to include sexual intimacy. He subsequently felt valuable once again to himself and to the world.

Through the experience of this patient and others, I came to realize that sexual counseling is yet another aspect of health care—another way of helping people restore the richness of life, despite chronic disease. Sexual counseling is not easy; there have been many times when a frank over-the-desk conversation about a patient's private life has sent a flush creeping up my neck or perspiration running down my forehead. But there have been many more times when I have seen patients relax and smile, relieved to have been able to share a deep, private concern and anxious to make progress toward a more fulfilling life. Clearly, we are not sex therapists and should not attempt to be. But we do our patients a disservice unless we are open to their sexual concerns and are able to address those concerns, or refer them to someone who is.

THE LANGUAGE OF THE BODY

In *The Ability to Love*,[2] Dr. Allan Fromme wrote,

> The language of the body has a quality of unmatched validity. Words, on the contrary, lend themselves to easy corruption. Not only is it easy to say things we do not mean, but it is even easier to say things the meaning of which we do not know. The body has a more primitive unsophisticated mode of expression.

Many of our patients who have had long-term intimate relationships have developed a body language of love that their partners understand and share. However, chronic lung disease can cut the conversation tragically short. The partners, fearing that intercourse may harm the patient, rule that part of intimacy out. If in their earlier patterns of lovemaking, touching always led to intercourse, they are likely to rule out touching as well. What results is a behavior that reinforces the patient's suspicions that he or she is unlovable.

Our role as rehabilitators is to help our patients understand that chronic lung disease does not have to eliminate the body language of love. It merely requires that the partners learn a new vocabulary—perhaps new approaches to intimacy, new timing, new positions—and the communication may well be as full and satisfying as before.

What follows is a summary of the male and female sexual anatomy, the male and female sexual responses, and the effects of aging. This review may seem basic, but even we health care professionals can benefit from revisiting the anatomy and physiology of sexuality so we can be more comfortable conversing with our patients. All lung disease patients should have the benefit of this knowledge, so they have a baseline of understanding against which they can measure their own personal experience. This knowledge will help partners estranged by lung disease to rewrite their lexicon of love.

THE MALE SEX ORGANS

The External Organs

The external male organs consist of the penis and the scrotum. The testicles, even though they are contained inside the scrotum and are, therefore, outside the abdominal cavity, are generally regarded as internal organs and are discussed in the next section.

The Penis

The most apparent external male sex organ is the penis (Latin for *tail*). It contains spongy erectile tissue, laced by heavy arteries. When these arteries fill with blood quickly, usually in response to sexual excitement, the penis stiffens and becomes erect. The erection will subside when the blood leaves the spongy tissue.

The tip of the penis, the glans (Latin for *acorn*), is served by multiple nerve endings. Therefore, it is extremely sensitive to touch and is an important source of sexual pleasure for men. A duct called the urethra, which releases urine or semen, runs along the underside of the penis. Its opening is in the glans.

The skin covering the penis is very loose to accommodate the penis's increase in size during an erection. When flaccid, the average length of an adult man's penis is between 3 and 4 in.; when erect, the length is between 5 and 7 in. Despite popular myths, a man's body build or race have little to do with the length of his erect penis. Furthermore, length is irrelevant to function or sexual pleasure.

The Scrotum

The scrotum is a sac that hangs outside the man's body at the base of the penis between the thighs. The scrotum contains a pair of testicles (the male gonads), each in its separate compartment. The testicles are the site of sperm production, a process that requires an even temperature, slightly below body temperature; hence, the scrotum is outside the body where ideal temperatures can be maintained.

The Internal Organs

The male internal organs include the testicles, which produce hormones and sperm; a network of ducts for transporting and storing sperm; and secretory organs involved in semen production and ejaculation.

The Testicles

In addition to manufacturing sperm, the testicles produce two kinds of gonadal hormones: male hormones called *androgens* and female hormones called *estrogens*. (The female gonads, the ovaries, also produce both male and female hormones.) It is the balance between these hormones achieved during puberty that bestown male or female sexual characteristics and functioning. At puberty, the level of androgen exceeds the level of estrogen in boys; in girls the level of estrogen is much higher than the level of androgens.

Although gonadal hormones are important during adolescence for sexual development, they are not as important for the continued sexual activity of adults. Contrary to widely held beliefs, castrated men can also be sexually responsive.

The Other Internal Male Organs

Space constraints do not allow a full discussion of the genital ducts and accessory secretary organs that are the other internal male organs, but we suggest that readers consult *The Sex Atlas,*[3] an excellent book by Haeberle.

THE FEMALE SEX ORGANS

The External Sex Organs

The external female sex organs include the mons veneris, the major and minor lips, the vaginal opening, and the clitoris. Sometimes all these organs as a group are referred to as the vulva (Latin for *covering*).

The Major Lips

The major lips are two folds of fatty skin, lying close together, keeping the rest of the vulva covered.

The Minor Lips

The minor lips lie just beneath the major lips. Richly innervated, they are sensitive to touch. At the top the minor lips merge, forming a cover (foreskin or clitoral hood) for the clitoris.

The Clitoris

The clitoris is a short, cylindrical, spongy organ composed mostly of erectile tissue. Richly endowed with nerve endings, it is sensitive to mechanical stimulation and plays a major role in female sexual excitement.

The Vaginal Opening

The vaginal opening lies opposite the clitoris, and may or may not be covered by a thin membrane called the hymen. The urethra, which in the female is used only for release of urine, lies halfway between the clitoris and the vaginal opening.

Bartholin's glands lie on each side of the vaginal opening, and they secrete a small amount of lubricating fluid during intercourse. However, most of the lubrication comes from the wall of the vagina itself.

The Internal Sex Organs

The female internal sex organs include the ovaries, fallopian tubes, uterus, and vagina.

The Ovaries
The ovaries (the female gonads) lie on both sides of the uterus inside the abdomen. They produce eggs, which are released into the fallopian tubes, and they produce hormones, which are released directly into the blood stream. Postmenopausal women, whose ovaries by definition are no longer producing hormones, can still enjoy sexual activity.

The Fallopian Tubes
The fallopian tubes (named after the 16th-century anatomist Fallopius) connect the ovaries to the uterus. They provide a tube through which the eggs can pass from the ovaries to the uterus and through which sperm can pass on the way to the egg. Fertilization of an egg normally takes place in the upper part of the fallopian tube.

The Uterus
The uterus, an organ measuring about 3 in. in length, but capable of great expansion during pregnancy, is located in the center of the lower abdomen. It is the site of implantation of the fertilized egg and development of the fetus. The uterus is very muscular, a fact that allows it to contract during the birth process. The uterine muscles also contract during orgasm.

The Vagina
The vagina is a muscular passageway joining the cervix (neck of the uterus) to an external opening in the vulva. It is about 3.5 in. long.

It serves three functions: It acts as a passageway allowing exit of the menstrual flow; it receives the male's penis and ejaculate and directs the sperm toward the cervix; and it is the birth canal.

MALE AND FEMALE SEXUAL RESPONSE

Sexual arousal is a complex phenomenon, which, in the human being, has a strong psychological component. Couples who feel enwrapped by an atmosphere of love and mutual respect have a much greater chance of achieving a fulfilling sexual experience. In the final analysis, it is the psychological richness of intimacy that elevates the human sexual experience above that of the animal. And it is the psychological richness of intimacy (with or without intercourse) that will bridge the isolation our patients so often experience.

As a result of their research, Masters and Johnson have proposed a four-phase model—excitement, plateau, orgasm, and resolution—to describe the human sexual response. The male and female responses are quite similar throughout these phases, so they will be discussed here jointly, with the differences noted.

Excitement

Individual men and women can both be aroused by certain sights, sounds, smells, or tastes that they have come to associate with a pleasurable sexual experience. One of the most powerful sexual stimuli is touch. Individuals vary a great deal in the places they like to touch and to be touched. One of the ways partners can improve their communication at both the physiologic and psychological levels is to explore those preferences together.

Many men can be aroused by mental images alone, whereas women generally are less likely to be aroused by mental images alone. Women are also more likely than men to become distracted after sexual activity has begun.

The signs of sexual arousal in men include erection of the penis and increased blood pressure and pulse rate. Some men also experience a "flush" that spreads from the abdomen to neck, and some also experience erection of the nipples.

The first sign of excitement in women is the release of lubricant in the vagina. Continued excitement changes the vagina from a collapsed tube to an open space owing to an increase in the length and width of the inner two-thirds of the vagina. The color of the vagina changes at this time from purple-red to deep purple. The major and minor lips swell and darken, the clitoris increases in size, and the uterus swells and is pulled up into the abdomen. Pulse rate and blood pressure rise.

During excitement, the woman's nipples become erect and remain so during intercourse. Most women also show the "sex flush" from abdomen to neck.

Plateau

As the name suggests, the plateau stage is a continuation of the excitement phase. Muscular tension increases and the individual is not easily distracted. The breathing rate, pulse rate, and blood pressure continue to rise in both men and women. In the healthy person, these blood pressure and respiratory rate increases are of little concern.

In men, the testicles swell and are drawn closer to the abdomen. A secretion (which may contain sperm) may appear at the tip of the penis.

In women, the lower third of the vagina tends to tighten; the minor lips darken in color and the clitoris retracts under its hood; the uterus expands and is pulled higher into the abdomen; vaginal secretions can be released; and the breasts expand in some women.

Orgasm

Orgasm is the sudden and powerful release of muscular and nervous tension generated by sexual excitement, and it involves virtually the entire body. During orgasm, breathing rate, pulse rate, and blood pressure can climb beyond that in the plateau stage. There is an intense sense of pleasure followed by complete relaxation.

Orgasm is fundamentally the same in man and women, with the major exception that sexually mature men ejaculate. It is important to note that orgasm and ejaculation are two distinct processes and do not always occur simultaneously in all men. Many women are capable of multiple orgasms within a short period. In contrast, only a very few men can experience multiple orgasms and usually only when they are young.

Resolution

During the resolution phase, the body returns to its original unexcited state. The length of time required for this return depends on the length of the excitement phase. Men, unlike many women, have a refractory period immediately following orgasm.

During this time, men are unable to have another erection or another orgasm. The refractory period tends to lengthen with age.

SEX AND AGING

The Effects of Aging on the Sexual Response

Despite popular belief to the contrary, men and women can continue to enjoy sexual activity far into their later years. There are a few changes in functioning, however, that seniors must acknowledge and recognize as normal (Table 16–1).

Older men often require a longer time to achieve an erection, and the erection may not be as firm as in younger years. In reality, older men can maintain their erections much longer than younger men and have more control over the timing of ejaculation. This gives them an advantage in being able to satisfy their partners. The older man can experience the sensation of orgasm without ejaculation. In some older men, orgasm can be as intense as in earlier years, but the ejaculate may be less in quantity.

Older women have long been victimized by the myth that sexual responsiveness disappears at menopause. To the contrary, postmenopausal women, whose ovaries by definition are no longer producing hormones, can still enjoy sexual activity. In

TABLE   16-1.   The Effects of Aging on the Sexual Response

Men and women can enjoy sexual intercourse well into old age. However, there are some normal changes in functioning:

Changes in Men

Functioning is no longer automatic.

It may take longer to achieve an erection, and the erection may not be as complete as before.

Older men can retain erections longer than younger men and have more control over the timing of ejaculation.

Orgasm is less forceful.

Ejaculations are weaker and the ejaculate may be less in quantity.

Erection is lost immediately after ejaculation.

The refractory period (time before another erection is possible) becomes longer.

Changes in Women

Vaginal lubrication appears later in the sexual excitement phase and is much less in quantity. (This can be overcome by using an artificial, water-soluble lubricant. A petroleum-based lubricant is not recommended because it is not easily expelled by the body.)

Because of loss of hormones after menopause, the vaginal walls become thinner and lose their elasticity. This may lead to bleeding and discomfort during intercourse. (This can be helped by hormone replacement, if not contraindicated.)

The contractions of orgasm are fewer and milder.

The resolution phase is much shorter.

(Adapted from Haeberle ER. The sex atlas. New York: Seabury Press, 1978)

fact, many women become more sexually responsive after menopause because they no longer need to consider the possibility of pregnancy. However, aging does bring women certain physiologic changes. Vaginal lubrication, for example, is less abundant and comes later in the excitement cycle. Vaginal walls become thinner and less elastic. Orgasmic contractions tend to be milder and fewer and the resolution phase is shorter.

As age advances, all the major organs lose their reserve capacity to perform. However, this does not mean that functioning should cease; instead, just a lower level of functioning should be expected. If people stay fit, the effects of aging can be slowed.

Intimate Relationships Among Older Patients

Intimacy is the communion of two hearts. Its expression is limited only by the creativity of those involved. Dancing, writing letters, stashing unexpected notes under the coffee cup, holding hands, sharing phone calls or over-the-dinner-table conversations can all be expressions of intimacy that bring a tremendous measure of shared joy to a couple no matter what their age or physical condition. In fact, patients should be encouraged to awaken to the possibilities for intimacy that abound.

Sexual intercourse is yet another form of intimacy, but many older patients do not allow themselves (or believe that society does not allow them) the right to express intimacy in this way. For some, there is the belief that older people just "don't do that anymore." For the many widowers and widows, especially, sexual intimacy outside of marriage is taboo. Yet, for many, the desire for sexual intimacy remains.

How do health care professionals help patients caught in this dilemma? They should suspend moral judgment and ask what is best for the patient. Giving the patient permission to acknowledge and possibly act on his or her own true feelings is a genuine service.

Patients can also be helped to overcome obstacles to communication with their partners. Many people, especially those at the age of most lung patients, are unable to talk to their partners about sexuality. They are afraid of what the other person might say or think if they expose their most personal feelings and desires. Health care professionals can help them set aside these concerns by underscoring the importance of honesty in the building and preservation of intimate relationships.

Some patients simply do not have a vocabulary for sexual matters. Reviewing sexual anatomy terms in the presence of both patient and partner not only legitimizes the discussion of sexuality, but establishes a vocabulary that both can use in the future.

HOW CHRONIC LUNG DISEASE COMPLICATES INTIMACY

Most COPD patients are middle-aged or older, so the effects of aging on intimacy and sexual response apply. But this group bears additional burdens. They must cope with fear, depression, and low self-esteem, along with altered lung function, pharmacologically induced effects, and the effect of their illness on their partner's mental state.

Fear

The fear of suffocation haunts most lung disease patients. They avoid any activity—walking, climbing stairs, sexual intercourse—that they believe might make the nightmare come true. Many patients with COPD have cardiac complications, and the fear of a sudden heart attack adds to their resolve to "take it easy" at all times.

Those who are willing to undertake lovemaking must sometimes stop because of an attack of dyspnea. They are left feeling defeated and "half a man" or "half a woman." Fear of failure becomes yet another reason to withdraw from intimacy toward isolation.

Fear is not solely the province of patients. Once partners have seen their loved ones suffer the agonies of acute shortness of breath, they are quite likely to settle for an activity level below the dyspnea threshold or what they perceive as the heart attack threshold. Both partner and patient are caught in a careful life, which often amounts to very little life at all. Sexual intercourse is often ruled out by one or the other partner for fear of morbid results. Robbed of this most basic function, male patients feel emasculated and female patients feel inadequate.

In her book *Heartsounds*,[4] Martha Weinman Lear captures a woman's pain when she believes her husband's life and self-esteem are at risk the first time they make love after his heart attack.

> It seemed crucial that he not know how scared I was. Lying there silently, as though my mind were on my pleasure. Watching him in the half-light that came from the bathroom, seeing the fingers pressed so slyly against his carotid artery, wondering what the pressure told him. Feeling his rhythm, the contact so sweet, and hearing him breathe heavily like that, and wondering if it was okay or too much. Then feeling his body go still. Was he all right? Did I dare ask?
>
> I felt poised at the edge of an irredeemable mistake. It would be dreadful to make him feel like an invalid here of all places, impulse gone, confidence gone, good-bye, and maybe for good.
>
> And yet it might be even more dangerous to say nothing. For his body was in motion again now, and what if he was feeling pain, denying it, pushing himself to perform?
>
> "Do you want to rest," I whispered.
>
> Wrong. He made a sound like a sob and fell away from me, and we lay silent, not touching in any way.

This is the anguish of a heart patient's wife, but it is not unlike the fear many lung patients' partners experience. When at the edge of lovemaking, they tread on a frightening mental landscape, wind-whipped by primeval opposing forces—life and death, love and rejection, ecstasy and pain. Few would venture willingly into that territory, but health care professionals must proceed gently with the information our patients and their partners desperately need. The rehabilitating patient and partner must be told that sexual intercourse is not any more stressful than climbing a flight of stairs. Specific suggestions (see the section on sexual counseling for the COPD patient below) to relieve anxiety and increase the likelihood of fulfilling lovemaking must be offered. And, above all else, loving partners must be encouraged to explore the full potential of intimacy at all its levels.

Depression

One of the hallmarks of chronic lung disease is depression. The past becomes the record of competence lost; it was when work was possible, jobs around the house were routine, and every day was different, or so it seemed. The future is at once both too short and too long; it is bound to stop disappointingly short of the normal life span yet, paradoxically, it is filled with too many years of fighting for breath. The present is quite simply a trap. It is an extended moment spent in a stooped, barrel-chested body that is constantly preoccupied with the business of breathing.

Overcoming depression requires a mental overhaul, something health care professionals can supervise. Depressed COPD patients need to step outside of themselves and become relinked with the environment. A health care professional can encourage this by helping patients reawaken their sensuality—their ability to smell, touch, taste, see, and hear their world. I sometimes suggest that my depressed patients take "smell walks" to detect whether a neighbor just cut the lawn, whether there is a new shrub in bloom, or whether the fall leaves are being burned. I suggest that they try wearing a new after-shave or a new perfume; it is amazing how many times the simple use of a fragrance gives them a psychic lift. The same strategy applies to redeveloping the other senses. Your patients will soon discover that they have certain vital capacities that lung disease has left untouched. They can still hear music and experience the inner stirrings it can create; they can still watch kids and puppies wrestle; they can still appreciate good food and good conversation. Perhaps the present is not quite the trap they had made it.

The sense of touch is an especially rich and powerful capacity for patients to rediscover. After all, it is the language of love. As Montague points out, touching is at the heart of the most fundamental animal and human relationships.[5] It establishes the bond between mother and offspring, and between mates. It is the first sense that is well developed, and perhaps the most important.

Low self-esteem and poor body image play prominently in many lung patients' depression. They feel old, wrinkled, stoop-shouldered—far from the Western concept of beauty and far from lovable. These people need to be reminded of "inner beauty." To some, that may seem a trite concept, but the recognition of inner beauty can provide great mental salvation. Beautiful and ageless are such attributes as a smile in the voice and a sparkle in the eye. Our patients can learn to search for and appreciate those things in themselves and in others.

Involvement in life is perhaps the best antidote to low self-esteem. For lung patients that may mean association with other patients in better-breathing clubs or rehabilitation programs. Many communities, especially those that have colleges or universities, also offer "elder hostels" where seniors can come together for learning and sociability.

The Partner

As discussed earlier, many partners become overzealous guardians, depleting the patient's life to mere existence. Other partners become resentful of the role changes forced by COPD. They are annoyed by the new demands of caretaking and, instead of blaming the disease, they blame the patient. This kind of attitude does not encourage a loving relationship and may be a real obstacle until the partner is able to work out his or her resentment and return to a positive respect for the patient.

Meanwhile, the patient becomes painfully aware of the role reversal that has taken place. The male patient is no longer able to bring home a paycheck, fix the car, even take out the garbage—tasks that he has come to associate with his masculinity. The female patient, who like most of her generation was a homemaker, can no longer do the housework or the grocery shopping. Self-esteem plummets, and the patient feels unworthy of a loving relationship.

Medications

By virtue of their age and disease, COPD patients typically take several prescription medications. If the patient has other medical conditions, there may be additional prescription drugs in the medicine chest. The patient needs to know whether or not sexual dysfunction may be related to the drugs he or she is taking (Table 16–2).

Some patients develop a dependency on sedatives and antidepressives to control anxiety. These drugs can reduce libido, a fact that produces anxiety for the patient. Unaware of the reason for lowered sex drive, the patient takes more medication, and a self-defeating cycle becomes established. The attending physician can break this cycle by prescribing only the lowest effective dose of the medication involved or by substituting an alternative drug.

TABLE   16-2.   Drugs that May Inhibit Sexual Performance

Antihypertensive Sexual Depressants
 Ganglionic blockers
 α-Adrenergic blockers (in high doses)
 β-Adrenergic blockers
 False sympathetic transmitters
 Clonidine
 Reserpine
 Diuretics

CNS Sexual Depressants
 Ethyl alcohol
 Narcotics
 Cholinergic blockers
 Monoamine oxidase inhibitors
 Tricyclic antidepressants
 Phenothiazines
 Haloperidol
 Benzodiazepines

(Adapted from Schochet BR. Medical aspects of sexual dysfunction. Drug Ther 1976; June: 37)

SEXUAL COUNSELING FOR THE PATIENT WITH
CHRONIC OBSTRUCTIVE PULMONARY DISEASE

Thus far, we have discussed why COPD patients have a special need to establish intimate relationships, yet, ironically, these relationships are especially difficult for them to acquire or sustain. We have suggested that health care professionals can do a great service to their patients by helping them mend or establish intimate relationships. But how?

Step one is to awaken patients and their partners to the many levels of intimacy. As stated earlier, a loving relationship includes many different forms of sharing and may or may not include intercourse. Encourage the partners to spend time alone together, to talk together, to experience life together. Help them find the words (or the courage required) to tell each other what they want from an intimate relationship at their stage of life.

If the couple wishes to include lovemaking in their intimate relationship, yet is having a "problem" with intercourse—perhaps fear or shortness of breath or rejection—you may wish to apply Annon's "P-LI-SS-IT" model for sexual counseling (Table 16–3).[6]

P-LI-SS-IT is an acronym for the four levels of intervention Annon describes: permission giving, limited information, specific suggestions, and intensive therapy. Some patients are adequately served by counseling at the first level, permission giving, whereas others must be guided through all the levels to the deepest one, intensive therapy.

The counselor who applies this model may be the attending physician, a nurse, or a respiratory care practitioner. Or, in some cases, a team approach in which the patient receives reinforcing messages from the various health care providers may be the most effective. The composition of the counseling team depends a great deal on the comfort level of the counselors and patients involved. In any event, the counselor does not need to be a sex therapist.

Counseling should always take place in an environment that respects the patient's privacy. Never attempt a discussion of the patient's sexual concerns in a ward or public area. The medical office is the most appropriate setting.

It is worthwhile mentioning that there are some patients who are simply not open to a discussion of sexuality, and their position must be respected. Sometimes these patients feel that revamping their intimate relationship is simply too much work and not worth the effort. Other patients, because of their cultural or religious heritage, simply cannot discuss sexuality. Health care professionals must be able to pick up and accept these cues or they risk endangering the whole of their relationship with the patient.

The P-LI-SS-IT Model

Permission Giving

About 7% of patients will volunteer information about their sexuality during an office visit; but when the conversation is invited by the physician, that number jumps to 14% or 15%.[8] Clearly, sexuality is a concern for patients, but less than half of them will raise the subject.

TABLE   16-3.   The P-LI-SS-IT Model

P—Giving Permission

Give the patient permission to have sexual thoughts, feelings, and fantasies and to engage in sexual behavior.

Suggested counseling approaches

- Include questions about sexual adjustment in the medical history.
- Ask open-ended questions.
- Avoid appearing judgmental.
- Convey the message that you believe sexual thoughts, feelings, and fantasies are normal, and that sexual activity is permissible.
- Follow up all indirect or partial responses.
- Use language the patient can understand.

LI—Providing Limited Information

Provide an overview of sexuality and how it is affected by lung disease and aging. Be sure to include the patient's partner in the counseling session.

Suggested counseling approaches

- Review those aspects of sexual anatomy and physiology that the patient does not seem to know.
- Review the normal changes in sexual functioning that accompany aging.
- Explain the energy requirements of intercourse and that shortness of breath during intercourse is normal and tolerable.
- Explain that intercourse will not harm the patient.
- Review the patient's medications and identify those that may be interfering with sexual functioning. Take steps to reduce or eliminate the effects of medication by adjusting dose or by substitution; explain to the patient how you are changing his or her medication and why.
- Remind the patient that alcohol consumption can affect sexual functioning.
- Encourage the couple to explore all levels of intimacy.

SS—Giving Specific Suggestions

Address the patient's specific concerns that have not been resolved by providing "limited information." Again, invite the patient's partner to the counseling session.

Suggested counseling approaches

- Identify intercourse positions that can reduce exertion and pressure on the patient's chest.
- If indicated, suggest the use of a metered-dose bronchodilator before intercourse.
- If indicated, suggest the use of oxygen during intercourse.
- Suggest that intercourse be planned for a time when the patient is rested.
- Suggest that the couple explore all aspects of intimacy.

IT—Providing Intensive Therapy

If the patient's sexual concerns still persist, refer the patient to a competent sex therapist for intensive therapy. Schedule follow-up appointments to assess the patient's response to intensive therapy.

(Adapted from Annon JS. The behavioral treatment of sexual problems. Honolulu: Enabling Systems, Inc., 1976)

The first task of the health care provider interested in sexual counseling is to establish a conversational climate that "gives the patient permission" to acknowledge sexual feelings and fantasies. This reassures the patient that he or she is normal, and that a discussion of private matters is routine.

The health care provider can broach the subject by asking open-ended questions like "How are things going at home?" or "Have you noticed any changes in your relations with your spouse?" If these questions are raised in the context of a medical history, the patient is more likely to be comfortable and willing to talk.

Recognize that comments like "I guess my age is catching up with me" or "Lately I just feel like half a man" are really the patient's attempt to open the door to a discussion of sexual adjustment to COPD.

It is important to project an attitude of acceptance. If the patient feels that he or she is being judged, the conversation will end abruptly and without benefit.

Avoid using technical language and labels such as frigid or impotent. Many patients dissipate the discomfort they feel while discussing sex by using slang, or sometimes they really do not know the correct terms. Be sure to discuss the facts in terms the patient can understand.

Do not hesitate to simply sit and listen. Time spent listening and pursuing incomplete or indirect responses is well spent.

Limited Information

If the patient appears to have a sexual problem you can progress to the next level of therapy—limited information. Whether or not a problem exists, of course, depends on the patient's definition. A man who is troubled by a drop in the frequency of intercourse after the onset of lung disease has a problem. One who may have experienced the same drop in frequency, but is not troubled, does not have a problem, and he is not an appropriate candidate for counseling.

Sometimes a patient's sexual problems can be remedied quite easily with simple factual information. If possible, the patient's partner should be present during this conversation, since some partners are overprotective and will block any physical activity, including lovemaking.

The first and most important point you should make is that shortness of breath during lovemaking is normal and is not particularly dangerous; anxiety, however, will increase shortness of breath. Repeat this statement during all counseling sessions, making sure that both patient and partner have assimilated the information. Emphasize that if a patient can tolerate walking up a flight of stairs—even slowly—then he or she should be able to tolerate sexual intercourse without ill effects.

Next, you should review the patient's medications and identify any that may be interfering with sexual performance. Most medications taken for the management of COPD will not interfere. Steroids and theophylline will have no effect on sexual performance, whereas oral sympathomimetic drugs may cause some urinary retention. β_2-Agonists prescribed for patients with asthma can make some men tremulous and may interfere with sexual arousal.

Many COPD patients take additional medications for the management of other medical conditions. Antihypertensive drugs that depress sexual functioning include ganglionic blockers, α-adrenergic blockers, β-adrenergic blockers, clonidine, and reserpine. Drugs that depress sexual functioning at the central nervous system level are ethyl alcohol, narcotics, cholinergic blockers, monoamine oxidase inhibitors, tricyclic antidepressants, phenothiazines, thioxanthines, haloperidol, and benzodiazepines. Antihistamines may reduce vaginal secretions in women. The patient should understand that drug-induced changes in sexual function are reversible. Use of an alternative drug or reduction of the dose will generally solve the problem.

Patients should also be told what changes in sexual performance they can expect with advancing age. Sometimes the simple knowledge that everyone is experiencing the same changes in function is enough to solve the problem and restore self-esteem.

Early in the counseling process, the counselor should attempt to discriminate between psychogenic and organic reasons for sexual problems. For many years, it was believed that 50% to 90% of impotence was psychogenic. Now, with the use of new diagnostic tests, some clinicians estimate that 50% to 75% of impotence can be attributed to organic causes.[8] A sexual history is important in determining whether impotence is psychogenic or organic. If the man has "wet dreams" or nocturnal erections, organic causes for dysfunction can generally be ruled out. Psychogenic reasons for sexual problems may be related or unrelated to lung disease. Those reasons unrelated to lung disease include anger or boredom with the sexual partner, preoccupation with work or lack of it, overeating, or alcoholism—all of which lead to a reduction in sex drive.

Specific Suggestions

If the patient appears to be having sexual problems that are related to lung disease, specific suggestions for overcoming these problems are in order. Again, the sexual partner should be present during these discussions.

HELP FOR THE PATIENT WHO IS FEARFUL OF DYSPNEA. There are a number of suggestions you can make to the patient who is afraid of acute dyspnea during lovemaking. Suggest using a metered-dose bronchodilator just before intercourse. Some patients can benefit from oxygen delivered via nasal prongs during intercourse. An exercise program that increases tolerance to activity can also be helpful.

There are certain positions for sexual intercourse that reduce pressure on the chest or allow the patient to be less active. Opting for these positions make acute shortness of breath less likely, and the patient is less likely to experience a sensation of suffocation. For the male patient, the female-superior position or intercourse with both standing and the woman doing most of the work can be helpful. Or the male patient can sit in a chair with his partner astride him. Waterbeds can also be useful, because the fluid movement can propel the patient without his or her own expenditure of energy.

Sometimes patients need to be reassured that variations from accustomed intercourse positions and oral sex are all right as long as both partners find them acceptable. In fact, experimentation with new approaches to sexual intercourse may introduce an element of excitement that can enhance the relationship.

HELP FOR THE PATIENT WHO IS AFRAID OF FAILURE. The most common cause of erectile problems is fear of failure. The patient who is afraid of failure can be helped if he is told that it is alright to stop making love when the first feelings of anxiety appear. That is the time to relax, talk, and touch his partner, thus preserving intimacy, but relieving anxiety. When confidence returns, the couple can resume lovemaking with the knowledge that it is alright to stop again.

Sometimes the patient who fears failure prefers to build confidence before facing a partner. The stop–start method during masturbation can help this patient realize that he can regain an erection after losing it.

HELP FOR THE FATIGUED PATIENT. The work of breathing requires a great energy expenditure from most COPD patients. There is frequently little energy in reserve for such "nonvital" functions as lovemaking. Patients can overcome this problem by having intercourse when they are most rested, be it in the morning or after a nap. Or they can make a daytime "date" for making love, a practice that allows pleasant anticipation and planning. Intercourse after a heavy meal should be avoided because extra energy is required for digestion.

Other suggestions for overcoming sexual problems related to COPD are offered in *A Visit with Helen* and *A Visit with Harry*, slide and tape shows produced for patient education. Physicians and other health providers can consult another slide and tape production entitled *Sexual Counseling for the COPD Patient.*[9]

Though the specific suggestions offered in this section have centered primarily on sexual intercourse, we must not forget that our objective is to help patients become reconnected with life through experiencing intimacy in its broadest sense. Suggesting that a patient rediscover the simple pleasures of holding hands, snuggling, and sharing food and conversation is certainly appropriate.

Intensive Therapy

Some patients' sexual problems persist even after limited information and specific suggestions have been offered. These patients need help beyond what is available from their concerned pulmonary physician, nurse, or respiratory care practitioner. These patients need referral to a trained sex therapist for intensive therapy.

INTIMACY AND THE YOUNG PATIENT

So far, our discussion has focused on the elderly COPD patient; but what problems do the young asthmatic patient or the cystic fibrosis patient face in achieving intimacy? How can the health care professional help?

Like COPD patients, many young asthmatics have a negative self-image. This is because our culture ascribes a great significance to the chest area. A man with broad shoulders is considered masculine, and a well-endowed woman is considered desirable. Lung patients, regardless of age, often have a negative self-image because their chest profiles are compromised.

Unlike COPD patients, young asthmatics and cystic fibrosis patients have had their lung disease all their life. They have never had the opportunity to develop an intimate relation that was not warped by disease. Therefore, a counselor cannot lead the patient to recall and duplicate old patterns of intimacy. Perhaps the health professional's greatest service to this kind of patient is to increase his or her confidence and encourage a more positive self-image.

In addition, young lung patients can benefit from a review of sexual anatomy and physiology, and the realization that their sexual functioning is normal, despite lung disease. Health care professionals can also remind these patients that many COPD patients are able to build satisfying intimate relationships, so the potential exists for them as well.

With the advent of the acquired immunodeficiency syndrome (AIDS), health professionals who offer sexual counseling have acquired another obligation. We must encourage people—young *and* old—who have decided to be sexually active to practice "safe" sex.

SUMMARY

Lifelong love is the human ideal. It is the hope of newlyweds; the flame that lights and warms the poet's verse; the essence of true happiness according to both the dialectics of the ancient philosophers and the down-to-earth instincts of the everyday man and woman. Everyone wants to love and be loved, yet many lung patients have difficulty feeling lovable and, in fact, acting lovably. It is our obligation, as rehabilitators, to pursue every means of restoring our patient's capacity for intimacy at all its levels, because the simple fact of loving attachment to another ennobles the human spirit to its fullest.

REFERENCES

1. Kolodny RC, Masters H, Johnson VE. Textbook of sexual medicine. Boston: Little, Brown & Co, 1979.

2. Fromme A. The ability to love. North Hollywood: Wilshire Book Company, 1971.

3. Haeberle EJ. The sex atlas. New York: Seabury Press, 1978.

4. Lear MW. Heartsounds. New York: Simon & Schuster, 1980:60.

5. Montagu A. Touching—the human significance of the skin. New York: Harper & Row, 1978.

6. Annon JS. The behavioral treatment of sexual problems. Honolulu: Enabling Systems, 1976.

7. Shochet BR. Medical aspects of sexual dysfunction. Drug Ther 1976; June:37.

8. Barber HR, Lewis M, Long J, Whitehead ED, Butler RN. Sexual problems in the elderly: I: The use and abuse of medications. Geriatrics 1989;44:61.

9. Kravetz HM. A visit with Harry. A visit with Helen. Sexual counseling for the COPD patient (slide and tape presentation). (Available from 1011 Ruth Street, Prescott, Arizona, 86301.)

BIBLIOGRAPHY

General for Health Care Professionals and Patients

Botwin C. Is there sex after marriage? New York: Pocket Books, 1985.

Comfort A. The joy of sex. New York: Crown Publishers, 1972.

Hite S. The Hite report (a nationwide study of female sexuality). New York: Dell Publishing, 1976.

Masters WH. Sex and aging—expectation and reality. Hosp Pract 1986;21:175.

Petty TL. Health, sex and better quality of life for your COPD patient. Med Aspects Hum Sex 1986;Aug:70.

Westheimer R. Dr. Ruth's guide for married lovers. New York: Warner Books, 1986.

Scientific

Agle DP, Baum GL. Psychological aspects of chronic obstructive pulmonary disease. Med Clin North Am 1977;61:749.

Fletcher E, Martin RJ. Sexual dysfunction and erectile impotence in chronic obstructive lung disease. Chest 1982;81:413.

Frank E, Anderson C, Rubenstein D. Frequency of sexual dysfunction in "normal" couples. N Engl J Med 1987;299:111.

Kass I, Updegraff K, Muffly RB. Sex in chronic obstructive pulmonary disease. Med Aspects Hum Sex 1972;6:33.

Kravetz HM. Sexual counseling for the COPD patient. Clinical challenge in cardiopulmonary medicine 1982;4:1. (Available from the American College of Chest Physicians, 911 Busse Highway, Park Ridge, IL 60068.)

Masters WH, Johnson VE. Human sexual response. Boston: Little, Brown & Co, 1976.

Sample PD, Beastall GH, Watson WS, Hume R. Hypothalamic–pituitary dysfunction in respiratory hypoxia. Thorax 1981;36:605.

Sample PD, Beastall GH, Hume R. Male sexual dysfunction, low serum testosterone and respiratory hypoxia. Br J Sex Med 1980;13:48.

Zilbergeld B. Male sexuality. Boston: Little, Brown & Co, 1978.

VITO A. ANGELILLO

Nutrition and the Pulmonary Patient

It has long been known that a change in body habitus accompanied far-advanced emphysema. Dornhorst[1] pointed this out in 1955, whereas Filley and coworkers[2] classified chronic obstructive pulmonary disease (COPD) patients on the basis of disease process and body habitus. From their observations came the blue bloater (bronchitic) and the pink puffer (emphysema) descriptions, with the pink puffer characterized by thinness and weight loss.

Subsequently, other studies recognized the association between increasing weight loss and severity of airflow limitation and between weight loss and mortality.[3,4] In the latter study, it was revealed that COPD patients with weight loss had a shorter survival rate than those patients without weight loss.[4] Driver and his coworkers found that patients with COPD who developed respiratory failure exhibited a higher degree of protein–calorie malnutrition, as manifested by lower body weight and anthropomorphic and visceral protein markers, than did those patients with COPD who were stable.[5] Finally, a study by Openbrier and colleagues[6] found that 43% of the emphysematous patients they studied showed evidence of malnutrition, whereas none of the bronchitics had any such evidence.

It appears, then, that evidence for malnutrition exists, especially in patients with emphysema. What is unclear, however, is whether malnutrition is the cause of deterioration in this disease state or whether it is a marker of deterioration that is caused by some other factor intrinsic to the disease process. What is also unclear is whether adequate nutrition can prevent deterioration of the lung disease, or whether it can reverse the deterioration once it has begun. These questions will be addressed later in this chapter.

Although most work done in nutrition and lung disease has been carried out primarily in patients with COPD, there are also important implications for the non-COPD patient. However, before discussing this in greater detail, it is important to review briefly malnutrition and its consequences.

MALNUTRITION

The healthy adult at stable body weight is in zero energy balance. When energy intake does not meet energy need, weight loss ensues. The reason for this weight loss is the result of an "autocannibalization" process. When food intake is decreased for any length of time, energy for metabolic processes is initially supplied from endogenous glycogen stores. Liver glycogen is broken down (*glycogenolysis*) and converted to glucose (*gluconeogenesis*), which is the primary energy substrate, especially for the central nervous system. Glycogen is also stored in muscle; however, muscle glycogen undergoing the same process as in the liver is available to only that particular muscle. This means that liver glycogen must supply glucose for all the other organ systems. However, the store of liver glycogen for gluconeogenesis is adequate for only approximately 24 hours.

If exogenous calories with a specified amount of glucose are not provided, then the various substrates necessary to meet energy requirements are derived from endogenous sources. The loss of weight that occurs is caused by the conversion of stored body fuels, such as fat, glycogen, and protein, into usable energy forms. Glycogen, as mentioned, is short-lived. From fats come fatty acids and ketone bodies. From body protein (lean body mass) comes the carbon chains (*proteolysis*) that are then processed into glucose (gluconeogenesis). If this process is not halted by the administration of exogenous calories, the end result of this autocannibalization is death caused by infection or multiple organ system failure. Ordinarily, supplying as little as 100 g of glucose will halt this process and, thereby, have a protein-sparing effect.

Whether the patient progresses to death is dependent on the severity and duration of the insult and when, in the course, refeeding is begun. Long before multiple organ system failure, a series of events takes place that has important pulmonary consequences (Table 17–1).

Malnutrition not only affects the integrity of the limb musculature, but also has a profound effect on the respiratory muscles (sternocleidomastoid and diaphragm). Both animal and human studies have shown this to be true. After a 3-day fast, young rats lost 28% of their initial weight, with a loss in diaphragm weight proportional to the loss in body mass.[7] Other investigators have shown a significant linear correlation between the weight of the diaphragm and body weight in humans.[8,9] Arora and Rochester noted that nutritionally depleted patients, none of whom had acute or chronic pulmonary disease, had significant reductions in respiratory muscle strength, as assessed by maximal static inspiratory and expiratory pressures.[10]

Malnutrition also has an adverse effect on the control of ventilation. Subjects fed a 500-kcal carbohydrate diet for 10 days showed a significantly decreased metabolic rate as well as a decreased hypoxic ventilatory response, which returned to normal after 5 days of refeeding.[11] A similar study revealed a decrease in the hypercapneic response that was increased when a total parenteral nutrition (TPN) diet high in amino acids was administered.[12]

Malnourished patients have an increased incidence of infection in general, with pneumonia being a leading cause of death. Numerous studies have shown that malnutrition leads to a loss of structural integrity of the lung. This includes a decrease in ciliary activity and macrophage function, as well as increased incidences of bacterial colonization, especially by *Pseudomonas* species.[13] In addition, animal studies

TABLE 17-1. Nutritional Concerns in the Pulmonary Patient

Consequences of malnutrition

Respiratory muscle dysfunction

  Loss of diaphragmatic mass and function

  Loss of accessory muscle mass and function

Effect on control of ventilation

  Decreased hypoxic and hypercapnic response

Increased incidence of respiratory infections

  Decreased lung clearance mechanisms

  Decreased secretory IgA

  Increased bacterial colonization

Changes in lung parenchymal structure

  Unopposed enzymatic digestion

  Loss of surfactant

Consequences of nutritional supplementation

Increased CO_2 production

  Excessive glucose calories

Increased respiratory drive

  Increased amino acid administration

---

have shown that enzymatic destruction of lung tissue may take place and that a decreased capacity to synthesize and secrete surfactant can exist during short periods of starvation.[13]

From the foregoing, it should be obvious that these consequences can take on greater significance in patients with preexisting lung disease.

There are two aspects of refeeding that may pose a problem for the respiratory-compromised patient. Ordinarily, refeeding is undertaken to stop protein (lean body mass) depletion and to promote weight gain. If excessive calories are given, they then are stored as fat. This process of fat formation, known as lipogenesis, is associated with a significant amount of carbon dioxide (CO_2) production per minute ($\dot{V}CO_2$). If the patient has a limited ability to increase ventilation, as exists in certain types of lung disease, then respiratory failure may ensue.

Since lean body mass has been lost, it is important to replace protein. As alluded to earlier, replacement of amino acids is associated with an increased ventilatory drive.[12] Although this is a desirable objective, increased amino acids could result in an increased work of breathing, with subsequent fatigue and respiratory failure, again in the patient with limited pulmonary reserve.

THE PATIENT WITH CHRONIC OBSTRUCTIVE PULMONARY DISEASE

It has long been known that as little as a 10% loss in ideal body weight is associated with considerable morbidity and in loss of adaptive ability.[14] Weight loss and deteriorating pulmonary function are closely related, specifically in patients with emphysema.[3,4–6] It has been estimated that more than 40% of patients with COPD have lost 10% or more of their ideal body weight.[15] The magnitude of the problem, then, is considerable.

The strongest evidence for the relation between body weight, pulmonary function, and survival was gathered recently from the National Institutes of Health (NIH)-sponsored intermittent positive-pressure breathing (IPPB) clinical trial involving 779 men with COPD.[16] Wilson and associates reported that mortality in this group was influenced by body weight, independent of the 1-second forced expiratory volume (FEV_1).[17] Although they felt the results of this study supported the hypothesis that factors related to nutritional status are an independent influence in the course of COPD, the possibility exists that weight loss is really a marker of disease severity, rather than the cause of deterioration. Additional studies are necessary to answer this question.

If weight loss is a significant factor in the morbidity and mortality of patients with COPD, then finding and correcting the cause may have a tremendous influence on this disease entity. Table 17–2 lists possible reasons for weight loss in COPD patients.

Several studies have shown that the resting energy expenditure, based on oxygen consumption, for patients with COPD is as high as 140% of predicted values for height, weight, and age (energy expenditure derived from the Harris–Benedict equation).[18–21] The increased oxygen consumption of the respiratory muscles (increased work of breathing) has been thought to be the primary reason for the increased energy demands.[22] For weight loss to occur under this scenario, caloric intake would have to be inadequate. Table 17–2 lists two reasons for inadequate caloric intake, both of which are speculative. Only one study has documented hypoxemia during meals.[23]

It has been thought that the flattened diaphragm impinges on the stomach, limiting the volume of food that can be eaten. However, several studies have shown calorie intake to be adequate when based on predicted needs, and that COPD patients can increase their caloric intake when encouraged to do so.[18–20] Other factors, such as malabsorption and psychosocial problems, have been studied and have either been disproved or inconsistently present.[13,24]

TABLE 17-2. Possible Causes for Weight Loss in COPD Patients

Increased energy expenditure
  Increased work of breathing

Inadequate caloric intake
  Dyspnea while eating
  Gastrointestinal symptoms while eating
  Suppressed appetite from medications (e.g., theophylline)

Poor utilization of calories—malabsorption

Psychosocial factors
  Depression
  Poverty
  Cigarette smoking
  Eating and living arrangements

It is obvious that the exact mechanism for weight loss is not easily understood. It may be multifactorial, as listed in Table 17–2, or there may be a simple unifying concept in which weight loss and decreasing pulmonary function are the clinical manifestations.

An important question that needs to be answered is whether or not adequate refeeding can halt or improve the downward spiral of COPD.

Efthimiou and associates carried out a prospective, randomized, controlled trial to investigate the effect of a 3-month period of a supplementary oral nutrition on 14 poorly nourished outpatients with COPD.[25] Seven patients were randomized to receive their normal diet during months 1 to 3, a supplemental diet during months 4 to 6, and their normal diet during months 7 to 9 (group 1). The other seven patients received their normal diet for the entire 9-month period (group 2). Seven well-nourished patients matched for age and severity of airflow obstruction served as control subjects and received their normal diets (group 3). At the end of the 3 months of supplementary oral nutrition, there was a significant improvement in the nutritional status of group 1 patients, as evidenced by an increase in body weight, triceps skin-fold thickness, midarm muscle circumference, respiratory muscle and handgrip strength. There was no change in pulmonary function or in actual blood gas concentrations. This 3-month supplementary period was sandwiched between two normal dietary intake periods so that, in a sense, this supplemental group of seven patients served as its own control, while still being compared with the other two groups. This study design allowed the degree of improvement to stand out more than it otherwise would have. Wilson and coworkers studied six malnourished patients with emphysema during a 3-week admission to a research unit.[20] The calories ingested were over and above energy requirements and, at the end of 3 weeks, there was a statistically significant improvement in body weight, anthropometric measurements, handgrip and respiratory muscle strength. Importantly, other attempts to improve nutritional status have been carried out with little or no success.[26–28] However, baseline caloric intakes were much higher than in the two malnourished groups of Efthimiou, and the mean increase in calories was less. These studies also were of shorter duration.[26–28]

It appears then, that providing calories well above requirements and of sufficient duration can improve nutritional status. Whether or not an adequate nutritional regimen can prevent long-term deterioration will require studies of much longer duration.

Nutritional Assessment and Management of Patients with Chronic Obstructive Pulmonary Disease

The application of nutritional principles applies to all patients with COPD, whether they are ambulatory, hospitalized with an exacerbation, or are in respiratory failure. Feeding methods will obviously differ, and whether a full nutritional assessment, as listed in Table 17–3, is performed depends both on the ability to make these measurements and the limited usefulness when nutritional support is of short duration.

Table 17–3 includes the nutritional, metabolic, and pulmonary characteristics of a complete evaluation. Probably the most useful screening tool to assess nutritional status is the percentage of ideal body weight. Ideal body weight (IBW) is determined

---

TABLE   17-3.   **Nutritional Assessment Profile**

Diet and weight history
  Dietary habits
  Usual weight
  History of weight loss
Anthropometrics
  Actual weight
  Ideal weight, % difference from actual weight (% ideal body
    weight)
  Triceps skin fold
  Midarm muscle circumference
  Creatinine height index
Visceral protein status
  Albumin
  Transferrin
  Thyroxine-binding prealbumin
  Retinol-binding protein
  Immunologic status
  Total lymphocyte count
  Delayed hypersensitivity with skin tests
  Nitrogen balance studies
  24-hour urine urea nitrogen
Pulmonary function parameters
  FVC, FEV_1
  Maximum inspiratory and expiratory pressures
  Exercise testing
    $\dot{V}O_{2max}$
    12-minute walk
    Diaphragmatic studies
Resting energy expenditure (REE)
  Prediction equation
  Indirect calorimetry
Total caloric requirements
  REE × stress factor
Diet design

---

from standrard weight-for-height reference tables (such as Metropolitan Life Insurance Company Weight Standards) by taking the midpoint of the weight range for a given height. Actual body weight less than 90% of IBW is significant, as has been alluded to previously.

Anthropometric measurements are a way of estimating the body's basic fuel reserves by measuring. Triceps skin-fold (TSF) to represent fat stores and arm muscle circumference and creatinine height index (CHI) to estimate skeletal (lean) muscle mass. The method has been well described,[14] but the interpretation of the measurements is less well standardized. Different values exist for different patient populations, and the measurements are not sensitive to short-term changes. Their value rests with epidemiologic surveys and to serially follow the nutritional status of individual patients over long periods. In patients with COPD, anthropometric measures could be useful in serial assessments when beginning a rehabilitation and nutrition program or in collecting data for a nutritional study. They are not an absolute necessity for a refeeding program.

The same can be said of measurements of visceral protein status. In the absence of parenchymal liver disease and protein-losing states, they reflect a decrease in protein synthesis because of limited substrate availability.[29] Their value is limited by their half-lives, with albumin having a half-life of 21 days, transferrin of 10 days, thyroxine-binding prealbumin of 2 days, and retinol-binding protein of 12 hours. This means that it not only takes at least 3 weeks of protein depletion to see a fall in serum albumin, but it also may take just as long a repletion period before seeing an increase in its level. Retinol-binding protein, on the other hand, is extremely sensitive, but not readily available, which limits its usefulness.

Depressed total lymphocyte counts and delayed hypersensitivity skin testing are also reflections of poor protein–calorie intake, but they are affected by numerous other factors, limiting their usefulness.

Determination of 24-hour urine urea nitrogen (UUN) is a good indicator of lean body mass breakdown and can serve to assess whether an anabolic state has been achieved in response to therapy.[30] The following formula provides an estimation of the total nitrogen turned over.

$$\text{Nitrogen excretion (g)} = \text{24-h UUN} + 4$$

A comparison can then be made by converting the amount of protein (g) being given in the diet to grams of nitrogen by dividing by 6.25.

$$\text{Nitrogen balance} = \text{Nitrogen intake} - \text{Nitrogen excretion}$$

The goal is to attempt to maintain the nitrogen intake 4 to 7 g ahead of the nitrogen loss. The main value of measuring the nitrogen balance probably lies in the assessment of nutritional states in more acute clinical situations.

Pulmonary function measurements consist of routine studies, such as spirometry and those to assess respiratory muscle strength, because of the effect of malnutrition on the diaphragm and accessory muscles. Which exercise test to perform depends on the patient's ability and what has been established as protocol by the pulmonary laboratory or rehabilitation program. Diaphragmatic studies, such as transdiaphragmatic pressures or electromyographic (EMG) studies are more appropriate for research purposes than for clinical management.

Determination of resting energy expenditure (REE) serves as a baseline for design of the patient's actual diet. The REE can be determined from prediction equations or by indirect calorimetry with measurments of oxygen consumption ($\dot{V}O_2$) and CO_2 production ($\dot{V}CO_2$).

The most common equation used is the Harris–Benedict equation (HBE).

$$\text{REE (male): } 66.4 + [13.7 \times \text{wt (kg)}] + [5 \times \text{ht (cm)}] - 6.75 \times \text{age}$$
$$\text{REE (female): } 655 + [9.5 \times \text{wt (kg)}] + [1.8 \times \text{ht (cm)}] - 4.67 \times \text{age}$$

Studies that have compared the HBE with indirect calorimetry have found the HBE to underestimate REE by as much as 40%.[18-21] A prediction equation derived from an ambulatory (Amb) COPD population has been published.[21]

Amb-COPD formula:
REE (male) = 11.5 × wt (kg) + 952
REE (female) = 14.1 × wt (kg) + 515

This formula was applied prospectively to ambulatory patients with COPD who were stable and to COPD patients with an exacerbation of their disease, including some receiving mechanical ventilation. The mean difference of the formula compared with indirect calorimetry was 75 ± 279 kcal and 108 ± 297 kcal, respectively.[21]

The most accurate method to determine REE is by indirect calorimetry. This requires the measurement of $\dot{V}o_2$ and $\dot{V}co_2$ in the patient after a rest period of at least 2 hours.[31] The values are then used in the Weir formula to determine REE.[32]

Abbreviated Weir formula
REE = $[3.9(\dot{V}o_2) + 1.1\ (\dot{V}co_2)]\ 1.44$

Several devices, ranging from a Douglas bag collection system to a computerized metabolic cart are available. With sophistication comes an added expense that not all hospitals can afford. In addition, expensive and frequent repairs, calibration difficulties, and technical limitations, especially in ventilated patients, has resulted in a 40% nonuse rate among a survey of nutritional support teams.[33]

Once the REE has been obtained, then total calories needed can be determined by multiplying the REE by a stress factor.

Total calories = REE × stress factor

No studies have been done to determine an appropriate stress factor for COPD patients, but extrapolating from studies mentioned earlier,[18-21] it appears reasonable to use a stress factor of 1.5 to 1.7 when the HBE is used and 1.2 to 1.3 when the Amb-COPD formula or indirect calorimetry is used.

The final task in feeding the patient is designing the diet and deciding the percentages of the various substrates that should be used. It may not be necessary to revamp the patient's entire diet. If an accurate diet history can be obtained, it would help to have a dietitian review it for actual content and total caloric value. It may be that no significant change in the basic diet is necessary, and all that is needed is the addition of a few high-calorie snacks or commercially prepared enteral products.

The diet history also is helpful to see if any of the factors listed in Table 17–2 are present, such as bloating or early satiety. These might require the change to more frequent meals of smaller volume and the avoidance of foods that cause increased bloating or gas.

Much of the work done on the effect of carbohydrate on CO_2 production ($\dot{V}co_2$) was done with patients receiving total parenteral nutrition. When excessive carbohydrate is given, the respiratory quotient exceeds 1.0, indicating an increase in CO_2 load for the patient. Clearly, this has caused or prolonged respiratory failure in critically ill patients. Few studies have been done in the ambulatory COPD population.

Gieske and colleagues evaluated a single carbohydrate load of 1000 kcal in

COPD patients with and without hypercapnia and found no significant rise in PCO_2.[34] On the other hand, Angelillo and associates found statistically significant elevations in $\dot{V}CO_2$ and PCO_2 when hypercapnic patients were given high carbohydrate loads over 5 days.[35] Brown and coworkers found that a large carbohydrate load adversely affected walking performance in stable COPD patients.[36]

Currently, it is unclear what recommendation to make in ambulatory patients with COPD. It does appear that most patients will be able to tolerate carbohydrate loads, but individualization, with a reduction in carbohydrates, may be necessary when dyspnea or hypercapnia is increasing, as occurs in respiratory failure.

Protein and amino acids can strongly affect ventilatory drive. Here again the studies have been done with the intravenous (IV) administration of amino acids. Although no studies have been done, it is doubtful that proteins administered in standard amounts (0.5 to 1.5 mg/kg) to ambulatory COPD patients will have any significant adverse effect. If a great deal of concern exists, or if the patient has lost considerable lean body mass, nitrogen balance studies would be helpful to determine actual protein requirements.

It is also unclear about the exact amount of fat that should be administered to COPD patients. Most studies that have dealt with adverse effects have involved the IV administration of lipid, usually to critically ill patients. Hypoxemia has been demonstrated and was felt to be due to a diffusion defect.[37] However, a recent review points out that hypoxemia, when it occurs with IV lipids is due to prostaglandin-stimulated ventilation–perfusion mismatch.[37] It is doubtful, that the oral administration of fats in standard amounts will have an adverse effect. However, the oral administration of a high-fat diet to hypercapneic COPD patients can reduce $\dot{V}CO_2$ and PCO_2.[35]

Although certain trace minerals and vitamins are necessary from an immunologic standpoint, no specific data is available in COPD patients. It is important to realize, however, that chronic protein–caloric malnutrition is usually not associated with significant vitamin or trace mineral deficiencies until the terminal stages.[38]

It is difficult to make definitive recommendations on the optimal form of nutritional support for patients with COPD because of insufficient data. In general, it appears most COPD patients will tolerate most feeding regimens. Where necessary, individualization will help for specific substrates. Many questions remain concerning nutrition and the patient with COPD. Is there a unifying concept to explain both progressive weight loss and functional deterioration? Will improving the nutritional status of COPD patients improve their clinical outcome? Only further investigation will help answer these questions.

REFERENCES

1. Dornhorst A. Respiratory insufficiency. Lancet 1955; 268:1185.

2. Filley G, Beckwitt H, Reeves J, Mitchell R. Chronic obstructive bronchopulmonary disease. Am J Med 1968;44:26.

3. Renzetti AD, McClement JH, Litt BD. The Veterans Administration cooperative study of pulmonary function. Mortality in relation to respiratory function in chronic obstructive pulmonary disease. Am J Med 1966;41:115.

4. Vandenbrug E, Van de Woestigne K, Gyselen A. Weight changes in the terminal stages of chronic obstructive lung disease. Am Rev Respir Dis 1967;96:556.

5. Driver AG, McAlevy MT, Smith VL. Nutritional assessment of patients with chronic obstructive pulmonary disease and acute respiratory failure. Chest 1982;82:568.

6. Openbrier D, Irwin M, Rogers RM, et al. Nutritional status and lung function in patients with emphysema and chronic bronchitis. Chest 1983;83:17.

7. Goldberg AL, Odessey R. Oxidation of amino acids by diaphragms from fed and fasted rats. Am J Physiol 1972;223:1384.

8. Thurlbeck WM. Diaphragm and body weight in emphysema. Thorax 1978;33:383.

9. Arora NS, Rochester DF. Effects of body weight and muscularity on human diaphragm muscle mass, thickness and area. J Appl Physiol 1982;52:64.

10. Arora NS, Rochester DF. Respiratory muscle strength and maximal voluntary ventilation in undernourished patients. Am Rev Respir Dis 1981;126:5.

11. Doekel RC Jr, Zwillich CW, Scoggin CH, Kryger M, Weil JV. Clinical semi-starvation: depression of hypoxic ventilatory response. N Engl J Med 1976;295:358.

12. Askanazi J, Weissman C, La Sala PA, Milic-Emili J, Kinney JM. Effect of protein intake on ventilatory drive. Anesthesiology 1984;60:106.

13. Wilson DO, Rogers RM, Hoffman RM. Nutrition and chronic lung disease: state of the art. Am Rev Respir Dis 1985;132:1347.

14. Blackburn GL, Bistrian BR, Maini BS, Schlamm HT, Smith MF. Nutritional and metabolic assessment of the hospitalized patient. JPEN 1977;1:11.

15. Hunter AM, Carry MA, Larsh HW. The nutritional status of patients with chronic obstructive pulmonary disease. Am Rev Respir Dis 1981;124:376.

16. Intermittent Positive Pressure Breathing Trial Group. Intermittent positive pressure breathing therapy of chronic obstructive pulmonary disease: a clinical trial. Ann Intern Med 1983;99:612.

17. Wilson DO, Rogers RM, Wright EC, Anthonisen NR. Body weight in chronic obstructive pulmonary disease. The National Institutes of Health intermittent positive-pressure breathing trial. Am Rev Respir Dis 1989;139:1435.

18. Openbrier DR, Irwin MN, Dauber JH, Owens GR, Rogers RM. Factors affecting nutritional status and the impact of nutritional support in patients with emphysema. Chest 1984;85 (suppl):67.

19. Braun SR, Keim NL, Dixon RM, Claganz P, Anderegg A, Shrago ES. The prevalence and determinants of nutritional changes in chronic obstructive pulmonary disease. Chest 1984;86:558.

20. Wilson DO, Rogers RM, Pennock BE, Keilly J. Nutritional intervention in malnourished emphysema patients. Am Rev Respir Dis 1985;131(part 2):61.

21. Moore JA, Angelillo VA. Equations for the prediction of resting energy expenditure in chronic obstructive lung disease. Chest 1988;94:1260.

22. Rochester DF. Body weight and respiratory muscle function in COPD. Am Rev Respir Dis 1986;134:646.

23. Brown SE, Casctari RJ, Light RW. Arterial oxygen desaturation during meals in patients with severe chronic obstructive pulmonary disease. South Med J 1983;76:194.

24. Brown SE, Light RW. When COPD patients are malnourished. J Respir Dis 1983:4:36.

25. Efthimiou J, Fleming J, Gomes C, Spiro SG. The effect of supplementary oral nutrition in poorly nourished patients with chronic obstructive pulmonary disease. Am Rev Respir Dis 1988;137:1075.

26. Lewis MI, Belman MJ, Dorr-Uyemura L. Nutritional supplementation in ambulatory patients with COPD. Am Rev Respir Dis 1987;135:1062.

27. Stauffer JL, Carbone JE, Bendoski MT. Effect of diet supplementation on anthropometric and laboratory nutritional parameters in malnourished ambulatory patients with severe COPD. Am Rev Respir Dis 1986;133:A204.

28. Knowles JB, Fairbarn MS, Wiggs BJ, Clan-Yan C, Pardy RL. Dietary supplementation and respiratory muscle performance in patients with COPD. Chest 1988;93;977.

29. Tavill AS. The synthesis and degradation of liver produced proteins. Gut 1972;13:225.

30. Long CL, Schoffer N, Geiger J, Schuler WR, Blackmore AS. Metabolic response to injury and illness estimation of energy and protein needs from indirect calorimetry and nitrogen balance. J Parenter Enteral Nutri 1979;3:452.

31. Feurer I, Mullen JL. Bedside measurement of resting energy expenditure and respiratory quotient via indirect calorimetry. Nutr Clin Pract 1981;1:43.

32. Weir JB. New methods of calculating metabolic rate with special reference to protein metabolism. J Physiol 1949;109:1.

33. Campbell SW, Kudsk KA. "High tech" metabolic measurements: useful in daily clinical practice. JPEN 1988;12:610.

34. Gieske T, Gunjiganur G, Glauser FL. Effects of carbohydrate on carbon dioxide excretion in patients with airway disease. Chest 1977;71:55.

35. Angelillo VA, Bedi S, Durfee D, Dahl J, Patterson AJ, O'Donohue WJ. Effects of low and high carbohydrate feedings in ambulatory patients with COPD and hypercapnia. Ann Intern Med 1985;103:883.

36. Brown SE, Nagendran RC, McHugh JW, Stanbury DW, Fischer CE, Light RW. Effects of a large carbohydrate load in walking performance in chronic air-flow obstruction. Am Rev Respir Dis 1985;132:960.

37. Skeie B, Askanazi J, Rothkopf MM, Rosenbaum SH, Kvetan V, Thomashaw B. Intravenous fat emulsions and lung function: a review. Crit Care Med 1988;16:183.

38. Keys A, Brozek J, Henschel A, Michelsen O, Taylor H. The biology of human starvation. Minneapolis: University of Minnesota Press, 1950.

RICHARD E. KANNER

Evaluation of Impairment
for Disability Determination

Respiratory diseases are the fifth leading cause of permanent disability in the United States. Approximately 123,000 workers received benefits from the Social Security Administration (SSA) in December of 1987 through the Old Age, Survivors, and Disability Insurance (OASDI) program as a result of having respiratory disease. This represents 4.8% of all disabled workers and in the 55- to 64-year-old group, the percentage is 7% to 7.5% of the total.[1] As of January 1989, monthly benefits averaged over 540 dollars per disabled worker[2] so that OASDI was paying out about 66.5 million dollars/month for disability caused by respiratory disease. Although OASDI is the largest program covering workers in the United States, there are other governmental programs, such as Supplemental Security Income (SSI) which is part of the SSA, the Black Lung Program, the Veterans Administration, the military, and others. State and local governments also are paying benefits and, in the private sector, many insurance companies provide disability coverage. Thus, disability caused by respiratory disease is a very serious and significant problem in terms of human suffering, lost productivity, and the total cost of the various involved programs.

The determination of impairment and disability is often a difficult and imprecise process. Approaches vary from country to country and even from region to region. In the United States, there are differences in methodology from program to program.[3] The lack of standardization is, in part, the result of an inability to determine who is truly incapable of working. It is not uncommon to see a patient who has, according to the various tests available to us, severe lung disease, and yet, that individual is gainfully employed and performing well on the job. At the other extreme, we may see another patient who appears to be essentially normal when assessed by our current methods, and yet, that person insists that he or she is incapable of doing a day's work. Another reason for differences among the various disability programs is that certain types of work (e.g., coal mining, the military) require a higher level of physical performance than sedentary occupations, and the program is designed to meet the needs of a specific group. Until methodology is developed that is acceptable to all, that could be adapted to all types of occupations, and that is better than current guidelines at predicting who can and cannot work, we will have to tolerate the present suboptimal situation. Thus, when we evaluate a worker, we will have to follow the guidelines

322

required by the particular insurance program that covers that person, and not be concerned with how it differs from the recommendations of other programs.

When evaluating a person, we must keep in mind that one person's minor annoyance is another's loss of ability to earn a living. Asthma caused by exposure to various wood dusts is of little consequence to an office worker, or a hospital worker, but can mean the loss of one's livelihood to a carpenter. Although it may have little bearing on the evaluting physician, the variability in guidelines and the benefits paid to the impaired worker can be the difference between living in poverty or being able to support oneself and family. The level of impairment that provides disability payments differs from program to program. The problem of different outcomes using different schemes to rate partial disability has been discussed in the medical literature.[4] Also, benefits differ with some programs paying much more or less than others.

In performing evaluations for impairment and disability, the tendency is to look at the functional abnormalities that are present. The guidelines stress pathologic and pathophysiologic criteria. What is more important to the person being evaluated is how much function remains. This is what determines the person's quality of life. The SSA uses the term *residual functional capacity* for this. Residual function is what determines who can and cannot benefit from a rehabilitation program.

There is often confusion and misunderstanding about the terms *impairment* and *disability*. The World Health Organization (WHO) terminology differs to some extent from that used in the United States. American usage defines *impairment*, as being

> . . . purely a medical condition. Most impairments result from a functional abnor-
> mality, which may or may not be stable at the time the evaluation is made, and may be
> temporary or permanent. . . . Impairments of lung function may be of varying
> degrees of severity, ranging from those that preclude some types of labor to those that
> ordinarily preclude any gainful employment. Some impairments are not dependent
> on lung function and result from an environmentally related diagnosis (e.g., occupa-
> tional asthma warrants proscription of continuing exposure to the inciting agents),
> from the prognosis (e.g., unresectable lung cancer), or from public health consider-
> ations (e.g., tuberculosis).[5]

Thus, this definition indicates that it is the physician's responsibility to determine if an impairment is present and if so, to quantitate it.

Disability, according to American usage, is

> . . . a term that indicates the total effect of impairment on a patient's life. It is affected
> by such diverse factors as age, gender, education, economic and social environment,
> and energy requirements of the occupation.[5]

Disability determination is an administrative, rather than a medical decision. Physicians have a say in the process, primarily by providing data on the person's impairment and residual abilities. An administrative law judge or a panel of persons will then relate the claimant's medical information to other factors to decide if benefits should be paid. Two people with identical impairments may be treated very differently by a disability panel or judge. A highly educated individual (with the ability to learn new skills that will not be affected by his or her medical problem) may be required to learn a new trade, whereas another claimant with minimal schooling may be deemed unable to be retrained to do any form of work that will be compatible with his or her residual capacity.

The terms recommended by the WHO[6] have been adapted for usage in many European countries. This terminology takes into account the lack of a strong correlation between the function of a particular organ system and the overall ability of the individual to perform. *Impairment* is used in terms of organ system impairment so that abnormalities, as defined by spirometry or the pulmonary diffusing capacity, would be considered a respiratory impairment. *Disablement* is the word used to describe the loss in exercise capacity caused by the particular organ system (or systems) impairment. It is quantitated (for the cardiac and pulmonary organ systems) by an exercise study on a treadmill or cycle ergometer. The total effect of the disablement on the ability of the person to function in society is called *handicap* and this term is similar to American usage of the word *disability*.

In the evaluation for impairment and disability the physician must follow the guidelines of the particular agency or insurance company responsible for awarding benefits. Governmental agencies have each developed their own methods for the evaluation. Private insurance companies usually ask that the American Medical Association (AMA) Guides[7] or the American Thoracic Society (ATS) Statement[5] be used, although they may leave this up to the evaluating physician. All guidelines require some quality control. There must be evidence that the spirometer has been properly calibrated and arterial blood gas laboratories will eventually be required to do the same. With the advent of standardization of pulmonary function laboratories, interlaboratory variation should decrease. This is important, as most guidelines require objective evidence of loss of function, as is quantitated in the pulmonary function laboratory. Benefits should not be awarded or denied as a result of poor quality control in a particular laboratory.

Some agencies, such as SSA, require total disability before benefits are awarded, whereas others, such as the AMA guides, allow partial as well as a total inability to work. The SSA considers the claimant's age in its guidelines and allows for the normal physiologic decline that is part of the aging process. Thus, the SSA uses a 55-year-old man as the standard for comparison. As a result, an older (more than 55 years of age) woman has an advantage in terms of receiving benefits, as women normally have lower spirometric values than men and there is a decline in function with age. The AMA and ATS methods compare a person with the reference values for their own gender and age. Thus, the same percentage loss in function compared with the reference value puts the younger person, who will have more residual function, as they have higher predicted values, on the same level as an elderly claimant. One hopes that the administrative part of the process, which determines disability on the basis of the impairment and the residual function plus other factors helps to keep the system fair.

At present, none of the schemes used to evaluate subjects with respiratory disease consider psychological factors or the effects of secondary gain. Obviously, this is not easy to accomplish. However, when symptoms are compared with objective physiologic measurements, those applying for disability benefits have better lung function than nonapplicants for the same degree of respiratory complaints. Of interest is that

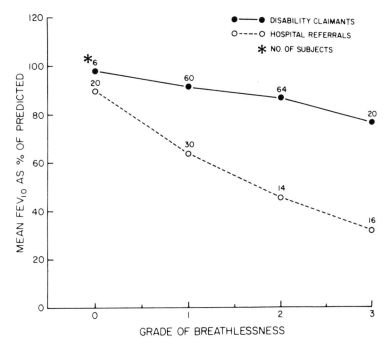

FIGURE   18-1   The relation between the grade of breathlessness and FEV_1 in subjects applying for black lung benefits and in hospital patients. (From Morgan WKC. Disability or disinclination? Impairment or importuning? Chest 1979;75:712, with permission)

in both applicants and nonapplicants there is a good relation between symptoms and quantitative function, but those seeking benefits have better pulmonary function values for the same degree of dyspnea (Fig. 18–1).[8–10]

Some forms of respiratory impairment cannot be easily quantitated by physiologic measurements. The presence of lung bullae, even with all pulmonary function measurements being normal, would preclude the individual from employment that would require being at very low or high atmospheric pressures (aviation or deep-sea diving). Asthma caused by a specific agent in the workplace (western red cedar, toluene diisocyanate, animal danders, or other) would cause on-the-job problems, but if symptomatic exposure has not been prolonged, the subject might have normal function when evaluated in the laboratory. This might also be true with hypersensitivity pneumonitis.

Asthma, in general, is difficult to quantitate for disability purposes. Most guidelines follow the precedent set by SSA.[11] This states that total disability is present if the subject, in spite of prescribed treatment, can document at least six asthmatic episodes during the year severe enough to require hospitalization or emergency room therapy and, in addition, demonstrate wheezing between acute episodes. Obviously, this guideline has weaknesses as it does not take into account those taking high doses of medications with potential toxicity and those who cannot hold down a job because of frequent mild exacerbations that cause them to miss more days of work than would be acceptable to their employer. The AMA guidelines in 1988 decided to try a different approach that uses objective measurements. Severe impairment caused by asthma is present if an individual, despite optimal medical therapy, has physiologic studies meeting the definition of severe impairment on three successive tests, performed at least 1 week apart.[7] Until we have a better understanding of the disorder (or group of disorders) we label asthma, we will be left with these less-than-ideal guidelines.

We do not know what are the best physiologic tests to use to determine disability. In the United States, we tend to favor simpler and less expensive studies such as spirometry and the single-breath carbon monoxide diffusing capacity. In select situations, exercise studies are requested. Many European countries prefer exercise testing. The correlation between spirometry and exercise testing is fairly good, but is far from perfect. Without a "gold standard" we cannot say how each compares with a person's ability to earn a living. The different approaches have been discussed and compared at a workshop sponsored by the National Heart, Lung and Blood Institute.[3]

The SSA administers the largest disability program in the United States. The primary program, which is for individuals who are entitled to Social Security benefits as a result of working a sufficient period and paying into the system, is OASDI. In part, this is paid for by the portion of your paycheck that goes to Federal Insurance Contribution Administration (FICA). There is also SSI, which is for individuals who have not paid into the system because of a lifelong inability to work, such as those with mental retardation, the blind, and such. The SSA publishes its guidelines, and copies are readily available from SSA or the local disability determination service (DDS). It is entitled *Disability Evaluation Under Social Security*.[11] When evaluating subjects for SSA, these guidelines must be followed, including documenting that the spirometer has been calibrated as well as other quality control measures. The local DDS is usually the office that requests medical evaluations. Also, they make the initial disability determination, using the guidelines set by SSA.

In the SSA manual are tables that list the criteria for severe impairment. The pulmonary function criteria are based on 40% of predicted, using the reference values of Kory and associates[12] for a 55-year-old man. The use of this standard is expected to remain, except that SSA is considering changing the reference equations to those of Crapo and colleagues.[13] If this occurs, it will be a little easier to qualify, as the Crapo equations provide higher reference values. Currently, the maximal voluntary ventilation (MVV) is required as part of the evaluation for chronic obstructive pulmonary disease (COPD), but this may be dropped in the future. The 1-second forced expiratory volume (FEV_1) is the primary measurement used for COPD. Vital capacity is the measurement used for restrictive ventilatory disorders. Chronic impairment of gas exchange from any cause is evaluated by either arterial blood gas analysis or the diffusing capacity. The arterial blood gas specimens should be drawn while the subject is exercising in a steady state for a period of 6 minutes at a workload requiring an oxygen uptake ($\dot{V}o_2$) of approximately 17 mL/kg per minute on a treadmill. If a cycle ergometer is used, an exercise equivalent of 450 kg/min or 75 W of energy should be expended. The tables relate the PO_2 to the PCO_2 to account for potential changes caused by hyper- and hypoventilation. Also, the tables stratify the values for fewer than 3000 ft in altitude, 3000 to 6000 ft, and over 6000 ft above sea level. The diffusing capacity methodology is vague, and subsequent editions are expected to recommend the standardized technique that has been proposed by the American Thoracic Society.[14] Although the SSA manual gives values only for severe impairment, benefits can be awarded to subjects with less than severe impairment. The DDS or an administrative law judge can take into account the presence of disease in multiple organ systems, none of which by itself meet the criteria for severe impairment, or factors such as educational level, age, and previous employment history.

The ATS has developed an official statement entitled *Evaluation of Impairment/ Disability Secondary to Respiratory Disorders*, which was published in 1986.[5] This was a refinement of a 1982 version. The ATS guidelines require a medical diagnostic evaluation, in addition to physiologic studies. The recommended primary measurements are the FEV_1, FVC, FEV_1/FVC, and the single-breath carbon monoxide diffusing capacity ($DLCO_{sb}$). Spirometry should be performed only after making an accurate diagnosis and while receiving optimal therapy. Standardized methodology[15] must be used. Reference values are from the equations of Crapo and associates.[13] The $DLCO_{sb}$ also should be carried out according to ATS standardized methodology,[14] but these were published a year after the impairment/disability statement and thus are not mentioned in this statement. The $DLCO_{sb}$ reference values of Crapo and Morris[16] are used with a correction factor to adjust the measured value to a standard hemoglobin concentration. In selected subjects, exercise testing should be carried out.

The ATS categorizes subjects as being normal, mildly impaired, moderately impaired, and severely impaired. *Mild impairment* is when the FVC or the FEV_1 or the $DLCO_{sb}$ is 60% to 79% of predicted, or the $FEV_1/FVCx100$ is 60% to 74% (if these are abnormal values for that person). *Moderate impairment* is when the FVC is 51% to 59% of predicted or the FEV_1 or $DLCO_{sb}$ is 41% to 59% of predicted or the $FEV_1/FVCx100$ is 41% to 59%. *Severe impairment* occurs when values are equal to, or less than 50% predicted for the FVC or 40% or less than predicted for the FEV_1 and/or $DLCO_{sb}$ or the $FEV_1/FVCx100$ is 40% or less. When using exercise studies, there are three categories. *Normal* is a maximal $\dot{V}O_2$ equal to or greater than 25 mL/kg per minute (7.1 METS); a *less-than-severe impairment* occurs when the $\dot{V}O_2$ is between 15 and 25 mL/kg per minute and *severe impairment* occurs when the $\dot{V}O_2$ is equal to or less than 15 mL/kg per minute (4.3 METS). Situations not directly related to lung function measurements are discussed in the ATS statement.[5] Arterial blood gas analysis is not given much emphasis in the ATS statement, which considers cor pulmonale a more reliable predictor of severe impairment than an arterial blood gas measurement.

The AMA is constantly revising their *Guides to the Evaluation of Permanent Impairment*.[7] The current third edition was published in 1988 and can be purchased directly from the AMA. The respiratory system chapter has features in common with the ATS guidelines. A medical history and physical examination are part of the evaluation, as is a chest radiograph. The equipment calibration and methodology for spirometry should follow the ATS recommendation,[15] as should the methodology for performing the diffusing capacity.[14] The recommended reference values are those of Crapo and coworkers for spirometry[13] and Crapo and Morris for the diffusing capacity.[16] Exercise testing is indicated when (1) the person's symptoms of dyspnea

	Class 1 0% No Impairment of the Whole Person	Class 2 10-25% Mild Impairment of the Whole Person	Class 3 30-45% Moderate Impairment of the Whole Person	Class 4 50-100% Severe Impairment of the Whole Person
FVC FEV_1 FEV_1/FVC (as percent) DCO	FVC ≥ 80% of predicted, *and* FEV_1 ≥ 80% of predicted, *and* FEV1/FVC ≥ 70% *and* DCO ≥ 80% of predicted.	FVC between 60% and 79% of predicted, *or* FEV_1 between 60% and 79% of predicted, *or* FEV_1/FVC between 60% and 69%, *or* DCO between 60% and 79% of predicted.	FVC between 51% and 59% of predicted, *or* FEV_1 between 41% and 59% of predicted, *or* FEV_1/FVC between 41% and 59%, *or* DCO between 41% and 59% of predicted.	FVC ≤ 50% of predicted, *or* FEV_1 ≤ 40% of predicted, *or* FEV_1/FVC ≤ 40% *or* DCO ≤ 40% of predicted.
	or	**or**	**or**	**or**
$\dot{V}o_2$Max	> 25 mL/(kg · min)	Between 20 and 25 mL/(kg · min)	Between 15 and 20 mL/(kg · min)	< 15 mL/(kg · min)

FVC is Forced Vital Capacity, FEV_1 is Forced Expiratory Volume in the first second, DCO is diffusing capacity of carbon monoxide. The DCO is primarily of value for persons with restrictive lung disease. In Classes 2 and 3, if the FVC, FEV_1 and FEV_1/FVC ratio are normal and the DCO is between 41% and 79%, then an exercise test is required.

$\dot{V}o_2$ Max, or measured exercise capacity, is useful in assessing whether a person's complaint of dyspnea (see Table 1) is a result of respiratory or other conditions. A person's cardiac and conditioning status must be considered in performing the test and in interpreting the results.

FIGURE 18-2 American Medical Association classes of respiratory impairment. (From Engelberg AL, ed. Guides to the evaluation of permanent impairment. 3rd ed. Chicago: American Medical Association, 1988:117)

are more severe than spirometry or the diffusing capacity would indicate; or (2) the subject states that he or she cannot perform his or her job because of breathlessness; or (3) the person does not perform maximally or correctly during spirometry or the diffusing capacity measurement. The AMA classes of respiratory impairment are shown in Figure 18–2.

Arterial blood gas analysis is usually not indicated in the AMA approach, as it is felt that, in general, in patients with airway obstruction, the FEV_1 correlates better with exercise capacity than does the PaO_2. However, if the PaO_2 is less than 60 mm Hg when breathing room air, a person may be considered severely impaired if the sequeallae of hypoxemia are present. These include cor pulmonale and erythrocytosis. A PaO_2 of less than 50 mm Hg by itself is considered disabling.

Conditions causing impairment that may not be directly related to the measurement of physiologic lung function are also part of the AMA guides. These are presented in Figure 18–3.

Coal miners are covered under a separate program that is administered by the Department of Labor.[17] This is based on the *Black Lung Benefits Reform Act* of 1977. This program applies only to disability or death caused by pneumoconiosis in workers employed in the coal-mining industry. In this context, the definition of pneumoconiosis is fairly broad. If complicated pneumoconiosis is present on the chest radiograph (ILO/UC classification of category A, B, or C), there is an irrefutable presumption of total disability. Some of these miners, especially those with category A pneumoconiosis, can have normal or almost normal lung function. Although these individuals should not return to work where there will be further exposure to coal

Condition	Comment
Asthma	An asthmatic person, who despite optimum medical therapy, including daily administration of a bronchodilator under regular physician care, and whose physiologic tests of impairment fall under Class 4 (Table 2) after administration of an inhaled bronchodilator in a laboratory, is considered to be severely impaired. This level of impairment should be found on three successive tests, performed at least one week apart. (It is recognized that persons whose asthma causes less-than-severe impairment, or whose asthma is related directly to a job-related exposure (such as toluene diisocyanate) may occasionally be evaluated for the purposes of determining employability or employment-related disability. The final determination, which is a nonmedical decision, relies in part on medical evidence. The physician's thorough documentation of the nature of the asthmatic condition, as well as nonmedical evidence, such as exposure data and reports of supervisors or fellow employees, are crucial to this determination.)
Hypersensitivity pneumonitis	A person with this condition may need to be removed from exposure to the causative agent or other agents with similar sensitizing properties, in order to avoid future attacks and chronic sequelae.
Pneumoconiosis	Although pneumoconiosis may cause no physiologic impairment, its presence usually requires removal from exposure to the dust that caused the condition.
Sleep disorders	Obstructive sleep apnea, central sleep apnea and Cheyne-Stokes respiration may prevent progression through normal stages of sleep, and may lead to hypersomnolence, hypoxia, hemodynamic changes and personality disorders. Impairment due to sleep disorders should be evaluated according to criteria in Chapters 4, 6 and 14, and combined using the Combined Values Chart.
Lung cancers	All persons with lung cancers are to be considered severely impaired at the time of diagnosis. At are-evaluation at one year after the diagnosis is established, if the person is found to be free of all evidence of tumor recurrence, then he or she should be rated according to physiologic parameters in Table 8. If there is evidence of tumor, the person remains severely impaired. If the tumor recurs at a later date, the person immediately is considered to be severely impaired.

FIGURE   18-3   American Medical Association scheme for evaluation of respiratory impairment not directly related to lung function. (From Engelberg AL ed. Guides to the evaluation of permanent impairment. 3rd ed. Chicago: American Medical Association. 1988:118)

dust, they can, if so motivated, find other types of employment. It is also possible to receive benefits if spirometry, including the MVV, is less than 60% of predicted using the reference values of Knudson and associates.[18] Thus, these individuals have more remaining lung function than workers who qualify for total disability, using guidelines requiring values less than 40% of predicted. Arterial blood gas tables are also used to determine total impairment–disability with PaO_2 values that are much higher than those used by SSA. So again, significant residual lung function can be present. Total disability, as determined by spirometry and arterial blood gas analysis, can be rebutted if it can be demonstrated that the cause of these abnormalities is not due to coal mine employment. In evaluating coal miners, the examining physician should follow the procedures outlined in the *Federal Register*.[17]

Federal programs, such as SSA and the *Black Lung Benefits Reform Act* of 1977 have specific directions for the evaluating physician to follow. Private insurance companies may give the physician lattitude in selecting which guideline to use or may specify that they want a particular guideline, usually the AMA or ATS. A requesting agency or insurance company may ask for only one or two physiologic studies, or they may want a complete medical evaluation. The government program or insurance company will not reimburse the physician for studies they have not requested. However, if the physician believes additional studies would be helpful he or she can negotiate this with the requesting company or agency. The physician's report should, whenever possible, follow the language of the guideline being followed.

Although the primary responsibility of physicians is to evaluate claimants for impairment, at times they are involved in disability determination as well. An insurance company, or other agency, may request that the physician assign a percentage disability on the basis of the impairment evaluation. This is often an uncomfortable position for the physician to be in. For example, one would hesitate to offend a claimant if that person was also one's private patient. Also, the physician may not have other nonmedical data that would help in such a determination. Finally, physicians usually do not know what rehabilitation programs are available to a particular claimant and, accordingly, could not determine if the subject was a suitable candidate for one of these programs.

The evaluating physician may be asked to present the findings to a board or administrative law judge. This could be in the form of a written report, a deposition, or live testimony in the courtroom. Since nonmedical personnel have little understanding of medical terminology, the data should be presented in words all can understand. Always avoid jargon. It helps to work with the lawyer who can teach the physician what certain legal terms mean and vice versa. A good lawyer can make this part of the process easy for the physician.

REFERENCES

1. OASDI current-pay benefits: disabled workers. Soc Sec Bull Ann Stat Suppl, SSA Publ 13-11700, 1988:198.

2. OASDI cash benefits: average amount of monthly benefits by type of beneficiary, 1940–89. Soc Sec Bull 1989;52(3):57.

3. Becklake MR, Rodarte JR, Kalica AR. Scientific issues in the assessment of respiratory impairment. NHLBI workshop summary. Am Rev Respir Dis, 1988;137:1505.

4. Harber P. Alternate partial respiratory disability rating schemes. Am Rev Respir Dis 1986;134:481.

5. American Thoracic Society. Evaluation of impairment/disability secondary to respiratory disorders. Am Rev Respir Dis 1986;133:1205.

6. World Health Organization. International classification of impairments, disabilities and handicaps. Geneva: World Health Organization, 1980.

7. Engleberg AL, ed. Guides to the evaluation of permanent impairment. 3rd ed. Chicago: American Medical Association, 1988:107.

8. Morgan WKC. Disability or disinclination? Impairment or importuning? Chest 1979;75:712.

9. Morgan WKC, Seaton A. Pulmonary physiology. Its application to the determination of respiratory impairment and disability in industrial lung disease. In: Morgan WKC, Seaton A, eds. Occupational lung disease. Philadelphia: WB Saunders, 1984:18.

10. Cotes JE. Assessment of disablement due to impaired respiratory function. Bull Physiopathol Respir 1975;11:210.

11. Social Security Administration. Disability evaluation under Social Security. U.S. Department of Health and Human Services, Social Security Administration. SSA Publ 05-10089, 1986:28.

12. Kory RE, Callahan R, Boren HG, Syner JC, The Veterans Administration–Army cooperative study of pulmonary function. I. Clinical spirometry in normal men. Am J Med 1961;30:243.

13. Crapo RO, Morris AH, Gardner RM. Reference spirometric values using techniques and equipment that meet ATS recommendations. Am Rev Respir Dis 1981;123:659.

14. American Thoracic Society. Single breath carbon monoxide diffusing capacity (transfer factor). Recommendations for a standard technique. Am Rev Respir Dis 1987;136:1299.

15. American Thoracic Society. Standardization for spirometry 1987 update. Am Rev Respir Dis 1987;136:1285.

16. Crapo RO, Morris AH. Standardized single breath normal values for carbon monoxide diffusing capacity. Am Rev Respir Dis 1981;123:185.

17. Department of Labor, Employment Standards Administration. Standards for determining coal miners' total disability or death due to pneumoconiosis. Fed Reg 1980; 45 (20 CFR Part 718):13678, Feb 29.

18. Knudson RJ, Slatin RC, Lebowitz MD, Burrows B. The maximal expiratory flow–volume curve: normal standards, variability, and effects of age. Am Rev Respir Dis 1976;113:587.

PATRICK J. DUNNE

SUSAN L. McINTURFF

CELE DARR

The Role of Home Care

An important aspect of comprehensive respiratory care takes place away from the classroom, the physician's office, and the hospital. It involves a multidisciplinary team that provides continuity to the services of a pulmonary rehabilitation program. Home care is somewhat self-defining, as it does take place in the patient's own home; however, there is a great deal involved in developing a home care program for your patient.

With the advent of Medicare reimbursement based on diagnosis-related groups (DRGs) and prospective payment systems, hospitals are attempting to limit costs, with the potential for discharging patients "quicker and sicker." These patients will often have continued medical needs that were formerly met by keeping them in the hospital for several additional days. Balinsky and Starkman, in their article on the effect of DRGs on the health care industry state: ". . . one might reasonably predict that the post-hospital care needs of patients are becoming more acute and that the number of actual placements in home health agencies is growing."[1] What happens to those patients who have continued medical needs or who have been released from their inpatient program before they have all the information and skills they need to care for themselves? Home care is the answer to this question.

A well-structured home care program will allow the continued treatment of the patient with nearly any known illness and with most of the therapeutic modalities available in the acute care setting, such as intravenous (IV) therapy, wound care, oxygen and nebulizer therapy, mechanical ventilator care, or for needs as basic as postdischarge follow-up to assess progress. It will allow continued education and evaluation of the practices learned during the pulmonary rehabilitation program or during the acute admission. For many patients, a good home care program is vital to their long-term survival.

This chapter will describe how to develop a total program for the patient who goes home, and it will discuss the roles of the members of the home care team. How home medical equipment suppliers can achieve home care accreditation and reimbursement by third-party payers will also be covered, as these are vital issues in providing quality care to patients.

BENEFITS OF HOME CARE

The goal of any outpatient treatment program is to perform a medical service outside the hospital. Home care permits these medical services to be rendered in the comfort and convenience of the patient's own home. A large and varied population of patients exist who can be considered candidates for the benefits of home care, most of them elderly and many of them inflicted with pulmonary diseases. Table 19–1 reviews the types of patients who would be considered potential candidates for home care.

The primary goal of home care is to prevent or reduce acute care hospitalizations. This is accomplished by an ongoing assessment by the members of the home care team for problems, progress, and compliance with the physician's plan of treatment. For example, a competent home care practitioner can assess the patient for such factors as a change in the amount or color of sputum, edema, tachycardia, abnormal breath sounds, or rapid respiratory rate; can communicate this to the physician; and can assist in initiating treatment. Early identification of problems that the patient may not perceive and treating them quickly can prevent admissions to the hospital.

The patient's home environment may enhance learning and compliance and provide a sense of control that is lost in the acute care setting. Patients are happier when they are at home and may be more willing to cooperate with planning their medical program when they feel they have some control and input into it.

It should also be apparent that a reduction in total hospital days, either by discharging the patient early to a structured home care program or by preventing future hospital admissions, will create a significant cost savings. This is particularly important in this day and age, when health care expenditures consume upward of 12% of the gross national product and is estimated to reach 15% by the year 2000.[2] Third-party payers are continually looking for ways to cut back their medical expenditures, and home care is an excellent way to achieve this.

THE HOME CARE TEAM

A multidisciplinary team is involved in providing home care services. This team includes the patient and family members or other caregivers, the physician, the

---

TABLE   19-1.   Potential Candidates for Home Care

- Have repeated hospitalizations, the "revolving door" patients
- Newly diagnosed or hospitalized for the first time
- Patients who are anxious, confused, or forgetful and who require medications or treatments
- Going home with new respiratory equipment, especially oxygen, ventilators, or tracheostomy tubes
- Stable patients who develop an exacerbation of their condition that the physician wants to manage at home
- Patients requiring brief follow-up after a formal rehabilitation program
- End-stage terminal patients who want to remain at home

(Meany-Handy J, Lareau SC. The role of home care. In: Hodgkin JE, Zorn EG, Connors GL, eds. Pulmonary rehabilitation: guidelines to success. 1st ed. Boston: Butterworths, 1984, with permission)

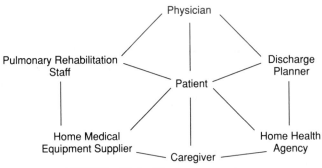

FIGURE   19-1   The home care team.

pulmonary rehabilitation staff, the hospital discharge planner, the home health agency, and the home medical equipment (HME) supplier. Each member serves an integral part, and all members must interact cooperatively (Fig. 19–1).

DELIVERY OF HOME CARE SERVICES

Identification of the need for home care is the first step in providing services. The patient's physician, pulmonary rehabilitation team, and discharge planner all may be responsible for assessing the patient and determining what type of home care program is necessary.

The physician may be advised by the pulmonary rehabilitation team or discharge planner that home care is indicated; all three entities must possess a good working knowledge of the availability of services. It must be determined if home services are covered by the patient's medical insurance. There are "qualifying criteria" for most home care services, and the medical need must be justified according to these qualifying criteria before payment will be made by the insurance company. This applies to home medical equipment, oxygen services, IV services, and wound care, as well as home visits by nurses, nursing aides, and physical and occupational therapists. The physician usually relies on the discharge planner or pulmonary rehabilitation staff to understand the qualifying criteria when home care services are ordered.

Once the decision has been made that the patient requires home care as part of his or her overall plan of treatment, a home care program is developed. Multiple factors need to be considered when developing the program. Patients must be involved in developing the program and be willing to allow team members into their homes; some patients do not feel they need this service or are uncomfortable with their privacy being "invaded" by strangers. Sometimes the patient has no intention of being compliant with the prescribed home care regimen, and in this case, attempts to provide home care will be in vain.

Another factor to consider is whether the patient's home environment is conducive to a home care program. The home may not have adequate electrical wiring to power medical devices safely. The home may be so unkempt that it poses a health or fire risk. Perhaps the home may be too small to accept a hospital bed or wheelchair when those items are deemed necessary, or there may be stairs that pose an obstacle for access to continuous oxygen therapy. It must be determined where to locate a stationary oxygen system in a two-storied home, or even a home longer than 100 ft (30 m).

The patient's geographical location must also be considered; for example, the patient may live in a remote area that is not readily serviced by an HME company or home health agency. In these situations, special arrangements need to be made for temporary living quarters until the patient no longer requires home care services and can return home.

Although it is advisable to assess for these potential problems before discharge to the home care program, some of these impediments to successful home care may be discovered during the initial visit by home care practitioners from the home health agency or HME supplier. At that time, the home care professional can work with the patient and his or her physician to facilitate the prescribed program within the confines of the problems discovered. An extremely useful publication, *Safety for Older Consumers* is a checklist outlining safety guidelines for all the rooms in a home.[3] This checklist can be used by the discharge planner and the other members of the home care team to assess the patient's home and identify areas needing modification to promote safety and health.

Once the need for home care has been identified, referrals are made to the appropriate members of the home care team. One of the most beneficial aspects of home care is the opportunity for visits by several different specialty practitioners employed by the home health agency that receives the referral. At the time of discharge, or during the initial home visit by the nurse it may be determined that the patient needs the services of a physical or occupational therapist, for example, to assess the effectiveness of an exercise program or to train the patient in energy conservation during activities of daily living. It may be determined that the patient needs visits by an aide to assist with bathing, or a chore-worker to help with cleaning or cooking while the patient recuperates. All services must be justified by a detailed plan of treatment and are limited to finite amounts of time; for example, following a discharge from an acute care hospital, nursing services are covered for a certain number of visits, depending on the diagnosis. When the home health program is designed for the patient it should be with these time limits in mind to ensure that the goals of therapy are reached before further reimbursement is denied. Table 19–2

TABLE 19-2. Medical Specialists Employed by Home Health Agencies

Registered nurses
Licensed vocational nurses
Nursing aides
Physical therapists
Respiratory care practitioners
Occupational therapists
Speech therapists
Social workers

outlines the types of medical specialists frequently employed by home health agencies who can be used in the plan of treatment.

PROVISION OF HOME MEDICAL EQUIPMENT SERVICES

One of the major components of a home care program is the provision of medical equipment. Technology allows almost any type of equipment that is used in the hospital to also function at home. It is not uncommon to see patients who need ventilators, IV pumps, enteral or parenteral nutritional therapy, continuous passive motion therapy, or oxygen therapy through a tracheostomy in the home. The challenge is to determine the most appropriate device to meet the patient's medical needs within the boundaries of the third-party payer's guidelines.

Once the physician has determined that the patient needs medical equipment at home, the referral source (e.g., the discharge planner or pulmonary rehabilitation staff) will contact an HME supplier to arrange for delivery of the equipment. Table 19–3 is a listing of some specific pieces of information the referral source will need to provide when placing an equipment order. The HME supplier may assist in determining the type of equipment needed. However, if the physician desires a specific piece of equipment, such as a liquid oxygen system, it will be necessary to ensure that the patient is not provided a substitute piece of equipment in an attempt to reduce costs to the supplier.

The HME supplier has certain responsibilities to the patient. The supplier is responsible for placing equipment in a timely manner; for example, oxygen ordered

TABLE   19-3.   Information Required When Ordering Home Medical Equipment

Personal Information
 Name
 Address
 Telephone number
 Date of birth
 Diagnosis
 Ordering physician
 Place of service

Billing Information
 Insurance name
 Policy or HIC number
 Insurance address
 Secondary insurance

Medical Equipment
 Type of equipment
 Frequency of use
 Qualifying medical criteria

for a patient being discharged should be delivered within a stated number of hours, not days. In fact, the oxygen may need to be in place in the patient's home before the patient's arrival, and a portable system may need to be delivered to the patient's hospital room for use during transport home. The HME company is also responsible for educating all concerned persons on the safe and proper use and maintenance of the equipment. This training is particularly important for the patient and their primary caregiver, but education and training may also involve the nursing staff or extended family members. Training may be ongoing, depending on the needs of the patient and caregivers, as for the patient requiring ventilator assistance who may have new nurses from time to time.

The HME company is also responsible for the routine and ongoing maintenance of all equipment placed on rental. Such maintenance should be performed at the frequency recommended by the manufacturer or more frequently as needed. This service should be at no charge to the patient when the equipment is being rented; third-party payers such as Medicare consider that the parts and labor involved in maintenance and repair are covered in the monthly rental fee.

Many HME companies employ respiratory care practitioners (RCPs) to oversee the needs of those patients with pulmonary impairment. The RCP will assist in the development of a plan of treatment and help establish goals of therapy for patients with home oxygen or other respiratory care equipment. Given the clinical evaluation, the RCP will determine a follow-up schedule to assess the appropriateness of therapy for the patient and to ensure that the goals of therapy are being met. There are some patients who may not need follow-up visits except for equipment maintenance. There are also patients who may need almost daily visits until the therapist is comfortable that the home situation is stable. Visits should be based on the initial clinical evaluation and subsequent visits should be tailored to changing medical needs.

There are several physiologic criteria the clinician will assess when doing an evaluation. This assessment may include auscultation, blood pressure, heart rate, respiratory rate, lower extremities check for peripheral edema, and O_2 saturation by pulse oximetry.

An evaluation of the home should be done to determine the appropriateness of the environment for access to the equipment, electrical hookups, and cleanliness. Modifications may need to be made to permit improved access to the equipment, such as moving the equipment or placing additional systems, as for the patient with a large home. Adaptation of electrical cords or outlets may be necessary to prevent electrical hazards. Devices may need modification to prevent tampering should there be small children in the home, or patients who change settings on their equipment against medical advice.

The RCP will also assess the patient's compliance with the physician's orders for respiratory care. Assessment for compliance may be difficult, since the patient's memory may be cloudy, or the patient may just not be truthful. Patients on oxygen therapy frequently overestimate the amount of time they are using oxygen, or will increase their oxygen flow rate above what the physician has ordered. Content gauges and hour meters are helpful tools to determine actual use and allow positive feedback to patients when you are evaluating them for compliance. Patients who have problems with their bronchodilator therapy may need additional instruction or unit-dose medications to increase compliance. Sometimes they cannot open the bottles holding the bronchodilator, or cannot read the scale on the dropper included with the medication. Frequently, patients will take abbreviated treatments until they feel an abatement of their dyspnea and not get the full dose of medication that is ordered. Overuse of metered-dose inhalers and medication nebulizers is also fairly common-place, requiring the RCP to inform the patient of the hazards of abuse and reinforce proper use and technique.

When inquiring about the patient's use of bronchodilators, the home care RCP may discover that the patient is having trouble with his or her other medications. It is helpful to request the assistance of the home health agency or pulmonary rehabilitation team when dealing with medication problems. The home health nurse may have a greater knowledge of the medications used for treatment of the patient's medical problems and can help in educating the patient. The pulmonary rehabilitation staff will have instructed the patient before discharge from the program about their medication schedule and may be able to help reinstruct the patient or revise the schedule to increase compliance.

Other areas that can be assessed by the home care practitioner include nutrition, activities of daily living, exercise, and psychosocial issues. The RCP may recognize that the patient is losing weight, not eating properly, is depressed or, possibly, even suicidal. These observations should be reported to the physician and the home health agency so that they can be addressed by the appropriate specialist.

COMMUNICATION AMONG THE TEAM MEMBERS

Each member of the team serves as the "eyes and ears" of the physician, and communication with the physician and among the team members is essential. Assessment of the items previously discussed is of little value unless that information is properly interpreted and relayed to the physician for his or her evaluation. As stated by Meany-Handy and Lareau in the previous edition of this book, "physicians should be able to rely on the clinical judgment and recommendations of qualified home care staff."[4] When the home care professional makes a visit to the patient, the findings are documented on a follow-up form, along with the plan of treatment and any other pertinent information. This information may be called to the physician during the patient visit for immediate attention; it should also be forwarded in its written form to the physician and, when appropriate, to other members of the team. Most HME companies will send copies of visit records not only to the physician, but also to the nursing agency and the referral source. Team conferences on patients with very complicated needs are particularly valuable before discharge and can be repeated as often as deemed necessary to address problems once the patient is home. It is helpful to include the home care practitioner from the HME company when scheduling team conferences to discuss medical needs that involve equipment. Documentation of problems should be shared with all appropriate team members; however, the patient's right to confidentiality should always be kept in mind.

It may also be necessary to communicate with the insurance company to advise them of the patient's progress. Many insurance companies have case managers who want an update on the patient's progress and goals of therapy to continue reimbursement. Insurance companies must also be contacted to verify coverage when the patient has additional equipment or supply needs. Supportive documentation is usually requested for continued reimbursement.

TYPES OF HOME CARE EQUIPMENT

Patients afflicted with chronic lung disease and resultant chronic hypoxemia represent one of the largest single population groups using home care equipment. A patient may need any number of pieces of durable medical equipment, such as a hospital bed, walker, wheelchair, enteral and IV pumps, oxygen devices, and home ventilators. Devices used to provide oxygen and aerosol therapy constitute the largest category of respiratory equipment.

Oxygen Therapy Devices

There are three distinct types of stationary systems available to provide continuous in-home oxygen therapy:

- High-pressure cylinders
- Oxygen concentrators
- Liquid oxygen systems

There are two distinct types of portable oxygen systems used to provide ambulation:

- Lightweight smaller-sized cylinders
- Portable liquid oxygen

High-Pressure Cylinders

The use of seamless steel cylinders to contain gaseous oxygen under high pressure is the oldest and most reliable method of storing oxygen for subsequent administration. Oxygen is compressed to pressures of 2200 to 2400 psi (15,169 to 16,548 kPa) in cylinders of various sizes. The larger the cylinder the more cubic feet (liters) of oxygen can be contained at the filling pressure of 2200 psi (15,169 kPa). The most common sizes seen in the home are H-tanks containing 244 cubic feet (6910L) of oxygen, and E-tanks, containing 22 cubic feet (623L). Table 19–4 lists the estimated lengths of time these tanks will last at particular flow rates.

TABLE 19-4. Estimated Time Remaining when Using an H-Cylinder at Certain Flow Rates and Pressures

Tank Pressure (psi)	1	2	3	4	5
2200 (full)	115 h	$57\frac{1}{2}$ h	$38\frac{1}{2}$ h	$28\frac{1}{2}$ h	23 h
1500 (3/4)	$73\frac{1}{2}$ h	$36\frac{1}{2}$ h	$24\frac{1}{2}$ h	18 h	$14\frac{1}{2}$ h
1100 (1/2)	$52\frac{1}{4}$ h	26 h	$17\frac{1}{2}$ h	13 h	10 h
500 (1/4)	21 h	$10\frac{1}{2}$ h	7 h	$5\frac{1}{4}$ h	$4\frac{1}{4}$ h

The high-pressure stationary oxygen system has several advantages: no external power supply is required for operation; there is no loss of oxygen when the system is not in use; high-pressure stationary systems can also be used to power other pieces of respiratory equipment such as nebulizers, blenders, or ventilators. There are, however, several disadvantages to this type of stationary system: each cylinder has a fixed capacity necessitating frequent changes and refills; high-pressure oxygen cylinders pose a safety risk and must be properly secured; moderate hand strength and dexterity are needed to open valves; patients or caregivers must be capable of reading gauges and meters, connecting regulators, and observing strict safety guidelines.

Perhaps most important, high-pressure gaseous systems are useful in providing a backup to other stationary oxygen systems at risk for breakdown. This backup system is an important requirement by many organizations accrediting home care equipment providers.[5]

Oxygen Concentrators

An oxygen concentrator is an electrically powered device capable of removing nitrogen from atmospheric gas (Fig. 19–2). Oxygen concentrators employ a molecular sieve (zeolite) to absorb nitrogen from room air gas that is drawn into a compressor, pressurized to a relatively low level of 4 to 10 psi (27.6 to 69 kPa), and directed through the sieve bed. As the gas passes through the sieve bed, nitrogen is absorbed by the zeolite, and the remaining oxygen is collected, concentrated, and passed through a flowmeter, where it is then delivered to the patient. Oxygen concentrators are capable of providing flow rates of up to 5 L/minute at concentrations of 90% or more. Generally, the lower the flow rate, the higher the oxygen concentration.

Oxygen concentrators offer many advantages when used as a stationary oxygen system. The concentrator has the ability to provide oxygen without resupply; concentrators are designed to run continuously and, when properly maintained, do so with minimum interruption; the console itself has an aesthetically pleasing appearance; the device is easy to operate for the patient or caregiver; concentrators have casters and weigh approximately 50 lb (22.5 kg), facilitating relocation about the home. There are several disadvantages with the use of an oxygen concentrator. The unit requires an adequate electrical power source (115 VAC) and, depending on the model, can consume up to 450 W/hour (many power companies allow special price breaks to patients using electrically powered life-support devices such as concentrators); any interruption of electrical power obviously renders the unit inoperable; concentrators also produce extraneous noise in the 50 to 60 decible range, which some patients find quite bothersome; there is a modest amount of heat generated by the unit.

Since concentrators are low-pressure systems, they cannot power other respiratory equipment, such as nebulizers and blenders, necessitating additional devices for these purposes. Concentrators are sophisticated pieces of equipment and require periodic and routine preventative maintenance to ensure optimal operation. The HME suppliers are responsible for providing this service at no additional charge to the patient when that equipment is being rented, and it should be done at a frequency specified by the manufacturer. For a concentrator patient requiring portability for

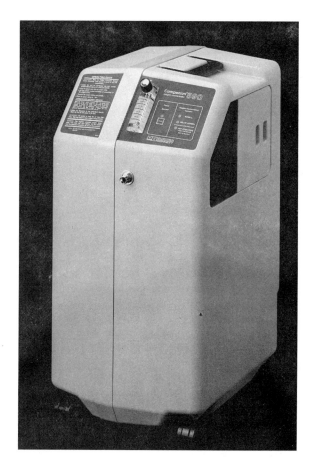

FIGURE 19-2 One type of oxygen concentrator. (Courtesy of Puritan-Bennett Corp.)

ambulation, a lightweight gaseous system is used. Steel or aluminum E- or D-cylinders in a carrying pouch or cart permit several hours of time away from the stationary source. Table 19-5 shows a time chart on E-cylinders.

Since their introduction in 1974, oxygen concentrators have become very popular and well accepted as a stationary in-home oxygen system. The HME suppliers have successfully worked around the problems associated with concentrators, and newer technology should only increase their reliability and performance.

TABLE 19-5. Estimated Time Remaining when Using an E-Cylinder at Certain Flow Rates

Tank Pressure (psi)	1	2	3	4	5
2200 (full)	12 h	6 h	4 h	3 h	$2\frac{1}{2}$ h
1500 (3/4)	8 h	4 h	$2\frac{1}{2}$ h	2 h	$1\frac{1}{2}$ h
1100 (1/2)	6 h	3 h	2 h	$1\frac{1}{2}$ h	1 h
500 (1/4)	$2\frac{1}{2}$ h	$1\frac{1}{2}$ h	1 h	$\frac{1}{2}$ h	$\frac{1}{4}$ h

Liquid Oxygen Systems

The third method of providing continuous oxygen therapy in the home is the liquid oxygen system (LOX). Oxygen is stored in its liquid state at $-297.3°F$ ($-182.9°C$), in specially manufactured containers that are in essence very sophisticated thermos bottles. These containers, called "Dewars," keep the oxygen in its liquid state and control the rate of evaporation through warming coils to provide sufficient gaseous oxygen for administration.

The primary advantage associated with the LOX system is portability. Most stationary LOX doers can be used to refill a smaller, lightweight version of the larger stationary unit. Figure 19–3 is an example of a stationary and portable liquid oxygen system. Portable LOX units, when filled with 1 to 2 lb (0.45 to 0.49 kg) of liquid oxygen, weigh approximately 8 to 10 lb (3.6 to 4.5 kg) and can provide continuous oxygen at 2 L/minute for up to 8 hours. There is no limit to the number of times a portable LOX unit can be refilled from a stationary LOX system, as long as there is an ample quantity of liquid oxygen in the stationary unit. Other favorable features associated with LOX include no need for external electrical power, availability of

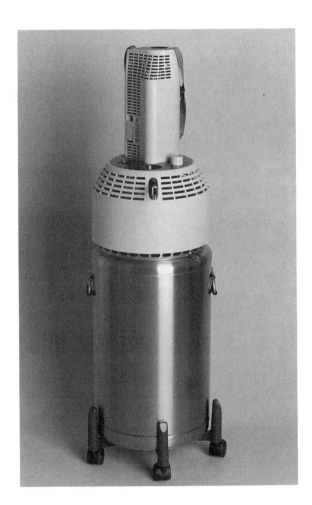

FIGURE 19-3 Stationary and portable liquid oxygen system. (Courtesy of Puritan-Bennett Corp.)

flow rates up to 10 L/minute, and the ability to power other respiratory equipment, provided the LOX system is pressured to 50 psi (this depends on the LOX system manufacturer). The biggest disadvantage of LOX is the "use-it or lose-it" feature. Simply stated, doers are not capable of maintaining oxygen in the liquid state for an extended time. Under normal conditions, the amount of evaporation is controlled and immediately made available for administration. However, if there is no flow, as happens when the system is not being used, evaporation still occurs at a rate of approximately 250 L of gaseous oxygen every 12 hours. The LOX system not used for days may run dry, solely through evaporative loss.

To reiterate, the most convenient feature of the LOX system is that is allows patients to transfill a small portable unit from the stationary unit on an as-needed basis. Transfilling of both the portable and stationary units warrant careful attention to detail. Liquid oxygen, because of its extremely cold temperature, if inadvertently allowed to come in contact with human skin, can result in severe burns.

From the HME supplier's perspective, LOX systems represent the most costly of the three systems described. Not only are capital acquisition costs much higher than for cylinders and concentrators, but special delivery and storage equipment are also required to provide refills. However, for the chronically hypoxemic patient with high ambulation needs (6 to 8 hours/week away from home), LOX is the system of choice, regardless of its shortcomings.

Determining the most appropriate oxygen delivery system for an oxygen patient is a very controversial issue. Table 19–6 outlines criteria to help determine what system will be most appropriate for the patient. Although the system may be selected before referral to the HME supplier, the supplier can provide information to help in decision making.

The most frequently used criteria for determining oxygen therapy needs is based on results of arterial blood gas analyses or on an O_2 saturation measured by pulse oximetry. Medicare, the third-party payer for most patients who require oxygen therapy will reimburse for oxygen therapy when there is a primary diagnosis of chronic lung disease and the PaO_2 is 55 mm Hg or less (O_2 saturation $\leq 88\%$), or 56

TABLE   19-6.   Criteria to Select the Most Appropriate Oxygen Delivery System*

	Ambulation Time			
Flow (L)	8 h or less	8–15 h/wk	15–30 h/wk	30 h or more
1/2	C w/P	C w/P	C w/P	C w/P
1	C w/P	C w/P	C w/P	LOX
2	C w/P	C w/P	LOX	LOX
3	C w/P	LOX	LOX	LOX
4	C w/P	LOX	LOX	LOX
5	LOX	LOX	LOX	LOX

C, concentrator; P, portable gas; LOX, liquid O_2 with portable.
* For nonambulatory patients it may be advisable to use a concentrator.

to 59 mm Hg (O_2 saturation 89%) when one of the following secondary conditions also exists: erythrocytosis, congestive heart failure, or cor pulmonale.[6] The oxygen prescription must be specific for liter flow, hours of use (e.g., during sleep, during exercise periods, or continuously), and for the type of system. Moreover, the prescribing physician must also indicate that the chronic hypoxemia has not responded to other therapeutic interventions. Oxygen ordered for as-needed (PRN) use is no longer reimbursable and, at the time of this writing, PO_2 or O_2 saturation measurements made more than 90 days before the order for oxygen and measurements made while the patient is breathing supplemental oxygen are unacceptable to qualify for Medicare reimbursement for oxygen therapy services. Many insurance companies follow the Medicare guidelines for payment; however, it is always wise to check with the carrier to determine coverage criteria.

Once it has been determined that the patient qualifies for oxygen, based on reimbursement criteria, the patient's oxygen use must be calculated. This calculation is based on flow rate and hours of use (e.g., 2 L/minute 24 hours a day, 1 L/minute during sleep, or 2 L/minute during approximately 6 hours of activities during the day). Generally, patients who qualify under Medicare guidelines will require more oxygen than a stationary gaseous system can deliver cost effectively, so H-tank systems as the primary source are rarely placed. Patients who qualify under Medicare guidelines will generally be using 10 to 24 hours of oxygen per day, so the decision to place a concentrator or liquid system as the primary stationary source will almost always depend on the patient's need for portability. As stated earlier, patients who are away from home for more than 8 hours/week would benefit from a liquid system. It does not make much sense to place a liquid system on a patient who seldom leaves the home, although there may be times when it would be necessary, such as when the patient's source of electricity is very unstable and a concentrator would be contraindicated.

Oxygen Conservation Devices

Oxygen conserving devices are a somewhat recent addition to domiciliary oxygen therapy. Employing either a passive reservoir system or electronic technology, these devices help extend the useful life of an oxygen canister (gaseous or liquid) through conservation. Instead of the continuous flow of oxygen throughout the entire breathing pattern, as occurs with traditional nasal cannulae, oxygen-conserving devices deliver a bolus of oxygen intermittently at the initial part of the inspiratory phase of breathing. Reservoir-type devices, such as the Oxymizer pendant, are in essence a continuous flow system running at a significantly reduced flow rate, passively collecting and storing oxygen during the expiratory phase of breathing. This allows a bolus of oxygen (approximately 35 mL) to be made available at the beginning of inhalation. Although reservoir-type devices are continuous flow systems, they accomplish oxygenation goals at substantially lower flow rates than would otherwise be required of a conventional cannula. For example, a reservoir device operating at 0.5 L/minute can usually match the oxygenation levels attained with a conventional cannula operating at 2 L/minute, assuming there is no increased demand for oxygen (e.g., with exercise). The major disadvantage to the reservoir-type cannula is that it is

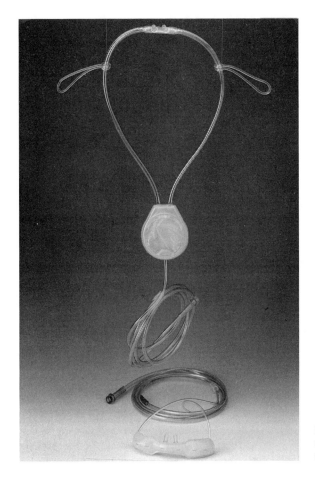

FIGURE   19-4   Reservoir-type oxygen-conserving device. (Courtesy of Chad Therapeutics)

rather unsightly to wear. For patients who dislike wearing nasal cannulae for cosmetic reasons, this device will be even more unacceptable (Fig. 19–4).

Electronic devices obtain their net effect by "pulsing" the oxygen bolus to the nasal pharynx in response to a sensor detecting the beginning of the inspiratory effort through a conventional cannula. Unlike their reservoir-type counterparts, electronic conserving devices, whether AC or DC powered, are not continuous flow systems. However, the end results, in terms of conservation, are remarkably similar for all such devices. A disadvantage of the pulsing device is that because it is delivered on-demand, a patient will not receive oxygen should there be periodic interruptions in breathing, such as during sleep. Some units also tend to be noisy when the demand valve opens, which can make the patient feel conspicuous. Figure 19–5 is an example of an electronic oxygen-conservation device currently available.

Oxygen-conserving devices have found their greatest acceptance when used to prolong the duration of portable oxygen systems. Newer iterations of the technology may make their use more commonplace with stationary systems, especially those requiring periodic resupply. However, although oxygen conservation makes sense,

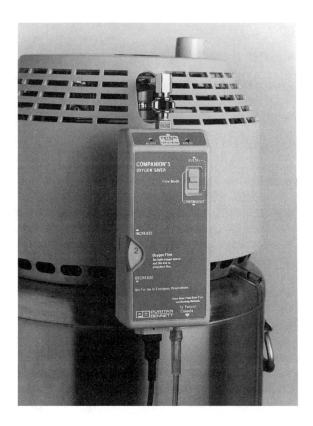

FIGURE 19-5 Electronic-type oxygen-conserving device. (Courtesy of Puritan-Bennett Corp.)

current reimbursement policies of Medicare have regrettably created a disincentive for the HME supplier. The supplier has to purchase a fairly expensive device to loan the patient for which there will be no reimbursement.

Transtracheal Oxygen Therapy

The development of the transtracheal oxygen catheter in the 1980s occurred as a result of the desire to increase patient compliance when continuous oxygen therapy is ordered. Patients taking oxygen through nasal prongs tend to remove them because of discomfort around the ears and nares, the feeling of restricted mobility, or because of the cosmetic disadvantage of the prongs. It is difficult to keep the nasal prongs in place during sleep, contributing to noncontinuous use and concomitant desaturation.

The original transtracheal catheter consisted of a 16-gauge angiocatheter and a pediatric tracheostomy tube that had been reversed. Today's catheter is a high-tech biopolymer tubing, approximately 20 cm in length with a 9-French tract; these dimensions will vary, to some degree, depending on the manufacturer (Fig. 19–6). This catheter is inserted somewhere between the cricothyroid membrane and the notch of the manubrium. The transtracheal catheter bypasses a considerable volume of anatomical deadspace (e.g., the hypopharynx), thereby reducing the amount of oxygen flow necessary to achieve desired oxygenation. These flow rates have been reported to be 25% to 50% less than with the conventional nasal cannula.[7]

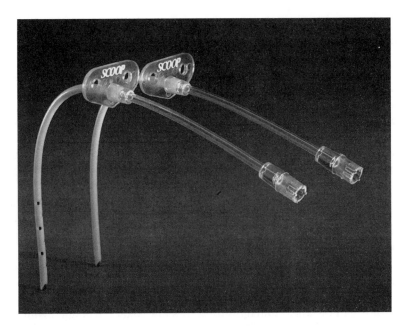

FIGURE   19-6   Transtracheal catheters. (Courtesy of Transtracheal Oxygen Systems)

The oxygen-conserving and aesthetic benefits of transtracheal oxygen therapy must be balanced with other aspects of a less desirable nature. Problems reported include stomal site infection, stoma maintenance, inadvertent catheter displacement, kinking, and mucous plugs adhering to the catheter partially obstructing the trachea. Other less prevalent complications include subcutaneous emphysema, mild hoarseness, and tract discomfort. However, with the proper patient selection, education and follow up, the side-effects of transtracheal oxygen therapy can be markedly reduced.[8]

Another consideration is the current reimbursement policies of third-party payers, particularly Medicare, for the catheter. Under Part A Medicare coverage, insertion of the catheter is reimbursable; however, the replacement catheters, which are billed under Part B, are to be replaced every 3 to 6 months and are reimbursable only under the following conditions: (1) the patient must have a medical problem related to nasal cannula use (e.g., the patient who remains severely hypoxemic at the highest tolerable nasal oxygen flow rate); or (2) the patient must derive a significant increase in ambulation through use of transtracheal oxygen; and (3) the prescribing physician's prescription must document the medical problem or increase in ambulation.[9] Prior authorization by other insurances is advisable. If a private pay arrangement is to be established with the patient, he or she should be aware of all the expenses before being accepted into the transtracheal program.

Traveling with Oxygen

Many patients who use oxygen express the feeling that they are tethered to their oxygen tank and cannot leave their home. We have described several portable systems to allow patients to do just that, but what about the patient who wishes to travel while using oxygen?

It is certainly possible to do long-distance traveling with oxygen. Car trips, train and bus travel, and commercial air travel, all are available to the pulmonary patient. There are details that must be considered before traveling to make it a safe and positive experience.

Normal, healthy persons maintain a PaO_2 between 50 and 60 mm Hg at elevations of about 8000 to 10,000 ft (2440 to 3050 m). Patients with COPD whose normal PaO_2 is 60 have been shown to maintain PaO_2s in the 30s at these altitudes.[10] Consequently, it is important to carefully assess the patient for general health and to identify contraindications before attempting air travel. The normal response to hypoxemia is to increase ventilation, which may be difficult or impossible for a patient with severe pulmonary disease, and the patient may be unable to compensate for the resultant drop in arterial PO_2. In-flight oxygen administration can assist the patient in managing the "acute altitude stress."

Most domestic airlines can supply oxygen at 2 to 4 L/minute by mask to patients requiring it. They will not allow patients to carry their own oxygen on board, but will allow empty oxygen containers to be checked as baggage. They will not supply oxygen for use in the air terminal, so it is advisable to fly direct and avoid having to make connecting flights. Airlines will require a medical certificate from the physician along with 24- to 72-hours notice. The airlines will also charge fees for the oxygen, which may not be reimbursable to the patient. Therefore, one must be aware of the additional costs involved in flying with oxygen. Prior arrangements must be made to have oxygen delivered to the arriving airport, if it is necessary, and to the traveler's final destination. The HME companies can help make the oxygen arrangements for the patient and may have helpful printed material to assist the patient in deciding the ideal method of travel.[11]

Traveling by bus or train is also possible. Greyhound will allow a portable oxygen container on its buses; however, the patient's stationary system cannot be checked as baggage, so prior arrangements for delivery of oxygen to the bus terminal and the traveler's final destination need to be made well in advance. Check ahead with private bus lines for their policies on allowing oxygen on board. Patients traveling on AMTRAK can bring their stationary liquid unit on board, but they must travel in the nonsmoking sections of the train. Again, arrangements must be made for oxygen at the final destination.

Travel by car is an easy way for a patient to make trips. Liquid oxygen systems can be secured by a seat belt into the back seat of the car, allowing continuous oxygen use if necessary. The stationary system must be removed from the car before transfilling the small portable unit, and both stationary and portable units must be kept upright at all times (allowing them to fall over will result in the venting of the liquid oxygen, posing a safety hazard). The patient's HME company can identify other suppliers along the patient's itinerary who can fill the stationary unit. It is essential that these locations are identified and contacted before travel; however, it must never be assumed that all suppliers carry the same types of equipment. With a little planning ahead, almost any type of travel is possible.

Aerosol Therapy Devices

Many patients with chronic lung disease require bronchodilator therapy as part of their plan of treatment when they are discharged to home. There are several options available for inhalation of medications. These include inhalers, compressor nebulizers, and bland aerosol delivery devices.

Metered-Dose Inhalers

The metered-dose inhaler (MDI) is the most cost-effective, most convenient, and most routinely prescribed method of delivery for home bronchodilator therapy. Its small size and ease of use make it an ideal device for the patient; however, there are patients who are unable to use MDIs owing to their inability to coordinate the breathing technique. It has been estimated that 10% to 20% of patients fail to receive optimal aerosol deposition.[12] Adjuncts, such as spacer devices, can help facilitate aerosol administration by eliminating the need to coordinate inhalation with activation of the MDI (Fig. 19–7). Third-party payers often require that patients be tried on MDIs before initiation of other modes of aerosolization (e.g., compressor nebulizers).

Compressor Nebulizers

When a patient is unsuccessful at using an MDI, a compressor nebulizer is a relatively inexpensive and simple way for the patient to have home bronchodilator therapy. Small oil-free compressors with outputs of 7 to 10 L/minute are used to power hand-held nebulizers. Current technology allows portability of these devices: internal batteries allowing approximately 60 total minutes of treatment time and DC

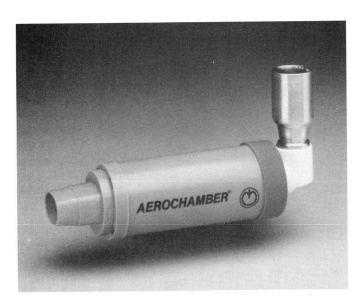

FIGURE 19-7 Aerochamber spacer device. (Courtesy of Monaghan Medical Corporation)

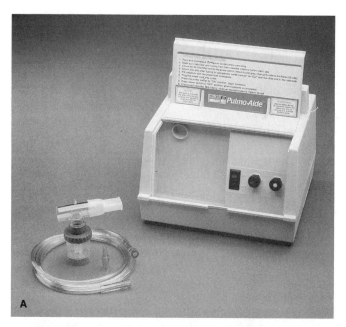

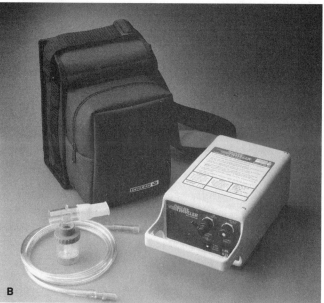

FIGURE 19-8 (**A**) One brand of compressor nebulizer and (**B**) battery-operated compressor nebulizer (Courtesy of Devilbiss Corp.)

adapters allow the patient to take treatments while in a vehicle (Fig. 19–8). Options such as these may enhance patient compliance to their overall home respiratory therapy program.

Bland Aerosol Therapy

Patients with artificial airways who receive aerosol therapy in the hospital can continue to receive it when they are discharged. Large-volume nebulizers can be driven by electrically powered high-output compressors and delivered through large-bore tubing to a tracheostomy mask (Fig. 19–9). Oxygen can be entrained into the circuit for those patients requiring it, and the mist can also be heated if desired. This type of treatment is beneficial for upper airway inflammation and management of secretion problems. Setup and maintenance of this type of equipment in the home is not difficult for the patient or caregiver; however, cleaning the equipment is of the utmost importance for infection control.

Home Ventilator Systems

The subject of home care is not complete without a discussion of the management of patients using home mechanical ventilators. The use of home ventilators has greatly increased owing to a larger patient population with more varied disease states and advanced technology. Ventilatory support can be given to patients whose needs are continuous and also for nocturnal support.

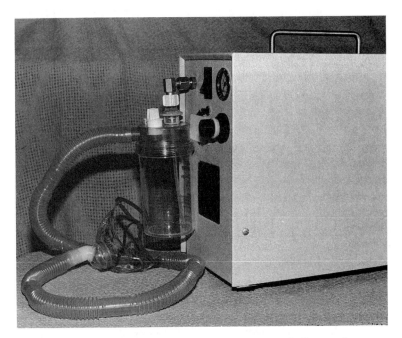

FIGURE 19-9 Tracheostomy mask with aerosol nebulizer and compressor.

There are three basic types of mechanical ventilators used in the home:

- Positive-pressure ventilators, including nasal mask, nasal pillows, and endotracheal delivery
- Negative-pressure ventilators, including iron lung, chest shell, or body wrap
- Pressure support devices, including CPAP and BiPAP.

The entire home care team is involved in the discharge and care of the patient requiring mechanical ventilation in the home. Scrupulous patient selection, dedication from all caregivers, and extensive education before discharge are essential elements for a successful home ventilator program.

Many third-party payers recognize the significant cost savings of managing a ventilator at home, as opposed to a skilled nursing facility or acute care facility; however, they will not reimburse for nursing services on a daily basis in many instances. It is vital to determine eligibility for nursing services before admitting the patient into a home ventilator program; it is extremely difficult for a family alone to care for the patient 24 hours a day, 7 days a week without them suffering exhaustion. For a continuous ventilator patient, it is ideal to have up to 16 to 24 hours of nursing, with the family supplementing noncovered shifts. Patients with Medicare as their only health insurance do not have the benefit of continuous nursing services, and might not be ideal candidates for continuous home ventilator care.[13] State-funded health insurance programs such as Medicaid often have waiver or in-home care programs allowing up to 16 hours of nursing care per day, as do some private insurance companies. Experience has shown that patients who have the benefit of nursing care supplemented by family involvement have a safer, more positive home ventilator program.

Planning the discharge of a patient to a home ventilator program is quite complicated and requires attention to many details. For a more complete view of the aspects of ventilator care in alternative sites, see Chapter 20.

REIMBURSEMENT ISSUES

We have referred to insurance and reimbursement issues repeatedly in this chapter. A home care program is not feasible without reimbursement for services rendered. It is vital to determine which aspects of the developed homecare program are reimbursable before initiation of services. Seldom can a patient or family assume the financial burden of medical equipment and home care services on a private pay basis. It is not fair to the patient nor the provider of the service to find out, after the fact, that a service is not covered.

Third-Party Payers

Medicare, the federally funded health insurance program, is probably the most commonly billed insurance carrier. Its beneficiaries include people 65 and over and people who have been 100% medically disabled for 2 consecutive years, regardless of their age. Most of the clientele receiving home care benefits are covered by Medicare. Coverage guidelines are established by the Health Care Financing Administration (HCFA).

Medicaid is a state-funded health insurance program for persons with very limited financial resources. Eligibility and coverage vary from state to state, but payment is generally at a reduced level compared with other health insurance reimbursement for the same service. For this reason, some providers of home care services are unwilling to accept Medicaid referrals. However, Medicaid may have waiver programs to provide extensive home care services that Medicare will not cover. Additionally, Medicaid will often reimburse for supplies and equipment not available to the Medicare patient.

Private insurances are another source of reimbursement for home care services. They generally follow Medicare guidelines for defining their coverage; however, policy coverage varies for each beneficiary, so it is always a good idea to verify coverage before providing the service. It should never be assumed that an item is covered by a third-party payer just because the patient received that same service in the acute care hospital.

It is important to know where to locate information detailing items covered by insurances, specifically Medicare. Your local Social Security office will have booklets available that explain both hospital and medical coverage policies (Part A and Part B, respectively) for Medicare.[14] You may also consult the white pages of your local telephone directory under the *Medicare Part B Claim Information* listing for the telephone number of your state's Medicare carrier. Your carrier can inform you of coverage guidelines. Many HME suppliers have printed materials available that list equipment and supplies that are covered and diagnoses that are acceptable to justify medical equipment under the Part B Medicare benefit that can serve as an excellent resource for the physician and discharge planner.

Documentation of Medical Necessity

Contrary to popular belief, a prescription written for a service does not automatically guarantee coverage for that service. For example, a prescription stating "oxygen 2 lpm" will not qualify for Medicare reimbursement without adequate documentation of medical necessity. This is also true for prescriptions for any medical equipment supplies and services. Third-party payers, especially Medicare, require justification that services are medically necessary and reasonable. In this day of escalating health care costs, insurance carriers will only pay for services the patient truly needs, not what is convenient to the patient or family, and not necessarily what the patient or physician may desire.

Medical necessity is established taking into consideration the patient's diagnosis and plan of treatment. The goals of therapy must be determined and any medical services required must be medically justified relative to those goals. For example, the use of a front-wheeled walker might be ordered for a pulmonary rehabilitation patient with a goal of increasing ambulation. Common requirements when documenting medical necessity are diagnosis, prognosis, length of need, and goals of therapy, and these must be established before service.

The physician must be very concise when writing a prescription for medical services or equipment and should avoid ambiguous statements such as "PRN" or "length of need: lifetime." Neither Medicare or Medicaid will pay for home medical services ordered for PRN use. Specific verbiage, such as "length of need: 3 months or until patient recovers from acute exacerbation" is most helpful, since it shows that a plan of treatment exists and that the physician has made the determination that the service is an essential part of the goals of therapy. Filling in the certifications of medical necessity as completely as possible ensures that the service will be reimbursed, provided that such service is included as a benefit of the insurance policy.

Medicare now requires the completion of a very specific document, the *Attending Physician's Certification of Medical Necessity for Home Oxygen Therapy*, form HCFA 484, when the physician orders home oxygen therapy.[6] This form can be completed only by the physician or someone on his or her immediate staff. It is also permissible for a hospital discharge planner to complete the form, but the physician must ultimately verify the accuracy of the information and sign the completed document. It is no longer acceptable for the HME supplier to complete the form and forward it to the physician for signature. The HCFA 484 form requires information to be filled in for diagnosis, arterial blood gas results on room air, type of system, and other items pertinent to qualification. It is a somewhat cumbersome form which, if not completed entirely, can result in the denial of payment for oxygen therapy services.

Reimbursement for Respiratory Therapy Services

Much discussion has been given to the home care team and the professional services provided by various professional entities. Unfortunately, professional services provided by respiratory care practitioners in the home are not now covered by Medicare or Medicaid. Some private insurance companies will reimburse RCPs on a fee-for-service basis, but the level of authorized services is generally very limited. In spite of this limited reimbursement, many HME companies still have RCPs on staff to follow their pulmonary patients, and absorb the related expense as part of the reimbursement provided for the equipment.

There is a current movement to obtain reimbursement from Medicare for services provided by respiratory care practitioners in the home. The *Medicare Home Respiratory Care Act* of 1991, S1120, was introduced to the U.S. Senate in May of 1991 to establish a respiratory home care demonstration project.[15] This project is designed to examine whether having a respiratory care practitioner provide services in the home would reduce the overall Medicare cost of pulmonary disease patients who need respiratory care hospitalization for an acute illness. The demonstration project proposes to use a select study group of patients and will compare total Medicare Part A and B costs for patients who use home respiratory equipment and have RCPs involved in their home care-treatment program with patients who use home respiratory equipment without the services of the RCP. The premise is that total Medicare dollars spent will be reduced when patients receive respiratory therapy services provided by RCPs at home because of reductions in the length of hospital stay, in hospital admissions, and in hospital readmissions. Once funded, the project would last 3 years and would involve hospital-based RCPs as well as those employed by HME companies accredited by the Joint Commission on Accreditation of Healthcare Organizations (JCAHO) as a supplier of both equipment management services and clinical respiratory services.

JOINT COMMISSION ON ACCREDITATION OF HEALTHCARE ORGANIZATIONS

Just as hospitals apply for accreditation through the JCAHO, accreditation was expanded in June of 1988 to include home care organizations.[16] This accreditation is available to providers of home health, private duty, personal care and support services, home pharmaceuticals, and home medical equipment. The home care accreditation program has quickly become the second largest within the JCAHO, with hospitals remaining the largest. This process is not without controversy, as many providers feel it is "voluntarily mandatory" to become accredited.

The JCAHO home care accreditation program evaluates the provider in six key areas to determine if certain standards are being met:[17]

1. What is the involvement of the patient and the family in the care process.
2. Is there timely access to needed services.
3. Is care effectively coordinated.
4. Are sound decisions made that are appropriate to the patient's needs.
5. Are staff decisions effectively executed.
6. Does the organization monitor and evaluate care on an ongoing basis?

The HME companies can apply for accreditation for equipment management services only; however, companies that provide clinical respiratory services are also surveyed for these respiratory services in addition to equipment management services. Clinical respiratory services may include ongoing clinical assessments (e.g., monitoring vital signs and auscultation of the lungs), periodic laboratory testing (e.g., oximetry), and the administration of therapeutic treatments or medications.

Once the decision has been made to pursue JCAHO accreditation, the HME company makes formal application to be surveyed. The survey is conducted by home care professionals who have administrative and clinical experience in the delivery of home care services. The cost and duration of the survey are dependent on the type of accreditation applied for (e.g., an HME company will have a minimum 2-day survey). After receiving the completed application and appropriate fees, the JCAHO will notify the applicant of the scheduled date of the survey. This notification occurs approximately 4 to 6 weeks before the scheduled survey date.

The survey process will identify the HME company's degree of compliance with the Standards for the Accreditation of Home Care (SAHC). These standards relate to the six key areas outlined previously. The surveyor will interview patients, staff, and management, review documents, such as clinical charts and company policies and procedures, and conduct an extensive site review.

Upon completion of the survey, the JCAHO will award one of four categories of accreditation:

- Accreditation with commendation
- Accreditation
- Conditional accreditation
- Not accredited

Although accreditation remains a controversial issue with some home care dealers, proponents argue accreditation promotes quality care and cloaks the HME industry with credibility and respect. It is believed that, at some point in the future, Medicare and other payers will require accreditation as a precondition to HME reimbursement. Certain private insurance carriers, in fact, do already require JCAHO accreditation for home care reimbursement.

DISCONTINUANCE OF THE HOME CARE PROGRAM

Patients receiving home care services will, at some point, need to be evaluated for continued services. Unless the patient is receiving home ventilator therapy, there is a finite amount of time for which home care services are going to be indicated and reimbursed. There are several areas that can be reviewed to determine when the patient is ready for "discharge."

Diagnosis is a primary indicator for determining the length of time home care services should be available to a patient. As stated earlier, home health agencies are allowed a certain number of professional visits over a certain time, depending on the diagnosis (e.g., Medicare will reimburse for home health services for an average of 6 weeks after hospital discharge for most diagnoses). Therefore, the original plan of treatment is usually developed with this in mind.

Another factor that can be measured is the ability of a patient to achieve improved health and comfort. It may not be possible to reverse the disease process in a patient, but it is possible to improve his or her day-to-day existence. Working with a patient on a prescribed exercise regimen, increasing activity levels, and easing activities of daily living will make the patient's life at home more enjoyable. Healed wounds, management of peripheral edema, improved oxygenation, or resolved pneumonia are other examples of improved status that may contribute to a decision to discharge a patient from home care services.

Patients' ability to manage their own care is another goal that might be set at the initiation of a home care program. A satisfactory understanding of the medication schedule and the ability to take the medications as prescribed is a good indication that the home care professionals have accomplished their task. The ability to properly balance rest, nutrition, and exercise independently may show that a patient is ready to be discharged. The patient's improved daily health and the knowledge of how to maintain it can reduce the potential for hospital readmission.

Enhancing a patient's understanding and acceptance of his or her condition is also a goal of home care. Patients must have a realistic view of their disease process, including the final outcome. Patients with chronic pulmonary disease, because of its debilitating nature and poor prognosis, will often display anger and depression over their condition.

Emotional counseling and motivational support are vital areas for which to provide before discontinuing a home care program. Frustration over their disease and the fear of dyspnea may keep patients from making progress or from even complying with the physician's prescribed program. A patient's physician should provide counseling about prognosis and treatment options. The home care team can evaluate the patient for acceptance and understanding of the prognosis, and watch for signs of anxiety, depression, and lack of realistic expectations.

An example of this would be an elderly woman with COPD who is sent home on a therapeutic regimen of continuous oxygen therapy, medications, and an exercise program. Unable to accept the realization that her disease is in its end stages, the patient becomes very depressed and refuses to get out of bed. She wants to get well, but if she cannot get well, she wants to die. Her shortness of breath is exacerbated by her weakened muscles because she will not move about in bed or get up in a chair. The plan of treatment may need to include treatment for her depression.

This patient should be counseled by her physician about her prognosis, which, even if it is poor, allows her some options. It is important to discuss whether she wants life-support devices employed when she reaches that stage in her disease. For some patients, using oxygen will be considered "life support" and they may not wish to use it. She should be counseled concerning the positive actions she can take. She may not "get well" but she can work at improving her quality of life. The patient's perception of his or her disease state should be clear and realistic.

At home, the patient can be assessed by the nurse, social worker, and other professionals to determine the most appropriate strategies to achieve compliance and provide emotional support. Viewing the patient's daily routine will identify the areas that are open for change as well as those the patient refuses to change. Reinforcing any positive activity is very important. Perhaps she will not get out of bed, but the patient is willing to learn upper body strengthening exercises. Maybe she is willing to dangle at the side of the bed while practicing pursed-lips or diaphragmatic breathing. By allowing her to express her fears of dyspnea, those activities she is most afraid of doing may be identified.

Although it is important to continue to work toward the physical goals of therapy, it is also important to address the psychologic aspect. Ongoing assessment for depression along with emotional counseling for the patient and caregivers are frequently required. Some patients may require medical intervention to relieve anxiety and depression to allow them to be more relaxed and cooperative with their plan of treatment. Patients need to have some degree of motivation to improve their situation once home care has been discontinued.

There are services that can be employed to help a patient once the formalized home care program has been discontinued. Referral of the patient to support groups, such as local "Better Breathers" clubs or outpatient pulmonary rehabilitation classes can be helpful. Local seniors' organizations or church groups may have volunteers who will make visits to the home to help with cooking, shopping, or just to pay a social call. The local county health department may provide ongoing home nursing visits and chore-workers for extended periods. Having meals brought in, such as provided by "Meals on Wheels" programs, can assist patients who may be too debilitated to prepare their own. Those HME suppliers who employ RCPs can be used for long-term follow-up and assessment, since those professional services receive no reimbursement that can be terminated. As long as patients have a continued need for medical equipment, RCPs can follow them.

Hospice programs should be made available to the patient who is in the terminal stages of illness. Most hospice programs will require that the patient's life expectancy be 6 months or fewer. Admittance to a hospice program will avail the patient and their caregivers to ongoing nursing visits, counseling, and respite care up until the patient's death and for a brief period afterward.

SUMMARY

The need for home care is well established and will continue to grow in the future. With the elderly population increasing and with the emphasis being placed on providing care in less costly settings, the comprehensive home care program will be an essential part of the overall reduction in health care expenditures. Moreover, as technology changes, our ability to treat more complicated health problems in the home setting will increase. Keeping abreast of the rapid changes in the home care industry and the array of services poses a formidable challenge to home care providers. One hopes that reimbursement for home care services will foster an environment wherein high-quality and accessible home care services continue to be the rule, rather than the exception.

REFERENCES

1. Balinsky W, Starkman JL. The impact of DRG's on the health care industry. Home Care Manage Rev 1987;12:61.

2. White J. Skyrocketing costs—what can be done? Independent Living 1991;6(4):13.

3. US Consumer Product Safety Commission. Safety for older consumers: Home safety checklist. June 1986.

4. Meany-Handy J, Lareau SC. The role of home care. In: Hodgkin JE, Zorn EG, Connors GL, eds. Pulmonary rehabilitation: guidelines to success. 1st ed. Boston: Butterworths, 1984.

5. Joint Commission on Accreditation of Healthcare Organizations. Accreditation manual for home care. Vol 1. July 1991.

6. Oxygen used in a beneficiaries home, revised coverage guidelines and documentation requirements. Medicare Bull Aug 1991;91;3.

7. Hoffman L, Johnson JT, Wesmiller SW, et al. Transtracheal delivery of oxygen: efficacy and safety for long term continuous therapy. Ann Oto 1991;100:108.

8. Spofford B, Christopher K, McCarty D, Goodman J. Transtracheal oxygen therapy: a guide for the respiratory therapist. Respir Care 1987;32:345.

9. Transtracheal oxygen therapy supplies. Medicare Bull 1991;91:2.

10. Gong H. Advising pulmonary patients about commercial air travel. J Respir Dis 1990;2:484.

11. Maguire J, Lundstedt D, Randazzo J, Bobeck J. Requirements for traveling with oxygen. AARC 1988.

12. Ward JJ, Helmholz HF. Applied humidity and aerosol therapy. In: Burton GG, Hodgkin JE, Ward JJ, eds. Respiratory care: a guide to clinical practice. 3rd ed. Philadelphia: JB Lippincott, 1991:381.

13. Medical denials threaten the health of home care. Hospitals 1987;61:58.

14. Medicare handbook 1991. US Dept of Health and Human Services: Health Care Financing Administration, 1991.

15. Cathcart M. AARC introduces home care bill. AARC Times 1991;15:44.

16. Novoselski D. Reshaping the face of home care. Homecare 1991;13:346.

17. Home care accreditation services: key questions of the standards and surveying process. JCAHO 1991;Jul.

BARRY J. MAKE

MARY E. GILMARTIN

Care of Ventilator-Assisted Individuals in the Home and in Alternative Community Sites

The concept of home care for individuals requiring mechanical assistance to ventilation was originally pioneered in the 1940s and 1950s in patients suffering from poliomyelitis.[1-6] Those patients used respiratory-assist devices, such as the iron lung,[7,8] chest cuirass,[9] rocking bed,[10,11] and pneumobelt,[12] which were developed earlier in the 20th century, but today are considered crude and ineffective by intensivists caring for critically ill patients in modern critical care units. Nevertheless, respiratory care practitioners in the late 1980s rediscovered both the concepts and the equipment of the polio era and applied them to the care of the rapidly increasing number of ventilator-assisted patients managed outside the acute care hospital setting.[13-15] This chapter will address the management of ventilator-assisted persons cared for in the home and other locations in the community, such as long-term care hospitals and skilled nursing facilities, where the goals are different from those for patients receiving mechanical ventilation in an intensive care unit (ICU). The goals of home care for this population are the following:[15]

- Reduce mortality
- Decrease morbidity
- Improve the quality of life
- Improve physical and physiologic function
- Provide an environment that will enhance individual potential
- Be cost-effective

EXTENT OF THE PROBLEM

Three major factors have led to an increased interest in home care for ventilator-assisted persons: (1) an increase in the number of candidates for home ventilation; (2) improvements in respiratory care in the home; and (3) increased societal awareness of the potential of handicapped individuals. The rapid increase in knowledge about respiratory disorders over the last two decades has been followed by an expansion of the number of training programs for all types of respiratory care practitioners (respiratory therapists, nurses, and pulmonary physicians). As a result of the widespread implementation of improved respiratory care techniques by an increased number of skilled professionals, there has been increased survival not only of seriously ill hospitalized patients, but also of individuals with chronic progressive respiratory and neurologic disorders. This, in turn, has led to an increase in the number of candidates for mechanical assistance to ventilation in the home. Increasing emphasis on reducing hospital costs has also created a greater demand for home care.

Two studies have documented inequities in Medicare's medical diagnosis related group (DRG) prospective payment system for prolonged ventilator care.[16,17] Douglas and associates found that costs exceeded reimbursement by an average of 23,129 dollars per case in 95 nonsurgical Medicare patients receiving mechanical ventilation for 3 or more days in a Chicago teaching hospital.[16] The average cost for hospital care was 38,486 dollars per patient, and each day on a ventilator added 439 dollars for respiratory-related services. The magnitude of the problem appears to be similar in community hospitals.[17] These findings led to a change in the DRG classification of ventilator patients in 1987.

Although prospective payment systems have encouraged hospitals to discharge patients earlier, pressures placed upon respiratory practitioners by hospital administrators should not be the prime motivation for discharging ventilator-assisted individuals. Rather, medical professionals should act as patient advocates and place the interests of their patients foremost in determining the optimal location for continued care of ventilator-assisted individuals. Potential candidates for mechanical ventilation in the home or alternative site in the community should be carefully screened to assure that they are appropriate for such care and will thrive in the nonhospital environment. Moreover, patients should not be sent home until they and the personnel participating in their care are appropiately trained in the necessary respiratory care.

Several studies[18-20] have reported a substantial number of ventilator-assisted individuals in acute care hospitals, many of whom cannot be discharged because of lack of community resources, both in less acute institutions, such as skilled nursing facilities, and in the home. In 1983, a study in Massachusetts identified 143 individuals who had been ventilator-dependent for more than 3 weeks.[18] Most (60%) were in acute care hospitals, and 60% of hospitalized patients were in intensive care units. Twenty-four percent of patients were in long-term care hospitals (a setting more readily available in southeastern Massachusetts than in many other areas of the United States), and two patients were in a skilled nursing facility. The most common diagnoses of these ventilator-assisted individuals were chronic obstructive pulmonary disease (20%), amyotrophic lateral sclerosis (13%), other neuromuscular disorders (13%), central nervous system diseases (8%), and spinal cord injury (5%). Given the prevalence of ventilator-assisted individuals (3 : 100,000 population) in this study, the authors estimated there were at least 6800 long-term ventilator-assisted individuals in the United States. The cost of caring for hospitalized long-term ventilator-assisted individuals was estimated at 1.7 billion dollars yearly, about 1.5% of the total hospital costs for the United States in 1983. The results of the Massachusetts study suggested that up to 40% of acute care hospital patients were candidates for transfer to chronic care hospitals, and 15% were candidates for home care, with a potential cost reduction of 251 million dollars/year in medical costs. A follow-up study 6 months later showed that 35% of the patients had died; 81% of patients still alive remained ventilator-dependent.

A 1983 survey conducted by the American Association of Respiratory Care (AARC) identified 2272 ventilator-dependent individuals in 106 hospitals in 21 states, 13% of whom were "deemed medically able to go home," but remained in acute care hospitals, presumably because of lack of third-party payment for other types of care or because of fewer acute care community facilities capable of caring for ventilator-assisted patients.[19] The AARC estimated the mean cost of hospital care per patient was 270,830 dollars/year, but only 21,192 dollars for home care. Although the number of patients is small, the cost savings of home care compared with hospital care was estimated to be over 64 million dollars/year.

As documented by Bone,[20] there are inadequate resources in chronic care facilities to appropriately manage patients requiring prolonged ventilatory assistance. In the metropolitan Chicago area, there is a 50 to 80 patient waiting list for the 33 available beds in two chronic care facilities.[20] In the Boston area, there is a waiting list of 25 to 50 patients for the 25 available beds in chronic care hospitals.

BENEFICIAL EFFECTS OF PROLONGED MECHANICAL VENTILATION

The benefits of mechanical ventilation when employed over an extended period in the home include (1) reduction of $PaCO_2$ and often maintenance of eucapnia during periods off the ventilator; (2) improved oxygenation; (3) improved ability to perform activities; (4) decrease in hospitalizations; (5) decreased respiratory symptoms, dyspnea, and cor pulmonale; (6) increased respiratory muscle strength; and (7) decreased mortality.[21–25]

Garay and coauthors reported the course of eight patients with alveolar hypoventilation, without parenchymal lung disease, who were treated with "noninvasive" forms of ventilatory assistance not requiring a tracheostomy.[21] Ventilatory assistance was required because of muscular dystrophy, kyphoscoliosis, postpolio muscular weakness, post-thoracic surgery and phrenic nerve crush, and primary alveolar hypoventilation. These patients were leading active lives, but were unable to maintain normal alveolar ventilation outside the hospital; they were begun on home ventilatory assistance only after repeated hospital admissions for carbon dioxide narcosis, hypersomnolence, or coma. Patients successfully received ventilatory assistance in the home, using negative-pressure ventilators or positive-pressure ventilation by mouthpiece for 3 to 14 years, with sustained reversal of hypercapnia and a decrease in hospital admissions to 1.5 per patient during a mean follow-up of 10.6 years. Pulmonary function studies were stable or showed mild improvement in some cases, and pulmonary hypertension resolved in three patients who had repeat cardiac catheterization.

Similarly, Hoeppner and associates described four patients with symptomatic chronic respiratory failure with secondary kyphoscoliosis caused by polio who did not respond to supplementary oxygen, diuretics, intermittent positive-pressure breathing treatments, and tracheostomy.[22] Within 3 days of institution of positive-pressure ventilation for 12 hours at night through a tracheostomy, symptoms of dyspnea and restless sleep improved. Within 1 to 3 weeks, the $PaCO_2$ during the day while breathing spontaneously had decreased from 60 to 38 mm Hg, and the PaO_2 increased from 38 to 68 mm Hg. In addition, vital capacity, erythrocytosis, and right heart failure improved, allowing an almost normal pattern over a mean follow-up of 3.4 years.

Studies of the effect of negative-pressure ventilation electively employed in patients with chronic obstructive pulmonary disease (COPD) have produced conflicting results. Braun and Marino tested the hypothesis that respiratory muscle rest could alleviate chronic respiratory failure by electively using external negative-pressure ventilators (the Pulmowrap, or poncho, from J. H. Emerson Co., Cambridge, MA) in 35 patients with a variety of thoracic and extrathoracic disorders.[23] After 5 months of 4 to 10 hours of daily ventilator use, the mean PCO_2 decreased from 54 to 43 mm Hg, with improvement in vital capacity; inspiratory and expiratory muscle strength, measured by maximal mouth pressures; endurance, measured by maximal voluntary ventilation; and functional activity, with a subsequent reduction in hospitalizations. Cropp and associates showed similar results in a group of nine COPD patients after only 3 days of negative-pressure ventilator use for 4 to 8 hours daily,[24] and Gutierrez and coauthors reported improvement in five patients ventilated 8 hours, once a week.[25] On the other hand, Pluto and associates[26] and Zibrak and colleagues[27] could not demonstrate improvement in similar patients. In addition, Celli and coworkers failed to show an improvement in diaphragm strength or exercise tolerance with negative-pressure ventilation in COPD patients randomized to receive either negative-pressure ventilation plus rehabilitation or rehabilitation alone.[28] All patients received rehabilitation, including exercise training, which resulted in improved exercise endurance and clinical status, with decreased respiratory muscle work and improved efficiency. In general, COPD patients with hypercapnia seem to demonstrate improvement following use of negative-pressure ventilation, whereas eucapneic individuals experience no improvement.

Rochester and associates suggested that the beneficial effects of negative-pressure ventilation in patients with chronic hypercapnia secondary to obstructive lung disease and chest wall disorders were due to reduced activity of inspiratory muscles.[29] They demonstrated decreased diaphragmatic electrical activity and accessory muscle activity with consequent relief of dyspnea, with use of a tank ventilator. In contrast, body respirators were able to reduce diaphragmatic activity only when the subject's upper airway resistance was increased. It has been suggested that negative-pressure ventilation may be ineffective in some studies of patients with COPD because of failure to reduce respiratory muscle work. Rodenstein and coworkers have demonstrated that diaphragmatic electromyographic (EMG) activity is not initially reduced in untrained COPD subjects placed in a negative-pressure ventilator.[30] Only a 20% reduction in EMG activity was apparent after a 20- to 60-minute trial of ventilation in Rodenstein's patients. Further research is required to determine exactly which COPD patients are likely to benefit from elective use of negative-pressure ventilation.

Other respiratory-assist devices used in the home, including rocking beds and pneumobelts, may also be of benefit in patients with chronic respiratory failure.[31–37] Alexander and coworkers used these external respiratory-assist devices in ten patients with Duchenne muscular dystrophy, ranging in age from 10 to 20 years, for an average of 3.5 years at home.[35] Similarly, Curran used body respirators intermittently in nine patients with muscular dystrophy, for an average of 2 years, with reduction in $PaCO_2$.[31] Body respirators are also useful in patients with other chest wall disorders.[32,36,37]

INDICATIONS FOR HOME MECHANICAL VENTILATION

Medical Diagnosis

Mechanical ventilation is usually initiated in acute care settings for one of the following disorders: (1) the new onset of acute respiratory failure with severe hypoxia, such as in patients with adult respiratory distress syndrome (ARDS) following trauma or surgical procedures; (2) treatment of acute neurologic disorders; (3) management of progressive hypercapnia in patients with chronic, underlying neuromuscular or skeletal disorders; and (4) management of progressive hypercapnia in patients with COPD. In the first two situations, home mechanical ventilation is not appropriate. In the first situation, the expectation is that the application of ventilatory support is a temporary lifesaving measure and will be discontinued when the underlying pulmonary and systemic disorders are reversed. Owing to the inherent physiologic and clinical instability of these patients, home care is not appropriate. In the second situation, use of mechanical ventilation may be applied briefly in an emergency setting and may also be expected to be of only temporary duration in patients with reversible neurologic disorders of recent onset such as Guillain-Barré syndrome or an overdose of narcotic or sedative drugs.

As indicated in Table 20–1, home mechanical ventilation is appropriate for individuals with a variety of disorders.[15,38] In patients with chronic, irreversible neurologic or skeletal disorders such as amyotrophic lateral sclerosis, the use of mechanical ventilation to treat progressive hypercapnia or recurrent episodes of respiratory failure may be needed over a prolonged period as a life-supporting measure. In patients with COPD, mechanical ventilation has traditionally been reserved for patients who develop acute respiratory failure with respiratory acidosis unresponsive to intensive inpatient medical care. Although health professionals hope that the use of mechanical ventilation will be of only short duration, sometimes it is impossible to remove such patients from ventilatory assistance, despite advances in our understanding of the physiologic determinants of ventilator dependence.

Elective Initiation of Ventilation

Many times when respiratory failure can be anticipated in patients with chronic neuromuscular disorders and respiratory status is monitored sequentially over time, the decision to institute ventilatory support may be made electively with the input of the patient and family. In these situations, effective application of mechanical assistance to ventilation may be "noninvasive" (i.e., not require a tracheostomy).

TABLE 20-1. Disorders that May Benefit from
Home Mechanical Ventilation

NEUROMUSCULAR DISORDERS

Central nervous system
Idiopathic (Ondine's curse)
Acquired (Arnold–Chiari malformation)

Spinal cord
Traumatic injury
Syringomyelia

Anterior horn cell
Amyotrophic lateral sclerosis
Poliomyelitis
Spinal muscle atrophy (Werdig–Hoffman)

Peripheral nerve
Neuropathy (Charcot–Marie–Tooth, isolated phrenic
neuropathy)

Muscle
Muscular dystrophy
Myopathy

Chest wall disorders
Kyphoscoliosis
Postsurgical (thoracoplasty)

CHRONIC OBSTRUCTIVE LUNG DISEASE
Adult (emphysema, chronic bronchitis, bronchiectasis)
Child (bronchopulmonary dysplasia)

Negative-pressure external ventilation, rocking bed, pneumobelt, or positive-pressure ventilation through a nasal mask may be effective in patients with chronic neuromuscular disorders. In such instances, respiratory care professionals should educate the patient and family so that they understand the progressive nature of the disease and the eventual outcomes, with and without ventilatory support. Patients and families should be given a realistic view of the future and encouraged to speak with other persons receiving long-term ventilatory support; speaking with other patients is of great educational value and may allay patient and family anxiety. The patient and family should play an integral role in the process of making a decision about whether to institute ventilatory support, and these decisions should be made well in advance of an acute episode of respiratory failure.[13] Elective initiation of mechanical ventilation in patients with neuromuscular disorders should be strongly considered on the basis of clinical and physiologic factors in patients who have

- Repeated hospital admissions for respiratory failure
- Unexplained development of pneumonia in the setting of reduced ventilatory function
- Marked reduction in exercise capacity and functional ability

- Dyspnea with minimal activity, tachypnea > 30/minute, and thoracoabdominal inspiratory paradox
- Hypercapnia ($PaCO_2 > 45$ mm Hg)
- Marked reduction in vital capacity ($< 25\%$ predicted or < 600 to 900 mL)
- Severely decreased respiratory muscle strength ($PI_{max} < 25$ cm H_2O)

Failure to Wean

Individuals who cannot be successfully weaned from mechanical ventilation should be considered chronically ventilator-dependent. There is no uniformly accepted definition of *ventilator dependence*, but the following are key elements that must be met before home ventilation is considered:

1. Multiple attempts to completely wean the patient from the mechanical ventilator for 24 hours/day have been unsuccessful over a period of at least 1 month.
2. Weaning attempts have been performed when the patient's medical condition is optimal and when the acute illnesses that led to initiation of ventilatory assistance have been reversed, if possible.
3. Weaning attempts have occurred when the patient is receiving an adequate bronchodilator regimen.
4. Weaning has been attempted in a meticulous manner by a skilled, respiratory care team.

It is unreasonable to consider long-term home mechanical ventilation unless the patient is truly ventilator-dependent, because of the intense effort on the part of many health professionals and the great expense necessary to discharge a ventilator-assisted individual. Although there are anecdotal stories of patients weaning from ventilatory assistance after discharge home, implying psychological improvement related to the home setting, there are no clear indications that these patients would not have weaned in the hospital with additional time and effort. Patients who are truly ventilator-dependent may then be considered as potential candidates for home care. Children with bronchopulmonary dysplasia (BPD) do have a greater potential to eventually wean from the ventilator than adults. Controversy exists over whether or not unweanable COPD patients should be considered for home mechanical ventilation.[15,38–40]

PATIENT SELECTION

The most important factor in assuring the success of mechanical ventilation in the home is selection of patients who are appropriate for such care. However, determining that a patient is a candidate for ventilatory assistance in the home or alternative site is not a simple task. The guidelines for long-term ventilatory support developed by the American College of Chest Physicians,[15] large published series on home ventilation,[3,5,13,39,41,42] and other reports,[20,43,44] give some indications of the types of patient who can be successfully managed outside the acute care hospital. These may assist the physician and respiratory care health professional in making a decision about the feasibility for home or alternative site care.

TABLE 20-2. Factors Influencing the Decision for Home or Alternative Site Care

Medical diagnosis	Social support
Ventilator dependence	Psychological health
Clinical stability	Financial support
Physiologic stability	Home resources
Desires of the patient	Physical environment
Desires of the family	Health professional support
Patient and family ability to learn and perform	Technical support
necessary care	Community support

Factors other than the diagnosis that caused respiratory failure and the determination that, indeed, the patient is ventilator-dependent must be assessed before a decision is made to discharge a patient receiving ventilatory assistance (Table 20–2). The other important medical factors in selecting patients for home mechanical ventilation are clinical and physiologic stability (Tables 20–3 and 20–4). Patients who are not clinically or physiologically stable have a high incidence of readmission and require intensive resources in the home. Patients should be considered for home care only if it is expected that they can spend most their time at home, rather than in the hospital, in the years following discharge. Coexisting diseases of other organ systems should be stable and not interfere with the patient's progress through the discharge-planning phase, nor with care in the home.

Frequent changes in ventilatory settings should not be required. Patients who have recurring deterioration in blood gas concentrations, despite optimal medical management, should be cared for in a hospital setting. Such unstable patients may need frequent medical, nursing, and respiratory therapy interventions that are unavailable in the home. Table 20–4 lists the criteria for physiologic stability of the

TABLE 20-3. Criteria for Clinical Stability

Absence of significant sustained dyspnea or severe dyspneic episodes or tachypnea
Absence of intercostal retractions (child)
Acceptable arterial blood gas levels, with $FiO_2 \leq 0.40$
Psychological stability
Progression on growth curve and developmental program (infants and children)
Absence of life-threatening cardiac dysfunction or arrhythmias
No major change in management requiring readmission to the hospital for 1 month
Ability to clear secretions
Evidence of gag/cough reflex or protected airway
Absence of significant aspiration
Presence of a tracheostomy (rather than an oral or nasal tracheal tube)

(O'Donohue WJ, et al. Long-term mechanical ventilation: guidelines for management in the home and at alternate community sites. Chest 1986; 90(suppl):1S; with permission)

TABLE   20-4.   Criteria for Physiologic Stability

Other organ systems stable
Absence of acute infections
Optimal acid–base and metabolic status
Ventilator parameters
   FiO_2 stable and < 0.40
   PEEP < 10 cmH$_2$O
   IMV not used
   Stable impedance
   Stable time on and off the ventilator

respiratory system necessary for successful home ventilatory support. Nevertheless, many children with BPD are managed with positive end-expiratory pressure (PEEP) in the home. The ventilator characteristics listed are necessary because of the increased complexity and difficulty inherent in delivering high inspired oxygen concentrations and PEEP with the current generation of small, home ventilators.

Ventilators used in the home are generally less sophisticated than those used in the intensive care setting. The addition of complex devices to the basic ventilator to provide more sophisticated care reduces the safety so important to successful home care. At times a hospital-type ventilator may be required in the home because the patient's needs exceed the capabilities of portable home ventilators. However, such ventilators are relatively large and stationary; a second portable ventilator may be necessary for mobility.[15,45] An important principle of home care is to employ as simple a technology as possible in the home, rather than attempting to recreate the intensive care unit environment.

Nonmedical factors are important and must be assessed when considering the feasibility of home ventilation. These factors include the desires of the patient and family and the presence of family to assist with care (see Table 20–2). Many family members may be fearful about their ability to provide all the care required in the home. These fears may be overcome by allowing them to meet other families involved in home care, read educational materials, or view audiovisual materials that provide a detailed description of the process of discharge planning, and participate in an extensive hands-on educational program designed to help them feel at ease and confident with their ability to perform the required tasks. The amount of support that patients and families will receive in the home should also be discussed in a realistic fashion, since the type of insurance and financial resources often dictate the amount of support that can be provided. The caretaker's physical health and age is crucial when making a decision about the feasibility of home care. The elderly potential caretaker may also have multiple medical problems, poor eyesight, or reduced eye–hand coordination, limiting ability to partake in the care, even when he or she is willing. The psychological health of the patient and family should be assessed before making a final decision because the stress involved in home care of a ventilator-assisted individual can unravel the structure and function of the family and, thereby, impair the safety of home care. The patient's coping mechanisms (i.e., optimism, resourcefulness, flexibility, and adaptability) and motivation should be assessed.[46]

Although the perfect patient is rare, it is important to have a model of the ideal home care candidate when assessing the patient and family.[46]

Payment sources available for home care should be determined for each individual; third-party payments are necessary for almost all patients. It should be determined early in the hospital course whether the patient can qualify for additional funding from alternative sources, such as a state Medicaid program. The amount of skilled health care professional services needed in the home is the major determinant of home care costs; in a patient who requires around-the-clock professional help, home care costs may exceed the cost of care in a hospital or chronic care facility.

EXPERIENCE WITH HOME MECHANICAL VENTILATION

Since 1980, there have been numerous reports of both adults and children successfully managed at home with mechanical ventilatory assistance.[3,5,18,22,23,35,39,41,42,44,47–60] Although many of these reports document the successful discharge of patients to the home, few have addressed the issue of maximizing the functional ability of patients receiving home ventilation. Garay mentioned that most of his patients were leading active, productive lives using body respirators for only a portion of each day.[21] When positive-pressure ventilators are used, patient activity has been more limited. Fischer and Prentice commented on the activity status of 6 of their 14 COPD patients and 11 of 15 patients with restrictive respiratory disorders.[3] Of the COPD patients, 1 was confined to bed, 2 were homebound, 1 occasionally traveled outside the home, and 2 were "independent." Of patients with restrictive disorders, 5 were occasionally able to perform outside activities, 1 was homebound, and 1 was confined to bed. Many patients mentioned in other reports have been confined to home or bed or require extensive home-nursing services because of inability to care for themselves. On the other hand, many patients who were ventilated during the polio epidemic have led productive lives.

It is interesting to note the relative paucity of COPD patients in the large series reports of patients receiving home ventilation (Table 20–5).[3,5,41,44,55,56,61] The reasons for the fewer COPD patients relate to their greater respiratory care requirements, such as suctioning, variability of airflow obstruction, and the progressive nature of the lung disease. Dull and Sadoul in France in followed eight COPD patients for over 1.5 years and demonstrated reduction in $PaCO_2$, but no decrease in hospitalization, after institution of home ventilation. They therefore suggested that quality of life may not be improved.[61] Robert and coworkers have followed a large group of ventilator-assisted individuals in the home in France and reported the survival rates of COPD patients as 55% at 3 years, 30% at 5 years, and 18% at 8 years, with substantially better survival rates for patients with neuromuscular disorders.[41]

Czorniak and associates reported the clinical course of 14 patients with COPD and 21 with neuromuscular disorders followed at home for an average of 31 months (range, 5 to 66 months) after hospital discharge.[62] The COPD patients had an average of 2.7 hospital admissions per patient per year at home and averaged 54 days in the hospital each year, whereas patients with neuromuscular disorders had significantly fewer hospitalizations (0.7 admissions and 9.8 hospital days per patient for

TABLE 20-5. Large Series of Ventilator-Assisted Patients in the Home

Author/Year	Restrictive Lung Disease Patients	COPD Patients	Positive-Pressure Ventilators	Years of Follow-up
Make, 1988	39	33	29	1–6
Sivak, 1986[42]	33	2	25	0.2–17
Ontario, 1985[55]	33	4	37	2
Kopacz, 1984[56]	14	4	18	0.2–3.6
Indihar, 1984[44]	11	3	14	0.1–2.1
Robert, 1983[41]	162	60	222	1–25
Splaingard, 1983[5]	47	0	47	1 day–11 yrs
Fischer, 1982[3]	15	14	29	0.1–5.5
Dull, 1981[61]	1	7	8	1–7
Total	355	127		

each year at home). Seven patients with neuromuscular diseases (33%) had no hospital admissions; these patients were generally younger and were receiving positive-pressure ventilation by tracheostomy, rather than noninvasive forms of ventilation. The reasons for hospitalization were similar in both COPD and neuromuscular patients. The most common reasons (54%) for admission were related to the lungs: 29% were for increased ventilatory requirements, 10% were related to pneumonia, and 9% were for bronchitis. Twenty-three percent of hospital admissions were for nonpulmonary problems unrelated to mechanical ventilation. Upper airway problems related to the tracheostomy (granulation tissue, stoma revision, cuff leak) led to 14% of the admissions. Hospitalization was uncommonly (9%) related to power failure or mechanical ventilation system malfunction. As shown in Figure 20–1, mortality in the COPD group was higher than in the neuromuscular group. Although the long-term survival of COPD patients is shorter than that of individuals with neuromuscular or skeletal disorders, our experience at Boston University suggests that physical capacity, independence, and possibly the quality of life may be greater in carefully selected COPD patients than in individuals with neurologic disorders.

Boston University Experience

Make and Gilmartin have shown that persons can be largely independent when a rehabilitation program is integrated into the to-home discharge of ventilator-assisted individuals, and have described the details of such a rehabilitation program.[39,60,63] From 1981 to 1988, 72 ventilator-assisted patients were admitted to the Respiratory Care Center at the University Hospital at the Boston University Medical Center. All patients were screened and thought to have a reasonable potential for discharge home. Characteristics of these patients are shown in Table 20–6. Of the patients with neuromuscular disorders, 8 had muscular dystrophy, 8 had sequelae of polio, 5 had spinal cord injury, 4 had amyotrophic lateral sclerosis, and 4 had kyphoscoliosis. All

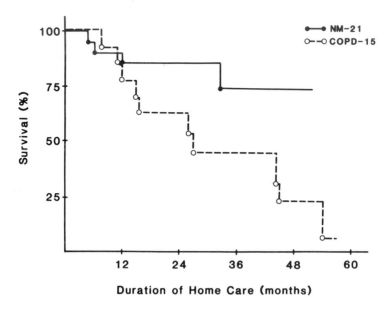

FIGURE   20-1   Survival of adults receiving mechanical assistance to ventilation in the home. NM, patients with neuromuscular disorders; COPD, patients with chronic obstructive pulmonary disease.

TABLE   20-6.   Outcomes of 72 Ventilator-Assisted Patients Admitted to Boston University Hospital (1981–1988)

	COPD	*Neuromuscular*
ADMISSIONS AGE	33	39
Mean	61.3	50.1
Range	46–78	22–81
OUTCOME		
Home care	23	35
Chronic hospital	2	4
Died in hospital	8	0
INDEPENDENCE*		
Maximal	6	13
Moderate	11	7
Minimal	16	10
None	0	9

* Maximal, performs own care independently; moderate, performs most of own care except for showering and meal preparation; minimal, can wash, dress, and eat at bedside once materials are set up; none, needs complete assistance with almost all personal care.

but 1 patient with COPD and 23 (59%) of the patients with neuromuscular disorders were initially placed on mechanical ventilation as an acute lifesaving procedure because of progressive hypercapnia, respiratory acidosis, and respiratory failure. The remaining patients were electively ventilated for gradually progressive hypercapnia, exercise intolerance, and dyspnea.

As shown in Table 20–6, all but 4 patients with neuromuscular disorders were successfully discharged home, but only 23 of 33 patients with COPD were discharged home. The COPD patients who did not go home included 2 who died in the hospital secondary to complications of abdominal surgery, 3 who died of cardiac disease, and 5 whose care was too complex to be managed independently or whose families were older and not physically capable of providing as much support as required. These results and those reported by others suggest that ventilator-assisted persons with neuromusculoskeletal disorders are strong candidates for discharge, whereas patients with COPD, even with careful screening and intensive rehabilitation efforts, may possibly not be successfully discharged home. We also found, as Table 20–6 shows, that many patients who are discharged can lead active, independent lives at home.

Complete "weaning" from mechanical ventilation was rarely possible in this patient population, but provision of as much "free time" off the ventilator as possible is an extremely useful goal. To attain this goal, weaning patients once or twice a day using a T-piece and gradually increasing the length of the wean is suggested. At the same time, increasing ventilator rate to minimize spontaneous respiratory efforts while receiving ventilatory assistance and, thereby, decreasing ventilatory work, has been effective. During ventilator-free time, patients can more easily perform activities of daily living (ADL) at home or participate in community activities. The amount of ventilator-free time tolerated by our 72 patients is shown in Table 20–7. For those patients discharged home, the amount of ventilator-free time that was tolerated at the time of discharge grew shorter during exacerbations of their disease, during respiratory infections, and as the disease progressed.

TABLE 20-7. Ventilatory Requirements* of Ventilator-Assisted Individuals in Boston University Hospital Program

	COPD	*Neuromuscular*
Positive-pressure ventilator		
Tracheostomy	33	29
Nasal	0	4
Negative-pressure ventilator	0	6
Ventilator-free time		
< 2 h	13	8
2–7 h	8	3
8–16 h	13	26
16–24 h	0	2

* At the time of discharge, transfer, or death.

VENTILATORS AND OTHER EQUIPMENT

Ventilatory support in the home has evolved from the polio era when patients were transferred home with simple equipment individualized for each patient. The patient and family became experts in the care and use of this equipment and generally were able to make modifications to suit their needs. They altered their equipment so they could travel, used batteries or generators in the event of power outages, and were well known to the ventilator companies. Negative-pressure ventilators were the main mode of ventilatory support, other forms of ventilatory assistance included rocking beds and pneumobelts. Many of these patients are still at home today and are using the equipment originally prescribed 30 years ago.

Because ventilator-assisted individuals discharged home today have a wider variety of medical disorders causing respiratory failure, different modes of therapy are often required. The three major types of mechanical ventilation used today are (1) positive-pressure ventilation provided through a tracheostomy or noninvasively through a nasal mask or mouthpiece, (2) negative-pressure ventilation provided by an iron lung or chest cuirass, and (3) other devices such as a pneumobelt or rocking bed. The type of device used will depend on the cause of respiratory failure, compliance of the lung and chest wall, and the presence of increased airway resistance. The ability of the patient to protect his or her airway and the presence of obstructive sleep apnea are also important determinants of the type of ventilatory support.

Positive-Pressure Ventilators

Positive-pressure ventilation is the most commonly used approach to ventilatory assistance in the home today.[33] Until recently, if patients had intrinsic lung or airway disease a more sophisticated hospital-type ventilator had to be used in the home.[33,34] These ventilators were reliable for long-term use and inspiratory flow rate could be altered for patients with severe airway or lung disease. The ability to provide supplemental oxygen was fairly simple, and the delivered inspired oxygen concentration (FIO_2) was usually constant. These ventilators usually had more than one alarm, important in the hospital, but unnecessary in the home environment.[33] The problem with using sophisticated ICU-type ventilators is that they are not "user friendly" to caregivers who have either no medical education or no education at all, and who may not be mechanically oriented. The most typical of the ICU ventilators used in the home were the Emerson Post-Op and 3MV (J. H. Emerson Co., Cambridge, MA), Bennett MA-1 and MA-2 (Puritan-Bennett Co., Overland Park, KS), and Bear 1 and 2 (Bourne Medical Systems, Riverside, CA) ventilators.

Today there are more home-style ventilators available, although many of their features are similar.[33,34,64] In general, when selecting a ventilator for the home the following features should be considered: reliability, portability, size, ease of operation, and ease of maintenance. The advantages of all of the home ventilators are their compact size and weight; they all weigh under 18 kg (40 lb). They can easily be placed on a cart or mounted on a motorized or manual wheelchair. They also can operate on normal household current, an internal DC battery, and an external DC battery. The internal battery is useful only as a very short-term power source in the event of power failure or for limited transportation. One major disadvantage of the small ventilators is that when operated in the intermittent mandatory ventilation (IMV) or synchronized IMV (SIMV) mode, the patient effort required for spontaneous breathing is very high.[65] Although work of breathing could be reduced by use of an external continuous-flow system for IMV, such systems add to the complexity of the ventilator. Simple methods to decrease the amount of patient effort are to (1) replace the filter at the air inlet on the back of the ventilator with a bacterial filter and add a bacterial filter at the outlet port, (2) remove the tower when using a cascade humidifier, (3) reduce patient spontaneous ventilatory effort by increasing the ventilator rate, and (4) use assist–control mode.

A potential drawback to small ventilators is the difficulty in delivering additional oxygen. Although a reservoir or accumulator may be added to the ventilator intake, oxygen may also be delivered through a small nipple adapter attached at the patient port proximal to the humidifer. With these latter methods, the oxygen flow will be constant, but the actual delivery to the patient may vary owing to changes in patient effort or respiratory rate. For most patients, this variability in the FiO_2 will not be of significance, since most home patients are receiving low oxygen concentrations. For those patients who require a precise FiO_2 or higher oxygen concentrations, a reservoir or accumulator might be appropriate. These systems add to the complexity of the ventilator and should be considered only when strict attention to oxygen delivery is mandatory. Table 20–8 lists some of the features of each of the currently available portable ventilators.

An increasingly popular and effective approach to home ventilation is the use of positive-pressure ventilation by a nasal mask, the origin of which can be traced to the use of nasal masks developed for continuous positive airway pressure (CPAP) in patients with obstructive sleep apnea. This form of ventilation is most appropriate for patients with neuromuscular disorders.[58,66,67] Positive-pressure ventilation with a mouthpiece has been used successfully for patients with polio.[57] Custom-made nasal masks and mouthpieces have been used at some centers to increase patient comfort.

Negative-Pressure Ventilation

Recently, there has been renewed interest in the use of negative-pressure ventilation for patients with neuromuscular disease faced with the need for ventilatory support; these patients would often rather use less invasive negative-pressure ventilation, rather than tracheostomy and positive-pressure devices. There has also been significant interest in this form of ventilatory assistance for patients with severe COPD, to provide elective rest of fatigued respiratory muscles. Negative-pressure ventilation can be accomplished with the use of an iron lung, a self-contained device that is an effective pressure generator and that can be manually operated during a power failure. The major disadvantage is the bulk and lack of portability of these machines and the difficulty of gaining access to the patient.

A portable version of the iron lung is available (Porta-Lung, W. W. Weingarten, Denver, CO). The chest cuirass ("turtle shell") is a much less confining negative-pressure ventilator chamber placed over the chest and abdomen. Ready-made shells are available, but custom-made shells are often necessary for patients who have kyphoscoliosis, protuberant abdomens, or thoracic deformity. A negative-pressure

TABLE 20-8. Features of Positive-Pressure Home Care Ventilators

Product	Mode	Tidal Volume	Rate	I/E Ratio	Alarms	Power Sources
Aequitron (Minn, MN) LP-6	C AC SIMV	100–2200 mL	1–38	Variable	Low-pressure, high-pressure, low-power, apnea, I/E ratio, power switchover, ventilator malfunction	AC DC Int.
Life Care (Lafeyette, CO) PVV	C	50–3000 mL	8–30	Fixed 1 : 1	Low-pressure, high-pressure, low-power, power failure	AC DC Int.
PLV-100	C AC SIMV Sigh	50–3000 mL	2–40	Variable	Low-pressure, high-pressure, low-power, power failure, apnea, I/E ratio, power switchover, inspiratory flow, ventilator malfunction, reverse battery cable connection	AC DC Int.
PLV-102	C AC SIMV	50–3000 mL	2–40	Variable	Low-pressure, high-pressure, low-power, apnea, I/E ratio, power switchover, inspiratory flow	AC DC Int.
Puritan-Bennett (Overland Park, KS) Companion 2800	C AC SIMV Sigh	50–2800 mL	1–69	Variable	Low-pressure, high-pressure, low-power, power failure, apnea, I/E ratio, power switchover, inspiratory flow, ventilator malfunction	AC DC Int.
Bear Medical Systems (Riverside, CA) Bear 33	C AC SIMV Sigh	100–2200 mL	2–40	Variable	Low-pressure, high-pressure, power failure, apnea, power switchover, inspiratory flow, I/E ratio, ventilator inoperable	AC DC Int.

generator is attached to the center of the shell by a flexible tubing. Even though these devices are well tolerated, as chest wall compliance worsens or skeletal deformity increases, adequate ventilation may not be possible, and other forms of ventilation may need to be considered. The Pulmowrap ("raincoat," pneumosuit) is made from nylon or other airtight material that surrounds the patient and requires the use of a negative-pressure generator. These are more cumbersome to get into for some patients, and the poncho type requires patience to reduce leaks around the arms and lower abdomen. A major complaint with some patients is back discomfort since a relatively hard surface is needed for the grid (which provides for maintenance of an air space inside the suit) to rest upon, thus requiring the patient to be in bed and limiting mobility.

A major contraindication to using negative-pressure ventilation is obstructive sleep apnea. If sleep-disordered breathing is a diagnostic consideration, a sleep study should be performed before instituting this form of ventilation. If there is objective or symptomatic deterioration without other explanation, a sleep study is indicated to evaluate the possibility of upper airway obstruction while the patient is using the negative-pressure device. A common complaint of patients using negative-pressure ventilators is that of being cold; this can be remedied by having the patient wear appropriate clothing.

Pneumobelt

The pneumobelt consists of a corset fitted around the abdomen and lower rib cage. Inflation of the "bladder" inside the corset by a positive-pressure ventilator compresses the abdominal contents, pushing the diaphragm cephalad and actively assisting expiration. When the "bladder" deflates, the diaphragm is allowed to descend, decreasing intrathoracic pressure and allowing gas to enter the lungs during inspiration.[12] The pneumobelt is most useful for patients who need some ventilatory support during the day and do not have significant airway or parenchymal disease. This assist device can be used during sleep, but the patient cannot lie flat. Patients with significant deformity of their thoracic or lumbar spine are unable to use this device, but patients with lower cervical spinal cord injury who do not require ventilatory support when lying flat may use this device to increase diaphragmatic motion when sitting upright.[68]

Rocking Bed

The rocking bed functions by alternately rotating the head of the bed down to shift the abdominal contents cephalad and assist expiration, and then rotating the foot of the bed down, to shift abdominal contents caudally and assist inspiration.[10,11] The rocking bed moves the diaphragm up and down, thereby assisting ventilation. The rate of the rocking motion and the pitch of the bed are adjustable. Generally, the tidal volume cannot be greatly enhanced, but it may be adequate for many patients with neuromuscular disease. The motion of the bed seems to mobilize secretions, which can be quite bothersome to some patients and interfere with sleep. It also takes up much more space than a regular bed, which is an important factor to consider when choosing a ventilatory-assist device for the home. The bed does have an automatic stop as a safety device if something interferes with its motion.

Accessory Equipment

The most important piece of accessory equipment needed in the home of a ventilator-assisted person is a self-inflating manual resuscitator and mask. This is necessary for several reasons. First, the resuscitator can provide ventilation, if there is a power failure or ventilator malfunction, as a short-term remedy until a battery or another ventilator is available. Second, the resuscitator can be used to assist ventilation when the patient is experiencing shortness of breath unrelieved by other modalities such as suctioning or bronchodilators. Third, during ventilator tubing changes, the resuscitator is helpful in patients who do not have free time from the ventilator. Furthermore, the resuscitator can assist in mobilizing secretions before or during suctioning. Finally, it may provide ventilation to the patient by face mask if the tracheostomy tube inadvertently falls out or during failure of noninvasive ventilatory equipment.

A second ventilator is necessary for any patient who has limited free time off the ventilator or who lives in a very rural area. As a general rule, a second ventilator should be considered if the patient requires 20 or more hours of mechanical assistance each day or if he or she cannot wean for 4 or more consecutive hours.[45] A second ventilator may also be helpful to improve mobility by permanently mounting it on a wheelchair.[15,45] Other accessory equipment used in the home is listed in Table 20–9.

Adaptive equipment useful for improving the patient's performance of ADL includes devices that help the caregivers, such as the Hoyer lift or hydraulic shower chair. Team members need to collaborate to decide what equipment is necessary and

TABLE 20-9.   Accessory Equipment Used In the Home

Self-inflating manual resuscitation face mask
Ventilator—backup
Ventilator filters
Humidifier
Water trap
Suction machines—electrical or battery powered
Oxygen source
Compressors—for medication delivery or aerosols
Battery—12-VDC
Battery charger
Battery cable
Mobility devices
Bathing and toileting devices
Environmental control unit
Bed
Safety devices

what will be reimbursed by third-party payers. Some adaptive devices may be funded through nonprofit agencies, such as the Muscular Dystrophy Association. A list of equipment and supplies[14,34] necessary for home care of ventilator-assisted patients should be developed before discharge, and the equipment should be made available for use by the patients and caregivers during their training. The necessary equipment and supplies should then be placed in the home before the patient is discharged.

AIRWAY MANAGEMENT

Maintenance of an adequate airway in the patient using positive-pressure ventilation by tracheostomy should be a top priority to the team caring for the patient. Potential problems to be anticipated by the discharge or home care team are (1) complications already encountered with the airway owing to a stormy and prolonged ICU course, (2) a poorly placed tracheostomy stoma, (3) an ill-fitting tracheostomy tube, (4) granulation tissue formation interfering with the patency of the airway associated with bleeding and increasing the difficulty of tube changes, (5) stomal infection of inflammation related to poor healing and continuous drainage of secretions around the stoma, and (6) peristomal fibrosis making tube changes difficult.

The airway complications associated with a prolonged ICU hospitalization include tracheomalacia, subglottic stenosis, tracheal stenosis, and poorly healed tracheal stomas. These may be related to prolonged endotracheal intubation; repeated endotracheal intubations before tracheostomy; relatively high ventilatory pressures, necessitating increasing amounts of air and pressure in the cuff to prevent a loss of ventilation; poor perfusion to the tracheal mucosa, secondary to low cardiac output or overinflation of the cuff; and poor healing related to chronic infection and nutritional deficits. At times, the tracheotomy stoma may be placed either too high or too low in the neck, causing problems with tube positioning. If the stoma is not placed centrally, the tip of the trachostomy tube may place constant pressure on the tracheal wall, causing erosion or scarring.

Many patients have tracheal tubes that are much too large, in which the angle of tube insertion is not appropriate for their anatomy. There is a tendency to place larger-diameter tubes when the cuff requires increasing amounts of air for a seal because of tracheomalacia, with the result that the patient ends up with a very large tube in place that still requires a large volume of air to create a seal. The patient with a thick neck often has tracheal tube positional problems, with the cuff bulging upward in the airway and the distal tip of the tube pressing on the posterior wall of the trachea, with potential erosion into the esophagus.

Granulation tissue formation at the stomal site may occur and is not always preventable. We have encountered granulation tissue inside the tracheal stoma of sufficient degree to impair spontaneous patient ventilation through a fenestrated tracheostomy tube. The presence of a foreign body constantly irritating the mucosa and skin surface causes formation of granulation tissue. If the patient is a candidate for long-term ventilation and the tracheostomy is not an emergency, then a permanent stoma may be created with skin flaps brought down to the level of the trachea; this may facilitate tube changes and reduce the frequency of problems with granulation tissue and bleeding. Inside the trachea, there may be granulation tissue at the subglottic level, at the superior aspect of the stoma, or at the tube tip site. If granulation tissue causes significant airflow obstruction, causes bleeding, or interferes with tube changes, it should be surgically removed.

Stomal infection or inflammation may be associated with repeated tracheobronchial infection, immunosuppression, and continuous drainage of upper airway secretions and saliva around the stoma. Loss of skin integrity secondary to maceration of the skin will also predispose to infection. Repeated use of antibiotics and the use of an antimicrobial ointment may predispose to a fungal infection.

When a patient enters a rehabilitation program or is being prepared for home, an assessment of the airway and tracheal tube should be made. Visual inspection of the stoma and tracheal tube should consist of an examination for skin breakdown around the stoma and under the tracheal tape or ties, type and amount of drainage, presence of granulation tissue, redness or swelling, shape of the neck, protrusion of the tube out of the neck, and relation of the neck plate or phalange of the tube to the neck itself. If the patient has a fenestrated tracheostomy tube that is used for phonation and spontaneous ventilation during free time from the ventilator, proper position of the fenestration must be assured. A limited examination can be performed by removing the inner cannula and inspecting the fenestration with a flashlight to determine if the fenestration is patent and positioned well in the airway lumen. An anteroposterior film of the neck or a well-positioned chest roentgenogram will show whether the cuff is bulging out the tracheal wall and whether the tube is midline. The lateral chest or neck film will show if the tip of the tube or cuff is bulging into the posterior wall of the trachea and toward the esophagus, which may impair swallowing and esophageal motility and increase the risk of aspiration.[69] The lateral film will also aid in determining the position of the fenestration.

A limited bronchoscopy can assess the presence of vocal cord edema, paralysis, or stenosis and determine subglottic abnormalities such as granulation tissue or stenosis. Direct visualization of the tube in the trachea can aid in properly placing the fenestration. Collapse or loss of support of the tracheal wall, especially at the level of the cuff site, may necessitate a longer tracheostomy tube, which can be placed under direct visualization to prevent inadvertent location in the right main stem bronchus. The position of the cuff can also be noted, and one can assess bulging into the proximal airway, which can decrease the adequacy of the seal with changes in patient position or movement of the tracheal tube. Not all tracheostomy problems can be corrected, but by using these assessment measures, at least the state of the airway can be observed, and further problems can be prevented.

Care of the stoma should consist of cleaning the stoma and surrounding skin as well as the portion of the tube that is visible. This should be done at least twice daily if there is minimal drainage, and the area should be kept dry to prevent maceration of the skin. Diluted hydrogen peroxide is generally used for cleaning the stoma and the inner cannula. An antiseptic ointment may also be used. The stoma should be observed for redness, swelling, itchiness, blisters, and signs of fungal infection. If any of these occur, procedures should be reviewed to make sure patients are properly caring for the stoma. If lack of care is not the problem, then altering the care may be necessary; omitting the hydrogen peroxide or stopping the antiseptic ointment may decrease irritation. If there is a fungal infection, an antifungal ointment combined with hydrocortisone will alleviate the problem. The patient should be taught to keep the inner cannulas and buttons clean and dry to prevent infection.

Cuff inflation, assessment of leaks in the system, and troubleshooting similar problems are a major part of home care and probably some of the hardest concepts for the patient and caretakers to learn. If the volume of air in the cuff cannot be maintained because of a leak, and the patient cannot tolerate the loss of ventilator volume, the patient or caregiver needs to know temporary measures to maintain ventilation, how to change the tube, or how to obtain care in a local emergency room for a tube change.

RESOURCES IN THE HOME

The discharge of a patient to home on a ventilator may seem relatively simple. However, if the patient is a key part of the team approach and if the goal of home care is to allow maximal patient self-responsibility and independence, then a comprehensive inpatient program of rehabilitation must be individualized for each patient. The process of discharging a patient home on life-support equipment requires the expertise and cooperation of many different people from different disciplines (Fig. 20–2). When many people are involved, communication may be enhanced and goals shared among personnel if they organize into a team.[15,45,63] The role of each team member should be defined, and the patient and family should be considered an integral part of the team and the discharge-planning effort.

In the home, many patients can provide much or all of their own care if their potential is maximized through a program of rehabilitation and education. Even patients who cannot physically participate in their own care may be able to direct their care providers. For other patients, family members or parents will provide the care or direct others in the delivery of care. Children represent a special case, since they require care totally given by others; in addition, children and neonates have special needs that are very different from those of adults.[49,54,70-75] The roles of the patient, family, and other home care providers should be clearly and precisely identified well in advance of discharge. Home care agencies should be integrated into discharge planning early in the hospitalization. If the patient and family will be providing most of the care, a community nursing agency may be involved to assess the patient in the home setting and to coordinate the functions of other allied health professionals when needed, such as physical or occupational therapists and social workers. If assistance with personal care, such as bathing, feeding, or meal preparation, is necessary, a home health aide or nursing assistant provided by a community nursing agency may be employed. Usually, these nonprofessionals cannot provide respiratory care, such as suctioning, bronchodilator treatments, or ventilator care, because of liability concerns of the home health care agencies. Some agencies allow their home health aides to administer chest physical therapy and assist with cleaning of ventilator circuits, but only after training and under supervision of a registered nurse. In the absence of a family member, chest physical therapy may be performed by nurses or physical therapists.

If the patient requires more comprehensive care in the home and is unable to physically provide his or her own care, then a personal care attendant (PCA) may be

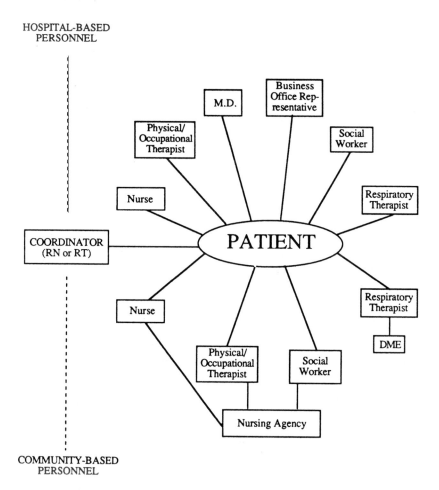

HOSPITAL-BASED
PERSONNEL

COMMUNITY-BASED
PERSONNEL

FIGURE   20-2   Members of the discharge-planning team for ventilator-assisted individuals.

helpful. The PCAs are generally lay people without prior experience who can be trained by the patient or family to provide the necessary care. In many areas, they are hired by the patient and, therefore, there is no liability to the home care agency. A PCA may cost much less than a home health aide, professional nurse, or therapist, and the cost may be reimbursed by a state Medicaid program or rehabilitation commission. They can be hired for day or night hours, and their salary may be supplemented with room and board. Many patients with neuromuscular disorders, such as polio, spinal cord injury, or muscular dystrophy, have employed such caregivers for years. An important point to remember about PCAs is that they are nonprofessional caregivers. Thus, the patient and family must be directive of the care, capable of providing the necessary education, and able to discipline the PCA if he or she is not providing the care as directed. State-funded "centers of independent living" can educate the patient and family in the methods of recruitment, reimbursement, and termination of a PCA.

Another option for short-term respite care or companionship is community volunteer organizations. If the patient needs continuous professional care, many factors may be considered, not the least of which is cost. Twenty-four-hour care by registered nurses may cost 500 to 800 dollars/day, which is unaffordable for most people. Some insurance plans cover this level of care, but the patient may have to pay the caregivers themselves and apply for reimbursement by the insurance carrier—a process that requires some financial resources. State and federal insurance programs may reimburse continuous skilled nursing care, but at a lower rate, thereby excluding participation by many nursing agencies. Other problems that must be considered with round-the-clock care are lack of coverage because of paucity of health professionals, availability of backup help in the event of illness or transportation problems, and inadequate training and experience of the caregivers.

It is important to stress that one of the most important resources necessary in home care is the emotional health of the patient and family and their ability to cope with changes in their lives that are imposed by chronic disease. The patient can be physically stable, but if there is deterioration in the psychological health of the patient or caretakers, home care will fail. Many patients and families will require a great deal of psychological support, and this can be provided by the referring institution or the home care agency. If respite care is available or if the family can afford to pay privately for respite care, it should become a routine part of the home program. If the caregiver does not get adequate sleep or rest, he or she will not be able to continue to provide optimal care, and his or her physical and psychological health may deteriorate, thereby placing the patient at risk, since an unhealthy caregiver makes mistakes.

Other types of community support may be necessary, such as transportation for medical care, meal preparation, homemaking, and shopping. Many communities have an emergency telephone service that connects directly to the local hospital; this service is particularly helpful for the ventilatory-assisted individual who may be alone during part of the day. The local utility company, ambulance service, and fire department should be aware of the patient at home on life-support equipment so that they can respond to emergency situations such as a power failure or need for transport to the hospital.

A home assessment should be performed by representatives from both the hospital team and the home respiratory care company, to determine if the home physical environment is adequate for the patient's needs and to make necessary modifications before the patient's hospital discharge. If the patient requires extensive adaptation to the physical layout because of wheelchair-dependence or because of severe functional impairments, a physical or occupational therapist should also be involved in the home assessment. The physical layout should be assessed for any barriers to mobility, such as narrow doorways, stairs, thick carpets, and thresholds. The patient's bedroom should not only be large enough to accommodate the required equipment, but also easily accessible to the rest of the house, so that the patient will not be isolated. If a hospital bed is required, the patient may not be able to remain in his or her own bedroom because of lack of space. There should be adequate ventilation and heat, and the electrical supply should be appropriate for the additional equipment. A separate electrical circuit for the ventilator and accessory equipment is preferable, but not mandatory, since all home care equipment will function with normal 110-VAC household current. Grounded outlets are preferable and should be available for such items as the ventilator, suction machine, humidifier, electric bed, and compressor. An evaluation by a licensed electrician is required for any patient that has a lot of electrical equipment and should be mandatory in older houses. Fortunately, the respiratory equipment does not draw much electrical power and will not usually exceed the capabilities of most homes. There should be a designated area to charge wheelchair and ventilator batteries; acid-filled batteries should not be charged in the patient's room because of potential danger from fumes emitted from the battery, sparks, and fire. Home modifications are not covered by third-party payment, but funding may be available through community agencies, such as the Muscular Dystrophy Association.

There must be space in the home for the cleaning, drying, and storage of equipment. Many patients use their kitchen sink for cleaning and then use a basin for the sterilizing process. A clothes rack placed in the bathtub is very useful for drying ventilatory tubing.

RESPIRATORY HOME CARE COMPANIES

One of the most important resources in the home is the respiratory care or durable medical equipment company (DME). Mechanical ventilators, other equipment, such as suction machines and wheelchairs, and disposable items are most often supplied to ventilator-assisted individuals in the home by respiratory home care companies. Many of these durable medical equipment vendors were founded in the 1970s to supply oxygen to patients at home. With the increased recognition of the importance of long-term oxygen therapy and subsequent reimbursement for this outpatient therapy, these local companies flourished and were merged with the several larger national concerns that currently dominate the marketplace. These larger vendors have the resources to provide any type of equipment or supply needed in the home and have expanded their personnel to satisfy the needs of the growing number of home ventilator patients. All the large national DMEs have developed written policies, procedures, and guidelines for home care of ventilator-assisted individuals and will gladly participate in the planning and education of caregivers before a patient's hospital discharge. However, the translation of such policies developed on a national level to care provided by local branches is not always optimal and depends heavily upon the expertise and experience of local branch personnel. There may be regional differences in home care techniques and equipment that are based upon common practice in the community. Competition among companies for a larger share of the home care market has traditionally been the motivating factor for development of a comprehensive, high-quality program by vendors.

The primary responsibility for planning and implementation of a comprehensive home care program for hospitalized ventilator-assisted persons should reside in the hands of a single, clearly designated, health care professional (usually either a respiratory therapist or clinical respiratory nurse specialist) who has the most knowledge and experience in respiratory home care. This discharge coordinator may be hospital- or community-based and should draw upon both hospital and community resources, as needed, to assure a smooth transition to the home.[45]

A reputable DME and community nursing agency should be involved early in the discharge process so that equipment needs can be determined and the necessary equipment provided for patient use and teaching before discharge. Backup equipment must be readily available in the event of equipment failure; consequently, a small company may not be the optimal choice for home care of ventilator-assisted individuals. Larger home care companies usually stock required home care equipment. The home care therapists may not be involved with the education of the patient and family in the hospital, but will definitely be involved with continuing education in the home setting. They may also be involved with the education of other home care providers such as community nursing agencies or PCAs. The hospital team and the respiratory home care company need to coordinate their efforts to provide optimal initial and continuing education for patients and caregivers. All educators must teach identical home care procedures and methods to avoid confusing patients and families. A comprehensive home management plan (Table 20–10) and specific respiratory care plan (Table 20–11) must be individualized for each patient before his or her hospital discharge, and the personnel responsible for each component must be adequately trained. The responsibilities of each person, as well as what procedures will be taught to the patient and family, need to be delineated well in advance of discharge; this will prevent confusion of the caregivers and assure a smooth transition from hospital to home.

Once the patient is stabilized in the home, the respiratory home care company should make periodic routine visits, at least monthly, to monitor the overall function of the ventilator and other accessory equipment, provide preventive maintenance, assess the patient's response to therapy, and assure compliance with the prescribed

TABLE 20-10. Comprehensive Management Plan

The written comprehensive management plan for a home ventilator patient should
- Identify primary and consulting physicians
- Identify local hospital emergency room
- Specify appropriate medical center for care re-evaluation
- Designate roles of health care providers
- Designate roles of patients and others in daily care
- Provide a method to select and train future caregivers
- Guarantee comprehensive funding
- Determine necessary modifications of the care environment
- Assess community resources to meet health, social, educational, and vocational needs
- Itemize equipment and supplies needed
- Identify equipment dealers and services they provide (maintenance, surveillance, and such)
- Outline alternative emergency and contingency plans

(O'Donohue WJ, et al. Long-term mechanical ventilation: guidelines for management in the home and at alternate community sites. Chest 1986; 90(suppl):1S; with permission)

TABLE 20-11. Respiratory Care Plan

Mechanical ventilator
  Type and characteristics (including backup when indicated)
Manual resuscitator
Ventilator power source
  Electrical requirements
  Battery or generator powered
Ventilator circuit
  Detailed description of circuits
  Description of alarms
  Instructions for cleaning, assembly, and use
  Documentation of the education of caregivers
Use of ventilators
  Specific times on and off the ventilator
  FiO_2 and range of oxygen
  Mode of ventilation
  Desired change with exercise or sleep
  Acceptable limits of dialed/measured exhaled volume
  Desired pressure ranges
Appropriate alarms and monitors
  For ventilator dysfunction, power failure
  For high and low pressure, exhaled volume
  Others as needed
Name and type of artificial airway
  Size and type
  Cuffed, uncuffed, fenestrated
  Double or single cannula
Instructions for care of artificial airway
  Cuff inflation (conditions for inflation/deflation)
  Airway care plan (tube changes, cleaning, problem solving)
  Airway suctioning
  Speaking tube operation, if appropriate
Adjunctive techniques
  Medications
  Aerosol (bronchodilator)
  Chest physiotherapy
  Oxygen therapy
Communication systems
  Intercom
  Physical sound (bell/siren)
  Telephone/beeper system

(O'Donohue WJ, et al. Long-term mechanical ventilation: guidelines for management in the home and at alternate community sites. Chest 1986; 90 (suppl):1S; with permission)

respiratory care plan. They may also participate in noninvasive monitoring to assure adequate oxygenation during various activities in the home. They usually provide disposable supplies, such as suction catheters, tubings, medication nebulizers, and gloves. The DME may also provide medications, a service that may be very helpful for the patient who is not mobile or does not have ready access to a pharmacy. The home care company should not be responsible for medical problems that occur in the home, but if the therapist determines that a medical problem or psychological deterioration is interfering with patient progress at home, the company should communicate with the referring physician or institution. At times, the patient or family may not be able to differentiate between a medical or equipment problem, and an on-site assessment should be performed by the home care therapist. Often, a telephone conversation between therapist and patient will provide important insight concerning the nature of the problem, but unscheduled home calls will also be necessary. Communication between the home care company, nursing agency, and referring physician is extremely important to ensure optimal continuing care in the home. Often the home health aide, nurse, or therapist is the first to notice increasing emotional problems that interfere with optimal delivery of care in the home; these problems may not be detected by the physician during a brief office visit.

It is imperative that the hospital discharge-planning team assure the presence of a comprehensive program for daily care in home. Because the respiratory home care vendor plays an important role in patient management, a company should be chosen on the basis of its ability to provide a continuous level of quality care—to deliver the necessary equipment and supplies to the patient in the home on a timely basis, provide experienced, qualified home care respiratory therapists, and to meet the Joint Commission on Accreditation of Healthcare Organizations (JCAHO) standards.

COSTS OF HOME VENTILATOR CARE

Although improved and more humane patient care, and not cost reduction, should be the motivating factor for home care,[76] costs cannot be completely overlooked. The Boston University program has evaluated the home care costs for ventilator-assisted individuals with COPD and with neuromuscular disorders.[77] The average cost of home care in 1987 for these patients was 2974 dollars a month, with a wide variation between individual patient costs. Figure 20–3 shows the costs of various components of care in the home. Other investigators have reported that substantial savings can be achieved by home care. The American Association for Respiratory Care[19] conducted a 20-state hospital survey in 1984 and estimated the cost of home care to be 1766 dollars per person per month and hospital care to be 22,569 dollars per patient per month. Giovannoni[52] reported an average hospital cost of 32,800 dollars a month for five ventilator-assisted patients in the hospital, compared with an average cost of 20,000 dollars for the first month at home for three patients successfully discharged. However, many chronic ventilator-dependent patients do not require the ICU level of care used by Giovannoni in her hospital cost estimates. Sivak and coworkers[78] estimated the average monthly cost of hospital care for ventilator-dependent patients to be 15,600 dollars (about half the cost estimated by Giovannoni), whereas the range of monthly costs for ten home care patients was 30 to 5673 dollars not including

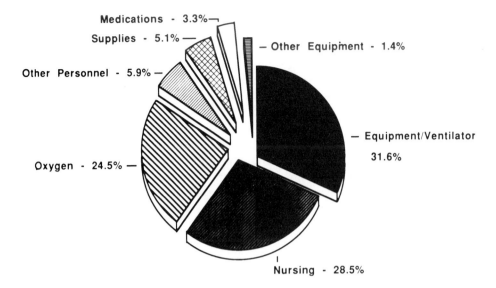

TOTAL MONTHLY COST - $2976

FIGURE 20-3 Average payments for home care for ventilator-assisted individuals in 1987 reported by the Boston University program. (LaFond L, et al. Home care costs for ventilator-assisted individuals. Ann Rev Respir Dis 1988; 137[4, part 2]:62)

equipment purchase. Unfortunately, home care equipment costs are often high, and equipment is often rented, rather than purchased, to ensure continued maintenance and home monitoring. In other reports, costs of home care have been reported to be as high as 16,000 dollars a month.[5,51]

It is clear that the single most expensive item in the home is the professional services of a nurse. If patients who are clinically stable are selected for home care, and if patients and families can become independent and self-sufficient through a comprehensive rehabilitation program, professional services required in the home may be reduced.

CARE IN ALTERNATIVE SITES

It is often difficult to determine the optimal site for continued care of ventilator-assisted individuals.[43,79] Unfortunately, all the options shown in Figure 20–4 are not available in all communities. Therefore, the decision to place a patient in a site outside the hospital is based upon the presence and availability of facilities and resources in the local community, as well as on the medical condition of the individual patient. All patients are managed in ICUs of acute care hospitals when positive-pressure mechanical ventilation is initiated on an emergency basis. Because many hospitals do not have other units with adequate skilled personnel and resources, ventilator-assisted patients often must remain in critical care units for the duration of their hospital stay. However, owing to the numerous ventilator patients, hospitals often develop step-

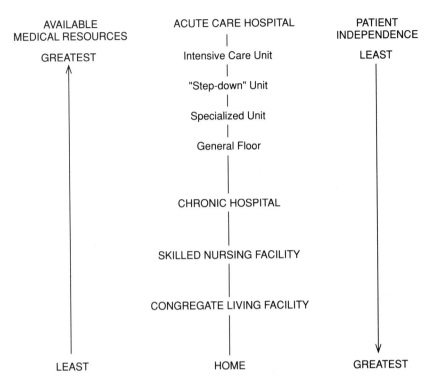

FIGURE   20-4   Sites for care of ventilator-assisted individuals. In general, facilities toward the bottom of the figure have fewer medical resources (physician, therapists, nurses, equipment), but show greater patient independence.

down units or other specialized areas to manage their patients, often with "noninvasive" monitoring.[44,80–82] In some regions of the United States, a limited number of beds are available in long-term care hospitals for patients.[20] Selected skilled nursing facilities (SNF) may admit such patients who are very stable, but SNF do not usually have 24-hour in-house physicians or therapists. Congregate living facilities are rarely available in the United States. Care for ventilator-assisted people is often more available and organized in a variety of nonhospital sites in other countries.[83]

Health care professionals must carefully assess the options for care available within their community and make the best choice of location, with patient safety as their foremost concern. Just as in home care, adequate skilled personnel, equipment, and supplies, sufficient to meet the needs of a comprehensive patient management plan must be available in an alternative care site.

REFERENCES

1. Affeldt JE, Bower AG, Dail CW, Aratan N. Prognosis for recovery in severe poliomyelitis. Arch Phys Med Rehabil 1957;38:290.

2. Alcock AJW, Hildelin H, Rasanen O, et al: Chronic respiratory paralysis. Acta Paediatr Scand 1972;228:1.

3. Fischer DA, Prentice WS. Feasibility of home care for certain respiratory-dependent restrictive or obstructive lung disease patients. Chest 1982;82:739.

4. Harrison GM, Mitchell MB. The medical and social outcome of 200 respirator and former respirator patients on home care. Arch Phys Med 1961;42:590.

5. Splaingard ML, Frates RC Jr, Harrison GM, et al: Home positive pressure ventilation: twenty year's experience. Chest 1983;84:376.

6. Christensen MS, Kristensen HS, Hansen EL. Artificial hyperventilation during 21 years in 3 cases of complete respiratory paralysis. Acta Med Scand 1975;198:409.

7. Drinker P, Shaw LA. An apparatus for the prolonged administration of artificial ventilation. J Clin Invest 1929;7:229.

8. Collier CR, Affeldt JE. Ventilatory efficiency of the cuirass respirator in totally paralyzed chronic poliomyelitis patients. J Appl Physiol 1954;6:531.

9. Flaum A. Experience in the use of a new respirator in the treatment of respiratory paralysis in poliomyelitis. Acta Med Scand Suppl 1936;78:849.

10. Eve FG. Activation of inert diaphragm by gravity method. Lancet 1932;2:995.

11. Plum F, Whedon GD. The rapid-rocking bed: its effect on the ventilation of poliomyelitis patients with respiratory paralysis. N Engl J Med 1951;245:235.

12. Adamson JP, Stein JD. Application of abdominal pressure for artificial respiration. JAMA 1959;169:1613.

13. Gilmartin ME, Make BJ, eds. Mechanical ventilation in the home—issues for health care providers. Probl Respir Care 1988;1:155.

14. Johnson DL, Giovannoni RM, Driscoll SA. Ventilator-assisted patient care: planning for hospital discharge and home care. Rockville, Md. Aspen, 1986

15. O'Donohue WJ, Giovannoni RM, Goldberg AF, et al. Long-term mechanical ventilation: guidelines for management in the home and at alternate community sites. Chest 1986;90(suppl):1S.

16. Douglas PS, Rosen RH, Butler PW, Bone RC. DRG payment for long-term ventilator patients: Implications and recommendations. Chest 1987;91:413.

17. Gracey DR, Gillespie D, Nobrega F, et al: Financial implications of prolonged ventilator care of Medicare patients under the prospective payment system. Chest 1987;91:424.

18. Make B, Dayno S, Gertman P. Prevalence of chronic ventilator-dependency. Am Rev Respir Dis 1986;132(4, part 2):A167.

19. Association holds press conferences on ventilator survey. AARTimes 1984;8(Apr):28.

20. Bone RC. Long-term ventilator care. A Chicago problem and a national problem. Chest 1987;92:536.

21. Garay SM, Turino GM, Goldring RM. Sustained reversal of chronic hypercapnia in patients with alveolar hypoventilation syndromes: long-term maintenance with noninvasive nocturnal mechanical ventilation. Am J Med 1981;70:269.

22. Hoeppner VH, Cockcroft DW, Dosman JA, et al: Nighttime ventilation improves respiratory failure in secondary kyphoscoliosis. Am Rev Respir Dis 1984;129:240.

23. Braun NMT, Marino WD. Effect of daily intermittent rest on respiratory muscles in patients with chronic airflow limitation. Chest 1984;85:595.

24. Cropp AJ, DiMarco AF, Altose MD. Effect of intermittent negative pressure on respiratory muscle function in patients with severe chronic obstructive pulmonary disease. Am Rev Respir Dis 1987;135:1056.

25. Gutierrez M, Beroiza T, Contreras G, et al. Weekly cuirass ventilation improves blood gases and inspiratory muscle strength in patients with chronic airflow limitation and hypercarbia. Am Rev Respir Dis 1988;138:617.

26. Pluto LA, Fahey PJ, Sorenson L, Chandrosekhar AJ. Effects of 8 weeks of INPV on

exercise parameters in patients with severe chronic obstructive lung disease. Am Rev Respir Dis 1985;131(4, part 2):64A.

27. Zibrak JD, Hill NS, Federman EC, O'Donnell C. Evaluation of intermittent long-term negative pressure ventilation in patients with severe chronic obstructive pulmonary disease. Am Rev Respir Dis 1988;138:1515.

28. Celli B, Lee H, Criner G, et al. Controlled trial of external negative pressure ventilation in patients with severe chronic airflow obstruction. Am Rev Respir Dis 1989;140:1251.

29. Rochester DF, Braun NMT, Laine S. Diaphragmatic energy expenditure in chronic respiratory failure. Am J Med 1977;63:223.

30. Rodenstein DO, Stanescu DC, Cuttita G, et al. Ventilatory and diaphragmatic EMG responses to negative pressure ventilation in airflow obstruction. J Appl Physiol 1988;65:1621.

31. Curran FJ. Night ventilation by body respirators for patients to chronic respiratory failure due to late-state Duchenne muscular dystrophy. Arch Phys Med Rehabil 1981;62:270.

32. Holtackers TR, Loosbrock LM, Gracey DR. The use of the chest cuirass in respiratory failure of neurologic origin. Respir Care 1982;27:271.

33. Kacmarek RM, Spearman CB. Equipment used for ventilatory support in the home. Respir Care 1986;31:311.

34. O'Donnell C, Gilmartin ME. Home mechanical ventilators and accessory equipment. Probl Respir Care 1988;1:217.

35. Alexander MA, Johnson EW, Petty J, et al. Mechanical ventilation of patients with late stage Duchenne muscular dystrophy: management in the home. Arch Phys Med Rehabil 1979;60:289.

36. Hill NS. Clinical application of body ventilators. Chest 1986;90:897.

37. Wiers PWJ, LeCoultre R, Dallingo OT, et al. Cuirass respirator treatment of chronic respiratory failure in scoliotic patients. Thorax 1977;32:221.

38. O'Donohue WJ Jr. Patient selection and discharge criteria for home ventilator care. Probl Respir Care 1988;1:167.

39. Make BJ. Long-term management of ventilator-assisted individuals: The Boston University experience. Respir Care 1986;31:303.

40. Davis PB, di Sant'Agnese PA. Assisted ventilation for patients with cystic fibrosis. JAMA 1978;239:1851.

41. Robert D, Gerard M, Leger P, et al. Domiciliary mechanical ventilation by tracheostomy for chronic respiratory failure. Rev Fr Mal Resp 1983;11:923.

42. Sivak ED, Cordasco EM, Gipson WT, et al. Home care ventilation: The Cleveland Clinic experience from 1977 to 1985. Respir Care 1986;31:294.

43. Prentice WS. Placement alternatives for long-term ventilator care. Respir Care 1986;31:288.

44. Indihar FJ, Walker NE. Experience with a prolonged respiratory care unit revisited. Chest 1984;86:616.

45. O'Donohue W, Petty TL, Plummer A, et al. Consensus conference on problems in home mechanical ventilation. Am Rev Respir Dis 1989;140:555.

46. LaFond L, Horner J. Psychological issues related to long-term ventilatory support. Probl Respir Care 1988;1:241.

47. Alba A, Pilkington LA, Kaplan E, et al. Long-term pulmonary care in amyotrophic lateral sclerosis. Respir Ther 1986;16:49.

48. Banaszak EF, Travers H, Fraizer M, et al. Home ventilator care. Respir Care 1981;26:1262.

49. Burr BH, Buyer B, Todres ID, et al. Home care for children on respirators. N Engl J Med 1983;309:1319.

50. Dunkin LJ. Home ventilatory assistance. Anaesthesia 1983;38:644.

51. Feldman J, Tuteur PG. Mechanical ventilation: from hospital intensive care to home. Heart Lung 1982;11:162.

52. Giovannoni R. Chronic ventilator care: from hospital to home. Respir Ther 1984;14:29.

53. Glover DW. Three years at home on an MA-1. Respir Ther 1981;11:69.

54. Goldberg AI, Kettrick R, Buzdygan D, et al. Home ventilation program for infants and children. Crit Care Med 1980;31:238.

55. Home ventilation: status in Ontario. Ont Med Rev 1986;(Jan):14.

56. Kopacz MA, Moriarty-Wright R. Multidisciplinary approach for the patient on a home ventilator. Heart Lung 1984;13:255.

57. Bach JR, Alba AS, Bohatuik G. Mouth intermittent positive pressure ventilation in the management of post polio respiratory insufficiency. Chest 1987;91:859.

58. Bach JR, Alba A, Mosher R. Intermittent positive pressure ventilation via nasal access in the management of respiratory insufficiency. Chest 1987;92:168.

59. Splaingard ML, Frates RC, Jefferson LS, et al. Home negative pressure ventilation: report of 20 years experience in patients with neuromuscular disease. Arch Phys Med Rehabil 1985;66:239.

60. Make B, Gilmartin M, Brody JS, et al. Rehabilitation of ventilator-dependent subjects with lung diseases: the concept and initial experience. Chest 1984;86:358.

61. Dull WL, Sadoul P. Home ventilators in patients with severe lung disease. Am Rev Respir Dis 1981;123(suppl):74.

62. Czorniak MA, Gilmartin ME, Make BJ. Home mechanical ventilation: clinical course of patients with neuromuscular disease (NMD) and chronic obstructive pulmonary disease (COPD). Am Rev Respir Dis 1987;135(4, part 2):194A.

63. Gilmartin M, Make B. Home care of ventilator-dependent persons. Respir Care 1983;28:1490.

64. McPherson SP: Respiratory home care equipment. Dubuque: Kendall/Hunt, 1988

65. Kacmarek RM, Stanck KS, McMahon K, et al. Improved work of breathing during synchronized intermittent mandatory ventilation (SIMV) via home care ventilators. Am Rev Respir Dis 1988;137(4, part 2):64.

66. Leger P, Jennequin J, Gerard M, Robert D. Home positive pressure ventilation via nasal mask for patients with neuromuscular weakness or restrictive lung or chest wall disease. Respir Care 1989;34:73.

67. Kerby GR, Mayer LS, Pingleton SK. Nocturnal positive pressure ventilation via nasal mask. Am Rev Respir Dis 1987;137:738.

68. Miller JH, Thomas E, Wilmont CB. Pneumobelt use among high quadriplegic population. Arch Phys Med Rehabil 1988;69:369.

69. Wilson DJ. Airway management of the ventilator-assisted individual. Probl Respir Care 1988;1:192.

70. Schreiner MS, Downes JJ, Kettrick RG, et al. Chronic respiratory failure in infants with prolonged ventilator failure. JAMA 1987;258:3398.

71. Lawrence PA. Home care for ventilator-dependent children: providing a chance to live a normal life. Dimens Crit Care Nurs 1984;3:42.

72. Report of the Brook Lodge symposium on the ventilator-dependent child: La Rabida Children's Hospital and Research Center, 1984. (Copies may be obtained from Children's Home Health Network of Illinois, East 56th Street, Chicago, IL 60649)

73. Report of the Surgeon General's workshop on children with handicaps and their families. Washington, DC: US Department of Health and Human Services, 1982

74. Kettrick RG, Donar ME. Ventilator-assisted infants and children. Probl Respir Care 1988;1:269.

75. Frates RC, Splaingard ML, Smith DO, et al: Outcome of home mechanical ventilation in children. J Pediatr 1985;106:850.

76. Moser KM. Home mechanical ventilation and the cost of humane care. J Respir Dis 1986;7(3):15.

77. LaFond L, Make BJ, Gilmartin ME. Home care costs for ventilator-assisted individuals. Am Rev Respir Dis 1988;137(4, part 2):62.

78. Sivak ED, Cordasco EM, Gipson WT. Pulmonary mechanical ventilation at home: a reasonable and less expensive alternative. Respir Care 1983;28:42.

79. Prentice WC. Transition from hospital to home. Probl Respir Care 1988;1:174.

80. Krieger BP, Ershowsky P, Spivack D, et al. Initial experience with a noninvasive respiratory monitoring unit as a cost-saving alternative to the intensive care unit for Medicare patients who require long-term ventilator support. Chest 1988;93:395.

81. Bone RC, Balk RA. The noninvasive respiratory care unit—a cost-effective solution for the future. Chest 1988;93:390.

82. O'Donohue WJ, Branson RD, Hoppough JM, Make BJ. Criteria for establishing units for chronic ventilator-dependent patients in hospitals. Respir Care 1988;33:1044.

83. Goldberg AI. Home care for life-supported persons: is a national approach the answer? Chest 1986;90:744.

MARY BURNS

21

Social and Recreational Support of the Pulmonary Patient

Graduation from pulmonary rehabilitation (PR) is like graduation from high school. Basic skills have been learned, physical conditioning has been improved, and there is hope for a better and brighter future. Graduation should mark the beginning of continued improvement in exercise tolerance and quality of life. Sometimes it does. More often we find that after a few months the patient begins to slide back into the old habits of inactivity, isolation, and depression so commonly seen in respiratory patients before PR. What can be done to prevent this when funding for maintenance outpatient (OP) visits is not available? You can offer your patients a support group.

NAME OF YOUR GROUP

Better Breathers Club (BBC) is adequate until you can come up with a name more meaningful to your patients. This may occur during organizational meetings of the group or perhaps not until the group has gotten together a few times.

The "Pulmonary Education Program," is the name of our program at Little Company of Mary Hospital in Torrance, California, and forms the acronym "PEP." Our graduates call themselves the PEP Pioneers because when the group started many years ago they were pioneering a new way of life. The name PEP Pioneer instills a sense of pride that BBC could probably never inspire in this group. Examples of other support group names include "The Inspirations," "The Huff and Puffers," "The Windpipers," and "The Pacers" to name a few.

JUSTIFICATION FOR SUPPORT GROUPS

Your BBC can be used to encourage continued involvement in activities outside the home and provide incentives for staying active. It offers your PR graduate continued updating of information and education begun in rehabilitation classes. It allows your hospital to maintain ties with increasingly loyal patients who will use your hospital for their continued care. And it allows your PR staff an inexpensive way of doing follow-up. Perhaps most important, it offers your patients friendship, encouragement, and caring from others who also understand what it is like to be short of breath.

It is very difficult for some respiratory patients to make the decision to start pulmonary rehabilitation. Attending BBC meetings may help prospective members make that decision. It also helps them start their PR classes with the positive attitude that they can be helped as much as other patients they have met. Notices of BBC meetings also provide publicity for your program and show your hospital's involvement in the community.

If you are thinking about starting a PR program you should seriously consider beginning a patient support group first. This could help you establish the need for PR in your area, develop community awareness of your program, and build a listing of patients to approach when you are able to start your program.

GETTING STARTED

A supportive pulmonary rehabilitation physician can help obtain permission and assistance from hospital administration in starting your support group and referring patients. A convenient place to meet on a regular basis is the first and perhaps most difficult challenge to overcome. Most hospitals have meeting rooms that can be used, but remember to take parking access into consideration. Parking should be convenient. Some hospitals have van pick ups. Our hospital provides valet parking just for our monthly meetings.

If there are no suitable meeting areas in your hospital, consider using a room at your local ALA, YMCA, or church.

Afternoon meetings work best for our pulmonary patients who have difficulty getting started in the morning and do not like to be out after dark. Timing your guest speaker between 1 and 2 PM avoids cutting into a physician's office hours and gets your patients home before rush-hour traffic. Let your meeting time be long enough to permit socialization. The PEP Pioneers have always had a luncheon meeting, but simple snacks work just as well.

The guest speaker, usually a physician or allied health professional, has a topic of specific interest to the patient with respiratory disease. Subjects that consistently draw a big crowd are asthma, medications, prednisone, and any title that includes the word *new*.

GETTING PATIENTS INVOLVED

Getting your BBC started is only half the battle. Now you have to get your patients involved. Remember that these often are people who have been inactive and isolated for years. They have experienced many "bad days" and are afraid of making a commitment they will not be able to fulfill.

Rule number one: Do not expect anyone to volunteer. Ask for help, but start with something easy that they are sure to do well. Requesting a member to sit next to a prospective member at a BBC meeting is a good beginning. Tell your patients you are counting on them to make nervous newcomers welcome. If a patient is too shy for even that, ask him or her to watch your camera, or your pen and note pad, so that you will not misplace them. Ask someone receiving oxygen if they will sit up front and tape the guest speaker. Your more outgoing patients might like to act as official hosts and hostesses, complete with badges to identify them. Find something that they can help you with to build up their confidence, for the more your patients are able to help, the more enthusiastic they become.

Even the most limited patient can be part of your phone committee. We assign ten names to each member. Calls are made every month to remind people about the upcoming meeting and to see how they are doing. This information, and any problems, are reported to the telephone chairperson. She or he, in turn, calls the PEP staff member with a synopsis of what has been going on. In this way the PR staff can keep posted on everything of importance, yet the time involved is limited to one or two phone calls.

Most people like being called and knowing that someone cares. Occasionally, we get requests for more frequent calls and find that our phone committee members are very pleased to know that they can help.

One very important contribution two or three PEP Pioneers make to each new PEP class is to be there the first day of the program to greet new students. The Pioneers give them a "PEP" talk about the value of PR, the value of exercise, and the impact it has in improving their lives. These testimonials profoundly effect everyone, including the staff. We start off on such a positive note that no one has ever dropped out of the program except for severe illness or injury.

On the last day of class the same Pioneers who welcomed the new group come again to officially make the graduates and their spouses PEP Pioneers. Along with a diploma from PEP they receive a PEP Pioneer badge with their name, and a list of all the members with their addresses and phone numbers. They also receive a free lunch certificate for the first meeting after graduation.

At their first PEP Pioneer luncheon meeting the new members have reserved seating front and center. They are individually introduced to the group with a short biography to help members find common bonds.

Patient Board of Directors

As your patient club grows and you succeed in getting patients involved, consider forming a Patient Board. This can be as simple or elaborate as you wish. We have co-officers for each position so that no one feels the burden of responsibility will be too much. Spouses are also considered vital members of the club and may hold office. At times when a patient might be reluctant to assume even a co-office, having the "better half" along may make the difference. This seems to strengthen the marriage and it also gives your club some members without respiratory disease. What this can translate into is as many as four people for one office. Although this rarely occurs, it is an asset, rather than a liability. Your board members become the strongest supporters of your BBC so the more you have the better your club will be.

Our board meetings are held once a month, the week before our patient luncheon meeting. During meetings a PR staff member, who is part of the board, keeps the board informed on what is going on with PR and gets board input on problems or policy changes. Upcoming social events are planned and the PR staff stays aware of new ways to meet the needs of the group.

Board members include two for each office of Co-chairman, Co-vice Chairman, Co-treasurer, Co-secretary, and Co-liaison officers, the latter being the board members who help the PEP staff with problems as they arise. Warning! Be very careful about who gets chosen as Treasurer. This needs to be someone who is reliable about finances and healthy enough to follow through with their responsibilities. The PR staff members who know patients' backgrounds can request a qualified patient or spouse to "volunteer" for this position.

Our board has rather informal meetings where Robert's Rules are not strictly enforced and the by-laws are simple.

Other Committees

Other important activities that your group can get involved with include a "Sunshine" committee that sends out birthday and get-well cards. Do not underestimate the value of this gesture. Sometimes this is the only card the patient receives, and it means a great deal to them.

The club historian keeps up the scrapbook of pictures and clippings. The librarian keeps track of tapes of guest speakers and books to be loaned. Having one or two people to write thank you notes to all guest speakers is also particularly helpful. Patients interested in crafts set up workshops for the Christmas Boutique or make favors for holiday luncheons.

Dues and Expenses

The PEP Pioneers have no dues. They raise money with an annual Christmas Boutique and a monthly White Elephant Raffle. Donations include fruit from trees and home-baked goods as well as white elephants. Ten dollars is taken out of the raffle money each month and used as a first prize.

Buffet luncheons are served by the hospital at their regular community charge. There is no charge for patients who come for the lecture, but do not eat.

The PEP Pioneer treasury is used to pay for an annual Christmas dinner for all Pioneers and a significant other if they do not have a spouse. At the Christmas party five or six winners are randomly picked to receive free luncheons for the year. The Pioneers also buy about 35 boxes of candy to be distributed around the hospital as thanks to people who have been helpful during the year. Distribution ranges from the emergency room to kitchen workers who serve their monthly luncheons.

During the year the board also occasionally arranges for "donations from Pioneers who have moved" to help out proud but needy Pioneers. When any Pioneers pass away a donation is made in their name to the hospital and to PERF, the Pulmonary Education and Research Foundation. [This is a small foundation that was started by patients, with the goal of using relatively small amounts of money where it will do the most good clinically. PERF has just produced two booklets for patients, *Essentials of Pulmonary Rehabilitation: A "Do it Yourself" Program*, Part I and Part II, available at no charge by writing to PERF, P.O. Box 1133, Lomita, CA 90717-5133.]

Newsletter

The PEP Pioneer newsletter, *The Second Wind*, started out as a 1-page typed summary of our monthly meeting. It now is a 14-page monthly newsletter that goes all over the country. A simple newsletter bringing members up to date about activities helps tie your group together. Many groups reprint a summary of monthly guest speakers' comments and Dr. Thomas Petty's letter. Dr. Petty's only stipulation is that his letter not be edited in any way, and our only wish is to have the original source of the summary acknowledged.

Folding, taping, and labeling the newsletter in preparation for mailing is another way to keep patients active. There is a lot of socialization in this group, and it is another good way to get patients started volunteering.

Walking Groups

Patients graduate from our PR walking an hour a day, but time, vacations, and illnesses often have a way of interfering with their daily walk. One of the prime objectives of your BBC should be to keep patients physically active. There are a variety of ways to accomplish this.

Contests

To give even your most limited patient an incentive, base the contest on time rather than distance. We consider one-half hour of walking or 15 minutes on the bike to equal 1 mile in our contests. Give out prizes for as many things as you can possibly think of and try to put a few patients in charge of keeping records. We once had a very successful "Walk to New York" for which mileage was posted each month on a large map. Our patient in charge of the walk wrote a page in the newsletter each month about the town where our mileage ended and even arranged to get letters of welcome from then Mayor Koch of New York and Mayor Clint Eastwood of Carmel. It was pretty hard to top that even by the Mayor of Torrance who arranged an official proclamation welcoming us back to Torrance and making it "PEP Pioneer Day."

Mall Walks

Malls are ideal for respiratory patients. They are air-conditioned, flat, and have seating and rest rooms. We were successful in getting one of the local malls to dedicate a measured walk to the PEP Pioneers, complete with a ribbon-cutting ceremony and newspaper coverage.

A group of our patients meet at the mall 1 day a week to walk, socialize, and eat. If you have a patient newly on oxygen who does not want to be seen in public this is the kind of group you can turn to for help.

Respiratory Rally

An Annual Respiratory Rally where patients, families, and staff from hospitals in your area can gather together for education, fellowship, and fun is the ultimate in support group meetings.

Drug companies and oxygen suppliers sponsor buses for groups from other hospitals and provide an honorarium for the guest speaker should you need one. Door prizes can be solicited from various businesses in the area.

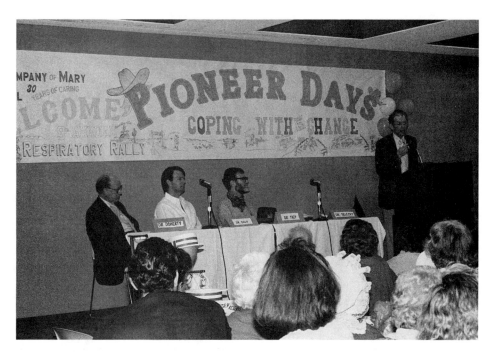

FIGURE 21-1 Annual Respiratory Rally meeting of the PEP Pioneers.

Highlights of our annual program include having a well-known pulmonary physician as guest speaker (Fig. 21–1) and the "Pace Race" (Fig. 21–2).

The object of the Pace Race is to estimate the time, within 0.01 minute, it takes to walk a measured area. The 3 to 7 minutes it takes to complete this short course makes it feasible for even the most limited of patients. An accurate stop watch can be borrowed from a local high school. Respiratory therapy students are great for cheering on the sidelines, while gifts for participants, with a certificate saying they completed a race, add to the fun. Someone on oxygen almost always comes in with first place, whereas one of the nurses or doctors is usually last, when it comes to pacing.

Bus Trips

Although completion of PR should enable patients to take trips on their own, many benefit by group support. A good way to start is a short day trip on a bus.

Be sure you get administrative approval, and see if your legal department wants passengers to sign a waiver. Make sure the trip you have planned does not require too much walking or too many stairs or hills. Accessible rest rooms are a must and that includes a bathroom in your air-conditioned bus. Once you find a bus company you like, continue to use it and request the same driver. We tip well and the drivers and bus company go out of their way to be helpful to us.

Provide a parking area for patients' cars during the day that has easy access to the bus. A footstool for getting in and out of the bus and a wheelchair for emergencies are

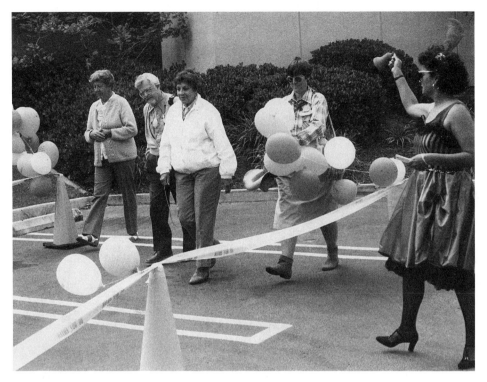

FIGURE   21-2   Participants in the Pace Race being encouraged on from the sidelines.

good to have along. The PR staff should note the number of passengers who will be on oxygen therapy, what their liter flow is, and what system they are using. The durable medical equipment (DME) supplier we use gives us a large container of oxygen for the back of the bus, along with a few portable units for emergencies. If the patient has a system incompatible with ours, or is using an E-cylinder, we lend them one of our portable units for the day. Sometimes patients also require an oxygen-conserving device, used with the permission of their physician.

Passengers should pay in advance. Giving full refunds for last minute cancellations is too hard on the club treasury. If patients get sick at the last minute they should be responsible for finding a replacement, although we do try to have a standby list for these occasions.

If your patient group is not large enough to fill a bus, ask other patient groups in the area to join you. Other alternatives are minivans or having patients drive themselves to your destination.

These bus trips are a lot of fun for everyone and build a real sense of friendship in the group.

Cruises

Cruises are the most glamorous of patient club activities and particularly appropriate for pulmonary patients. There are no problems with altitude and no pollens or pollutants to trigger bronchospasm. Our initial cruise in 1984 was historic in that it marked the first time oxygen-dependent patients were allowed on board a ship (Fig. 21–3).[1] Since then, other hospitals have sponsored cruises.

If your BBC wants you to arrange a cruise, the support of a physician, administrative approval, and waivers from the legal department are necessary before proceeding.

Cruises sound like a lot of fun, and they are. However, the staff arranging for the cruise should be prepared for many hours of work if they wish to have a safe and smooth voyage.[2] Do not depend on a travel agent to do the work for you. They are not accustomed to handling the special needs of our patients, especially arrangements for oxygen.

Although the Coast Guard and many cruise lines now allow passengers with medical oxygen on board, this is subject to change. It is essential that you have a clear understanding of the requirements and restrictions of the cruise line on which you wish to sail. There are some that still do not allow oxygen-dependent patients on board. Some ships allow concentrators, whereas others will refuse concentrators, but allow liquid oxygen to be stored in the individual cabins. If you are at all uneasy about the response you receive, especially second-hand from a travel agent, get permission in writing.

Refer to regulation DOT-E 9856 if you have a problem with oxygen use on board the ship. This can be obtained from the U.S. Department of Transportation, Office of

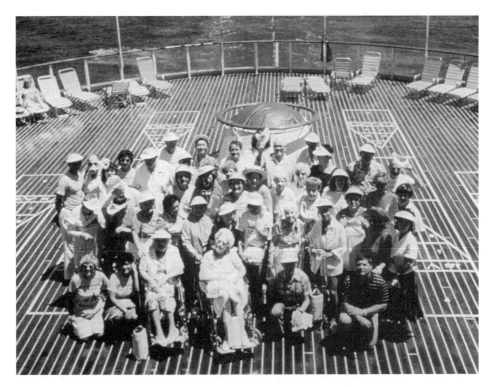

FIGURE   21-3   Patients on the deck of a cruise ship.

Hazardous Material Transportation, Exemptions and Approvals Division (DHM-30), 400 7th St., SW, Washington, DC 20590.[3,4] For specific questions concerning special provisions you can contact the Hazardous Materials Branch, U.S. Coast Guard Headquarters, Commandant (G-MTH-1), 2100 Second St. SW, Washington, DC 20593 or call (202) 267-1577. In my many contacts with the Coast Guard in both Los Angeles and Washington I have always found them to be helpful and very courteous.

When you know what your oxygen needs will be and what the cruise line restrictions are, you can contact your local DME to arrange for preboarding of oxygen and removal after disembarking. Store a few extra units in staff cabins, since valves can freeze open and vent off all the oxygen. Make sure all patients have portable units that can transfill from the unit stored in their cabin. To limit the amount of oxygen you need to bring along have patients use oxygen-conserving devices, especially when they are in their cabins. They will need the permission of their physician and an oximetry check if they have not previously used conserving devices, such as the Oxymizer or Pendant.

The amount of staff you need on the cruise will depend on how sick your patient group is and how many are your regular BBC members who are well known to you. Minimum staff would be a pulmonary rehabilitation or emergency room physician, a nurse, and a respiratory therapist. The physician's work on board should be minimal, since all calls can be triaged by the nurse or therapist.

In addition to a spouse, many patients wish to bring another couple with them. Since cruise line group discounts can be used to help pay for staff these extra "healthy" guests are most welcome. Some lines are more generous with discounts than others so shop around.

When booking rooms, try to have the sickest patients nearest the elevators or staff.

Screening patients is very important, especially if they are not graduates of your PR program. Checklists are very helpful in making sure you have not forgotten anything. All patients should have a history record and a physical examination, pulmonary function test (PFT), and arterial blood gas analysis (ABG), so that you can better know their condition. Patients also need to provide you with a list of their current medications. Although all your patients should have permission from their physician to sail with you, do not depend on this to give you a patient who will be safe to take along.

A preacceptance interview and a 6-minute walk on the oximeter are essential for patients who are not known to you. Some patients are so badly deconditioned that they cannot walk more than 1 or 2 minutes. If they wish to have a safe and enjoyable cruise they need to be started on a conditioning program of daily walking. We ask that everyone be able to walk a minimum of 15 minutes. With a cruise as a carrot, even a few bed-bound patients have achieved this goal for us.

Another potential problem to watch for in your interview is the confused patient. We have had far more difficulty with this than with respiratory exacerbations, especially in patients who were not part of our regular group. The stress of being in unfamiliar surroundings can cause patients to become bewildered and lost. Ships' physicians call it the "sundowner syndrome" because it gets worse in the evening.

Make sure that the supplies and medications you bring with you contain diuretics. Even anorexic patients gain weight on a cruise and, since large amounts of high-sodium foods are consumed, fluid retention is also a problem. Special diets can be arranged in advance.

Patients who are not part of your regular group benefit from attending a few BBC meetings before the cruise so that you start out with a group known to you and to each other.

On-board activities can be as structured or as casual as you wish. Patients form their own walking groups, but will also attend formal exercise sessions or lectures if you care to plan them. Staff responsibilities include helping fill portable oxygen units, making sure no one gets lost, and making sure that the shy patient is kept part of the group.

Patients and their spouses disembark from a cruise exhilarated, ready to plan their next trip.

Individual Travel

After successfully taking part in group travel, or sometimes after graduating from PR, patients are often ready to venture forth on their own.[5] An excellent reference would be the chapters on travel and altitude in *Portable Oxygen Therapy* by Tiep.[6] Although it is geared to the patient receiving oxygen, the principles apply to all patients.

Some general advice would be to allow lots of time to make plans and reservations well in advance of the travel date. The patient's physician should be consulted for advice, and a summary of his or her history and physical examination along with extra prescriptions should be given to the patient. If the trip is extended, the physician may wish to provide the patient with antibiotics and prednisone to take in the event of an exacerbation if this is part of the patient's usual regimen. Extra amounts of regularly taken medications are wise to have along in case of accidents. Stool softeners are also good to have on hand, since constipation is a frequent complication of travel. The patient's physician may be able to recommend a physician in the area of travel. Patients can of course call their own regular physician directly for advice.

Making arrangements with the local pharmacist to send medications by overnight mail is often easier than trying to refill prescriptions out of state or seeing a new doctor for a prescription.

Remind your patients to check on the altitude of their destination *and* of their itinerary.[7,8] Temperature, humidity, and air pollution should be taken into consideration. Traveling light is always good advice. Patients should also be reminded to stay well hydrated, well rested, and to interrupt long periods of sitting with movement of the feet and ankles to maintain circulation and prevent blood clots.

The patient receiving oxygen therapy needs to discuss the itinerary with his or her oxygen supplier, take along extra copies of the oxygen prescription, and be prepared to pay for oxygen in cash at companies other than the regular provider. Receipts should be kept so that reimbursement can be obtained when the patient returns home.

Further hints on travel can be obtained from travel books at the library. Lung associations and companies providing oxygen can be contacted for brochures specific to the needs of the respiratory patient.

Patients wishing to travel outside the United States need to plan carefully and, as a rule, avoid countries with primitive medical support systems. They need to be reminded to check their insurance coverage carefully and also trip cancellation clauses for pre-existing conditions. An excellent resource is Eurolung Assistance, which lists physicians, hospitals, and oxygen suppliers for travelers throughout the world.[9]

Travel adds zest to life and patients should be assisted and encouraged to expand their horizons.

SUMMARY

Social and recreational support of pulmonary patients is an important aspect of their care and well being. The BBCs provide educational updates, social support, and PR program follow-up. They are useful in maintaining patient activity levels and preventing withdrawal and social isolation. Obtaining patient support in achieving these goals helps control the amount of PR staff time and money expended but, more importantly, also benefits the pulmonary patient.

Acknowledgments

The author wishes to thank Betsy Barnes, Jackie Herrera, and the PEP Pioneers for their support and assistance.

REFERENCES

1. Burns M. Cruising with COPD. Am Jr Nurs 1987;87:479.

2. Burns M. Travel and the COPD patient: planning for problems. Respir Times 1988;4:10.

3. Olenik P. Planning a cruise? AARC Times 1988;4:24.

4. Maguire J, Randazzo J, Lundstedt D, Bobeck J. Requirements for traveling with oxygen. AARC Times 1988;4:31.

5. Burns M. Travel hints for the person with COPD. In: Petty T, Nett L, eds. Enjoying life with emphysema. 2nd ed. 1987:103.

6. Burns M. Travel with oxygen. In: Tiep BL, ed. Portable oxygen therapy. New York: Futura Press, 1991

7. Gong H. Guidelines for travel with oxygen in advanced COPD. Respir Times 1986;1:22.

8. Gong H, Tashkin D, Lee EY, Simmons MS. Hypoxemia-altitude simulation test. Am Rev Respir Dis 1984;130:980.

9. Eurolung Assistance. F. Smeets, M.D., Centre Hospitalier de Saint-Ode, 6970 Tenneville, Belgium, Tel.: 32-84-4554444.

BRIAN L. TIEP

Biofeedback and Respiratory Muscle Training

Pulmonary rehabilitation is the definitive approach to the long-term management of patients with chronic lung disease.[1-3] The essence of chronic lung disease *is* its chronicity. It is permanent—it will not go away, and it will probably get worse over time. Furthermore, chronic lung disease does not occur suddenly; it starts out slowly and progresses slowly and insidiously. In contrast with acute conditions, patients have time to adapt by slowly becoming less active. Their personalities become embodied in growing dependency, inactivity, disability, and giving up control of their lives to others. Consequently, chronic lung disease takes on not only a pathophysiologic structure, but a behavioral structure also.

Pulmonary rehabilitation teams assume the task of reversing this trend. The patient must become active and take control over his or her life and disease. The self-concept must once again be vital. When the patient looks in the mirror, the reflected image is that of a person who is active and in control.

In rehabilitation, patients become involved in their own care. The patient becomes an extension of the physician, carrying out daily bronchial hygiene, exercise to build strength and endurance, self-medication, and monitoring of health signs. Patients learn the important signs and symptoms that indicate the need for medical support, when to report to the physician, and how to effectively communicate changes in health status.

Both biofeedback training and ventilatory muscle training exemplify and contribute to the rehabilitation process—promoting patient self-management and independence. *Biofeedback* teaches self-control over physiologic functions, and *ventilatory muscle training* builds strength and endurance in the respiratory muscles. Since these therapeutic approaches are really separate issues, they will be described separately. Actually, ventilatory muscle training is increasingly employing threshold and goal-shaping techniques common to biofeedback training. Thus, these two modalities may compatibly intersect. Biofeedback will be presented first to establish some insight into its application in ventilatory muscle training.

403

BIOFEEDBACK

Inherent in biofeedback is the intriguing concept that people can be taught to willfully direct internal bodily functions to increase or decrease their activity. The most common application of biofeedback has been stress management by teaching major muscle groups to relax, but recently, the scope of biofeedback training has broadened to include a wider variety of physiologic functions. By using biofeedback, patients learn to modify such autonomically controlled functions as vasomotor activity, heart rate, blood pressure, and bronchomotor tone, as well as brain waves and electromyography. In many ways, biofeedback attempts to nonchemically emulate pharmacology. The implication emerges that successful biofeedback training might lead to a replacement for medications. Although such a goal is attractive, the effects of biofeedback tend to be mild, so that complete replacement of pharmaceuticals is rare. As biofeedback applications have increased, its role in medicine has been expanding; in fact, skin temperature biofeedback may be the treatment of choice for certain vascular headaches.

Biofeedback Training

Biofeedback is the training of physiologic control over body functions previously assumed to be out of reach of such willful control. These are usually autonomic functions that, in earlier times, were considered and assumed to be automatic—unconnected to centers in the brain where such learning takes place. Since people are unable to perceive the operation of these internal functions, the assumption of inaccessibility was reasonable. The missing ingredient was the ability to know either the status of the physiologic function or its relative change. Biofeedback came into being with the advent of physiologic instrumentation that could continuously monitor and feed back physiologic data to the patient. The patient can then learn to influence that function. The feedback presentation format can be *audio*, such as a variable-pitched tone, or *visual*, such as a voltmeter or light display. For training to be successful, absolute physiologic values are unnecessary; what is important is immediate and accurate representation of relative physiologic change (Fig. 22–1).

By using this continuous stream of data, the patient practices various strategies to influence the biofeedback monitor display. Since all biologic systems are dynamic (i.e., continuously changing), patients have the opportunity to learn to modify the direction and degree of that physiologic variation. Patients who are motivated can perfect biofeedback control through a system of trial and error, although, when questioned, they are rarely able to relate how they affect such control.

Thus, in principle, biofeedback blends learning theory with physiologic instrumentation. The patients in training hone their physiologic skills by a series of experimental trials. They attempt to vary their physiologic function while paying attention to the effect of each trial on the monitor display. The change in the monitor display will be encouraging or discouraging, depending on the biofeedback display's indication of success, or lack of success, of the given strategy; as a result, the patient may choose to continue that line of strategy or switch to another. A training session comprises many such trials.

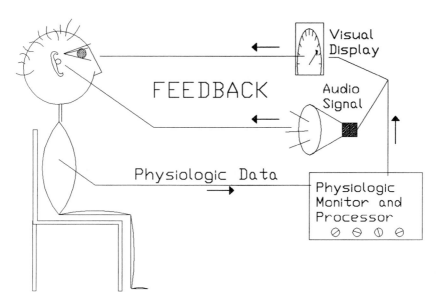

FIGURE   22-1   Biofeedback Loop: Physiologic function is monitored; displayed to the patient; patient attempts to modulate physiologic function; monitor display informs the patient if any change has occurred; the patient then modifies the intervention.

As one examines this process of biofeedback learning, it becomes obvious that there is very little that is unique about it. Most learning uses this principle of trial and error. Consider bicycle riding. The person attempts many strategies and is very clumsy at first, but eventually learns by trial and error. The difference in learning to ride a bicycle resides in the fact that all information is external. The person is immediately aware of the consequences of each trial and is thereby able to modify the next trial. In biofeedback, the patient is required to control an internal event; thus, the information must be externalized by a physiologic monitor so that control is possible. Otherwise, the approach to learning is the same.

Biofeedback techniques have been applied in many areas of medicine including neurology, cardiology, pulmonology, immunology, and gastroenterology. Most of these areas are just beginning to be explored.

Respiratory Biofeedback

Several biofeedback techniques have been applied to patients with pulmonary disorders, often within the purview of pulmonary rehabilitation. In pulmonary rehabilitation, patients are taught and encouraged to gain control over their lives. In respiratory biofeedback, a signal relating to some respiratory function is monitored and displayed to the patient, who attempts to modify that function in some useful fashion. Biofeedback has been used in patients with asthma, emphysema, and pulmonary fibrosis and has been used to improve gas exchange and reduce the work of breathing.

Asthma

Bronchial asthma is an inflammatory disease of the airways in which reversible airway obstruction is a major feature. Bronchospasm is probably the most immediately reversible component of asthma. Because the airways are enervated by a rich network of autonomic fibers, several biofeedback approaches are directed to relaxing bronchomotor tone, presumably through these neural pathways.[4] Many psychologists and physicians still envision asthma to be largely emotional or psychophysiologic in origin. Even though most experts do not now hold to that notion, that belief system led to the earliest nonpharmacologic approaches designed to control emotions and reduce stress. It is difficult to deny that among the many triggers emotional factors can precipitate asthmatic attacks. McFadden in 1969[5] and Spector and associates in 1976[6] demonstrated that suggestion, in the form of placebo aerosol challenges, can provoke and reverse asthma attacks. These responses can be blocked by atropine. These reports suggested that higher centers in the brain are capable of influencing bronchomotor tone in either direction, presumably through the vagus nerve.

ANXIOLYTIC THERAPY Anxiolytic methodologies have met with some success in many asthmatics because, in spite of little or no evidence for psychologic etiology, asthma itself is a stressor.[7] The effectiveness of relaxation as primary therapy is seriously questioned.[8] It may be useful in reducing spasms of the larger airways, but probably has little or no effect on smaller airways.[9] Sedatives, tranquilizers, and nonpharmacologic stress reduction techniques are not considered effective single asthma therapy. Despite this, techniques that relieve stress are logically adjunctive to any asthma self-management program. From the physiologist's standpoint, the best stress reduction is to maximize physiologic control over asthma.

ELECTROMYOGRAPHIC BIOFEEDBACK Electromyographic (EMG) biofeedback, a commonly employed biofeedback therapy for general relaxation and stress reduction, is gaining some participatory role in the treatment of asthma.[10] In most applications, EMG electrodes are positioned over the frontalis muscle and the patients are taught to relax these muscles with the assumption that many other muscles groups will follow suit, leading to general relaxation. This is a well-recognized form of relaxation training.

Glaus and Kotses have asserted that EMG biofeedback has a therapeutic benefit beyond that of relaxation; that facial muscle tension and bronchomotor tone are linked reflexively.[11-13] This contention will require further study. Moreover, further study is required to determine the efficacy of EMG feedback for asthma.

DIAPHRAGMATIC BREATHING Several methods have been used to encourage slow, deep breathing and diaphragmatic breathing in asthma. Diaphragmatic breathing generally is characterized by slower breath rates and larger tidal volumes. If we assume a stable deadspace volume (V_D) and a larger tidal volume (V_T) from deep diaphragmatic breathing, the V_D/V_T will become smaller. This should improve gas exchange by increasing alveolar ventilation. Also, slower breathing tends to reduce airways resistance by slowing airflow and decreasing turbulence. Patients generally report symptomatic benefit from diaphragmatic breathing, although there is little data confirming its gas exchange benefits.

INCENTIVE SPIROMETRY Peper and coworkers have used an incentive spirometer to facilitate diaphragmatic breathing training.[14–16] The goal is to encourage deep diaphragmatic breathing while decreasing upper thoracic efforts. Often these training approaches include hand-warming skills with skin temperature biofeedback and guided imagery, EMG training, and prolonged exhalation. Their patients were able to reduce their upper chest wall EMG voltages and increase their inhalation volumes by practicing these techniques. These changes were accompanied by an improvement in symptom score and reductions in breathlessness, medication use, and frequency of emergency room visits. One of their studies demonstrated 25% posttraining improvement in 1-second forced expiratory volume (FEV_1) and prevention of exercise bronchospasm.[16]

PEAK EXPIRATORY FLOW Patients are often taught to measure the status of their asthma using a peak expiratory flowmeter. Khan has taken peak flow measurement one step further by using the peak flowmeter as a biofeedback device.[17] The patient is trained to increase peak flow by multiple trials in a kind of peak flow exercise-training venture. The patient tries to improve peak flow performance on each succeeding trial. Khan reported that asthmatic children were able to improve their peak expiratory flows, but there is little data on the effect of this training on the clinical course of their asthma. Caution is advised to ensure that the forced expiratory maneuvers do not actually provoke bronchospasm.

AIRWAYS RESISTANCE Techniques that may more directly affect bronchomotor tone use noninvasive measures of airways resistance as the biofeedback monitor. Vachon[18] and Feldman[19] used forced oscillation to continuously monitor airways resistance. Early reports were optimistic that patients are able to dilate their airways with the guidance of an oscillatory airway-resistance monitor. This method requires that the patient use a mouthpiece, but in contrast with the previous method, the patient is able to breathe at normal tidal volumes, rather than performing forced expiratory maneuvers. Forced oscillation feedback appears promising and should be investigated more fully.

BREATH SOUNDS Consistent with the foregoing principle, a variation technique described by Tiep uses breath sound intensity to indicate bronchospasm.[20–22] A microphone is positioned on the neck at the trachea to sense the patient's breath sounds (Fig. 22–2). A tone is created that relates to the intensity of the patient's breath sounds. The patient is then guided by both the voltmeter display and the variable pitch tone to reduce the intensity of his or breath sounds.

In a preliminary study comparing breath sound intensity with FEV_1, decreases in FEV_1 were accompanied by increases in breath sound intensity. Conversely, decreases in breath sound intensity signaled an improvement in FEV_1. This was true for both inhalation and exhalation in mild to moderate asthma. The biofeedback study evaluated the use of breath sound intensity to train asthmatic subjects to reduce exercise bronchospasm.[22] Exercise bronchospasm was provoked by treadmill exercise challenge; the subjects alternately used isoproterenol inhalers, general relaxation (control), or biofeedback to abort the attack. With breath sounds biofeedback, patients were able to increase their FEV_1 to preexercise levels—similar to inhaled isoproterenol. This technique has been clinically useful as an adjunct to other therapies in pulmonary rehabilitation.

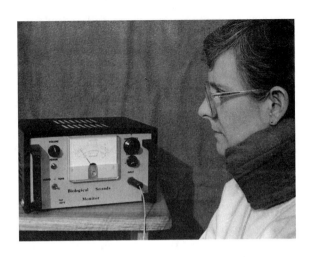

FIGURE 22-2 Breath sounds monitor: A microphone attaches to the neck; breath sounds are sensed; the module converts the breath sounds into a tone and varies the meter display; the patient attempts to influence the monitor; the display informs the patient if the intervention is successful; the patient modifies the intervention.

Emphysema

Stress reduction techniques, including EMG biofeedback, have been employed in the management of patients with emphysema. Patients with advanced disease tend to develop panic, as reflected in their breathing patterns becoming less efficient, leading to increased work of breathing. By relieving panic and inspiring the feeling of control, patients should be able to cope better. Whether relaxation and stress reduction techniques actually reduce the work or energy cost of breathing has not yet been determined.

Several biofeedback techniques have been specifically designed to reduce the work of breathing in emphysema patients.[21,22] In measuring the work of breathing, the two major components are *intrathoracic pressure* and *tidal volume*. For similar tidal volumes, a reduction in intrathoracic pressure for each breath would be expected to reduce the work of breathing.

Two work-of-breathing biofeedback techniques, focusing on variations in intrathoracic pressure, have been studied.[21,23] The first is a noninvasive respiratory pressure monitor that attaches to the upper sternum and directs a transducer into the soft tissue of the suprasternal notch. The suprasternal surface retracts on inspiration and bulges on expiration, as directly influenced by variation in intrathoracic pressure. In fact, it is possible to calibrate suprasternal displacement to alveolar pressure. Patients attempt to minimize these fluctuations. Assuming no increase in tidal volume and breath rate, a reduction in intrathoracic pressure fluctuation would be expected to reduce the work of breathing. In this method, the positioning of the transducer is critical to accuracy; neither the neck nor the transducer may be allowed to shift, otherwise recalibration will be necessary. By this technique, some patients are able to reduce their intrathoracic pressures partly by changing their respiratory patterns. They learn to breathe smoothly, rather than impulsively, to avoid airway collapse.

The second approach uses an indirect indicator of intrathoracic pressure that is expressed as variation in the height of the pressure pulse of the finger plethysmograph.[21] As the patient breathes, changes in intrathoracic pressure cause the peaks of the pulses to vary, similar to the paradoxical pulse. The information that is fed back

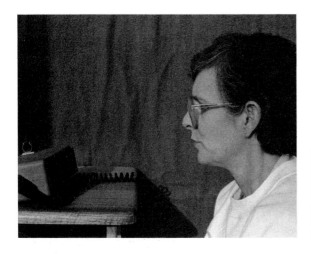

FIGURE 22-3 Pursed-lips breathing training with oximetry biofeedback: The patient is taught pursed-lips breathing and practices it using the oximeter as a guide to increase oxygen saturation.

to the patient relates to only the respiratory pressure fluctuations; pulse is factored out. Much further study is required to determine both accuracy of the theory behind these devices and their efficacy in treating patients with chronic lung disease.

Biofeedback to Increase Oxygen Saturation

Patients derive two benefits from pursed-lips breathing: it relieves dyspnea, and it improves gas exchange.[24,25] Until recently, pursed-lips breathing retraining completely focused on relieving dyspnea. However, Tiep and colleagues demonstrated that pursed-lips breathing retraining could be directed to increasing oxygen saturation.[26] They used the pulse oximeter as a biofeedback guide to teach patients to increase their oxygen saturation (Fig. 22–3). They, as others before them, found that pursed-lip breathing is accompanied by substantial increases in tidal volume and decreases in ventilatory rate.[24,25] The exhalation phase is prolonged, and the minute volume does not change appreciably. Oximetry-guided pursed-lips–breathing training has now been employed in patients with chronic obstructive pulmonary disease (COPD) and restrictive lung disease during rest and exercise and in persons with normal lungs at high altitude.[27,28]

In patients who require oxygen only during exercise, pursed-lips breathing may prevent exercise desaturation. Thus, a few patients may be able to completely avoid the use of supplemental oxygen by practicing pursed-lips breathing during exercise while using a small portable pulse oximeter. The fact that oximetry biofeedback guided pursed-lips training has been demonstrated effective in increasing oxygen saturation in patients with restrictive lung disease and normal individuals at high altitude, poses new questions regarding the physiologic basis for its efficacy (Fig. 22–4).

Recommendations for Clinical Application

Biofeedback directed to relaxation may be useful in a rehabilitation setting to assist in stress management training. It is important for the reader to recognize that biofeedback is only one of several approaches to relaxation and stress management. Other

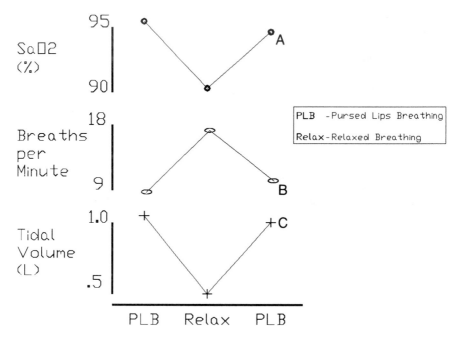

FIGURE   22-4   Oximetry-guided pursed-lips–breathing training causes (A) increase in oxygen saturation, (B) decrease in respiratory rate, (C) increase in tidal volume. There is usually little or no change in minute volume.

stress management techniques, such as jacobsonian tension–release methods and autogenic training are also quite effective.

The asthma training techniques using respiratory sounds and the work of breathing techniques cannot be recommended for general use because equipment is not generally available. Also, further study is required to examine long-term efficacy.

Biofeedback using incentive spirometry is standard for postoperative application, where it is desirable for patients to take deep breaths. Its application in asthma will require further study, although initial results appear promising.

The oximetry biofeedback-augmented pursed-lips–breathing training can be recommended. Pursed-lips breathing is well accepted by both patient and therapist, and there is a firm scientific basis for its use, despite our incomplete knowledge of the physiologic mechanisms involved. Also, pulse oximetry is commonly available.

CONCLUSION

Several biofeedback techniques have been employed in pulmonary rehabilitation. These techniques vary from relaxation and stress management to patient self-control of specific physiologic functions. Electromyographic feedback has been used for stress management and treatment of asthma. More specific areas include incentive spirometry to assist in high-volume diaphragmatic breathing, airway resistance indicators for treatment of asthma, and pulse oximetry for improving gas exchange. Biofeedback is being applied adjunctively to other therapeutic approaches. Training the patient in pursed-lips breathing guided by oximetry is only one example. Other examples will be described in the following section in which threshold techniques are used to guide ventilatory muscle exercise training. The future of biofeedback will depend on our improved ability to monitor the patient's physiologic actions and optimize patient–instrument interface.

VENTILATORY MUSCLE TRAINING

The ventilatory muscles and the chest structure constitute the *ventilatory pump*, the pulmonary analogue of the heart. In recent years, increased attention has been paid to the ventilatory muscles and the possibility that weakness and fatigue in this muscle group could contribute to respiratory failure.[29] Also, inspiratory muscle fatigue may limit exercise tolerance in patients with chronic lung disease.[30–34] Defects in the following factors can predispose patients with chronic lung disease to ventilatory muscle fatigue: performance factors, including work of breathing, and strength and efficiency of muscle contraction, and muscle energy factors, including nutritional stores, tissue oxygen availability, and metabolic processes.[29] The clinician should be cognizant of these variables and attempt to rectify as many of them as feasible. In any attempt to improve the performance side of ventilatory muscle activity, an obvious approach is to exercise those muscles specifically.

The muscles of inhalation perform most of the work of breathing, particularly during quiet respiration. Exhalation passively expends the elastic recoil energy stored during the previous inhalation. Since the diaphragm is the strongest muscle of inhalation, most ventilatory muscle training is directed toward building that muscle group.

The ventilatory muscles, being skeletal muscles, are subject to length–tension relations. As such, a stretched muscle is able to muster a greater force of contraction. The diaphragm of a patient with COPD is flattened; hence, nonstretched. Therefore, it operates at a mechanical disadvantage and thereby is unable to efficiently generate inspiratory forces.[29,33,34]

Ventilatory muscle training has been used to selectively build endurance and strength in these muscles. In the next sections, ventilatory muscle exercise training will be presented. First, some general considerations may add perspective to the clinical application of ventilatory muscle training in patients.

The Training Effect

Many patients with chronic lung disease can achieve a greater level of physical functioning from an exercise program.[1–3] When the exercise program consists of progressive walking, patients increase their ability to walk longer, farther, and with less dyspnea. The same benefits are obtained from upper extremity bicycle ergometry.[35,36] Patients can improve their ability to perform their self-care functions as they increase strength and endurance in the upper extremities. What is *not* clear is the mechanism for these desirable exercise responses. In the past, attempts to observe an anaerobic threshold in severely impaired COPD patients have not met with success. Consequently, it has been tempting to accept the notion that patients with severe respiratory impairments become so limited by their ventilatory mechanics that they are unable to reach a work load level sufficient for aerobic training.

Recent studies have suggested that even severely impaired chronic lung disease patients actually reach an anaerobic threshold, as indicated by an end-exercise rise in their serum lactate levels.[37-39] That even severely impaired COPD patients may attain an anaerobic threshold adds physiologic justification for the low-level exercise training that is so central to pulmonary rehabilitation programs. This concept is tantalizing because it opens the possibility that low-level exercise such as ventilatory muscle training may be sufficient to improve general conditioning.

Alternative mechanisms also contribute to the benefits of exercise training in patients with COPD. Patients improve their skill of performance, their tolerance to dyspnea, and they increase their motivation and incentive to become active.[36] All of these factors have a favorable effect on reversing disability, without changing muscle physiology.

Endurance Training

The ventilatory muscles are muscles of endurance, beginning their activity before birth and ceasing at the time of death. It is logical that endurance training would be the choice of some investigators. In contrast with strength training, which requires a high work load, endurance is improved by having the patient exercise repeatedly against a submaximal work load over some time period (15 to 30 minutes). One such training protocol would have the patient hyperventilate, by breathing rapidly and deeply into a device that prevents hypocapnia by returning some of the patient's CO_2 (Fig. 22–5). This is termed *isocapneic hyperpnea.*[40]

Ventilatory muscle endurance can be expressed as the *maximum sustained ventilatory capacity* (MSVC), which is the maximum ventilation that can be sustained for 15 minutes. Alternatively, there are two simpler methods for measuring endurance: either as the *maximum time* that the patient is able to exert an inspiratory pressure or

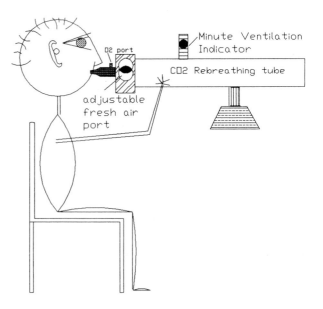

FIGURE 22-5 Isocapnea–hyperpnea trainer: The patient hyperventilates into a tube that has an adjustable opening for fresh air. Some of the expired CO_2 is returned to the patient so that the PCO_2 can remain constant. Thus, patients can hyperventilate for 15 to 30 minutes without suffering respiratory alkalosis.

the *maximum work load* that a patient can tolerate for a given time period. General conditioning is measured by incremental treadmill or bicycle ergometry tests or by the 12-minute walking distance test.

Leith and Bradley in 1976[40] studied persons with normal lungs and determined that they were able to increase their MSVC by isocapneic hyperpnea training.[40] Meanwhile, Keens determined that normal subjects and patients with cystic fibrosis could increase their ventilatory muscle endurance through a vigorous training program of swimming and canoeing.[41] None of these subjects trained ventilatory muscles specifically; however, they were able to raise their MSVC by 57%. Orenstein, evaluating cystic fibrosis patients in a program of supervised running, demonstrated increased exercise tolerance, cardiorespiratory fitness, and ventilatory muscle endurance.[42] However, there is no evidence that submaximal exercise can have the same effect on the ventilatory muscles, particularly in COPD patients.[43]

Belman and Mittman in 1980[44] instituted isocapneic hyperpnea training in COPD patients who had no demonstrable bronchodilator reversibility.[44] Their protocol included two daily 15-minute isocapneic hyperpnea training sessions. They demonstrated increases in MSVC and oxygen uptake along with improvements in arm and leg submaximal exercise endurance. These studies lend support to the contention that ventilatory muscle training can increase general exercise capacity in patients with chronic lung disease.

Strength Training

Another approach to ventilatory muscle training is to selectively increase muscle strength. Ventilatory muscle strength is measured as the maximum inspiratory pressure that can be exerted against a meter at zero (or near zero) airflow (PI_{max}). The PI_{max} measurements are taken at either residual volume or functional residual capacity. At residual volume the diaphragm is more stretched, thereby enabling a stronger force of contraction. Patients trained specifically to increase ventilatory muscle strength are instructed to inspire against high work loads that approach their PI_{max}. At very high work loads, patients cannot endure more than a few repetitions, as they are limited by ventilatory muscle fatigue.

Strength and Endurance Training

It is probably apparent that strength and endurance training need not be mutually exclusive, rather they are at opposite poles of a training continuum. The work load of inspiratory resistance training may be set to 15%, 30%, or 60% of PI_{max} and training schedules could be designed to meet goals that include both strength and endurance. Training protocols may lean toward higher work loads for shorter durations or lower work loads for longer durations. The ideal training protocol has yet to be established.

Sonne and Davis trained COPD patients using an inspiratory resistance device (similar to P-Flex, HealthScan Products Inc., Cedar Grove, NJ) and were able to increase the maximum work rate by 37%.[45] They demonstrated an increase in their maximum $\dot{V}O_2$ of 15%. Chen and associates, using resistive load training, discovered substantial increases in inspiratory muscle endurance and small increases in inspiratory muscle strength, but no increase in exercise conditioning measured by bicycle ergometry.[46] Because the devices used in these studies were simple resistive devices, the actual inspiratory work loads are unknown.

Nickerson and Keens introduced the concept of inspiratory pressure threshold training, using a weighted plunger that serves as an inspiratory valve.[47] The subjects had to exceed a specified negative pressure to release inspiratory airflow. They were able to demonstrate an improvement in ventilatory muscle strength and endurance, measured as sustained inspiratory pressure. Clanton and coworkers,[48] using the foregoing weighted valve technique[47] combined with an oscilloscope visual feedback display for breathing pattern guidance, tested the effects of varying the breathing pattern on endurance time. Since the mouth pressure remained constant, they were able to alter the inspiratory flow rate, expressed as the percentage of the ventilatory cycle spent in inspiration (T_I/T_{tot}). They determined that tension and time were the major determinants of ventilatory muscle endurance, independent of breath rate. These findings have been confirmed by Morrison and colleagues, who found that the testing of ventilatory muscle endurance, using a 2-minute threshold incremental loading test, was reproducible and independent of breathing rate.[49]

Clanton and associates, training normal subjects, demonstrated that relatively short bursts of higher-intensity exercise could increase ventilatory muscle endurance.[50] They trained subjects three times a week for 2 weeks. Each session lasted 2.5 minutes, beginning at 50% of each subject's PI_{max} and increasing the work load each session toward ventilatory muscle fatigue. Strength increased by 34% and endurance, as measured by the time that they could tolerate breathing against 85% and 100% of their PI_{max}, was increased to 5 and 10 minutes, respectively.

In Normal Subjects and Chronic Obstructive Pulmonary Disease Patients

Studies have been performed on healthy subjects and patients with COPD, neuromuscular disease, quadriplegia, and cystic fibrosis.[40–64] In general, these studies have demonstrated some effect of training, such as increased ventilatory muscle endurance, strength, or general conditioning, or a combination thereof. Among these variables there is some disagreement. Also, the studies using nonventilatory muscle training have not uniformly demonstrated improvement in the ventilatory muscles.

One might expect that any exercise that entails prolonged panting, will increase ventilatory muscle endurance, if not strength. This hypothesis is supported by Keens and coworkers in normal subjects and cystic fibrosis patients, who demonstrated that canoeing and swimming can increase ventilatory muscle endurance.[41] Also, cystic fibrosis patients naturally had 36% greater ventilatory muscle endurance than their normal counterparts, reflecting chronic resistance breathing by virtue of their lung disease. Orenstein demonstrated that a running program could increase ventilatory muscle endurance in cystic fibrosis patients.[42] However, Belman and Kendregan found that arm and leg endurance exercises, although increasing exercise conditioning, had no effect on MSVC.[37] Ries and colleagues determined that isocapneic hyperpnea training increased ventilatory performance as well as general walking performance, but walking improved only walking, not ventilatory muscle performance.[53] Thus, it appears that the submaximal work loads of other types of exercises may not sufficiently challenge the ventilatory muscles.

Larson and coworkers compared patients training with an inspiratory pressure threshold device at 15% and 30% of PI_{max}.[54] They trained COPD patients for 15 minutes initially and worked them up to 30 minutes. They found that the patients training at the higher work load improved their ventilatory muscle strength, endurance, and 12-minute walking distance (general conditioning), whereas the lower work load patients did not improve any of these variables. A recent study evaluated inspiratory muscle training using a weighted incentive spirometer in COPD patients.[55] The experimental group worked against more weight than the control group. Most patients in both groups increased their PI_{max}, although neither the intragroup nor intergroup difference in performance achieved significance. However, the actual inspiratory pressures exerted were *not* different between groups, despite the differences in spirometer weights. Interestingly, the mean changes, although insignificant, were similar in degree to the Larson study.[54] Thus, the important variable in their training scheme is the inspiratory pressure work load, independently of how that exerted pressure was reached.

Few studies have addressed symptomatology. Harver and associates, in a recent study, used a pressure target device adaptation of the P-Flex. They studied symptomatic COPD subjects and found that ventilatory muscle exercise not only increased ventilatory muscle strength and endurance, but it significantly reduced dyspnea in COPD patients.[56] They quantified dyspnea based on magnitude of effort, magnitude of task, and functional impairment.

For Neuromuscular Deficits

Quadriplegic patients and patients with neuromuscular deficits are likely to be exceptionally deconditioned. One can speculate that their physical deconditioning could be so extreme that even small endurance exercises might be rewarded with a training effect. Ventilatory muscle training may present these patients, who are unable to exercise any other muscle groups, an opportunity to develop better general conditioning. In fact, some studies involving these patient populations have demonstrated increases in PI_{max}, MSVC, and general endurance.[57,58]

Patients with muscular dystrophy have increased their ventilatory muscle endurance, but not strength.[59] Another study on the same population failed to demonstrate a training benefit.[60] Patients with multiple sclerosis were able to increase ventilatory muscle strength and endurance. In addition, training was accompanied by increases in vital capacity.[61]

For Ventilator Weaning

One exciting application of ventilatory muscle training is in the process of weaning patients from mechanical ventilation. Belman introduced this concept when he successfully weaned two COPD patients using isocapneic hyperpnea training through the ventilator at the zero pressure continuous positive airway pressure (CPAP) mode.[62] Both patients had failed previous attempts at weaning. Aldrich and associates used inspiratory resistance training to wean patients from the ventilator who were unresponsive to the usual methods.[63] Of the 27 patients, 63% with primary lung disease and neuromuscular disease were successfully weaned. Inspiratory muscle training was accompanied by large and significant improvements in vital capacity and other weaning parameters.

Expiratory Muscle Training

Practically all of the ventilatory muscle training described in this chapter has focused on exercising inhalatory muscles, but what about the muscles of exhalation? There is a logic to training that muscle group as well. Although it is true that the muscles of exhalation are only minimally active during quiet breathing in normal individuals, they are recruited in patients with severe COPD, particularly during respiratory distress and exertion. It is then possible that expiratory muscle fatigue could add to an already tenuous inspiratory muscle fatigue.

In another consideration for COPD patients, perhaps efficient recruitment and employment of exhalatory muscles could move the diaphragm from its flattened and inefficient posture to a more stretched and rounded position. This could render the diaphragm more efficient and able to exert stronger inspiratory forces. Thus, expiratory muscle training appears to merit greater scientific attention.

Commercially Available Training Devices

Unfortunately, isocapneic hyperpnea devices have never become commercially available as such, probably because of their greater complexity relative to other available devices. However, as previously mentioned, the mechanical ventilator, set to the CPAP mode, serves as an isocapneic hyperpnea trainer by returning some of the CO_2 and providing feedback of minute ventilation. Such ventilatory endurance training may be a useful adjunct in weaning refractory patients from the ventilator.[62,63]

The P-Flex (HealthScan Inc, Cedar Grove, New Jersey) (Fig. 22–6) is a commercially available device for training inspiratory muscles.[45] It incorporates a dialable menu of orifices, each offering specific resistance, providing the patient expends adequate effort. On exhalation, an expiratory valve permits nonobstructed, free flow of expired air. It is a simple portable device that is easily learned. Since the work load imposed by the P-Flex is accomplished by breathing through simple orifices, the pattern or strategy of breathing has a direct effect on the actual work load.[64] Inspiring slowly through the orifice creates little resistance, whereas aggressive inspiratory efforts impose disproportionately greater resistances and, consequently, higher work

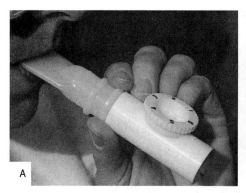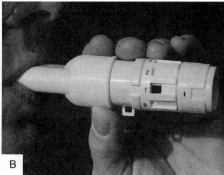

FIGURE   22-6   (**A**) P-Flex and (**B**) Aerobica ventilatory resistance trainers.

loads. Therefore, patients must be instructed to maximize their inspiratory effort to achieve sufficient work load to benefit from the training. To circumvent the patient's tendency to exert minimal inspiratory effort, we designed an electronic threshold biofeedback monitor that attaches to the P-Flex.[65] It has a timer that cues the patient when to inhale. If the patient meets criterion pressure, he or she is able to avoid the sounding of an irritating feedback tone. The P-Flex with the attached threshold device is used to set the exact work load and training schedule. There are several strategies of training; for example, high work load for short periods such as 2 to 3 minutes, or lower work loads for 15 to 30 minutes. The threshold attachment is not commercially available.

Another resistance training device similar to P-Flex, Aerobica (MBA Health Care Products Inc., Fayetteville, New York), incorporates an adjustable resistive work load that can be set for either inspiratory or expiratory muscle training. No patient studies have been performed with this device, but inspiratory muscle training should be similar to the P-Flex for comparable resistances. The concept of expiratory muscle training is interesting and, unfortunately, untested. Again, because of the increased recruitment of expiratory muscles during respiratory distress, studies examining expiratory muscle training are needed.

A spring-loaded device, Threshold (HealthScan Inc, Cedar Grove, New Jersey), (Fig. 22–7) was designed, based on the Nickerson–Keens technique for inspiratory pressure threshold training.[54] The Threshold can be set to specific inspiratory pressures, which the patient must exceed before inspiratory airflow is released. The Threshold incorporates a spring, its tension being adjustable to set different workloads. Thus, the passage or nonpassage of air, indicating that the threshold criterion has or has not been met, serves as a biofeedback signal to the patient.

Recommendations for Clinical Application

The appropriate clinical application of ventilatory muscle training is not obvious. Patients with COPD participating in a rehabilitation program have not been shown to derive *additional* benefit from ventilatory muscle training. However, patients too weak to begin a pulmonary rehabilitation program, might be able to gain enough

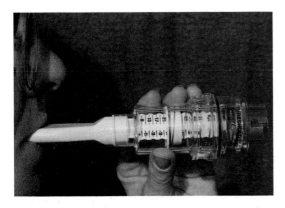

FIGURE 22-7 Threshold inspiratory pressure threshold trainer.

strength from ventilatory muscle training to improve their candidacy for rehabilitation.

Patients with neuromuscular deficits, such as those with quadriplegia or muscular dystrophy, are, by the nature of their diseases, denied the opportunity for arm- or leg-based cardiovascular training. As it appears that ventilatory muscle exercise training can improve general exercise conditioning and increase the vital capacity, it is reasonable to provide these patients with that opportunity.

In another application, patients in respiratory failure, who are difficult to wean from the mechanical ventilator, might be more successful with adjunctive ventilatory muscle training.

Important exercise variables include the work load, duration of training, pattern of training, frequency of training, and adequate instructions to the patient. All of these factors should be considered and in place before embarking on a ventilatory muscle exercise prescription and program.

SUMMARY

Ventilatory muscle training has repeatedly been shown to increase ventilatory muscle strength and endurance. Several studies have demonstrated that ventilatory muscle training improves general exercise conditioning, whereas other studies are in conflict. On the other hand, normal subjects and cystic fibrosis patients, who have undergone *vigorous nonventilatory* muscle training, were able to increase their ventilatory muscle strength and endurance. However, submaximal general exercise failed to increase ventilatory muscle strength or endurance.

Thus, if the clinical goal is to increase ventilatory muscle strength and endurance, ventilatory muscle training should meet that goal. If the goal is to reverse ventilatory muscle fatigue and avoid ventilatory muscle failure, some evidence suggests that ventilatory muscle training could be beneficial. Certainly, other factors must be considered in the treatment of respiratory failure, such as gas exchange status, nutritional status, and adequate oxygenation.

Finally, ventilatory muscle training may be applicable in weaning patients from the mechanical ventilator.

REFERENCES

1. Hodgkin JE, Petty TL, eds. Chronic obstructive pulmonary disease: current concepts. Philadelphia: WB Saunders, 1987.

2. Hodgkin JE, Zorn EG, Connors GL, eds. Pulmonary rehabilitation: guidelines to success. Stoneham, MA: Butterworth Publishers, 1984.

3. Tiep BL, Lewis Y, Branum N, Chow MT, Walsh RL, Servetto E. Respiratory management at home. In: Portnow J, ed. Physical medicine and rehabilitation: state of the art reviews. 1988:385.

4. Nadel JA. Airways: autonomic regulation and airway responsiveness. In: Bronchial asthma. Mechanisms and therapeutics. Boston: Little, Brown & Co, 1976:155.

5. McFadden ER, Luparello T, Lyons HA, Bleecker E. The mechanism of action of suggestion in the induction of acute asthma attacks. Psychosom Med 1969;31:134.

6. Spector S, Luparello TJ, Kopetzky MT, Souhrada J, Kinsman RA. Response of asthmatics to methacholine and suggestion. Am Rev Respir Dis 1976;12:43.

7. Davis MH, Saunders DR, Creer TL, Chai H. Relaxation training facilitated by biofeedback apparatus as a supplemental treatment in bronchial asthma. J Psychosom Res 1973;17:121.

8. Alexander AB, Cropp GJA, Chai H. Effects of relaxation training on pulmonary mechanics in children with asthma. J Appl Behav Anal 1979;12:27.

9. Lehrer PM, Hochron SM, McCann B, Swartzman L, Reba P. Relaxation decreases large-airway but not small-airway asthma. J Psychosom Res 1986;30:13.

10. Scherr MS, Crawford PL, Sergent CB, Scherr CA. Effect of biofeedback techniques on chronic asthma in a summer camp environment. Ann Allergy 1975;35:289.

11. Kotses H, Glaus KD, Crawford PL, Edwards JE, Scherr MS. Operant reduction of frontalis EMG activity in the treatment of children in asthma. J Psychosom Res 1976;20:453.

12. Kotses H, Glaus KD, Bricel SK, Edwards JE, Crawford PL. Operant muscular relaxation and peak expiratory flow rate in asthmatic children. J Psychosom Res 1978;22:17.

13. Glaus KD, Kotses H. Facial muscle tension influences lung airway resistance; limb muscle tension does not. Biol Psychol 1983;17:105.

14. Peper E, Smith K, Wadell D. Voluntary wheezing versus diaphragmatic breathing and Voldyne feedback: a clinical intervention in the treatment of asthma. Clin Biofeedback Health 1987;10:83.

15. Roland M, Peper E. Inhalation volume changes with inspirometer feedback and diaphragmatic breathing coaching. Clin Biofeedback Health 1987;10:89.

16. Peper E. Strategies to reduce the effort of breathing: electromyographic and inspirometry biofeedback. In: Von Euler C, Katz-Salamon M, eds. Respiratory psychophysiology. London: Macmillan 1988:113.

17. Khan A, Staerk M, Bonk C. Role of counter conditioning in the treatment of asthma. J Asthma Res 1973;11:57.

18. Vachon L, Rich ES. Visceral learning in asthma. Psychosom Med 1976;38:122–130.

19. Feldman GM. The effect of biofeedback training on respiratory resistance of asthmatic children. Psychosom Med 1976;38:27.

20. Tiep BL. Biofeedback in pulmonary rehabilitation. In: Biofeedback and family practice medicine. New York: Plenum Publishing, 1983:29.

21. Tiep BL, Alaniz J, Cordell J. Respiratory feedback: two non-invasive approaches in the treatment of patients with chronic obstructive lung disease. Proc San Diego Biomed Symp 1976;15:372.

22. Tiep BL, Belman MJ, Trippe M. Wheeze biofeedback in exercise induced bronchospasm. Am Rev Respir Dis 1980;121:A200.

23. Tiep BL, Mittman C, Trippe M. A new biofeedback technique for controlling intrathoracic pressure in patients with pulmonary emphysema. Proc San Diego Biomed Symp 1977;16:215.

24. Ingram RH, Schilder DP. Effect of pursed lips expiration on the pulmonary pressure–flow relationship in obstructive lung disease. Am Rev Respir Dis 1967;96:381.

25. Mueller RE, Petty TL, Filley GF. Ventilation and arterial blood gas changes induced by pursed lips breathing. J Appl Physiol 1970;28:784.

26. Tiep BL, Burns M, Kao D, Hererra J, Madison R. Pursed lips breathing training using ear oximetry. Chest 1986;90:218.

27. Tiep BL, Burns M, Walsh L, Chow M. Pursed lips breathing in normal subjects at modest altitude. Am Rev Respir Dis 1987;135:A410.

28. Tiep B, Burns M, Chow M, Hererra J, Madorsky A. Pursed lips breathing increases oxygen saturation in restrictive lung disease patients. Chest 1989;96:205S.

29. Roussos C. The failing ventilatory pump. Lung 1982;160:59.

30. Bye PTP, Esau SA, Walley KR, Macklem PT, Pardy RL. Ventilatory muscles during exercise in air and oxygen in normal men. J Appl Physiol 1984;56:464.

31. Grassino A, Gross D, Macklem PT, Roussos C, Zagelbaum G. Inspiratory muscle fatigue as a factor limiting exercise. Bull Eur Physiopathol Respir 1979;15:105.

32. Martin B, Heintzelman M, Chen H-I. Exercise performance after ventilatory work. J Appl Physiol 1982;52:1581.

33. Carter R, Nicotra B. Recognition and management of respiratory muscle fatigue in chronic obstructive pulmonary disease. Int Med Spec 1988;9:171.

34. Bellemere F, Grassino A. Effect of pressure and timing of contraction on human diaphragm fatigue. J Appl Physiol 1982;53:1190.

35. Wasserman K, Hansen J. In: Principles of exercise testing and interpretation. Philadelphia: Lea & Febiger, 1987:3.

36. Belman MJ, Wasserman K. Exercise training and testing in patients with chronic obstructive pulmonary disease. Basics RD 1981;10(2):1.

37. Hodgkin JE, Litzau KL. Exercise training target heart rates in chronic obstructive pulmonary disease. Chest 1988;94:30S.

38. Casaburi R, Patessio A, Ioli F, Zanaboni S, Donner DF, Wasserman K. Reductions in exercise lactic acidosis and ventilation after exercise training in obstructive lung disease patients. Am Rev Respir Dis 1989;139:A330.

39. Daly J, Cooper C, Casaburi R, Burns M, Chang R, Wasserman K. Exercise training as a mediator of increased exercise performance in COPD patients undergoing rehabilitation. Am Rev Respir Dis 1989;139:A330.

40. Leith DE, Bradley M. Ventilatory muscle strength and endurance training. J Appl Physiol 1976;41:508.

41. Keens TG, Krastens JR, Wannamaker EM, Levison H, Crozier DN, Bryan AC. Ventilatory muscle endurance training in normal subjects and patients with cystic fibrosis. Am Rev Respir Dis 1977;116:853.

42. Orenstein DM, Franklin BA, Doershuk cf, et al. Exercise conditioning and cardiopulmonary fitness in cystic fibrosis. The effects of a three-month supervised running program. Chest 1981;80:392.

43. Belman MJ, Kendregan BA. Physical training fails to improve ventilatory muscle endurance in patients with chronic obstructive pulmonary disease. Chest 1982;81:440.

44. Belman MJ, Mittman C. Ventilatory muscle training improves exercise capacity in chronic obstructive pulmonary disease patients. Am Rev Respir Dis 1980;121:273.

45. Sonne LJ, Davis JA. Increased exercise performance in patients with severe COPD following inspiratory resistive training. Chest 1982;81:436.

46. Chen H-I, Dukes R, Martin BJ. Inspiratory muscle training in patients with chronic obstructive pulmonary disease. Am Rev Respir Dis 1985;131:251.

47. Nickerson BG, Keens TG. Measuring ventilatory muscle endurance in humans as sustainable inspiratory pressure. J Appl Physiol 1982;52:768.

48. Clanton TL, Dixon GF, Drake J, Gadek JE. Effects of breathing pattern on inspiratory muscle endurance in humans. J Appl Physiol 1985;59:1.

49. Morrison NJ, Fairbarn MS, Pardy RL. The effect of breathing frequency on inspiratory muscle endurance during incremental threshold loading. Chest 1989;96:85.

50. Clanton TL, Dixon GF, Drake J, Gadek J. Inspiratory muscle conditioning using a threshold loading device. Chest 1985;87:62.

51. Pardy RL, Rivington RN, Despas PJ, Macklem PT. The effect of inspiratory muscle training on exercise performance in patients with chronic airflow limitation. Am Rev Respir Dis 1981;123:426.

52. Asher MI, Pardy RL, Coates AL, Thomas E, Macklem PT. The effects of inspiratory muscle training in patients with cystic fibrosis. Am Rev Respir Dis 1982;126:855.

53. Ries AL, Moser KM. Comparison of isocapneic hyperventilation and walking exercise training at home in pulmonary rehabilitation. Chest 1986;90:285.

54. Larson JL, Kim, MJ, Sharp JT, Larson DA. Inspiratory muscle training with a pressure

threshold breathing device in patients with chronic obstructive pulmonary disease. Am Rev Respir Dis 1988;138:689.

55. Gregg BL. Inspiratory muscle training with a weighted incentive spirometer in subjects with chronic airways obstruction. Resp Care 1989;34:860.

56. Harver A, Mahler DA, Daubenspeck A. Targeted inspiratory muscle training improves respiratory muscle function and reduces dyspnea in patients with chronic obstructive pulmonary disease. Ann Intern Med 1989;111:117.

57. Gross D, Ladd HW, Riley EJ, Macklem PT, Grassino A. The effect of training on strength and endurance of the diaphragm in quadriplegia. Am J Med 1980;68:27.

58. Estrup C, Lyager S, Noerea N, Olsen C. Effect of respiratory muscle training in patients with neuromuscular diseases and in normals. Respiration 1986;50:36.

59. Martin AJ, Stern L, Yeates J, Lepp D, Little J. Respiratory muscle training in Duchenne muscular dystrophy. Dev Med Child Neurol 1986;28:314.

60. Rodillo E, Noble-Jamieson CM, Aber V, Heckmatt JZ, Muntoni F, Dubowitz V. Respiratory muscle training in Duchenne muscular dystrophy. Arch Dis Child 1989;64:736.

61. Olgiati R, Girr A, Hugi L, Haegi V. Respiratory muscle training in multiple sclerosis: a pilot study. Schweiz Arch Neurol Psychiatr 1989;140:46.

62. Belman MJ. Respiratory failure treated by ventilatory muscle training. A report of two cases. Eur J Respir Dis 1981; 62:391.

63. Aldrich TK, Karpel JP, Uhrlass RM, Sparapani MA, Eramo D, Ferranti R. Weaning from mechanical ventilation: adjunctive use of inspiratory muscle resistive training. Crit Care Med 1989;17:143.

64. Belman MJ, Thomas SG, Lewis MI. Resistive breathing training in patients with chronic obstructive lung disease. Chest 1986;90:662.

65. Belman MJ, Shadmehr R. A target device for ventilatory muscle training. J Appl Physiol 1988;2726.

PATTY WOOTEN

Laughter as Therapy for Patient and Caregiver

A merry heart does good like a medicine, but a broken spirit
dries the bones
   —Proverbs 17:22

Laughter can be a powerful therapy for both the patient and the caregiver. This chapter will examine the beneficial effect of humor and laughter on the body, mind, and spirit; for the patient during recovery from illness; and for the health professional during delivery of care. Most experienced caregivers have discovered that attention to only the physical body during treatment will yield a partial or temporary recovery. The patient's emotional responses, belief system, support network, and such, all can affect compliance with treatment and the ability to cope with fear, pain, and loss.

   The ability to laugh at a situation or problem gives us a feeling of superiority and power. Humor and laughter can foster a positive and hopeful attitude. We are less likely to succumb to feelings of depression and helplessness if we are able to laugh at what is troubling us. Humor gives us a sense of perspective on our problems. Laughter provides an opportunity for the release of those uncomfortable emotions that, if held inside, may create biochemical changes that are harmful to the body.

   Caregivers, as well as patients are in need of the therapeutic effects of humor and laughter. Most caregivers are compassionate persons who choose to work in a profession that places them at risk for their physical, emotional, and spiritual well-being. Because of our sympathetic tendencies we may feel the same emotions that our patients feel, such as fear, anger, helplessness, and depression. We can experience feelings of failure when our efforts are ineffective. We feel anger and frustration when a patient rejects our care or is noncompliant with treatment. We may feel grief when patients die or families mourn. Caregivers are at risk physically too (e.g., exhaustion from long shifts with inadequate staffing, exposure to infectious organisms, and physical abuse from combative patients). Health professionals working in a stress-filled environment are at risk for burnout and stress-related illness. Our ability to see the humor in a situation and to laugh freely with our coworkers can be an effective way to take care of our own body, mind, and spirit.

   For thousands of years, the human race has extolled the health-enhancing benefits of laughter. Current research by Lefcourt, Ader, and Fry in the areas of psychology, physiology, and psychoneuroimmunology is defining the specific changes effected by the experience of mirthful laughter.[1-7] *Therapy* is defined as "an activity or treatment intended to alleviate an undesirable condition." With that in mind, let us explore the therapeutic benefit of laughter for the body, mind, and spirit.

A PATIENT RESPONDS TO HUMOR

During the last 20 years, I have been active in the profession of nursing. Most of those years have been spent at the bedside in intensive care units; I have also worked in home care, hospice, and cardiac rehabilitation. I can remember many situations during which humor and laughter made a significant difference in a patient's response to care, but none as profound as this story. Fred was 60 years old and recovering from a mitral valve replacement. During his immediate postoperative recovery, Fred experienced a mild psychosis and severe depression. The acute psychotic episode resolved before discharge, but the profound depression continued for many weeks. Fred lacked enthusiasm for anything. He refused to eat, to walk, and even refused to wear anything but pajamas. His surgeon referred him to our outpatient cardiac rehabilitation program. Upon entry into our program, Fred walked with a shuffling gait, responded to questions with one or two words, and was unable to make eye contact. His wife was exhausted and discouraged. For several weeks we saw little improvement in his depression, in spite of antidepressant drugs and psychological counseling. One day, about a month after beginning rehabilitation, he was walking on the treadmill, his 11 ¼ kg (25 lb) weight loss noticeable as his sweat pants hung loosely over his hips. After about 6 minutes of walking, his sweat pants suddenly fell down around his ankles, revealing bright red boxer shorts. We hit the emergency stop button in time to prevent his falling and went to assist him. He was looking down at his dropped drawers and when he lifted his head we could see a big grin starting, and he began to laugh. We smiled and joined him in the laughter, grateful for the permission to respond by laughing at the ridiculous situation. Our mutual embarrassment and tension was released through laughing. From that moment on Fred's depression continued to resolve, he became involved in his recovery process and was able to regain his strength, and he eventually returned to an active involvement in his church and community. Recalling this story reminds me of this popular folk poem:

> It's easy enough to smile when the world goes round and round but the man worthwhile is the man who can smile when his pants are falling down.
> —Anonymous

LAUGHTER SUPPORTS RECOVERY
FROM ILLNESS

Norman Cousins, former editor for *Saturday Review,* brought the attention of the medical community to the possibility that laughter may have a healing potential. In 1964, Cousins was diagnosed with ankylosing spondylitis, a progressive degenerative disease of the collagen tissue. His physicians gave him little hope for recovery, indicating that a possible cause of his illness was due to heavy-metal poisoning. Recalling his activities in the month before the onset of symptoms, he remembered frequent exposure to diesel exhaust fumes during his travel in Russia. He suspected that a condition of adrenal exhaustion weakened his ability to tolerate the toxic exposure. From his reading of Hans Selye's 1956 book about the body's response to stress, Cousins recalled that research had shown that negative emotions could create chemical changes that would eventually lead to adrenal exhaustion. He suspected that the positive emotions (such as faith, hope, confidence, and joy) might create changes within the body that would enhance his recovery process. Since the behavior of laughing tends to open one to these positive emotions, Cousins began viewing amusing films to stimulate laughter. After each laughing episode he noted that he could sleep comfortably without the need for analgesia or sedation. He also discovered that laughter also stimulated a decrease in his sedimentation rate, indicating a reversal of the inflammatory response.[9] After his recovery, Cousins spent the last 10 years of his life as an adjunct professor at UCLA Medical School where he established a Humor Task Force to coordinate and support clinical research.[10] Today, 25 years after Cousins' experience, we have the scientific research to explain the specific physiologic changes that his anecdotal story suggested. Laughter does affect the body, mind, and spirit. Perhaps Mark Twain captured the relation most succinctly when he wrote:

> The human race has only one really effective weapon, and that's laughter. The moment it arises, all our hardnesses yield, all our irritations and resentments slip away, and a sunny spirit takes their place.
> —Mark Twain

PHYSIOLOGIC RESPONSE

Humor is a perceptual process, whereas laughter is a behavioral response. This behavior creates predictable physiologic changes within the body. As with other exercise, we see two stages of the body's response, the arousal phase when the physiologic parameters increase, and the resolution phase when they return to resting rate or lower. With vigorous sustained laughter, the heart rate is stimulated, sometimes reaching rates of about 120 beats per minute; the normal respiratory pattern becomes chaotic; respiratory rate and depth are increased, whereas residual volume is decreased. Coughing and hiccups are often triggered by phrenic nerve irritation or the dislodging of mucous plugs. Oxygen saturation of peripheral blood does not significantly change during the increased ventilation occurring with laughter. Conditions such as asthma or bronchitis may be irritated by vigorous laughter. Peripheral vascular flow is increased because of vasodilation. A variety of muscle groups become active during laughter—diaphragm, abdominal, intercostal, respiratory accessory, facial, and occasionally muscles in the arms, legs, and back.[1-3]

Some of the most exciting research exploring the potential healing value of laughter is in the area of psychoneuroimmunology (also referred to as neuroendocrinology or neuroimmunology). *Psychoneuroimmunology* is an area of research that explores the connections between the nervous system (the seat of thought, memory, and emotion), the endocrine system (which secretes powerful hormones), and the immune system (which defends the body from microbial invasions). Loma Linda University Medical Center has recently completed research showing that the neuroendocrine system is affected during the experience of mirthful laughter.[11] This work has shown that serum cortisol levels decreased with laughter. Also, the experimental group demonstrated a lower baseline epinephrine level than the control group (possibly because of their relaxed status in anticipation of the laughter experience). Levels of cortisol and epinephrine (known to be immunosuppressive) are elevated during the stress response. Therefore, Berk and Tan conclude that by decreasing these levels we can diminish the suppression of the respective immune components. Other research has demonstrated that mirthful laughter increases the spontaneous lymphocyte blastogenesis and the natural killer (NK) cell activity. Natural killer cells are a type of lymphocyte that has a spontaneous cytolytic activity against tumor cells.[12]

Frequency of stressful life changes, severity of depression, and coping styles, all have been shown to affect the immune response. Locke of Harvard has shown that the activity of natural killer cells is decreased during periods of increased life change accompanied by severe emotional disturbances, whereas subjects with similar patterns of life change and less emotional disturbances had more normal levels of NK cell activity.[13] Similar findings were confirmed by Irwin in 1987 at the VA Medical Center in San Diego, noting that NK cell activity decreased during depressive reaction to life changes.[14] Janice and Ronald Glaser of Ohio State University School of Medicine studied the cellular immunity response patterns of medical students before examinations. Their work showed a reduction in the number of helper T cells and a lowered activity of the NK cell just before the examination.[15,16] In 1985, Stein, at Mt. Sinai School of Medicine in New York, looked at the effect of conjugal bereavement by studying men whose wives had advanced breast cancer. His work showed that the lymphocyte response pattern in his subjects dropped significantly within 1 month after the death of their wives.[17] This finding was also confirmed by the research of Schleifer[18] and Bartrop[19].

Research by Stone of the State University of New York (SUNY) has revealed that salivary immunoglobulin A (our first-line defense against the entry of infectious organisms through the respiratory tract) response was lower on days of negative mood and higher on days with positive mood.[20] This finding was duplicated by Dillon at Western New England College, showing an increased concentration of salivary IgA after viewing a humorous video.[21] The research in the field of psychoneuroimmunology continues to prove that the mind (emotions) and the body (immune system) are interrelated. Positive emotions seem to enhance the immune response, whereas negative emotions suppress it.[22,20] Current research seems to be confirming what Sir William Osler, a physician and pioneer of modern medicine, stated years ago:[23]

> It is more important to know what sort of patient has the disease, than what sort of disease the patient has.
> —W. Osler

HUMOR AND ILLNESS

How then, may the behavior of laughter be therapeutic to the body of both patient and caregiver? Laughter is a pleasurable experience; it momentarily banishes feelings of anger and fear. It gives us a feeling of power and control; we feel carefree, lighthearted, and hopeful during the moments of laughter. These feelings may have therapeutic benefits by reversing the immunosuppressive effects of the emotions of anger, fear, or loneliness that often accompany hospitalization and recovery from illness.

Illness, either acute onset or exacerbation of a chronic illness, can be a stressful event. Hospitalization, separation from family, invasive procedures, complex technology, or unfamiliar caregivers, all can create feelings of anxiety, loneliness, discomfort, anger, panic, and depression for the patient. These emotions are known to produce physiologic changes that are harmful to the body; changes that the use of humor and laughter can ease. Shared laughter is a uniquely human bond and serves as an equalizer and "social lubricant."

Caregivers can express their understanding and appreciation of the patient's struggle through the use of humor. For example, when a patient complains about the inadequate length or coverage of their gown we could respond with: "Well, now you *know* your doctor admitted you for observation." or "It's a designer creation by Seymor Butts." Humor can also help to reframe a situation by creating a context suggesting a more pleasant environment. As you instruct in the use of the call light: "Now I'm going to place your room service button right here." Or after completing an uncomfortable procedure, smile and say: "I bet it's hard for you to believe I'm on your side right now." When you've completed a ventilator check, blood gas analysis, or vital sign check, smile and say: "Well, you look good on paper. How does it feel on the inside?" Each of these statements, while not profoundly funny, will communicate a gentle awareness of the patient's dilemma and express a relaxed and lighthearted attitude by the caregiver—giving the subtle message that the caregiver is confident and in control of the situation.

But it is extremely important that the patient first be convinced of the health professional's competence and ability to deliver expert clinical care. A carefree, joking demeanor can be used to cover up inept skills or to deflect and ignore the importance of a patient's feelings. The appreciation of humor is highly individual, and there are no guarantees that your attempts will be successful; therefore, one must be observant of the patient's response. Sometimes the response may be subtle, a glistening of the eyes or flushing of the cheeks. Of course we all hope for the big smile, chuckle, or playful retort; but if you suspect that the patient felt insulted or misunderstood your intention, it is helpful to say something like: "Gee, I sure hope you weren't offended by that. I was just trying to lighten up the situation and help you to relax. I didn't mean to upset you, sorry." If the humorous attempts are not working with that patient, then quit. Always remember, *never* use sexual, ethnic, or racial material with patients or their families. It is unprofessional, and you risk offending them and losing rapport and respect.[24]

PSYCHOLOGICAL EFFECTS OF HUMOR

Humor and laughter affect how we perceive and respond to change. Herbert Lefcourt, a noted psychologist from the University of Waterloo in Canada has explored the possibility that a sense of humor and its use can change our emotional response to stress. In this study, subjects were asked to review the frequency and severity of stressful life changes occurring to them over the previous 6 months, and their recent negative mood disturbances were evaluated. Lefcourt then administered tests to evaluate use of humor, perception of humor, appreciation of laughter, and efforts to include opportunities for humor and laughter into each subject's life-style. Results of this study have shown that the ability to sense and appreciate humor can buffer the mood disturbances that occur in response to negative life events.[5,6]

Humor gives us a change of perspective on our problems and, with an attitude of detachment, we feel a sense of self-protection and control in our environment. Freud[25] noted the powerful psychologic influence of humor stating:

> Like wit and the comic, humor has a liberating element. It is the triumph of narcissism, the ego's victorious assertion of its own invulnerability. It refuses to suffer the slings and arrows of reality.
> —Freud, 1905

Some of the best humor about illness and recovery has been written by former patients. My favorites are *Surviving the Cure* by Janet Henry,[26] *They Tore Out my Heart and Stomped the Sucker Flat* by Lewis Grizzard,[27] *Patients at Large* by cartoonist Tom Jackson,[28] *Please Don't Stand on my Catheter* by T. Duncan Stewart,[29] and *Have a Heart* by Wilford Nehmer Jr.[30] Each of these authors reveals some of the absurdity, irony, and incongruity of being a patient under care. When we choose to laugh at or about a situation, we give ourselves the subtle message: "This is not so threatening; look, it's amusing and absurd sometimes. I can't take it too seriously."

Humor can also influence the mind by enhancing the ability to learn. Health professionals spend considerable time educating the patient and family about drugs, diet, life-style change, and treatment benefits. Delivering the information with humor will improve the communication in three ways:

- It will capture the attention of the learner.
- It will enhance retention of the material.
- It will help release the tension that blocks learning.

The use of cartoons or funny stories can be an effective way to add humor.[31–33] Shown in Figure 23-1 are four cartoons, drawn by Tom Jackson, based on real-life situations.[28]

Caregivers work in a stress-filled environment and are prone to professional burnout. A major causative factor in burnout is powerlessness. Hans Selye, (physician, physiologist, and pioneer in the field of stress research) noted in 1954: "Stress is not the event, it's our perception of it."[8] Kobassa clarifies this concept even further with her research into personal hardiness factors. She found that some personality types seem resilient to the harmful effects of stress because they possess three traits:

- Commitment to self and work
- A sense of control within their environment
- A feeling of challenge rather than threat when events change

Kobassa discusses the importance of "cognitive control". Control of events in your external world may not be possible, but we all have the ability to control how we view these and the emotional response to them we choose to have.[34]

(*Text continues on p. 430*)

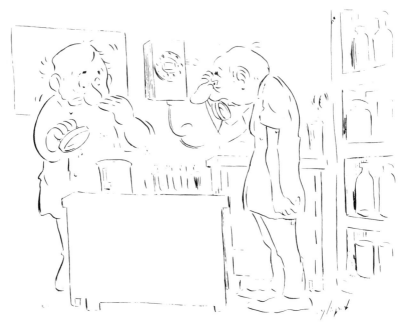

"Would you tell the patient in 605 that we asked for a stool 'culture' not 'sculpture'."

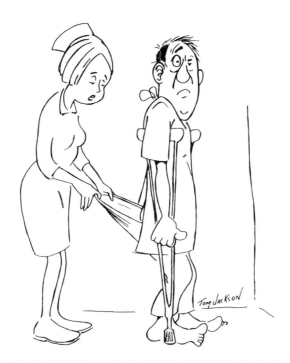

"Yep! You sure did! That's enough exercise for today."

FIGURE   23-1

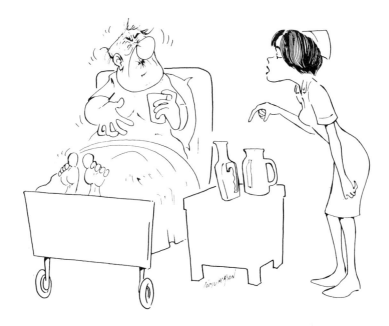

"One more time, 'this is the water, this is not'—"

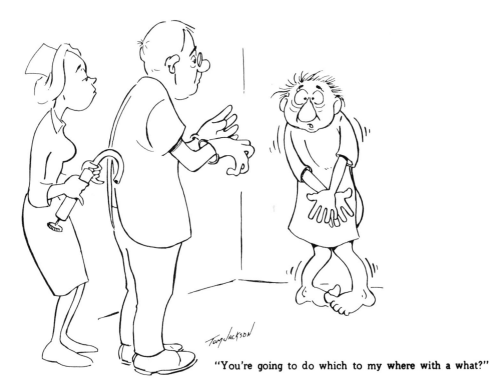

"You're going to do which to my **where** with a what?"

FIGURE   23-1   (*continued*)

Humor gives us perceptual flexibility and, thus, can increase our cognitive control. One nurse used her perceptual flexibility to help her cope with a demanding patient who frequently interrupted the nurse's busy schedule with minor complaints and requests. The nurse's patience and tolerance were wearing thin. It was lunchtime and the patients were eating when again the nurse was called to this patient's room. Upon entering, the patient indignantly pointed to her tray and told the nurse, "This is a bad potato!" The nurse then picked up the potato and began spanking it, saying "Bad potato! Bad potato!" The patient and nurse both laughed and the tension of the moment was dissolved.

Any thorough discussion of caregiver's use of humor must include a style called "gallows humor." Freud named it when he reported an incident of joking that occurred on the gallows by a man about to be hung. It refers to the style of humor that laughs directly at tragedy or death, as if it were amusing. Gallows humor is unique to caregivers or any professional who deals directly with the gruesome reality of pain, suffering, and death. Police, social workers, news reporters, psychologists, and workers in all areas of the health professions use this style of humor to help them cope with the sympathetic tendencies they feel when working with those who suffer. William McDougall,[35] professor of psychology at Harvard wrote:

> The possession of this peculiar disposition shields us from the depressing influence which the many minor mishaps and shortcomings of our fellows would exert upon us if we did not possess it . . . It not only prevents our minds from dwelling upon these depressing objects, but it actually converts these objects into stimulants that promote our well being, both bodily and mentally, instead of depressing us through sympathetic pain or distress. Laughter is primarily and fundamentally the antidote of sympathetic pain."
> —William McDougall, 1922

This type of humor is most often misunderstood or unappreciated by those who do not work closely with the suffering client or who are perhaps new to the profession. One often develops an appreciation for this humor when the tension is so great that one must release it or begin to feel crushed from the pressure. Freud describes the use of this humor as the caregiver's self-care technique that attempts to convert unpleasant feelings into pleasant ones.[25] Some of the best collections of gallows humor for the health professions can be found in *A Chance to Cut Is a Chance to Cure*[36] and *Journal of Nursing Jocularity* (see list of Humor Resources at end of chapter).

Samuel Shem's book *House of God*, gives classic examples of gallows humor.[37] One of my favorites is the "Gomer Assessment Scale—how do you know someone is a G.O.M.E.R.?" (a definition from Shem's book that stands for *Get Out of My Emergency Room*)

1. Old chart weighs more than 5 pounds
2. Ties Foley catheter into pajama strings
3. Has seizure and never drops his cigarette
4. Asks for cigarette during pulmonary function test
5. BUN is higher than IQ
6. PO_2 is less than respiratory rate

Perhaps one of the most accurate, poignant, and personal discussions of the importance of gallows humor for the caregiver was written by a nurse anesthetist working in an emergency room in Illinois. Wayne Johnston shares his personal experience and viewpoint in *To the Ones Left Behind*.[38]

> You saw me laugh after your father died . . . to you I must have appeared calloused and uncaring . . . Please understand, much of the stress health care workers suffer comes about because we do care . . . Sooner or later we will all laugh at the wrong time, I hope your father would understand, my laugh meant no disrespect, it was a grab at balance. I knew there was another patient who needed my full care and attention . . . my laugh was no less cleansing for me than your tears were for you.
> —Wayne Johnston

We have discussed the beneficial physiological changes that laughter creates within the body—offsetting the harmful biochemical changes that occur during stress. We have explored how humor gives us a change of perspective and a sense of control within our environment, thus increasing our resilience to stress and burnout. We will now look at the effect of humor and laughter on the spirit.

SPIRITUAL EFFECTS OF HUMOR

Spirit can be defined as the vital essence or animating force of a living organism, often considered divine in origin. Spirit can also be regarded as vivacity or energy. Or it can refer to a characteristic temper or disposition (the spirit of the group was hostile). The word *humor* itself is a word of many meanings. The root of the word is *umor* meaning liquid, fluid. In the Middle Ages and Renaissance, humor was one of the four principal body fluids thought to determine human health and dispositions (sanguine, phlegmatic, choleric, melancholic). One dictionary defines humor as "the quality of being laughable or comical" or "a state of mind, mood, spirit." Humor, on all levels, therefore, is something that flows, involving basic characteristics of the individual that express themselves in the body, in moods and emotional reactions, and in qualities of feeling, of mind and of spirit. The qualities of humor and spirit are similar and, I believe, interdependent. As caregivers we offer therapy to facilitate the healing processes within the body. To be most effective, we must direct our efforts to touch the body, mind, and spirit. The root of the word *heal* is *haelen*, meaning to make whole. Commenting on the medical theories of his day, Socrates noted (in Moody[39]):

> As it is not proper to cure the eyes without the head, nor the head without the body, so neither is it proper to cure the body without the soul.
> —Socrates

During the Middle Ages, Henri de Mondeville, professor of surgery wrote (in Walsh[40]):

> Let the surgeon take care to regulate the whole regimen of the patient's life for joy and happiness, allowing his relatives and special friends to cheer him, and by having some one tell him jokes. The surgeon must forbid anger, hatred and sadness in the patient and remind him that the body grows fat from joy and thin from sadness.
> —Henri de Mondeville

Throughout the history of medicine, we have discussed the importance of attending to the body, mind, and spirit. Humor is one of the pleasures of life. To dispense laughter will directly enhance the quality of life and perhaps the will to live—this may be the most important result of all. The will to live is a force that is very difficult to define, but can be a powerful influence in the patient's recovery process. Many of us have witnessed the patient who asserts that he or she is going to die, despite a fairly normal physical examination and laboratory results; and then proceeds to do so, often surprising the professional staff. The opposite can also be true. A patient is given a grim prognosis by his or her physicians, but announces that he or she will overcome the condition, and then lives for many years beyond the predicted demise. Sometimes mobilizing the will to live can be the most powerful influence one human can offer another.[41] Humor and laughter can create an environment in which hope can flourish because it provides a sense of joy, helps us connect with family and friends, and inspires an appreciation and gratitude for life.

SUMMARY

I have attempted to provide information, qualifications, and inspiration for the possibility that laughter and humor can be a source of therapy for both the patient and the caregiver. My intent was to answer the questions: "Why are humor and laughter important? What happens to the body, mind, and spirit when we laugh?" You are now probably wondering: "How can I get myself and others to laugh more? When is humor appropriate to use? Who is most likely to laugh?" For help in finding answers to these questions, consult the resource list and references that follow.

Begin to explore your own style and appreciation of humor. Find what works for you and your patients. Remember, the shortest distance between two people is a shared laugh.

REFERENCES

1. Fry W. Mirth and oxygen saturation of peripheral blood. Psychother Psychosom 1971;19:76.
2. Fry W. Mirth and the human cardiovascular system. In: Mindess and Turek, eds. The study of humor. Yellow Springs, OH: Antioch University Press, 1979.
3. Fry W. The respiratory components of mirthful laughter. J Biol Psychol 1977;19:39.
4. Ader R. Psychoneuroimmunology. New York: Academic Press, 1991.
5. Lefcourt H. Humor and life stress. New York: Springer-Verlag, 1986.
6. Lefcourt H. Humor and immune system functioning. Int J Humor Res 1990;3(3).
7. McGhee P, ed. The handbook of humor research, vols. 1 and 2. New York: Springer-Verlag, 1983.
8. Selye H. The stress of life. New York: McGraw-Hill, 1956.
9. Cousins N. Anatomy of an illness. New York: WW Norton & Co, 1979.
10. Cousins N. Head first—the biology of hope. New York: Dutton, 1989.
11. Berk L. Neuroendocrine influences of mirthful laughter. Am J Med Sci 1989;298:390.
12. Berk L. Eustress of mirthful laughter modifies natural killer cell activity. Clin Res 1989;37:115A.
13. Locke S. Life change stress, psychiatric symptoms, and natural killer cell activity. Psychosom Med 1984;46(5).
14. Irwin M. Life events, depressive symptoms and immune function. Am J Psychiatry 1987;144:4.

15. Glaser J. Psychosocial moderators of immune function. J Behav Med 1987;9:16.

16. Glaser R. et al. Stress-related impairments in cellular immunity. Psychiatry Resident 1985;16:233.

17. Stein M. Stress and immunomodulation: the role of depression and neuroendocrine function. J Immunol 1985;135:827.

18. Schleifer S. Suppression of lymphocyte stimulation following bereavement. JAMA 1983;250:374.

19. Bartrop R. Depressed lymphocyte function after bereavement. Lancet 1977;1:834.

20. Stone A. Evidence that IgA antibody is associated with daily mood. J Personal Soc Psychol 1987;52(5).

21. Dillon K. Positive emotional states and enhancement of the immune system. Int J Psychiatry Med 1985;15:1.

22. Martin R. Sense of humor, hassles, and immunoglobulin A: evidence for a stress-moderating effect of humor. I J Psychiatry Med 1988;18:93.

23. Cushing J. The life of Sir William Osler. New York: Oxford University Press, 1940.

24. Robinson V. Humor and the health professions. Thorofare, NJ: CB Slack, 1990.

25. Freud S. Jokes and their relation to the unconscious. (J Strachey, trans; 1960), New York: WW Norton, 1905.

26. Henry J. Surviving the cure. Cope Inc., Cleveland, (216) 663-0855, 1984.

27. Grizzard L. They tore out my heart and stomped that sucker flat. New York: Warner Books, 1982.

28. Jackson T. Patient's at large. Jackson's Corner, P.O. Box 504, Pacifica, CA 94044, 1984.

29. Stewart D. Please don't stand on my catheter. (Sponsored by Orange Co. Chapter of American Heart Assoc) Fullerton, CA: Sultana Press, 1982.

30. Nehmer W. Have a heart. Cudahy, WI: Reminder Enterprise Printing, 1988. [or write to author at: 5362 Cedardale Dr., West Bend, WI 53095].

31. Parfitt JM. Humorous preoperative teaching: effect on recall of postoperative exercise routines. AORN 1990; 52(1).

32. Kelly W. Laughter and learning: humor in the classroom. Portland, ME: J Weston Walsh, 1988.

33. Parkins C. Humor, health, and higher education: laughing matters. J Nurs Educ 1989;28:229.

34. Kobassa S. Personality and social resources in stress resistance. J Personal Soc Psychol 1983;45:839.

35. McDougall W. A new theory of laughter. Psyche 922;2:298.

36. Pfeiffer R. A chance to cut is a chance to cure. 1983. [A funny book about medicine, surgery, hospitals, and patients; written by a cardiovascular surgeon. To order, send check for $5.00 to: Rip Pfeiffer, M.D., 171 Louiselle St., Mobile, AL 36607]

37. Shem S. The house of God. New York: Dell Publishing, 1978.

38. Johnston W. To the ones left behind. Am J Nurs 1985; A pp. 936.

39. Moody R. Laugh after laugh. Jacksonville, FL: Headwaters Press, 1978.

40. Walsh J. Laughter and health. New York: D Appleton & Co, 1928;147.

41. Klein A. Healing power of humor. Los Angeles, Tarcher, 1989

BIBLIOGRAPHY

Humor Resources

Jest for the Health of It workshops. [Presentations about humor and laughter for health professionals. Consultation for creating humor carts, humor rooms, and hospital clowning programs.] Patty Wooten, BSN, CCRN (a.k.a. "Nancy Nurse"), P.O. Box 4040, Davis, CA 95617-4040. (916) 758-3826].

American Association for Therapeutic Humor. [Quarterly newsletter and networking source for humor authors, researchers etc. $ 35/yr.] 1163 Shermer Road, Northbrook, IL 60062-4538. (708)291-0211.

J Nurs Jocularity. [A hilarious quarterly publication, written by nurses, for nurses, about the funny side of the nursing profession.] Send $12.00 to: JNJ dept FKOX 5615 W. Cermak Rd. Cicero, IL 60650-2290. Send contributions for publication to: Doug Fletcher RN-editor, P.O. Box 40416, Mesa, AZ 85274.]

Laughter Therapy. [Candid Camera Video films for free rental to use for stimulating laughter for recovery from illness.] Send letter explaining plans for use to: P.O. Box 827, Monterey, CA 93942.

Humor Project. [Sponsors Humor and Creativity conference biannually. Also excellent humor book catalogue. Publishes *Laughing Matters* a quarterly journal with ideas on how to bring humor into your life.] Order: 110 Spring St., Saratoga Springs, NY 12866. (518) 587-8770.

Laughter Works. [Quarterly newsletter of helpful tips, articles, funny items, jokes, book review, upcoming humor events;] $15/yr. Order: P.O. Box 1076, Fair Oaks, CA 95628. (916) 863-1592.

Whole Mirth Catalog. [Access to many humorous items, toys, gags, books.] Order: 1034 Page Street, San Francisco, CA 94117.

Medical Antics. ["Stat" and "Code" T-shirts, hats, mugs, and much more.] Order from: 99 Kinderkamack Rd., Westwood, NJ 07675. (201) 666-1558.

Anatomical Chart Company. [Mail order for anatomical body suit] 8221 N. Kimball, Skokie, IL 60076. (800) 621-7500.

Funny Times. [Monthly newspaper with cartoons and funny articles about current events; $17.50/yr.] Order from P.O. Box 18530, Cleveland Heights, OH. 44118. (216) 371-8600.

THOMAS L. PETTY

24

Ethical Considerations in the Care of Advanced and Final Stages of Chronic Obstructive Pulmonary Disease

The past quarter of a century has resulted in better drugs and improved technologies for the care of patients with advanced chronic obstructive pulmonary disease (COPD). Also better understanding of the disease process itself has created a remarkable improvement in the lives and happiness of large numbers of patients with advanced COPD. Together, pharmacologic agents, rehabilitative techniques, and oxygen therapy have improved survival and reduced hospital needs for many patients. Today almost all patients with COPD live into their late 60s or even 70s and 80s, but most finally die of their disease.

Pulmonary rehabilitation, described elsewhere in this monograph, should be considered preventive therapy. It is designed to forestall and prevent premature morbidity and mortality. The Nocturnal Oxygen Therapy Trial (NOTT) strongly suggested that oxygen "buys" approximately 3 1/2 years of happy life for patients on continuous oxygen therapy.[1,2] Thus, the course of advanced disease can be altered by systemized, comprehensive care.

METHODS OF DEALING WITH ADVANCED DISEASE

Chronic Compensated Carbon Dioxide Retention

Although acute CO_2 retention is a mark of exacerbation when acidemia is present, slow, chronic, and compensated CO_2 retention can be considered adaptive in advanced COPD.[3] When the CO_2 tension rises slowly in the face of advancing airflow obstruction and renal reclamation or generation of bicarbonate maintains isohydria (i.e., a normal pH), an adaptive state can be reached.[3,4] This phenomenon allows

435

CO_2 homeostasis to occur at a lower level of minute ventilation and thus with less work of breathing. Often this is translated into a reduction in dyspnea. Indeed, some patients have diminishing dyspnea as their carbon dioxide level rises. Patients may live at home for months or years with carbon dioxide tensions higher than 90.[4] Thus, chronic compensated CO_2 retention should be allowed to occur naturally or even encouraged with the use of opioids or anxiolytics when appropriate (see later discussion).

Other Methods of Reducing Dyspnea

Adaptation to advancing dyspnea is probably largely mediated by endogenous endorphins. Consequently, it makes sense to provide exogenous opioids for the same purpose. Modest amounts of codeine have reduced breathlessness in patients with advanced COPD. Opioids can be used to encourage compensated CO_2 retention. Anxiolytic drugs, such as benzodiazepine[6] and a nonbenzodiazepine preparation, Buspirone, may often relieve dyspnea and also help promote chronic-compensated CO_2 retention.

Considerations for Mechanical Ventilation

Mechanical ventilation can be used to buy time to help patients recover from exacerbations of disease. Intubation and mechanical ventilation may be quite appropriate, even in older individuals who suffer pneumonia, influenza, episodes of purulent bronchitis, and heart failure, when there is the possibility of further meaningful recovery. By contrast, when it is likely that patients will have their death only extended by the use of intubation and mechanical ventilation, it follows that this approach would be inappropriate.

Ethical Considerations in Final Care

Most patients with advanced COPD recognize that they will die, not only with their disease, but of their disease. My own experiences with hundreds of such patients has clearly taught that these patients do not particularly care that they will die of their disease; they are panicked over how they might die. They often have fantasies of suffocating, "climbing the walls," and being generally miserable. When it can be understood that CO_2 retention is rather pleasant and the patients simply go to sleep, reassurance can often be a great solace to patients and their families.

The President's Commission has clearly stated that there is no difference between withdrawing or withholding any therapy that is otherwise only a futile gesture, at best, or something that extends the dying process.[7] These principles were reevaluated and expanded at a National Institutes of Health (NIH) workshop on withholding and withdrawing mechanical ventilation held in Washington DC in October 1985.[8] Thus mechanical ventilation, oxygen, parenteral nutrition, ordinary foods and fluids can be withdrawn by a physician upon directive of a patient or even on the request of families when there is a clear advance directive from the patient that such therapy is not desired.

Ethical Principles

I have published the following ethical principles elsewhere.[9] In my opinion, they remain fundamental to decision-making in patients with advanced COPD.

Beneficence

There is a long history in the medical and nursing professions dealing with beneficence to the patient. These begin with the oath of Hippocrates: ". . . I will come for the benefit of the sick." The Florence Nightingale pledge includes the phrase ". . . and devote myself to the welfare of those committed to my care." These guiding principles, so simply stated, must be not only forever remembered, but practiced daily by the entire health care team.

Autonomy

The autonomy of the individual is guaranteed by fundamental legal principles. These include the United States Constitution, which guarantees the right to privacy; and the common law, which determines the right to bodily self-determination. The principle of autonomy includes the fundamental right of confidentiality. Accordingly, all decision-making concerning resuscitation or withdrawing life support must consider these established legal and moral obligations.

Informed Consent

Informed consent is a fundamental matter that deals with a clear understanding and, indeed, a contract between patient and physician about the patient's wishes and desires about his or her care during any medical circumstance, be it a procedure or the conduct of long-term care. In the opinion of many experts, the "do not resuscitate" decision or order becomes part of the doctrine of informed consent. The patient consents to be treated or not, and the patient can demand that life-support systems be withdrawn. How this informed consent is documented is another matter. Written informed consent is largely mechanical and ceremonial, but it also carries some weight. Oral informed consent is a far deeper human process, implying a level of trust and understanding that often goes beyond the record of the written word. Yet when informed consent for life-and-death medical decisions is achieved and fully understood by all parties, this fact should be recorded somewhere, particularly on the official medical record, for possible later reference. The principle of informed consent embodies the fundamental of truth-telling.

Advanced Directives

Today most states have living-will legislation with the rights of the individual and directives to physicians written in somewhat different language. There is a great need for a uniform rights act throughout the United States. All 50 states embrace the principle of durable power of attorney. A durable power of attorney permits surrogate decision-making, even in the case of incompetence of the person who gives this legal power. Although living wills are perhaps better known to the public through publicity, the durable power of attorney principle is more powerful and permits flexibility. Yet it must go without saying that living wills and the durable power relationship are subject to constant review, revision, and possible revocation.

Substituted Judgment

The process of substituted judgment embodies the determination of evidence that a patient who no longer can articulate, write, or otherwise communicate his or her wishes has left written and verbal instructions to a "substitute" who can convey these wishes and make decisions.

The living will and durable power of attorney provide for surrogate decision-making in the event of an incompetent or unconscious patient. The goal is to carry out the final wishes of the patient in the most dignified and humane way. In the absence of provision for substituted judgment, the next best approach is to invoke the principle of the patient's best interests.

The Patient's Best Interests

Much of this principle or, rather, a method of arriving at a decision, is embodied in the foregoing paragraphs. It includes the principles of beneficence and individual autonomy as well as substituted judgment. The problem here is that opinions differ at times over what the patient's best interests may be. This occurs when families come into conflict or there is a difference of opinion between the caregiver and one or more family members. If there is a disagreement, negotiation and final reconciliation are required. This may be aided materially by an Ethics Committee. Ethics committees do not make decisions, but rather serve as a board of review where all parties can express their opinions and feelings. Often an open airing of a dispute results in reconciliation. In the final analysis, it must be agreed by all parties that the patient is or was the only one who really knew how he or she felt and what life meant. The burdens of illness and therapy and the patient's hopes and expectations for the future must dictate the final decision-making, whether the patient is in a competent state or whether the surrogate decision-maker has the final responsibility.

Reason

Human beings are endowed with various levels of reason and judgment. The issues of beneficence, autonomy, confidentiality, informed consent, best interests, and substituted judgment must be aired, reviewed, and rereviewed. At this point, it becomes obvious that what is considered reasonable to one may be thought folly to someone else. Here again the process of reconciliation must apply.

Medical Decisions Concerning Resuscitation

The Decision not to Resuscitate in Chronic Obstructive Pulmonary Disease

Sudden death in or out of the hospital almost always calls for a rush of emergency medical teams for the purpose of reestablishing respiration and circulation. Although few would question that useful lives have been saved, there is also the nagging feeling that many should have been allowed to die without resuscitative efforts. It is inherently wrong to deny human beings one of nature's most fundamental events, life's transition into death at the appropriate time. More than a decade ago I wrote an editorial designed to help guide decision-making in the event of sudden cardiopulmonary arrest.[10] This has been widely quoted, but I have taken the liberty of reproducing this commentary as follows:

> Faced with a patient with sudden cessation of respiration and cardiac function, how does one decide whether intubation, mechanical ventilatory support, and reestablishment of cardiac function with closed chest massage and/or pharmacologic agents should be instituted? The systematic review of four basic questions provides major assistance in this important decision. These questions are as follows:
>
> 1. Do I know the patient's underlying disease process and its course and prognosis?
> 2. Do I know the patient's quality of life in the context of his [or her] disease process? [I now must add and reemphasize, Do I know the patient's wishes for the future?]
> 3. Do I have anything more to offer the patient by resuscitative efforts designed to gain more time?
> 4. Do I wish to gain more time through resuscitative efforts to resolve these other questions? [Now I must add, wish on behalf of my patients.]

The physician and nurse (or therapist) should be able quickly to answer these questions to determine if the patient is best served by initiating respiratory or cardiac support. If one is unable to answer the first two questions in the affirmative, it is still highly likely that support should be offered until the answers become clearer. One should not fear making a mistake in the direction of vigorous support, for certain patients will be saved to lead meaningful lives once again. If "yes" is the clear answer to the first two questions and the third and fourth are "no," then the physician, nurse, or allied health worker should simply stand by and offer whatever comfort and assistance he or she can to the patient or the family, or both. When the patient's life is known to be miserable at best, and when the patient has indicated no wish to have his or her suffering extended by technological means—in short, when there is nothing to be gained by the additional hours, days, or weeks one might achieve by supporting respiration and circulation—the interventions such as tracheal intubation, mechanical assistance, and cardiopulmonary support should be set aside on behalf of the patient with advancing, disabling emphysema with no hopes of recovery from respiratory failure.

Today I would add to this list a fifth question:

> 5. Do I have a verbal or written contract with my patient about how I should handle situations when further medical care to sustain life is not appropriate?

The Decision not to Ventilate

One could use approximately the same check list to make the decision not to ventilate, when such intervention would only create pain and sorrow or postpone an otherwise inevitable death.

The Decision to Discontinue Ventilatory Support

As stated earlier, there is no fundamental moral or ethical difference between withholding or withdrawing life support. The decision to discontinue ventilatory or circulatory support in cases of certain hopelessness are governed by the same principles as those that govern not initiating support. It is reemphasized that the same principles apply to withdrawing supplemental oxygen, food, electrolytes, fluids, and pharmacologic agents.

The Decision to Continue Ventilatory Support in Patients Destined to Become Ventilator-Bound

These are perhaps the most difficult situations because they usually involve patients who are awake and alert and whose life clearly can be sustained with mechanical ventilatory support, but who are destined to be tethered to their life support system for prolonged periods. There are patients who can enjoy life in such situations, and their rights must be recognized. It must also be recognized by patient and family that living in a hospital or today, more commonly, in the person's own home for months or years supported by a mechanical ventilator creates its own burdens. There can be no clear-cut guidelines in this difficult medical decision because the considerations are almost endless and the complexities profound, but the rights of the individual to self-determination must be the overriding consideration, and more and more people will have life sustained hopefully, happily, and productively with mechanical ventilatory support in extended care facilities or, preferably, in the home.

CASE EXAMPLES Some aspects of the ethical and moral principles involved in continued life support of patients with advanced COPD are cited in the following two case examples.

Case 1

FC was a 72-year-old retired businessman who had enjoyed life until disabling emphysema first limited his activities at age 62. He retired from his successful business at age 65 and entered a pulmonary rehabilitation program. His exercise tolerance improved only slightly following breathing training and physical conditioning. Because of severe sustained hypoxemia and congestive right heart failure from cor pulmonale, he was given continuous ambulatory oxygen. This caused a dramatic improvement in his ability to participate in activities of daily living and in his mood and quality of life. He traveled extensively with his wife and visited his children and grandchildren. However, as the years passed he became progressively dyspneic on exertion and, finally, at rest. Ultimately, he was housebound because of unrelenting dyspnea, in spite of continuous oxygen and other pharmacologic therapy. He and I (his personal physician) had an excellent relationship; and the wife, patient, and I often discussed the future, that resuscitation would not be appropriate should death occur at home, and that the patient should not enter a hospital during final stages of disease.

The patient became progressively forgetful as chronic CO_2 retention emerged. His dyspnea nearly disappeared when the arterial PCO_2 gradually became elevated above 80 with appropriate serum bicarbonate compensation. Following a very mild upper respiratory illness, the patient became semistuporous. I made a house call and determined that death was probably imminent, but not certain. Again, the patient and wife stated that transfer to the hospital and intubation with mechanical ventilation was not the wish of the patient because of the verbal contract made on numerous occasions by meaningful discussions when the patient was totally lucid.

The patient was maintained at home with oxygen. He remained comatose for approximately 24 hours with his wife in attendance. After approximately 36 hours of "deep sleep," the patient awakened gradually one morning and asked for some breakfast. He then rapidly emerged from a stuporous state and felt relaxed and at ease. He had nothing but pleasant recollections of his emergence into the CO_2 narcosis. It was springtime and he took an interest in sitting out in the sunshine on the patio and even puttering a little bit with the flowers. After several visits from his children and grandchildren in the fall of that same year, his wife realized one morning that her husband had died in bed during the night.

COMMENT This is an example of ideal preparation for death and a clear directive against intervention. This man died at age 73 in peace and the quiet of his own home. The interesting rally from a comatose state is not unusual in advanced emphysema. The late Alvan Barach even termed this "sleep therapy." The gradual buildup of carbon dioxide, a potent smooth-muscle relaxant, may well provide some bronchodilatation, and it probably engenders an outpouring of brain endorphins that blunt respiratory drives and counter dyspnea. Whatever the mechanism, I have seen numerous patients such as this private patient of mine emerge through "the short sleep" into a period of detente with death. At times, the period of detente may be 6 to 24 months of meaningful life. The detente, of course, is followed by what I describe to my patients as "the long sleep." Indeed, sleep and death have often been equated:

> O sleep, thou ape of death, lie dull upon her and be her sense but as a monument.
>   —Shakespeare, Cymbeline Act II, Scene 2

and:

> How wonderful is Death,
> Death and his Brother Sleep!
>   —Shelley

Family Conflicts

Withdrawing care and providing comfort such as the use of intravenous morphine, often as a drip, to ease suffering during the final hours is legally, morally, and ethically appropriate. However, there may be emotional considerations. Sometimes family members do not recognize the patient's rights or the legal, ethical, and moral principles described herein. In fact, often the medical and nursing professions may not recognize these principles. Some of these problems are illustrated in the following case example, which is a true story depicting the delicate and beautiful relation that may occur between patient, physician, and the patient's family.

Case 2

RK first came to me at age 48 because of worsening cough, wheeze, and dyspnea. He had smoked extremely heavily and had consumed the equivalent of 37 pack years at the time he was first seen. He expressed a desire to be able to live to the age of 60, which would be about the time that all of his children would be grown. He followed every detail of my medical advice and counseling, including stopping smoking and the systematic use of bronchodilating agents. Since he was responsive to corticosteroids and had marked improvement, he frequently took these drugs on my advice and, at times, on his own with permission. At age 60, the patient had deteriorated to the point that he was nearly housebound. At this time, he began to receive continuous portable oxygen by nasal cannulae. He had extremely high respiratory drives and often would use pursed-lips breathing to the extent that even the degree of hypoxemia required for reimbursement under Medicare could not be achieved. Said another way, he would often maintain an oxygen saturation higher than 88%, but with extreme dyspnea while pursed-lips breathing. On other occasions, while seated quietly, his oxygen saturation would fall to 78%. The patient was improved with oxygen and physical reconditioning as he participated in a pulmonary rehabilitation program. Later, however, dyspnea became intolerable. At this point I gave him codeine, 32 mg every 4 hours, and also as needed to help blunt dyspnea. This was only modestly effective. The patient freely used inhaled beta-agonists and anticholinergics, and increasing doses of corticosteroids were required. Two compression fractures occurred during the patient's last year of life. In an attempt to extend the patient's oxygen use and because of nasal complications, the patient received the insertion of a transtracheal oxygen catheter.[11] He felt that this helped relieve dyspnea. He was maintained on full pharmacologic management and oxygen by transtracheal catheter until dyspnea became overwhelming. At this point he requested a prescription of 40 ea. 100 mg secobarbital (Seconal) tablets, which he had read would be a lethal dose, should he decide to take the entire prescription. He wanted a method of "getting out," if he wished, and control of this decision. I gave him this prescription after full discussions with his wife and, at that time, a living will was signed. She was also designated durable power of attorney to help carry out the patient's wishes in the event that he would become incompetent and thus unable to express his wishes about further treatment. However, he never did take the Seconal, except on occasion, in individual capsules when overwhelming nocturnal anxiety and insomnia were present. He reported that it gave him great comfort to have the medication available in case he wanted or needed it. Finally, the patient deteriorated to the point at which he could not leave his house. Later, he could not leave his room or even get dressed without involuntary urination. He was miserable. Accordingly, he called me asking to be admitted to the hospital for morphine and to discontinue his oxygen. He felt his wife could not deal with death at home. It was agreed that this would be accomplished on the ward that cares for terminal cancer victims. Here it was commonplace to give sufficient morphine by intravenous administration to provide comfort. The patient's family was in general agreement, but a son-in-law struggled with anxieties over what he viewed as euthanasia. It was clearly discussed that relieving patients' suffering is something quite different from euthanasia. The patient became hungry on his last day of life. He had an abundant breakfast with scrambled eggs, bacon, and hash browns, and salt (which had previously been restricted from his diet because of right heart failure). He also wanted to watch a professional football game one more time. At this time he ordered a prime rib with plenty of salt, and he was jovial as he was surrounded by his family, and myself; he was now receiving a morphine drip. Casual observers could not believe that he was a dying man. After the meal and following the advice of the family, the patient stopped his oxygen and went to sleep. However, there were many anxieties on the part of the nursing support staff who felt that stopping oxygen was inappropriate. Indeed, they almost always used oxygen for the care of terminal cancer patients as a *comfort matter*. Finally, I had to write an order to discontinue oxygen, and the patient died quietly while morphine was running. This case was discussed at the Hospital Ethics Committee and all were in unanimous agreement that his care was proper.

This case illustrates many of the problems faced by health workers who care for terminal patients. The patient died at aged 63.5 years, which was longer than predicted or expected when I first saw him. His quality of life was excellent until his last year. Even his last few days of life were meaningful because of the discussions he could have with his family and the saying of goodbyes, and offering forgiveness for past transgressions.

Medical care is designed to relieve suffering, as well as to promote health, happiness, and longevity. These principles must be carefully considered and applied on an individual basis when one deals with advanced and final stages of COPD.

REFERENCES

1. Nocturnal oxygen therapy trial group. Continuous or nocturnal oxygen therapy in hypoxemic chronic obstructive lung disease: a clinical trial. Ann Intern Med 1980;93:391.

2. Roberts SD. Cost-effective oxygen therapy [editorial]. Ann Intern Med 1980;93:499.

3. Riley RL. The work of breathing and its relation to respiratory acidosis. Ann Intern Med 1954;41:172.

4. Neff TA, Petty TL. Tolerance and survival in severe chronic hypercapnia. Arch Intern Med 1972;129:591.

5. Stark RD, O'Neill PA. Dihydrocodeine for breathlessness in "pink puffers." Br Med J 1983;286:1280.

6. Stark RD, Gambles SA. Effects of diazepam and promethazine on breathlessness induced by exercise or raised CO_2 in healthy subjects. J Clin Respir Physiol 1980;16:220P.

7. President's Commission for the study of ethical problems in medicine and biomedical and behavioral research. Making health care decisions, vol 1. Washington DC. Government Printing Office, 1982.

8. National Institutes of Health workshop on withholding and withdrawing mechanical ventilation. Am Rev Respir Dis 1989;140(suppl 2):51.

9. Petty TL. Resuscitation decisions, ethical issues in the care of the elderly. Clin Geriat Med 1986;2:535.

10. Petty TL. Don't just do something—stand there! Arch Intern Med 1979;139:920.

11. Christopher KL, Spofford BT, Petrum MD, McCarty DC, Goodman JR, Petty TL. A program for transtracheal oxygen delivery. Ann Intern Med 1987;107:802.

25

DALE R. BERGREN

Respiratory Physiology in Health and Disease

THE PURPOSE OF RESPIRATION

In the past, *respiration* referred to the process of ventilation. Today the term respiration also includes the processes of gas exchange in the lungs and tissues as well as cellular metabolism involving the gases of respiration. Ventilation and gas exchange are termed *external respiration*, whereas cellular metabolism is termed *internal respiration*. The paramount purpose of the lung is to perform gas exchange. A continuous supply of oxygen is required to build or release stores of energy in most cells other than for short periods.

Carbohydrates are the major energy source for cellular functions. The oxidation of glucose and the reduction of O_2 can generate adenosine triphosphate (ATP) from ADP and inorganic phosphate. The energy is stored in its high-energy phosphate bonds. Oxidative phosphorylation occurs within the inner membrane of the mitochondria, the destination of oxygen. In the processes of glycolysis and oxidative phosphorylation a total of 38 molecules of ATP are formed from the oxidation of a single glucose molecule to carbon dioxide and water.

In the single-celled or smaller multicellular organism, O_2 is able to diffuse from the environment to the mitochondria of the cell to supply all the O_2 needed to sustain life. In larger organisms, the distance for O_2 to diffuse from the environment to the internal cells is inhibitory for survival. Therefore, a system must serve to supply these internal cells with O_2 from the environment as well as to remove metabolic waste products of oxidative metabolism, such as CO_2, from accumulating within the body.

The supply and delivery systems for the human body are the pulmonary and the cardiovascular systems. There are two basic problems these systems encounter to accomplish the delivery of O_2 from the atmosphere to the mitochondria: first, convection in the airways and in the circulation vasculature and, second, diffusion across the alveolar–capillary membrane and from the systemic capillaries to the mitochondria. The problems involved in convection can be simplified by examining Ohm's law, which we may modify to say $\dot{V} = \Delta P / R$. Therefore, in the respiratory system, air flow ($\dot{V}$) between two points is dependent on a difference in pressure (ΔP) between the points, but inversely affected by the existing resistance (R).

444

The process of diffusion can be understood in part by examining Fick's law which is expressed as: $\dot{V}_x = K(P_xA - P_xB) \cdot S/T$.

The rate of diffusion ($\dot{V}$) of gas X between two points or areas is directly proportional to the pressure or concentration difference across the diffusion barrier ($P_xA - P_xB$) and the surface area (S) of the barrier separating the two areas. The diffusion of gas X is inversely proportional to the thickness of the barrier or membrane (T). K (Krogh's constant) is equal to the diffusion coefficient multipled by the solubility coefficient of the gas under study. The diffusion coefficient (D) is inversely proportional to the square root of the molecular weight (MW) of the gas in accordance to Graham's law ($D = 1/\sqrt{MW}$). With the development of pulmonary disease, parameters of these two equations become altered. It is my purpose to review the processes involved in respiration in both health and disease.

A Review of Pulmonary Anatomy

In humans, beginning at about day 24, the human lungs develop as an endodermal bud of the primitive gut at the level of the upper esophagus.[1] During development, the lungs grow by a process of irregular dichotomous or paired branching. This branching continues for about 23 generations.[2] At birth, about 24 million alveoli exist in the lungs, which increases to about 300 million in adult lungs.

In the functioning lung, the first 16 generations serve to conduct air to the later generations where the surface area has dramatically increased. No significant gas exchange occurs within the first 16 generations. Air traveling through this *conducting zone* is warmed, humidified, and cleansed. From generation 17 until the 23rd generation, gas exchange occurs with increasing efficiency. Therefore, this area is termed the *respiratory zone* of the lung. The first alveoli may appear as early as the 17th generation. It is probable that these alveoli are the first to open and expand during the inspiratory cycle.[3]

During a ventilatory cycle of 500 mL, approximately 1 mL of air per pound (0.45 kg) of lean body weight (about 150 mL) must occupy the conducting zone after the initial ventilatory volume (about 350 mL) has reached the respiratory zone. The conducting zone (*anatomical dead space*) does increase somewhat as lung volume increases, owing to the traction tension of expanding alveoli surrounding the walls of the conducting airways. This increases airway diameter. The air that reaches the respiratory zone is exposed to a surface area of approximately 70 m² in the adult lung.[4,5]

In normal lungs, the histologic structure of the airway epithelium changes as a function of increasing airway generations. Ciliated, pseudostratified, columnar epithelium lines the trachea, which serves the purpose of lung defense. Distally, the cells become cuboidal. Squamous cells (alveolar type I cells) line the alveoli, which serves the purpose of gas exchange, having an average thickness of less than 0.5 μm.[6,7] The alveolar type I cells also present a formidable barrier to passage of fluids, large molecules, or other materials or cells, owing to the presence of tight junctions between cells.[8] These tight junctions extend from the terminal airways into the alveolus. Normal lung function is dependent on the integrity of the epithelial layer in the distal areas of the lung. The endothelial cells of the pulmonary capillaries, on the other hand, are quite porous.

About 95% of the alveolar surface is composed of these alveolar type I cells.[9] Because of this specialization to minimize the diffusion barrier, the alveolar type I cells cannot replicate.[10] After cellular injury and death in the alveoli of type I cells, the surface epithelium must be replenished by alveolar type II cells that cover approximately 5% of the alveolar surface under normal conditions. The cuboidal-shaped alveolar type II cells will with time then differentiate into type I cells.[11,12]

PULMONARY MECHANICS

Ventilation of the Lungs

The process of ventilating the lungs involves two phases: an inspiratory phase, which always involves muscular contraction (an active process), and an expiratory phase, which can either be an active or a passive process (no muscular contraction). The change in thoracic dimensions during inspiration occurs, in part, when the dome-shaped diaphragm, separating the thoracic cavity from the abdominal cavity, contracts to a more flattened position proportional to the amount of effort expended during the inspiratory process. The contraction of the diaphragm increases the craniosacral dimensions of the chest and increases the lateral dimensions of the chest somewhat by pushing the lower ribs outward. The diaphragm is assisted by the external intercostal muscles, which increase the circumference of the chest by pulling the sternum and ribs upward and outward, and by tensing the intercostal space, which increases the efficiency of the diaphragm. During dyspnea the scalene, the sternocleidomastoid, and the trapezius muscles may assist the respiratory effort by elevating the clavicle, sternum, and the upper ribs to increase the circumference of the upper chest.

The expiratory phase can use potential energy from the elastic recoil of the lung parenchyma, after relaxation of the inspiratory muscles, to induce airflow. This *passive* expiration will return the lungs to its functional residual capacity (see later discussion of lung capacities). An *active* expiration involves the contracting expiratory muscles to increase the rate of expiratory flow or to bring lung volume below that of the functional residual capacity (FRC). The major expiratory muscles are the internal intercostal muscles, which lower the ribs' position and pull the sternum inward, and the abdominal muscles, which compress the abdominal contents against the diaphragm, thereby reducing the craniosacral dimensions of the chest. Those muscles in the abdomen that can participate in expiration include the rectus abdominous, the transverse abdominous, and the internal and external oblique muscles.

Changes in chest dimensions caused by muscle contraction or relaxation change the pressure in the intrapleural space. This "space" contains only a few milliliters of fluid that separates the parietal pleura of the chest wall from the visceral pleura surrounding the lungs. An abnormal amount of fluid in this space is called a *pleural effusion* and decreases the volume the lung can occupy. During contraction of the inspiratory muscles from FRC, the chest cavity increases in size, which *decreases* the intrapleural pressure. As a result a traction tension is transduced to the lung parenchyma and intrapulmonary pressure also decreases. The air inside the expanded tissues, such as the alveoli, becomes subatmospheric (rarified). Air from the environment then flows into the airways and alveoli until there is no pressure gradient between the alveoli and the mouth. The process is reversed during the expiratory phase. The inspiratory muscles relax, the chest recoils, intrapleural pressure increases, and alveolar air is compressed. Air flows from the alveolus to the mouth.

The normal ventilation volume per breath of the lungs is called *tidal volume*. The tidal volume changes to meet the O_2 demands of the body (i.e., the current metabolic rate). At rest the tidal volume (TV), about 0.6 L, occupies about 10% of a person's total lung capacity (TLC), about 6 L. As metabolic demands cause ventilation to increase, tidal volume increases into the inspiratory reserve volume (IRV), about 3 L. This results from increased contractile action of the inspiratory muscles. Should ventilation still be inadequate to match metabolic demands, respiratory rate also increases. As can be seen in Figure 25–1 blood gas composition depends on "alveolar ventilation" and not on the absolute minute volume. *Alveolar ventilation* can be defined as the tidal volume minus the anatomical dead space. It would be possible to have a tidal volume such that there is no alveolar ventilation. This occurs when the tidal volume is smaller than the sum of the anatomic and alveolar dead space or when the anatomical dead space is increased by attempting to inhale and exhale through a long tube. By examining Figure 25–1, we see that increasing tidal volume, not rate, is initially the most efficient means to increase alveolar ventilation.

If further ventilation is needed, or if an individual coughs or sneezes, then ventilation may include the volume of air in the lungs below the normal starting point of a tidal volume, the expiratory reserve volume (ERV), about 1.2 L. This is accomplished only through the recruitment of expiratory muscles, such as the internal intercostal or abdominal muscles. Even with a maximal expiratory effort not all the air is removed from the lungs. This occurs because the expiratory muscles cannot compress the chest wall farther. The air remaining within the lungs is termed *residual volume* (RV), about 1.2 L.

The normal starting point for inspiration at rest is at a combination of the residual volume and the expiratory reserve volume and is called the *functional residual capacity* (FRC), about 2.4 L. The FRC is the natural balance between the elastic recoil of the lungs inward and that of the chest outward. Therefore, any change in the histologic structure or compliance of either system will alter the FRC.

Lung capacities are the combination of two or more of the four lung volumes. There are two capacities of the lungs in addition to FRC and TLC. *Inspiratory capacity* (IC) is the air that can be inspired from rest (FRC) to the total lung capacity (TLC) or tidal volume (TV) plus inspiratory reserve volume (IRV). *Vital capacity* (VC) is the total ventilatory capacity of the lungs and can be derived a number of ways: TLC − RV, ERV + TV +IRV, or IC + ERV. An update of standardized clinical spirometry has been prepared by the American Thoracic Society.[13]

Pressure–Volume Relations: Pulmonary Compliance

When the inspiratory muscles contract, energy is used to expand the tissues of the chest as well as the tissues of the lung parenchyma. The compliance of the respiratory system (Crs) is the resulting change in volume (ΔV) occuring in response to the

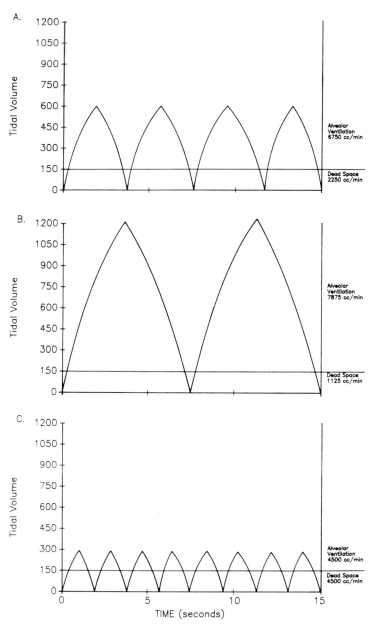

FIGURE   25-1   Relation between changes in tidal volume (TV) and alveolar ventilation (AV) when minute volume (MV) and dead space (DS) are constant. In each case MV = 9000 mL/minute and DS = 150 mL. (**A**) Typical breathing pattern: TV = 600 mL, breathing rate (BR) = 15.0/minute, AV = 6750 mL/minute. (**B**) Slow, deep-breathing pattern: TV = 1200 mL, BR = 7.5/minute, AV = 7875 mL/minute. (**C**) Rapid, shallow-breathing pattern: TV = 300 mL, BR = 30.0/minute, AV = 4500 mL/minute.

change of pressure (ΔP) and is usually described as the change in liters per centimeter of water ($Crs = \Delta V/\Delta P = L/cmH_2O$).

The Crs is affected by two "systems" in parallel: the thoracic cage and the lungs. Each has its own compliance profile. The lungs are surrounded by the chest wall and diaphragm. Muscular effort from the diaphragm and the external intercostal muscles changes the volume of the thoracic cage. If the thorax is either increased in mass, as it is in obesity, or deformed, as it is in kyphoscoliosis, then the thoracic cage resists changing its volume more so than when the thoracic cage has less mass or is not deformed. In other words, the chest is less compliant in these examples than in a normal condition. The compliance of the thorax for an adult at about FRC is approximately 0.2 L/cmH_2O.

As the chest wall and diaphragm increase thoracic volume, the lung tissue is "pulled along" because the parietal and visceral pleura adhere together, much like two glass microscope slides held together by a droplet of water. The lung responds to the pressure change surrounding it by expanding, but relative to its own compliance. The average compliance of the lung is also about 0.2 L/cmH_2O at FRC.

The compliance (C) of the lungs is affected by two major contributing factors: tissue elastance and surface tension. The tissue elastance (E or $1/C$) is a function of the tissue mass and its composition. Fluid accumulation within the lungs, such as vascular engorgement or interstitial edema, increases the mass of the lungs and requires more muscular effort to achieve a similar volume than that attained during normal conditions. Collagen invasion of the interstitial areas of the lung (interstitial lung disease; ILD) decreases tissue compliance and increases elastance.

Interstitial lung disease includes many disorders such as idiopathic pulmonary fibrosis, sarcoidosis, asbestosis, silicosis, pneumoconiosis, and extrinsic allergic alveolitis. The common features of these diseases is the increase in lung elasticity owing to fibrous and cellular accumulation in the lung parenchyma. As the work of breathing increases, the breathing pattern becomes rapid and shallow, which is the most efficient method of ventilation under these circumstances. There is little reserve ventilation capacity for these individuals upon exertion because of decreased IRV and ERV. Expiratory flow rates are characteristically high because of the increased elasticity of the lung tissue. Fibrotic tissue also tends to hold the airways open more than usual, which explains the higher than expected expiratory flow rates in ILD, because airway resistance is low. Although the rate of expiratory flow is high, the resulting volume is low. The high elastance and low compliance of the lung tissue decreases all lung volumes and capacities.

As the disease progresses and the alveolar membrane thickens, the diffusion capacity of the lungs decreases. Arterial PO_2 decreases and eventually the PCO_2 increases.[14] The pathologic progression of the disease is often not uniform throughout the lungs, resulting in mismatching of ventilation to perfusion (see the section on $\dot{V}/\dot{Q}$).

Currently the treatment of some interstitial lung diseases includes anti-inflammatory, glucocorticoid, and immunosuppressive agents to retard the progress of the disease. Supplemental O_2 is prescribed for significant hypoxemia. Vasodilators may counteract a proposed increase in thromboxanes in certain forms of ILD.[15]

Lung Surface Tension Forces

During normal conditions, tissue elasticity accounts for about 25% of the collapsing forces of the lungs, the remaining 75% of the collapsing forces of the lungs is attributable to surface tension forces. This can be demonstrated by comparing the pressure–volume curve of an air-filled with a saline-filled lung (Fig. 25–2). In an air-filled lung, surface tension occurs at the air–liquid interface, which tends to collapse the lung. This tension is eliminated in the saline-filled lung; therefore, less pressure is required to achieve the same volume.

Surface tension (T) and its effects on the collapsing pressure (P) in a one-sided structure such as an alveolus can be examined using the law of Laplace ($P = 2T/r$). This relation states that the collapsing pressure of an alveolus because of surface tension forces increases as its radius (r) decreases. However, agents are present on the alveolar surface that reduce the surface tension forces at low lung volumes sufficiently that the diameter of the small alveoli does not lead to alveolar collapse (*atelectasis*) as predicted by the law of Laplace. These agents are called *pulmonary surfactants*.

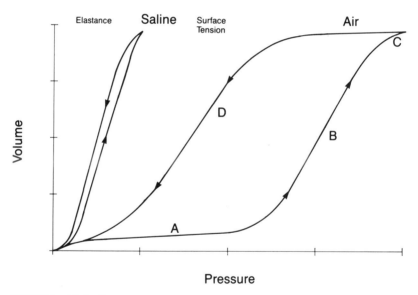

FIGURE   25-2   Pressure–volume relation in an isolated lung preparation inflated with air or saline. The difference between the two curves at any horizontal point is due to surface tension forces in the air-filled lung. The difference in the expansion and compression curve in the air-filled lung is called *hysteresis* and is due to changes in the characteristics of the surfactants: (**A**) Region of critical opening pressure of collapsed alveoli during inflation; (**B**) combination of inspirational surface tension and elastic forces; (**C**) upper elastic limit of the lungs; (**D**) combination expirational surface tension and elastic forces.

Pulmonary Surfactants

Function

Pulmonary surfactants reduce the surface tension between the air and liquid interface in the alveoli. Pure water has a surface tension of 72 dynes/cm when interfaced with air. This tension is constant, regardless of surface area. The surface tension of water can be reduced to near 0 dynes/cm when covered sufficiently by surfactants (Fig. 25–3). The surface tension of an alveolus near its total capacity has been reported to be 30 dynes/cm,[16] as compared with nearly 0 dynes/cm at its FRC.[17] When the surfactants present on the alveolar surface are either abnormal or absent, the minimum surface tension is higher than normal. Such is the case in infant respiratory distress syndrome (IRDS)[18] or adult respiratory distress syndrome (ARDS).[19]

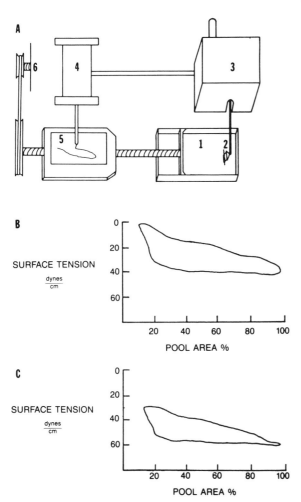

FIGURE 25-3 (A) Surfactometer which measures surface tension of lung fluids: *1*, trough with moving "barrier dam" holding lung lavage fluid; *2*, platinum flag that is pulled into lung lavage fluid as a function of increasing surface tension; *3*, force transducer; *4*, pneumatic recording stylus; *5*, graph of surface tension recorded as a function of trough surface area; *6*, Motor. **(B)** Surface tension record of normal lung lavage fluid. Minimum surface tension of near 0 dynes/cm occurs at minimal surface area (15% of pool surface area) when the surfactants are the most concentrated per unit surface area. **(C)** Surface tension record of abnormal lung lavage fluid (pulmonary edema). Minimum surface tension is near 30 dynes/cm at the minimal surface area.

Origin of Pulmonary Surfactants

The source of the surfactant complex is the alveolar type II pneumonocyte. The type II pneumonocyte has within its cytoplasm vesicles called lamellar bodies. The lamellar bodies contain the surface-active agents, primarily phospholipids, which are released by means of exocytosis into the alveolus.

The major surface active agent of the surfactant complex is dipalmitoyl phosphatidalcholine (DPPC), accounting for about 75% of the surfactant phospholipids. DPPC has both a hydrophobic end and hydrophilic end, which account for its ability to reduce the surface tension of an air–liquid interface. However, expansion and compression cycling of the alveolar surface is required to maintain a low surface tension.[20]

Control of Surfactant Secretion

The rate of production and secretion of pulmonary surfactants is affected by both physical conditions and chemical agents. Increased ventilation increases surfactant release.[21] β-Adrenergic agonists also increase surfactant production.[22,23] Certain prostaglandins may decrease surfactant secretion.[24] Exposure to high concentrations of O_2 also can inhibit surfactant production or physiologic function.[25]

Fate of Pulmonary Surfactants

The turnover rate of the surfactant complex is reported to be 3 to 11 hours.[16,26,27] Therefore, surfactants are continually synthesized and released from the type II pneumonocyte into the alveolar lumen. Surfactant is lost from the alveolus during the ventilatory cycle into the airways and is carried up the mucociliary escalator.[28,29] Some of the surfactant complex is cleared through the lymph or even the blood. The surfactant complex is also phagocytosed by alveolar macrophages that may have also undergone extracellular enzymatic degradation.[30] However, most of the surfactants are recycled and reconditioned by the alveolar type II cell for further use.[29,31] The amount of surfactant that is recycled decreases with age from about 90% in the young[27] to about 25% in the old.[32]

Airway Resistance

Frictional Forces and Airflow

The work of breathing includes overcoming not only viscoelastic resistance of the chest and lung tissue, but also frictional resistance of airflow throughout the tracheobronchial tree. The frictional resistance of airflow occurs primarily in the upper airways where air velocity is high. Although branching results in a decrease in individual airway diameter for each successive generation, after generation four or five the combined cross-sectional area of each generation increases markedly over the previous airway generation (Fig. 25–4). Air velocity must fall as the cross-sectional area increases; therefore, airway resistance tends to decrease with each subsequent generation in the lung periphery. As an example, the effectiveness of a cough with its explosively high airflow extends from the trachea (generation zero) down to only about generation 7 of the 23 generations of the airways.

If the velocity of air is constant in a certain airway, frictional forces increase as the airway diameter decreases. Frictional forces or airway pressure increases 16 times for

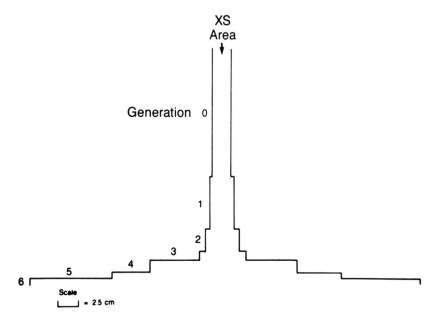

FIGURE   25-4   Scaled diagram of combined cross-sectional (*XS*) area of lung generations 0 to 6. As cross-sectional area increases, air velocity must decrease; therefore, small-airway disease is difficult to determine spirometrically.

every 50% decrease in the radius of the airway. The relation between pressure and airflow in an airway caused by friction when airflow is laminar is described by Poiseuille's law:

$$\Delta P = 8\mu l\dot{V}/\pi r^4, \text{ and since } R = \Delta P/\dot{V}, \text{ then } R = 8\mu l/\pi r^4$$

where ΔP = hydrostatic pressure drop, $\dot{V}$ = gas flow, μ = gas viscosity, l is tube length and r = tube radius.

Airway pressure increases linearly as air velocity increases as long as the airflow is laminar (streamlined). When airflow becomes turbulent, the frictional forces increase because vectors of airflow cross the mainstream of flow at various angles (i.e., eddies). During turbulent airflow, airway pressure (*P*) is proportional to the square of air velocity ($\dot{V}^2$), so that pressure in an airway is no longer linearly related to flow, but exponentially related. Reynold's number is used as a predictor of turbulent flow and is

$$N_R = \rho\dot{V}D/\mu A,$$

where N_R = Reynold's number, ρ = fluid density, μ = fluid viscosity, $\dot{V}$ = mean linear velocity, A = cross-sectional area, and D = tube diameter. When N_R exceeds 2000, turbulent flow occurs.

During ventilation at rest, when airflow is low, turbulence occurs within the trachea or perhaps in the primary bronchi after airway branching. However, turbulence occurs in more distal generations during higher airflow, such as during exercise.

Turbulence also occurs with localized airway constriction or the presence of mucus. The work of breathing increases as the result of air turbulence.

Resistance and Lung Volume

Lung volume itself affects resistance during airflow. As the lung volume increases, alveoli expand, including those surrounding the conducting airways. This physical situation produces a pulling or traction tension on the walls of the airways that increases the airway diameter. Airway expansion is a function of lung volume and the number and compliance of alveoli that exert traction tension. In emphysema, fewer alveoli exist, which also have higher compliance than normally encountered. This results in reduced traction tension on the airway so that the airway diameter is not as great as in the normal lung. Because there is less traction tension surrounding the airways in emphysema, for example, these airways are also more susceptible to expiratory compression, which increases airway resistance or even results in airways collapse during an expiratory effort. The air trapped within the lungs or the *closing volume* occurs sooner in emphysema. The closing volume occurs when intrapulmonary pressure overcomes airway pressure and the airway collapses, especially if the airway has lost its supporting structures through disease. Patients with emphysema often breath at higher lung volumes to overcome these effects.

The maximal expiratory airflow rate decreases as lung volume decreases in normal as well as diseased airways, owing to several factors, as demonstrated in Figure 25–5. Airway diameter decreases and airway resistance increases as lung volume decreases owing to a decline in traction tension of the surrounding alveoli on the conducting airways. However, the maximal expiratory airflow also decreases as lung volume decreases volume because the elastance of the pulmonary system is at its peak at total lung capacity. As the lung volume decreases, so does the elastic recoil of

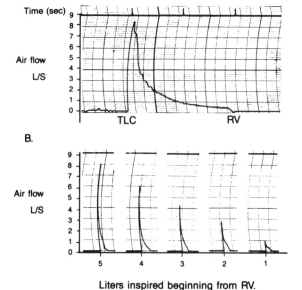

FIGURE 25-5 Relation between lung volume and maximal expiratory flow rate. Flow rate decreases as lung elasticity, inward chest recoil, airway diameter, and alveolar surface tension all decrease from *TLC* to *RV*: (**A**) forced expiratory flow from total lung capacity (*TLC*) to residual volume (*RV*); (**B**) maximal expiratory flow starting at various lung volumes.

the lung parenchyma and chest wall. At approximately 60% of the vital capacity, the "natural" volume of the chest wall is reached. Therefore, at 60% of the VC, chest wall elasticity or recoil no longer assists the expiratory process. At lower lung volumes, the chest actually recoils outward. Lung elastance still is capable of "drawing" the chest inward until FRC is reached. At FRC, which is the balance of the chest's tendency to expand and the lung's tendency to collapse, expiratory muscle contraction is necessary if lung volume is to be further reduced. In other words, this is the end of a passive expiration. Muscular effort during expiration, either before or after FRC is reached increases intrapulmonary pressure, which also reduces the diameter of the airway. This pressure of compression on the airways further increases resistance to airflow and increases the possibility of airway collapse.

With these factors in mind, the expiratory flow curve may be divided into *effort-dependent* and *effort-independent* zones. Starting at total lung capacity, increased expiratory effort increases expiratory flow to a limit of the muscular potential. From TLC and down to approximately 80% VC, an effort-dependent zone is said to exist. However, near and below 80% VC, there is observed a plateau in airflow after a certain level of muscular effort is reached. One may attempt to increase the expiratory effort to attain greater airflows after this critical point, but without success. Therefore, there is observed what is termed the effort-independent zone.

Modulating Airway Tone

Several neurotransmitters and neurohormones are now known to exist and function in the lungs. Many function to increase airway smooth-muscle tone, but several have the ability to decrease it. These agents may be released by several mechanisms.

Classic autonomic nervous control of organ systems in the body pits the adrenergic system against the cholinergic system. In the lungs, demonstrable autonomic innervation of the airways of smooth muscle and submucosal glands is dominated by cholinergic efferent nerves carried by the vagi.[33] A rich supply of motor fibers is demonstrable in the upper airways, but this diminishes toward the distal airways. An increase in cholinergic tone increases airway smooth-muscle tone. Little, if any, adrenergic innervation has been demonstrated to either the airway smooth muscle or the submucosal glands to oppose cholinergic motor tone.[33]

Although the airways do not contain classic sympathetic innervation of physiologic significance, normal airway smooth muscle is quite responsive to either circulating or aerosolized sympathomimetic agents. Naturally occurring catecholamines, such as epinephrine, released from the adrenal medulla and carried through the circulation to the lungs, act upon β_2-adrenergic receptors, causing airway smooth muscle to relax (i.e., bronchodilation).

A nonadrenergic, noncholinergic nervous system (NANC) exists in the airways as an inhibitory system to relax airway smooth muscle.[34] The primary neuropeptide released during this activation is vasoactive intestinal peptide (VIP) and is 50 to 100 times more potent to induce bronchodilation than is isoproterenol, a nonspecific β-adrenergic agonist. The NANC nervous system may not function properly in asthma and cystic fibrosis.[35,36] One study reports that VIP is absent in the airways of at least some patients with asthma.[37] Administration of VIP to asthmatic patients produces disappointedly minimal bronchodilation.[38] It appears the peptide is rapidly destroyed by the proteases in the airway secretions.

Throughout the airways are unmyelinated sensory endings that are called C-fiber endings.[39] These nerve endings contain several "tachykinins," including substance P, that cause bronchoconstriction.[40] Neuropeptides are released from the C-fiber endings in the vicinity of airway smooth muscle, blood vessels, the epithelium, and the mast cell by a mechanism called an *axon reflex*.[41] The C-fiber stimulation appears to cause the symptoms observed during allergic reactions, anaphylaxis, and asthma, such as bronchoconstriction, vasoconstriction in some systems and vasodilation in others, edema formation, and infiltration of inflammatory cells (chemotaxis).

Asthma

The influence of airway smooth muscle upon airway resistance, and therefore, on ventilation, is most dramatically apparent during acute episodes of asthma. Asthma has been a difficult disease to characterize, in part because of various and noninclusive causes of its symptoms. Asthma triggered by agents from the environment, such as pollens, molds, dander, and chemical irritants, is termed *allergic* or *extrinsic asthma*. Asthma resulting from altered conditions within the body that should not normally alter airway function is termed *intrinsic asthma*. Triggers of intrinsic asthma include changes in ventilation (exercise, laughter), changes in airway temperature, and changes in emotions. A fundamental definition of asthma was offered by a 1959 Ciba symposium stating *asthma* is "a widespread narrowing of the airways which changes in severity over short periods of time either spontaneously or under treatment and not due to cardiovascular disease."

The classic symptom of asthma is a marked and acute decrease in the expiratory flow rate. This decrease is caused, in part, by airway smooth-muscle contraction, which constricts the airways. The bronchoconstriction in allergic reactions is compounded by increased and thickened secretions in the airways, which can result in the mucus wedging in the airways (i.e., mucous plugs). Hypertrophy is seen in the airway muscle and the submucosal glands in asthma.[42,43]

The etiology of asthma has been intensely investigated, but is still poorly understood. There appears to be direct and reflex components of asthma. Possible explanations of airway hypersensitivity by direct mechanisms may include the down regulation of β_2-adrenergic receptors in the cellular membrane of airway smooth muscle.[44] It is possible that mechanisms within the cell connected to the expression of the β_2-adrenergic receptor are restricted. Either possibility would tip the balance in favor of parasympathetic mechanisms that increase airway smooth-muscle tone.

A second possible explanation of increased airway hypersensitivity may exist within the immune system involving participates such as macrophages, lymphocytes, leukocytes, and the mast cells. A heightened ability to react to antigenic challenge might result in massive production and release of the putative mediators that increase airway tone and secretions. Such mechanisms may account for the late-phase reaction seen with severe episodes of asthma.

A third possibility may involve reflex control of airway tone by the autonomic nervous system. Histamine was one of the first mediators to be shown to lead to reflex bronchoconstriction.[45] Antigenically induced bronchoconstriction in dogs has a dominant reflex component mediated by the vagus nerve.[46] However, other investigators have failed to generate significant reflex bronchoconstriction in their studies and have challenged its proposed contribution to the asthmatic episode.[47–49]

To establish a reflex mechanism of bronchoconstriction, it is important to determine the receptors in the lungs and the afferent pathway involved. There are now three accepted categories of afferent receptors in the lungs: slowly and rapidly adapting receptors and C-fiber endings. Although many have believed that the rapidly adapting or "irritant" receptors mediate reflex bronchoconstriction, it now appears that C-fibers produce reflex bronchoconstriction either mediated through the central nervous system[50] or through a more localized axon reflex.[51,52]

An intriguing mediator of asthma is platelet-activating factor (PAF), which is produced by alveolar macrophages and eosinophils. The actions of PAF include platelet chemotaxis from the circulation, bronchospasm, increased vascular permeability, and increased sensitivity to other agents that constrict the airways. Currently, PAF is the only mediator that causes sustained nonspecific airway hypersensitivity to histamine, methacholine, substance P, and $PGF_{2\alpha}$ for as long as 4 weeks after a single exposure.[53] Prostaglandin (PG) D_2 and the leukotrienes produce very short-lived nonspecific airway hypersensitivity.[54–57]

Ventilation/Perfusion Ratios

Neither ventilation nor perfusion is uniformly distributed within the lungs. Gravity affects both ventilation and perfusion relative to posture. Local factors affecting airflow and circulation also affect the ventilation/perfusion ($\dot{V}/\dot{Q}$) ratio in both the normal and, more importantly, the diseased lung. Measurement of $\dot{V}/\dot{Q}$ describes the efficiency and coordination of the pulmonary and cardiovascular system to perform gas exchange.

Ventilation increases from the lung's apex to its base. Anatomically, the lungs are pyramidal so that the cross-sectional area is greater at the base than at the apex. Therefore, the base of the lungs has greater potential ventilation. Second, at the lung's apex the ribs are in a more horizontal position and have less potential to move than the ribs toward the base of the lungs.

The lung parenchyma at the apex is physically subjected to a greater subatmospheric tension than lung parenchyma at the base in an upright position in a gravitational field. Gravity exerts a force of 9.8 m/sec^2 on mass in its field. The lungs have mass but only about one to five that of water (i.e., 0.2 g/cm^2 vs 1g/cm^2). The lungs also have height; therefore, intrapulmonary pressure becomes a function of height (P = height $\times$ density $\times$ gravity). As one descends in a pool of water, one becomes quickly aware of increased pressure owing to its effect on the ears. Similarly intrapleural pressure increases from the apex to the base in an upright lung. However, because the lungs' density is about 0.2 g/cm^2, a lung with a vertical height of 30 cm will have an intrapleural pressure difference of 6 cmH_2O between the apex and the base, (i.e., 0.2 $\times$ 30). If the intrapleural pressure is -9 cmH_2O at the apex in this case then intrapleural pressure must be -3 cmH_2O at the base.

Therefore, the alveoli at the apex are subjected to a greater negative pressure at FRC than the alveoli at the base. Since the alveoli have similar tissue density all over the lung, the alveoli at the apex must have a larger radius than those at the base (Fig. 25–6). The potential of alveoli to expand to total capacity is also similar throughout the lungs. This creates a situation in which the alveoli at the apex are already expanded closer to their total capacity than are those at the base. One must then realize that the potential for ventilation dictated by these physical circumstances is much greater at the base than at the apex. Zero gravity would cancel this factor affecting regional ventilation.

The same physical and anatomical factors affect lung perfusion. The heart is in the midthoracic region, so it must pump blood "uphill" to the apex and "downhill" to the base. The pulmonary vessels are thin walled and will collapse without adequate perfusion pressure. Gravity affects cardiac output to the lungs more than it affects regional ventilation; therefore, the $\dot{V}/\dot{Q}$ ratio becomes a function of lung position relative to gravity. This ratio becomes less than 1 at the base and greater than 3 at the apex. The ideal situation would be to have a 4 : 5 ratio in all areas of the lungs, 4 L/minute representing the average minute ventilation and 5 L/minute average cardiac output.

The $\dot{V}/\dot{Q}$ ratio at rest is useful in determining functional abnormalities in the lungs. When the $\dot{V}/\dot{Q}$ ratio approaches infinity in a certain region of the lungs, then there exists a probability that blood flow is being restricted, such as the presence of

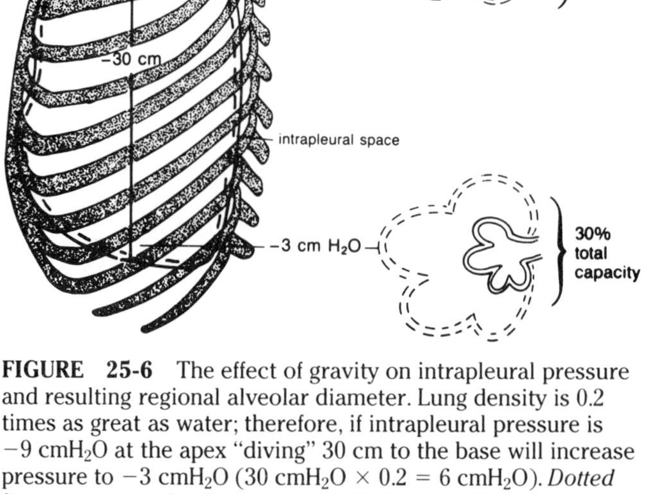

Alveolar Diameter at FRC

−9 cm H_2O — 80% total capacity

−30 cm

intrapleural space

−3 cm H_2O — 30% total capacity

FIGURE   25-6   The effect of gravity on intrapleural pressure and resulting regional alveolar diameter. Lung density is 0.2 times as great as water; therefore, if intrapleural pressure is −9 cmH_2O at the apex "diving" 30 cm to the base will increase pressure to −3 cmH_2O (30 cmH_2O × 0.2 = 6 cmH_2O). *Dotted line* represents alveolar volume at TLC versus that at FRC.

pulmonary shunts, thrombi, emboli, or perhaps heart failure. This situation results in *physiologic dead space* or wasted ventilation. When the V̇/Q̇ ratio approaches zero then there is the likelihood of airways obstruction, such as airway constriction or mucous plugging of asthma, or decreased ventilatory drive (i.e., with drug overdose from drugs such as morphine or barbiturates).

GAS TRANSPORT: THE LUNG TO THE TISSUES AND BACK AGAIN

The Respiratory Membrane and Gas Diffusion

The muscles of inspiration have completed their function of ventilation once the incoming air has reached the respiratory bronchioles. The process of air movement by convection ends here. Although some O_2 exchange takes place in the respiratory bronchioles, most of the influx of newly inspired O_2 molecules continue to diffuse down the concentration gradient toward the alveolar sacs. The respiratory membrane separates O_2 in the alveolar space from the blood in the pulmonary capillaries. Oxygen crosses this barrier by the process of diffusion, as described by Fick's law (as presented earlier).

The fraction of O_2 in our environment is about 21% of the ambient pressure. At sea level (760 mm Hg) and in dry air this pressure is about 160 mm Hg. This is in accordance with Dalton's law, which states that the total atmospheric pressure is equal to the sum of the partial pressure of the individual gases ($P_T = P_1 + P_2 + P_3 \cdots$).

The sum of the partial pressure of each component gas can never exceed the ambient pressure in an open system. As other gaseous components are added to an open system the partial pressures of the original components must decrease. As air enters the body it is quickly humidified until saturated. The vapor pressure of water is 47 mm Hg when it is 100% saturated at 37°C. As a result, nitrogen and oxygen, which constitute most of the inspired air, must then become diluted; nitrogen from approximately 600 mm Hg to 564 mm Hg and O_2 from 160 to 150 mm Hg. As CO_2 enters the alveolar lumen the partial pressure of O_2 drops further. The partial pressure of oxygen (PO_2) in the respiratory zone also falls because it is diffusing out of the alveoli into pulmonary capillaries. It is important to realize these values are affected by the alveolar ventilation and, therefore, represent an estimated mean pressure. Alveolar PO_2 averages 100 to 104 mm Hg during eupnea, but drops quickly with apnea or may increase with hyperpnea. The incoming partial pressure of O_2 in the pulmonary artery ($P\bar{v}O_2$) is near 40 mm Hg, so that the diffusion pressure for O_2 into the pulmonary capillary, therefore, is normally about 60 to 64 mm Hg. As the ambient or atmospheric pressure falls, so does the partial pressure of a gas, although its proportional contribution to the total atmospheric pressure remains the same. At an elevation of 3040 m (10,000 ft; Leadville, Colorado), the contribution of O_2 to the atmospheric pressure (about 524 mm Hg) is still about 21%, but PO_2 is now only about 110 mm Hg. Therefore, the driving pressure of O_2 across the respiratory membrane is decreased; accordingly, oxygen diffusion must also decrease.

The respiratory membrane is a heterogeneous barrier. Beginning at the alveolar lumen, O_2 must cross a monomolecular surfactant layer; a layer of fluid called the hypophase; the alveolar epithelium, which is primarily composed of type I pneumonocytes; an interstitial space, consisting primarily of collagen; the endothelial basement membrane; and the highly permeable endothelial cell, before reaching the plasma. Even the red blood cell (RBC) membrane presents a significant resistive barrier to diffusion.[58]

The rate at which O_2 diffuses across the respiratory membrane is dependent not only on a pressure gradient, but is also dependent on its surface area and thickness. It is said the surface area of the lungs is about the size of a tennis court. The respiratory membrane's thickness averages 0.5 μm, whereas the total distance to the RBC averages 0.77 μm.[7] A decrease in surface area (emphysema) or an increase in the thickness of the respiratory membrane (idiopathic pulmonary fibrosis) will affect the overall ability to exchange gases. When the respiratory membrane is increased in thickness, O_2 exchange is reduced before CO_2 exchange is reduced.[59]

Oxygen Transport

Oxygen diffusing across the respiratory membrane does so as a gas dissolved in a liquid. The net diffusion or movement of O_2 from the alveolar lumen to the capillary lumen continues until pressure equilibrium is reached.[60] Since the PO_2 in the alveolar lumen averages approximately 100 mm Hg, so too will be the PO_2 of the plasma as it leaves the pulmonary capillary in the normal lung if diffusion equilibrium is reached. At a PO_2 of 100 mm Hg, 3 mL of O_2 can dissolve in 1 L of plasma. At a cardiac output of 6 L/minute the amount of dissolved O_2 reaching the metabolizing tissues falls far short of even the basal metabolic needs of the body (i.e., 18 mL of O_2 per minute delivered, versus 250 to 300 mL of O_2 per minute needed).

The erythrocyte solves the problem of the dissolved O_2 being inadequate for the body's O_2 requirements through its chemical combination of O_2 with iron of the hemoglobin molecule. Any O_2 molecule that combines with the hemoglobin molecular no longer contributes to oxygen's partial pressure in the blood. As one O_2 molecule binds to hemoglobin, another O_2 molecule may dissolve into the plasma. The O_2 content of the blood is directly related to the hematocrit.

A normal hematocrit of 45% (i.e., 45% RBC and 55% plasma) contains a hemoglobin concentration of 150 g/L. Each gram of hemoglobin can combine with 1.34 to 1.39 mL of O_2. Therefore, each liter of blood can carry about 200 mL of O_2 combined with hemoglobin and 3 mL of dissolved O_2 when the PO_2 in the alveolus is 100 mm Hg. For a cardiac output of 5 L/minute, the O_2 carried in the blood is now far greater than the 250 to 300 mL/minute required for the process of basal metabolism (i.e., 1015 mL min^{-1}L^{-1}. Therefore, during basal metabolic conditions, only about 25% of the O_2 carried by the blood is used by the tissues.

Perfusion Versus Diffusion Limitations

An important physiologic and pathologic concern is whether or not the diffusion of O_2 has reached equilibrium across the respiratory membrane so that the PO_2 in the pulmonary capillary is roughly equal to that of the alveolar lumen. Factors that influence whether diffusion equilibrium occurs include the diffusion distance across the respiratory membrane and the transit time of blood as it passes through the pulmonary capillaries. The total diffusing distance across the respiratory membrane to the RBC averages 0.77 μm under normal conditions.[7] During "normal" resting conditions the transit time of blood through the pulmonary capillary is about 0.75 second. Under these conditions diffusion equilibrium occurs within about 0.25 second or by one-third the distance through the pulmonary capillary.

During exercise, with increased stroke volume and heart rate, the blood's velocity increases. Even so, gas exchange or diffusion equilibrium still occurs before the blood leaves the capillary because of the "extra" transit time through the normal alveolar capillary. Therefore, the normal lung is limited in its ability to oxygenate the blood by the cardiac output and it is said to be *perfusion limited* until extreme conditions exist.

If the respiratory membrane increases in thickness, then the diffusion of O_2 across the membrane requires more time. This occurs with pulmonary fibrosis and edema. As pathologic conditions worsen, diffusion equilibrium may not occur, ($T_D/T_T > 1$; time of gas diffusion equilibrium/capillary transit time). Since conditions within the lungs do not permit the equilibrium of diffusion, then a *diffusion limitation* to equilibrium exists within the lung. Arterial O_2 pressure (PaO_2) falls below alveolar O_2 pressure (PAO_2) as a function of the severity of the lung disease.

The Oxygen–Hemoglobin Dissociation Curve

How much oxygen is carried by the hemoglobin molecule depends on the physical and chemical conditions surrounding it that influence its structure. One may obtain an empirical relation of hemoglobin for the O_2 molecule by exposing known concentrations of hemoglobin to a known PO_2 (Fig. 25–7). The relation of O_2 bound to hemoglobin and its surrounding PO_2 results in an S-shaped curve with the steepest portion of the curve existing between a PO_2 of 10 and 40 mm Hg. This 30-mm Hg range of PO_2 accounts for about 60% of the saturation of the hemoglobin molecule. From a PO_2 of 60 mm Hg to 100 mm Hg the curve rapidly plateaus. In this range of 40 mm Hg PO_2, hemoglobin saturation increases only 7% more. During normal ventilation in environments containing a PO_2 of 150 to 160 mm Hg, the PO_2 in the pulmonary alveolus and capillary will average 100 mm Hg. The saturation of the hemoglobin molecule when the surrounding PO_2 is 100 mm Hg is 97% of its capacity.

Oxygenated blood of the pulmonary veins is mixed with deoxygenated blood coming from the heart and the bronchial circulation, about 2% of the cardiac output. The PaO_2 in the arterial blood as it travels to the metabolizing tissues is now about 97 mm Hg in the normal young adult. In the arteries the blood and the oxyhemoglobin molecule are protected from conditions that would cause oxygen's release. Once the blood enters the highly permeable systemic capillaries, various factors that reflect tissue metabolic rate, such as CO_2, come in contact with the incoming blood.

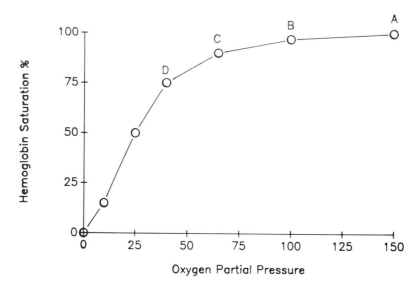

FIGURE   25-7   Oxygen–hemoglobin association versus varying partial pressures of oxygen. The difference between points B and D represent the amount of oxygen normally extracted by the tissues: (**A**) 100% saturation, an example is breathing air at 1.5 atm; (**B**) 97% saturation, an example is breathing air at 1 atm (sea level); (**C**) 90% saturation, an example is breathing air at 0.5 atm (3.5 km; 10,000 ft above sea level); (**D**) 75% saturation, an example of normal saturation of mixed venous blood at rest and at sea level.

The oxygen–hemoglobin dissociation curve is affected by these factors, which reflect the level of cellular metabolism. As CO_2 from the metabolizing cells increases in concentration within the capillary blood and then the RBC, the hemoglobin molecule has less affinity for O_2 (the Bohr effect). The binding of CO_2 with hemoglobin changes the configuration of the hemoglobin molecule, thereby decreasing its ability to hold on to O_2.

The binding of 2,3-diphosphoglycerate (DPG) to hemoglobin also changes the configuration of its molecular structure.[61] As a result hemoglobin has reduced affinity for O_2 and, like the effect of CO_2, the entire curve is shifted to the right. Carbon dioxide and 2,3-DPG apparently compete with each other for the binding to hemoglobin. The concentration of 2,3-DPG increases during anaerobic conditions and is an intermediary product of RBC glycolysis. The 2,3-DPG has greater affinity for deoxyhemoglobin than it does for oxyhemoglobin. As the RBC reaches the pulmonary capillary, increasing O_2 concentrations will increase the free concentration of 2,3-DPG.

Increases in either temperature or decreases in pH also decrease hemoglobin's affinity for O_2. The hemoglobin molecule is an important buffer of hydrogen ions. These changes normally occur within the systemic capillary network as the result of cellular metabolism. The degree of change reflects the level of ongoing metabolism.

The Tissue Capillary and Gas Exchange

The PO_2 in the interstitial fluid surrounding the tissue capillaries averages 40 mm Hg, whereas that of the metabolizing cell surrounding it is reported to average 5 mm Hg. If one begins with the O_2 that is physically dissolved in the plasma, a cascade of O_2 flows from the systemic capillary to the interstitial fluid, then into the cell, and finally to the mitochondria. Hemoglobin releases oxygen, maintaining equilibrium with the PaO_2. When the blood leaves the systemic capillary, it is no longer subjected to changes in the gas partial pressures or pH. The $P\bar{v}O_2$ is then about 40 mm Hg, reflecting the average PO_2 in the interstitial fluid.

Transportation and Excretion of Carbon Dioxide

The final end products of oxidative metabolism are water and CO_2. The lung is the ideal organ to accomplish CO_2 elimination because of its volume of ventilation. The CO_2 is produced in the cell's mitochondria (i.e., inner outer membrane) as the result of carbohydrate metabolism. The PCO_2 in the interstitial fluid is directly related to the cellular metabolic rate. During normal metabolism the interstitial fluid PCO_2 is reported to average 46 mm Hg. The incoming $PaCO_2$ averages 40 mm Hg. Therefore, the diffusion gradient of 6 mm Hg from the interstitial fluids surrounding the metabolizing cells to the capillary lumen results in a flow of CO_2 into the capillary. The diffusion of CO_2 is rapid, being 20 times that of O_2, which compensates for the smaller partial pressure gradient compared with that of O_2. The CO_2 enters the blood in the dissolved state. The $P\bar{v}CO_2$ averages 45 mm Hg, which corresponds to a CO_2 concentration of 29 mL/L of plasma. The reason for using mixed venous blood ($\bar{v}$) is that it is a mixture of blood returning from all vascular beds and, therefore, is not biased by the activity of only one organ system. Less than 10% of the CO_2 carried in the blood is dissolved gas. Slightly more CO_2 is transported in the blood as carbamino compounds. The amino group of the carbamino combination is supplied by proteins in the plasma, but particularly by hemoglobin in the RBC. As more CO_2 combines with hemoglobin in the systemic capillaries, the shape of the hemoglobin molecule changes (conformational change), which reduces its affinity for O_2 (the Bohr effect), thereby enhancing oxygen's release from hemoglobin to the tissue.

Most of the CO_2 is carried in the plasma as bicarbonate ions. The reaction of CO_2 with water to form carbonic acid occurs swiftly within the RBC owing to its high concentration of carbonic anhydrase. Carbonic anhydrase speeds this reaction 10,000 times faster than it would occur spontaneously. Carbonic acid rapidly dissociates to bicarbonate and hydrogen ions at normal body pH. Hydrogen ions within the RBC are buffered primarily by the hemoglobin molecule. Meanwhile the concentration of bicarbonate ions increases in the RBC as the blood travels through the tissue capillary. Bicarbonate ions maintain a concentration equilibrium with the plasma. Bicarbonate ion, being negatively charged, easily passes through the RBC membrane. Positively charged ions, such as hydrogen, cannot easily cross this membrane. To preserve isoelectrobalance within the RBC, chloride ion from the plasma crosses into the RBC as HCO_3^- passes out. This process is termed the *chloride shift;* it is reversed in the lungs. The mechanism of the chloride shift is still uncertain. There is an anionic membrane pump, which composes perhaps one-third the RBC membrane protein, that apparently requires an "exchange" of anions[62] (i.e., Cl^- and HCO_3^-). This pump may explain the mechanism of the chloride shift.

Disruption of Oxygen Supply

The O_2 content of the blood is dependent on the combined functions of the lungs, heart, and tissues. A PO_2 significantly lower than those described at any point from the environment to the mitochondria results in a condition called hypoxia (low O_2). There are four classifications of hypoxia based on its origin.

When the PaO_2 leaving the pulmonary capillary is lower than expected the classification of hypoxia is termed *hypoxic hypoxia.* Low PaO_2 causes both low PaO_2 and low arterial oxygen content (CaO_2) and occurs with high-altitude exposure, reduced ventilatory drive, suffocation, or airway obstruction. Increased resistance of the respiratory membrane to O_2 diffusion, as occurs with pulmonary edema or fibrosis, decreases PaO_2 despite an adequate PAO_2. Low PaO_2 occurs even with normal PAO_2 when ventilation and perfusion are not matched correctly (i.e., cardiovascular right-to-left shunts).

A second general classification of hypoxia is *anemic hypoxia.* Unlike hypoxic hypoxia, which is characterized by having a low PaO_2, with anemic hypoxia the PaO_2 is normal; however, the CaO_2 in the arterial blood is reduced. This is due to either a lower than normal concentration of hemoglobin in the blood, such as in acute hemolytic or primary anemia, or a decreased ability of the hemoglobin in the blood to carry O_2, such as in sickle cell anemia or carbon monoxide poisoning.

Cardiac output ultimately determines the quantity of blood and, therefore, that of O_2 traveling through the systemic capillaries. Because O_2 uptake corresponds to the ongoing cellular activity, the longer the blood remains in the systemic capillaries the greater the amount of O_2 extracted from the blood. As a result both the $P\bar{v}O_2$ and $C\bar{v}O_2$ become lower when blood flow is slowed, even though the PaO_2 entered the capillary within a normal range. The reduced delivery of blood supplied by the cardiovascular system to the tissues is referred to as *hypoperfusion hypoxia.* This occurs as the result of heart failure and certain forms of circulatory shock.

When the tissues do not accept the O_2 being supplied, despite a normal PO_2 surrounding it, a condition of *histotoxic hypoxia* results. When the enzymes of the respiratory chain are poisoned, with cyanide, for example, higher than expected $P\bar{v}O_2$ and $C\bar{v}O_2$ are found.

PULMONARY INVOLVEMENT IN BODY pH

To live is to produce hydrogen ions. In humans, the end product of anaerobic metabolism is lactic acid, whereas the end product of aerobic metabolism is CO_2 and water. Both can lower body pH. Changes in hydrogen ion concentration (pH) changes the efficiency of enzyme function. For example, lowering body pH encourages proton binding to the enzymatic proteins. At a plasma pH of 7.4 the normal hydrogen ion concentration is normally 40 mEq/L. A pH of 7.1 represents a doubling of the hydrogen ion content to 80 mEq/L, whereas a change of pH 0.3 pH units to 7.7 equals a reduction to 50% of the normal hydrogen ion content (20 mEq/L). Prolonged exposures to either pH value soon become incompatible with life.

Bicarbonate ions, phosphate ions, RBC and plasma proteins rapidly buffer hydrogen ions in the intra- and extracellular fluids. However, failure to actually eliminate the hydrogen ion quickly becomes a serious problem. The kidney normally excretes 50 to 70 mEq/day of hydrogen ions; however metabolism within the body produces over 20,000 mEq/day of hydrogen ions. Because most of the hydrogen ions in the body originate from carbonic acid, the lung's elimination of CO_2 plays a major role in maintaining the pH within normal limits. The level of ventilation is largely regulated by chemoreceptors acting on central respiratory centers as a function of the CO_2 concentration in the CSF and the plasma.

Until CO_2 is eliminated from the body, hydrogen ions resulting from its conversion with water to form carbonic acid must be buffered. The carbonic acid–bicarbonate buffering system is the primary buffering system of the plasma and is largely responsible for the resulting pH of the blood. Carbonic anhydrase in the RBC rapidly converts CO_2 and water to carbonic acid. Carbonic acid rapidly dissociates to a hydrogen and bicarbonate ion. The ratio of dissolved CO_2 to H_2CO_3 is very high, approximately 400 : 1 to 800 : 1. Plasma CO_2 concentration, rather than carbonic acid, is then used according to the Henderson–Hasselbalch equation to approximate the actual pH of plasma. The calculation of plasma pH is estimated by substituting into the Henderson–Hasselbalch equation the plasma bicarbonate concentration, which is normally 24 mEq/L, and the plasma concentration of CO_2, which is normally 1.2 mEq/L. The $PaCO_2$ in mm Hg is converted to milliequivalents per liter by the solubility coefficient of CO_2 in plasma which is 0.03 $mEqL^{-1}$ mm Hg^{-1}. Therefore: pH = pKa + log $[HCO_3^-]/[CO_2]$ and pH = 6.1 + log 24 mEq/L/(40 × 0.03) or 1.2 mEq/L = 7.4. Note, that the normal HCO_3^-/CO_2 ratio is 20 : 1; therefore, when one factor of the equation deviates from its normal value, the other factor can be changed to return the pH toward a value of 7.4. Although either the lungs or kidneys can compensate for changes in pH from 7.4, compensation by the lungs normally will be quite rapid (minutes), whereas that of the kidney may require days.

Disturbances in the body pH can occur with either hypoventilation or hyperventilation. Hypoventilation causes retention of CO_2 and, therefore, hydrogen ion concentration also increases within the plasma and throughout the body. This results in respiratory acidosis. Decreased ventilation may result from decreased ventilatory drive, such as depression or paralysis of the respiratory centers within the CNS (i.e., morphine overdose) or decreased ability to ventilate resulting from obstructive or restrictive problems of the lungs. Another mechanism by which respiratory acidosis develops is by a decrease in respiratory muscle strength. This occurs with myasthenia gravis, which is an autoimmune disease of the muscarinic receptors. As the number of functional muscarinic receptors associated with the respiratory muscles declines, so does the capability of ventilation. Therefore, the plasma not only becomes hypoxemic, but hypercapnic as well.[63] Respiratory acidosis quickly develops. The kidneys attempt to compensate by excreting hydrogen ions in exchange for sodium ions, which are reabsorbed with bicarbonate ions. Hypoventilation may also occur as a compensatory action to metabolic alkalosis in an attempt to lower plasma pH by retaining CO_2 and thereby hydrogen ions. This response is limited owing to stimulation of the central and peripheral chemoreceptors to increase ventilation.

On the other hand, hyperventilation results in the reduction of the plasma PCO_2 from 40 mm Hg to lower values, which thereby reduces the hydrogen ion content of the plasma, the intracellular fluids, and ultimately, the cells. Respiratory alkalosis results. Causes of hyperventilation include stimulation of the respiratory center either through cortical stimulation (excitement) or by direct action of certain stimulatory drugs (aspirin) on the respiratory center. The kidney will secrete more $NaHCO_3$ while reabsorbing more hydrogen ions in an attempt to lower pH. Hyperventilation may also occur in metabolic acidosis when increased hydrogen ion content increases ventilation through chemoreceptors stimulation.

CONTROLLING VENTILATION

The respiratory system must rapidly match ventilation with the current level of cellular respiration to maintain cellular and plasma pH at about 7.4. Although certain areas of the body sense changes in pH, PO_2, and PCO_2, only centers within the central nervous system can alter ventilation. Without communication from a central respiratory rhythm generator to the muscles of respiration, all ventilation ceases. Although the location of a central pattern generator is still uncertain, certain areas within the central nervous system are known to affect ventilation (Fig. 25–8).

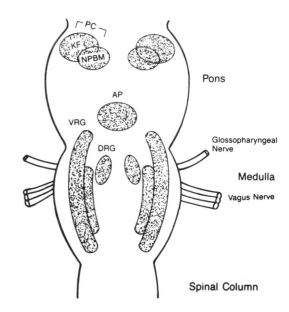

FIGURE   25-8   Location of "centers" of respiratory neurons in the central nervous system: *DRG,* dorsal respiratory group; *VRG,* ventral respiratory group; *AP,* apneustic center; *PC,* pneumotaxic center (*KF,* Kolliker–Fuse nuclei; *NPBM,* nucleus parabrachialis medius).

Central Control of Ventilation

One established nucleus is the dorsal respiratory group of neurons (DRG) in the medulla. Neurons in the DRG receive input from sensory receptors in the lungs and higher centers in the CNS. The DRG initiate inspiration through efferent nerve tracts of the phrenic nerve to the diaphragm and spinal nerves to the external intercostal muscles; accordingly, the neurons within the DRG may play an important role in respiratory rhythm generation.

Lateral to the DRG is the ventral respiratory group (VRG), which extends from the base of the medulla into the pons.[64–67] Both inspiratory and expiratory neurons populate the VRG. Neurons in the VRG also project to the diaphragm and the intercostal muscles,[68] but the VRG appears to be an accessory center for enhanced inspiratory or expiratory effort.

A group of respiratory-related neurons at the base of the pons is called the *apneustic center*. The function of this center is yet to be clearly defined. It has been called the apneustic center because tumors or lesions just cranially to this group of neurons results in prolonged apnea in the inspiratory position (inspiratory apneusis). Neurologic monitoring of this area has shown that primarily inspiratory neurons are present here.[69] The apneustic center has a stimulatory effect upon the DRG.

In the rostral pons are the nucleus parabrachialis medialis (NPBM) and the Kolliker–Fuse nucleus. Collectively, the two centers are termed the *pneumotaxic center* (PC). The PC receives input from both the peripheral and CNS. The function of the PC appears to be one of switching of the phase of ventilation.[70]

Other centers within the CNS influence the pattern of breathing through these ventilatory centers. For example, the cortex affects ventilation during vocalization, with changes in emotions, or during voluntary ventilatory maneuvers organized through the PC. The thalamus affects ventilation with fluctuations in temperature in many species, including humans. However, there are conditions in which the control of ventilation fails to function properly. Such conditions include sudden infant distress syndrome, Ondine's disease, and sleep apnea. Our knowledge of the mechanisms of these diseases is quite limited.

Central Chemoreceptors

Chemoreceptor input to ventilatory control also originates from within the CNS. In the floor of the fourth ventricle are neurons that sense the hydrogen ion content of the cerebral spinal fluid (CSF).[71] Carbonic anhydrase is present in the CSF, so the amount of hydrogen ions present also reflects its PCO_2. Carbon dioxide is lipid-soluble and rapidly diffuses across biological membranes, whereas positively charged ions, such as hydrogen, do not. Therefore, the PCO_2 in the CSF also reflects the PCO_2 in the cerebral circulation. It is assumed that this area is responsible for 70% or more of the respiratory drive during normal conditions. There is believed to be little or no response within the CNS to hypoxia. Furthermore, isocapneic hypoxia within the CNS results in central depression.

The ventilatory response to CO_2 can become depressed when one is exposed over an extended period to higher levels of CO_2, such as occurs during reduced ventilation (chronic obstructive pulmonary disease; COPD). Carbon dioxide can have an anesthetic action at higher than normal concentrations. Certain drugs, metabolic acidosis, and even sleep can result in higher tolerance for CO_2. This increased tolerance to higher plasma PCO_2 is due to an adjustment of the sensitivity of the chemoreceptors (carotid bodies included) to a higher PCO_2; therefore, ventilatory drive is reduced. On the other hand, exposure to low environmental PO_2 (hypoxic hypoxia) causes stimulation of the peripheral chemoreceptors through a decrease in PaO_2 and, therefore, increased ventilation. The $PaCO_2$ levels fall and, with time, cause the chemoreceptors to lower their PCO_2 threshold.

Reflexes from Outside the Lungs

Within the cardiovascular system located in the arch of the aorta (in animals) and near the bifurcation of the internal and external carotid arteries are "bodies" of chemoreceptors that sense changes in CO_2 and hydrogen ions with great sensitivity and changes in O_2 with comparatively less sensitivity.[72,73] At a $PaCO_2$ of 40 mm Hg the sensory receptor's impulses in the carotid and aortic bodies increase or decrease substantially with changes of only several mm Hg in PCO_2. On the other hand, when $PaCO_2$ is held constant, PaO_2 must fall from a normal value of near 100 mm Hg to nearly 60 mm Hg before the neuronal activity within these bodies increase ventilation. Once stimulated, these receptors reflexly increase ventilation and decrease heart rate.[75] In addition to the carotid and aortic bodies, the baroreceptors in the same general area also induce increased ventilation, when stimulated by low blood pressure, or decreased ventilation, when stimulated by high blood pressure.

Reflexes from Within the Lungs

Presently, there are but three major categories of sensory receptors accepted to exist within the lungs: slowly adapting pulmonary stretch receptors (SAR), rapidly adapting receptors (RAR, irritant receptors), and C-fiber endings associated with both the pulmonary and bronchial circulation. Table 25–1 summarizes the major characteristics of each category of receptor.

LUNG DEFENSE

Base-level metabolism requires lung ventilation of approximately 500 L/hour. The air inhaled during ventilation contains a suspension of numerous particles of both inorganic and organic nature. Although most of these particles are innocuous to the body and respiratory system, without a means to remove particulate matter from the airways, the sheer volume of particulates would soon present a formidable problem to continued ventilation and gas exchange. Some inhaled substances have the potential to induce injury or disease. Therefore, the lungs are also a major strategical site for the entrapment, detoxification, and elimination of inhaled substances and for the immune system to limit microorganism invasion to the body.

TABLE   25-1.   Major Characteristics of Sensory Receptors in the Lungs

Category	Afferent Fiber	Stimuli	Proposed Reflex
Slowly adapting receptor	Myelinated (fast)	Positive transmural pressure	Limited lung inflation, induce expiration, bronchodilation.
Rapidly adapting receptor	Myelinated (fast)	Rate change of transmural pressure	Gasp, sigh, restore lung compliance.
C-fiber Pulmonary Bronchial	Unmyelinated (slow)	Edema, putative mediators of inflammation, chemicals	Defense reflexes: decrease tidal volume, increase respiratory rate, bronchoconstriction, decrease heart rate, decrease blood pressure.

Mucociliary Escalator

The lung's first line of defense is a nonspecific mechanism for clearance called the *mucociliary escalator*. This system consists of a mucous layer that is propelled upward in the tracheobronchial tree by cilia of the respiratory epithelium. The daily volume of secretions range from 10 to 100 mL, but can increase to 200 to 300 mL when irritated.[76] There are approximately 200 cilia per epithelial cell that beat in a whiplike motion toward the mouth (cephalad). A mucous (gel) layer is suspended upon a serous (sol) layer that is less viscus. Most of the stroking action of the cilia takes place in this serous layer which conserves considerable energy for the cell. When the beating cilia reach maximal velocity they lengthen and come in contact with the mucous layer and, thereby, propel this layer toward the mouth. The cilia have hooked ends to increase the propulsion of the mucous layer.[77]

Particulate matter of both inorganic and organic nature, becomes trapped in the mucous layer once coming in contact with it. The contact may occur as the result of impaction of particles from the inertia of a particle propelling it into the wall of an airway, sedimentation of the particle once the kinetic energy of a particle fails to keep it suspended as air velocity falls, or diffusion of particles owing to the random Brownian motion, particularly for very small particulates when airflow is low, as in the terminal bronchioles.

There exists a potential problem in the lungs in that mucus is transported from a larger combined cross-sectional area to a smaller cross-sectional area with the ascent of each successive airway generation, until the trachea is reached having a diameter of 2 to 3 cm in the adult human (Fig. 25–9). This problem is solved because the frequency and, hence, the velocity of mucus increases from the distal to the proximal lung generations (i.e., from 300 to 1300 beats per minute and from 1 to 12 mm/min., respectively).

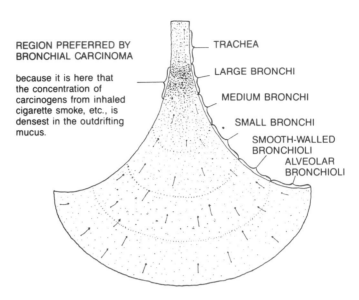

REGION PREFERRED BY
BRONCHIAL CARCINOMA

because it is here that
the concentration of
carcinogens from inhaled
cigarette smoke, etc., is
densest in the outdrifting
mucus.

TRACHEA

LARGE BRONCHI

MEDIUM BRONCHI

SMALL BRONCHI

SMOOTH-WALLED
BRONCHIOLI

ALVEOLAR
BRONCHIOLI

FIGURE   25-9   Diagram of the clearance of particulate matter
from the distal reaches of the lungs proceeding proximally to
the trachea. Particulate buildup is indicated in region of the
large bronchi, which is associated with a high incidence of
disease. (Modified from Macklin CC. Induction of bronchial
cancer by local massing of carcinogen concentrate in outdrifting
mucus. J Thorac Surg 1956;31:238, with permission)

Disturbances in the clearance of the lung also occur when there is a reduction
in the beating frequency of the cilia or the composition of the mucous layer is
altered. In the former, the frequency of ciliary beating decreases after exposure to
certain irritants, such as cigarette smoke, ozone, nitrogen dioxide, or sulfur dioxide,
or as the result of viral infection. The paralysis or impaired function of the cilia to
beat rhythmically is usually reversed during recovery from an illness or withdrawal
from the irritant exposure.[77] This may require at least 3 months.

When the composition of the mucous–serous layer is altered, then its removal
along with particulate matter, pathogens, and proteolytic enzymes from the lung, is
also affected. For example it has been proposed that the viscosity of the mucous
layer is increased in cystic fibrosis.[78] Ciliary activity is also impaired. Decreased
clearance of particles in the lungs increases the likelihood of pulmonary and systemic infection. This is especially true when there is a buildup of noxious substances within airways (see Fig. 25–9).

Because the lungs are continually exposed to the external environment, this
presents an opportunity for invading organisms to enter the body. Therefore, not
only does the mucociliary escalator act to nonspecifically remove particulate matter
from the lung, but it also serves as a medium for immunoglobulins, interleukins,
cytokines, and the complement system for antigen recognition and for certain enzymes that act to check the growth of invading organisms in the lungs. Enzymes,
including lactoferrin[79] and lysozyme,[80] attack the bacterial cell wall, causing lysis

of the invading cell. These enzymes are secreted in part by serous cells of the submucosal glands.[81] Although the systems of the complement and immunoglobulin proteins have been recognized for some time, functions of interleukins and cytokines in the lungs are largely unknown. Although vastly important, the immunology of the lung will not be discussed in this brief review of the respiratory system in health and disease.

The Alveolar Macrophage

The alveolar macrophage is vitally important in the defense of the lungs. There are an estimated 600 million macrophages in the lungs. This number increases in cigarette smokers as much as four times.[82] Monocytes,which enter the lungs from the circulation, differentiate into alveolar macrophages. A certain percentage of the macrophage population originates from resident cell division.[83]

Phagocytosis

Macrophages deactivate and remove microorganisms and particulate matter from the lungs by the processes of phagocytosis.[84,85] Lysosomes in the cell combine with the phagosome to form a phagolysosome. The contents of the newly formed phagolysosome are then degraded to basic components such as amino acids and simple sugars.[86,87] Matter that the macrophage cannot degrade remains within the cell. Certain microorganisms or particulates, such as mycobacteria, viruses, silicon, and asbestos, can be cytotoxic to the alveolar macrophage. These agents increase the number of macrophages in the lungs.[88] Dead and dying macrophages lose their membrane integrity and release their contents into the surrounding environment. Hydrolases, proteases, and superoxide radicals from the macrophage then cause the destruction of the lung tissue, resulting in tubercular cysts, silicosis, and asbestosis. Normally, however, the macrophages make their way into the interstitium and then into the lymphatic system or are carried up and out of the airways by the mucociliary escalator.

Role of Free Radicals

Macrophages manufacture and release over 100 different agents[88] that include free radicals, including the superoxide anion. Free radical production helps to maintain a nearly sterile environment in the airways. Free radicals in low concentrations are bacteriostatic and bactericidal in high concentration. The rate of superoxide anion radical production increases during respiratory bursts of macrophages, neutrophils, and eosinophils during immune response reactions and phagocytosis.

Much of the damage caused by free radicals is due to lipid peroxidation (abstraction of hydrogen), notably lipids in cell membranes. The membrane's decreased ability to function results in loss of its ability to function as a barrier. The cell then leaks. Unleashed enzymes further contribute to localized tissue destruction.

The lung has mechanisms to counter the effects of these free radicals that, if uncontrolled, can cause its own destruction. These mechanisms include free radical scavengers and enzymatic action. Scavengers include α-tocopherol (vitamin E) and

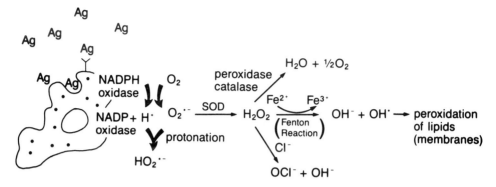

FIGURE   25-10   Generation of free radicals during the respiratory burst of an activated macrophage or neutrophil. NADPH oxidase is membrane-bound and acts on molecular oxygen to form the superoxide radical $O_2^{\cdot-}$. *SOD,* superoxide dismutase; *AG,* antigen; *Y,* antibody.

ascorbic acid (vitamin C). Enzymatic removal of superoxide anion radical begins with the action of superoxide dismutase (SOD) and is summarized in Figure 25–10. The increased free radical production of cigarette smoking, phagocytosis, or high O_2 environments, however, quickly overwhelms SODs ability to contain free radicals from causing lung tissue destruction. The role of free radicals in the lungs has been recently reviewed.[89,90]

Failure of the Lung Protective Mechanisms

Emphysema is a disease in which the lung's protective mechanisms have failed or are overcome. Proteolytic enzymes cause the destruction of tissues of the lung parenchyma. This tissue destruction results in an increase in lung compliance; accordingly, the chest recoils outward, increasing the functional residual capacity of the individual. With the destruction of lung tissue, the surface area for gas exchange decreases and the diameter of the conducting airways is reduced. Hypoxia and dyspnea result when the O_2 demand by the body's metabolism is not met.

The development of emphysema has been linked to the frequent exposure to certain irritants, such as cigarette smoke. Cigarette smoke adversely affects α_1-antitrypsin (AAT), a major enzyme protecting the lungs from proteases. Emphysema also develops because of genetic causes in certain individuals having low or abnormal serum AAT.[91–96]

Therapy in this disease has included β-adrenergic agents, O_2, and cardiovascular conditioning. Steroids have not been tested. Weekly intravenous injection of human AAT (Prolastin) is being used in an attempt to limit the progress of the hereditary form of this disease.[97] In the future, it may be possible to introduce to the lungs by aerosol the gene complement that has the ability to synthesize AAT from the patient's own cells.[98]

REFERENCES

1. Spooner BS, Wessells NK. Mammalian lung development: interactions in primordium formation and bronchial morphogenesis. J Exp Zool 1970;175:445.

2. Weibel ER. Morphometry of the human lung. Heidelberg: Springer-Verlag, 1963.

3. Scarpelli EM, Mautone AJ. The surfactant system and pulmonary mechanics. In: Robertson B, Van Golde LMG, Batenburg JJ, eds. Pulmonary surfactant. Amsterdam: Elsevier, 1984;119.

4. Burri PH. Development and growth of the human lung. In: Fishman AP, sect. ed. Handbook of physiology, the respiratory system, Bethesda, MD: American Physiology Society 1985;1(sect 3):1.

5. Radford EP Jr. Method for estimating respiratory surface area of mammalial lungs from their physical characteristics. Proc Soc Exp Biol Med 1954;87:58.

6. Weibel ER. Design and structure of the human lung. In: AP Fishman, ed. Pulmonary diseases and disorders. New York: McGraw-Hill, 1980:224.

7. Weibel ER. Morphometric estimation of pulmonary diffusion capacity. I. Model and method. Respir Physiol 1971;11:54.

8. Oliver RE, Schneeberger EE, Walters DV. Epithelial solute permeability, ion transport and tight junction morphology in the developing lung of the fetal lamb. J Physiol (Lond) 1981;315:395.

9. Van Golde LMG, Batenburg, JJ, Robertson B. The pulmonary surfactant system: biochemical aspects and functional significance. Physiol Rev 1988;68:374.

10. Weibel ER. A note on differentiation and divisability of alveolar epithelial cells. Chest 1974;65:195.

11. Adamson IYR, Bowden DH. The type 2 cell as progenitor of alveolar epithelial regeneration: a cytodynamic study in mice after exposure to oxygen. Lab Invest 1974;30:35.

12. Evans MJ, Cabral LJ, Stephens RJ, Freeman G. Transformation of alveolar type 2 cells to type I cells following exposure to NO_2. Exp Mol Pathol 1975;22:142.

13. American Thoracic Society committee on proficiency standards for clinical pulmonary function laboratories. Standardization of spirometry—1987 update. Am Rev Respir Dis 1987;136:1285.

14. Chung F, Dean E. Pathophysiology and cardiorespiratory consequences of interstitial lung disease—review and clinical implications: a special communication. Phys Ther 1989;69:956.

15. Risk C, Peterson M, Woods B, et al. Thromboxane and prostacyclin (epoprostenol) during exercise in diffuse pulmonary fibrosis. Lancet 1982;2:1183.

16. Schurch S, Goerke J, Clements JA. Direct determination of volume- and time-dependence of alveolar surface tension in excised lungs. Proc Natl Acad Sci USA 1978;75:3417.

17. Schurch S. Surface tension at low lung volumes: dependence on time and alveolar size. Respir Physiol 1982;48:339.

18. Robertson B. Neonatal respiratory distress syndrome and surfactant therapy; a brief review. Eur Respir J 1989;2(suppl 3):73s.

19. Lachmann B. Animal models and clinical pilot studies of surfactant replacement in adult respiratory distress syndrome. Eur Respir J 1989;2(suppl 3):98s.

20. Clements JA, Surface tension of lungs extracts. Proc Soc Exp Biol Med 1957;95:170.

21. Thet LA, Clerch L, Massaro GD, Massaro D. Changes in sedimentation of surfactant in ventilated excised rat lungs. Physical alterations in surfactant associated with the development and reversal of atelectasis. J Clin Invest 1979;64:600.

22. Oyarzun MJ, Clements JA. Control of lung surfactant by ventilation, adrenergic mediators, and prostaglandins in the rabbit. Am Rev Respir Dis 1978;117:879.

23. Brown LAS, Longmore WJ. Adrenergic and cholinergic regulation of lung surfactant secretion in the alveolar type II cell in culture. J Biol Chem 1981;256:66.

24. Hollingsworth M, Gilfillan AM. The pharmacology of lung surfactant secretion. Pharmacol Rev 1984;36:69.

25. King RJ, Coalson JJ, Seidenfeld JJ, Anzueto AR, Smith DB, Peters JI. O_2^- and pneumonia-induced lung injury. II. Properties of pulmonary surfactant. J Appl Physiol 1989;67:375.

26. Baritussio AG, Magoon MW, Goerke J, Clements JA. Precursor–product relationship between rabbit type II cell lamellar bodies and alveolar surface-active material. Surfactant turnover time. Biochim Biophys Acta 1981;666:382.

27. Jacobs H, Jobe A, Ikegami M, Jones S. Surfactant phosphatidylcholine source, fluxes, and turnover times in 3-day-old, 10-day-old and adult rabbits. J Biol Chem 1982;257:1805.

28. Fisher HK, Hyman MH, Ashcraft SJ. Alveolar surfactant phospholipids are not cleared via trachea [abstract]. Fed Proc 1979;38:1373.

29. Geiger K, Gallagher ML, Hedley-Whyte J. Cellular distribution and clearance of aerosolized dipalmitoyl lecithin. J Appl Physiol 1975;39:759.

30. Desai R, Tetley TD, Curtis G, Powell GM, Richards RJ. Studies on the fate of pulmonary surfactant in the lung. Biochem J 1978;176:455.

31. Chander A, Reicherter J, Fisher AB. Degradation of dipalmitoyl phosphatidylcholine by isolated rat granular pneumocytes and reutilization for surfactant synthesis. J Clin Invest 1987;79:1133.

32. Jacobs HC, Ikegami M, Jobe AH, Berry DD, Jones S. Reutilization of surfactant phosphatidylcholine in adult rabbits. Biochim Biophys Acta 1985;837:77.

33. Richardson JB. Nerve supply to the lungs. Am Rev Respir Dis 1979;119:785.

34. Said SI. Influence of neuropeptides on airway smooth muscle. Am Rev Respir Dis 1987;136:S52.

35. Said SI. Vasoactive peptides in the lung, with special reference to vasoactive intestinal peptide. Exp Lung Res 1982;3:343.

36. Matsuzaki Y, Hamasaki Y, Said SI. Vasoactive intestinal peptide: a possible transmitter of non-adrenergic relaxation of guinea pig airways. Science 1980;210:1252.

37. Ollerenshaw S, Jarvis D, Woolcock A, Sullivan C, Scheibner T. Absence of immunoreactive vasoactive intestinal polypeptide in tissue from the lungs of patients with asthma. N Engl J Med 1989;320:1244.

38. Morice A, Unwin RJ, Sever PS. Vasoactive intestinal peptide causes bronchodilation and protects against histamine-induced bronchoconstriction in asthmatic subjects. Lancet 1983;2:1225.

39. Coleridge JCG, Coleridge HM. Afferent vagal C fibre innervation of the lungs and airways and its functional significance. Rev Physiol Biochem Pharmacol 1984;99:1.

40. Said SI, Mutt V. Relationship of spasmogenic and smooth muscle relaxant peptide from normal lung to other vasoactive compounds. Nature 1977;265:84.

41. Lundblad L. Protective reflexes and vascular effects in the nasal mucosa elicited by activation of capsaicin sensitive substance P immunoreactive trigeminal neurons. Acta Physiol Scand [Suppl] 529:1.

42. Takizawa T, Thurlbeck WM. Muscle and mucous gland size in the major bronchi of patients with chronic bronchitis, asthma, and asthmatic bronchitis. Am Rev Respir Dis 1971;104:331.

43. Ebina M, Yaegashi H, Takahashi T, Masakichi M, Tanemura M. Distribution of smooth muscles along the bronchial tree. A morphometric study of ordinary autopsy lungs. Am Rev Respir Dis 1990;141:1322.

44. Fraser CM, Venter JC. Beta-adrenergic receptors: relationship of primary structure, receptor function, and regulation. Am Rev Respir Dis 1990;141:S22.

45. DeKock MA, Nadel JA, Zwi S, Colebatch HJH, Olsen CR. New method for perfusing bronchial arteries: histamine bronchoconstriction and apnea. J Appl Physiol 1966;21:185.

46. Gold WM, Kessler G-F, Yu DYC. Role of vagus nerves in experimental asthma in allergic dogs. J Appl Physiol 1972;33:719.

47. Kaplan J, Smaldone GC, Menkes HA, Swift DL, Traystman RJ. Response of collateral channels to histamine: lack of vagal effect. J Appl Physiol 1981;51:1314.

48. Loring SH, Drazen JM, Ingram RH Jr. Canine pulmonary response to aerosol histamine: direct versus vagal effects. J Appl Physiol 1977;42:946.

49. Snapper JR, Drazen JM, Loring SH, Braasch PS, Ingram RH Jr. Vagal effects on histamine, carbachol, and prostaglandin $F_{2\alpha}$ responsiveness in the dog. J Appl Physiol 1979;47:13.

50. Jammes Y, Mei N. Assessment of the pulmonary origin of bronchoconstrictor vagal tone. J Physiol (Lond) 1979;291:305.

51. Barnes PJ. Asthma as an axon reflex. Lancet 1986;1:242.

52. Lungdberg JM. Polypeptide-containing neurons in airway smooth muscle. Annu Rev Physiol 1987;49:557.

53. Cuss FM, Dixon CMS, Barnes PJ. Effect of inhaled platelet activating factor on pulmonary function and bronchoresponsiveness in man. Lancet 1986;2:189.

54. Rubin AE, Smith LJ, Roy Patterson. The bronchoconstrictor properties of platelet-activating factor in humans. Am Rev Respir Dis 1987;136:1145.

55. Kern R, Smith LJ, Patterson R, Krell RD, Bernstein PR. Characterization of the airway response to inhaled leukotriene D_4 in normal subjects. Am Rev Respir Dis 1986;133:1127.

56. Kaye MG, Smith LJ. Effects of inhaled leukotriene D_4 and platelet-activating factor on airway reactivity in normal subjects. Am Rev Respir Dis 1990;141:993.

57. Phillips GD, Holgate ST. Interaction of inhaled LTC_4 with histamine and PGD_2 on airway caliber in asthma. J Appl Physiol 1989;66:304.

58. Geiser J, Betticher DC. Gas transfer in isolated lungs perfused with red cell suspension or hemoglobin solution. Respir Physiol 1989;77:31.

59. Sharan M, Singh MP, Aminataei A. A numerical model for blood oxygenation in the pulmonary capillaries—effect of pulmonary membrane resistance. Biosystems 1987;20:355.

60. Federspiel WJ. Pulmonary diffusing capacity: implications of two-phase blood flow in capillaries. Respir Physiol 1989;77:119.

61. Duhm J. Effects of 2,3-diphosphoglycerate on functional properties of hemoglobin and on glycolysis of human erythrocytes. Adv Exp Med Biol 1976;75:81.

62. Gunn RB, Dalmark M, Tosteson DC, Wieth JO. Characteristics of chloride transport in human red blood cells. J Gen Physiol 1973;61:185.

63. Nishimura Y, Hida W, Taguchi O, et al. Respiratory muscle strength and gas exchange in neuromuscular diseases: comparison with chronic pulmonary emphysema and idiopathic pulmonary fibrosis. Tohoku J Exp Med 1989;259:57.

64. Merrill EG. The lateral respiratory neurones of the medulla: their associations with nucleus ambiguus, nucleus retroambigualis, the spinal accessory nucleus and the spinal cord. Brain Res 1970;24:11.

65. Merrill EG. Finding a respiratory function for the medullary respiratory neurons. In: Bellairs R, Gray EG, eds. Essays on the nervous system. Oxford: Clarendon, 1974:451.

66. Taylor EK, Duffin J, Vachon BR, McCracken DH. The recruitment times and firing patterns of the medullary respiratory neurones of the cat. Respir Physiol 1978;34:247.

67. Vibert JF, Bertrand F, Denavit-Saubie M, Hugelin A. Three dimensional representa-

tion of bulbopontine respiratory networks architecture from unit density maps. Brain Res 1976;114:227.

68. Hilaire G, Monteau R. Connexions entre les neurones inspiratoires bulbaires et les motoneurones phreniques et intercostaux. J Physiol (Paris) 1976;72:987.

69. Kahn N, Wang SC. Electrophysiologic basis for pontine apneustic center and its role in integration of the Hering–Breuer reflex. J Neurophysiol 1967;30:301.

70. St John WM, Glasser RL, King RA. Rhythmic respiration in awake vagotomized cats with chronic pneumotaxic area lesions. Respir Physiol 1972;15:233.

71. Mitchell RA. The regulation of respiration in metabolic acidosis and alkalosis. McC Brooks, Kao F, Lloyd BB, eds. In: Cerebrospinal fluid and the regulation of respiration. Oxford: Blackwell, 1965:109.

72. von Euler US, Liljestrand G, Zotterman Y. The excitation mechanism of the chemoreceptors of the carotid body. Scand Arch Physiol 1939;83:132.

73. Heymans C, Bouchaert JJ, Dautrebande L. Sinus carotidien et reflexes respiratoires. II. Influences respiratoires reflexes de l'acidose, de l'alcalose, de l'anhydride carbonique, de l'ion hydrogene et de l'anoxemie: sinus carotidiens et echanges respiratoires dans les poumons et au dela des poumons. Arch Int Pharmacodyn Ther 1930;39:400.

74. Fidone SJ, Sato A. A study of chemoreceptor and baroreceptor A and C-fibres in the cat carotid nerve. J Physiol (Lond) 1969;205:527.

75. Heymans CJF. The part played by vascular presso- and chemoreceptors in respiratory control. In: Nobel lectures—physiology or medicine (1922–1941). Amsterdam: Elsevier, 1965:460.

76. Toremalm NH. The daily amount of tracheo-bronchial secretions in man: a method of continuous tracheal aspiration in laryngectomized and tracheotomized patients. Acta Otolaryngol [suppl] (Stockh) 1960;158:43.

77. Pavia D, Agnew JE, Lopez-Vidriero MT, Clarke SW. General review of tracheobronchial clearance. Eur J Respir Dis 1987;71(suppl 153):123.

78. Reynolds HY. Identification and role of immunoglobulins in respiratory secretions. Eur J Respir Dis 1987;71(suppl 153):103.

79. Sertl K, Casale TB, Wescott SL, Lainer MA. Immunohistochemical localization of histamine-stimulated increases in cyclic GMP in guinea pig lung. Am Rev Respir Dis 1987;135:456.

80. Goldie RG, Spina D, Henry PJ, Lulich KM, Paterson JW. In vitro responsiveness of human asthmatic bronchus to carbachol, histamine, β-adrenoceptor agonists and theophylline. Br J Clin Pharmacol 1986;22:669.

81. Jeffery PK. The origins of secretions in the lower respiratory tract. Eur J Respir Dis 1987;71(suppl 153):34.

82. Harris JO, Swenson EW, Johnson JE. Human alveolar macrophages: comparison of phagocytic ability, glucose utilization, and ultrastructure in smokers and non-smokers. J Clin Invest 1970;69:2086.

83. Adamson IYR, Bowden D. Role of monocytes and interstitial cells in the generation of alveolar macrophages: kinetic studies after carbon loading. Lab Invest 1980;42:518.

84. Goldstein E, Lippert W, Warshauer D. Pulmonary alveolar macrophage, defender against bacterial infection of the lung. J Clin Invest 1974;54:519.

85. Green GM, Kass EH. The role of the alveolar macrophage in the clearance of bacteria from the lung. J Exp Med 1964;119:167.

86. Cohn ZA, Ehrenreich BA. The uptake, storage and intracellular hydrolysis of carbohydrates by macrophages. J Exp Med 1969;129:201.

87. Ehrenreich BA, Cohn ZA. The fate of peptides pinocytosed by macrophages in vitro. J Exp Med 1969;129:227.

88. Sibille Y, Reynolds HY. Macrophages and polymorphonuclear neutrophils in lung defense and injury. Am Rev Respir Dis 1990;141:471.

89. Blake DR, Allen RE, Lunec J. Free radicals in biological systems—a review orientated to inflammatory processes. Br Med Bull 1987;43:371.

90. Ward PA, Johnson KJ, Warren JS, Kunkel RG. Immune complexes, oxygen radicals, and lung injury. Oxygen radicals and tissue injury. Proc Upjohn Symp 1987:107.

91. Crystal RG, Brantly ML, Hubbard MD, Curiel DT, States DJ, Holmes MD. The alpha-1-antitrypsin gene and its mutations. Chest 1989;95:196.

92. Larsson C. Natural history and life expectancy in severe alpha-1-antitrypsin deficiency, piZ. Acta Med Scand 1978;204:345.

93. Erikkson S. Alpha-1-antitrypsin deficiency: lessons learned from the bedside to the gene and back again. Chest 1989;95:181.

94. Hutchison DCS. Natural history of alpha-1-protease inhibitor deficiency. Am J Med 1988;84(suppl 6A):3.

95. Laurell C-B, Eriksson A. The electrophoretic alpha 1-globulin pattern of serum in alpha-1-antitrypsin deficiency. Scand J Clin Lab Invest 1963;15:132.

96. Tobin MJ, Hutchison DCS. An overview of the pulmonary features of alpha-1-antitrypsin deficiency. Arch Intern Med 1982;142:1342.

97. American Thoracic Society Medical Section of American Lung Association. Guidelines for the approach to the patient with severe hereditary alpha-a-antitrypsin deficiency. Am Rev Respir Dis 1989;140:1494.

98. Rommens JA, Iannuzzi MC, Keren B-S, et al. Identification of the cystic fibrosis gene: chromosome walking and jumping. Science 1989;245:1059.

PHILIP C. WEISER

DONALD A. MAHLER

KEVIN P. RYAN

KAREN L. HILL

LEE W. GREENSPON

26

Dyspnea: Symptom Assessment and Management

Exertional dyspnea is one of the most common symptoms we hear about in clinical situations. Yet, its subjective nature leads it to be one of the most difficult symptoms for us to assess and manage. Commonly, individuals describe dyspnea as "being short-of-breath," "being breathless," or "having difficulty breathing"—feelings that limit their activities of daily living. As will be discussed later, dyspnea is more than increased breathing work and it is more than increased breathing effort. It is an uncomfortable feeling associated with daily physical activity.

We have four objectives in this chapter. First, dyspnea will be defined, and potential mechanisms will be briefly described. Second, the use of rating scales for the self-biofeedback monitoring of dyspnea will be detailed. Third, we will review the procedures used for the clinical assessment of dyspnea. Last, strategies and techniques for the management of dyspnea will be discussed.

BACKGROUND: WHAT IS DYSPNEA?

Symptoms such as dyspnea are vital perceptual "signals." All of us use these signals as part of our "self-biofeedback" system to enable us to appropriately react to the stresses of daily living. We use these signals as guides to achieve an acceptable level of intensity and quality for our life.

Definition of Dyspnea

In this chapter, *dyspnea* will be defined as labored or difficult breathing that is associated with an awareness of discomfort or distress.[1,2] The experience of dyspnea is multidimensional. The symptom represents a class of experiences that may not be precisely reported by each individual patient. Notice that the foregoing definition separates two dimensions[3] that are used to describe breathing discomfort. First, we can be aware of greater sensations indicating increased breathing activity, as increased respiratory rate or tidal volume. Second, we become aware of a heightened subjective appraisal of the discomfort of breathing, as increased breathing difficulty.

Mechanism of Dyspnea

Symptoms such as dyspnea are created from the functioning of our multilevel, perceptual, biofeedback system. Figure 26–1 shows a multilevel schema for dyspnea that was modified from a model originally described for bicycling fatigue.[4] The model has been modified to represent the symptomatology reported for dyspnea by patients with COPD[5,6] (Hill KL, Weiser PC, Bell CW, Kinsman RA, Greenspon L, unpublished observations). At the lowest level, our sensations are formed from input being sent from various peripheral physiologic processes. Next, as sensory signals are processed in the lower central nervous system (CNS) perceptual centers, they are reported as simple, discrete symptoms (e.g., breathing fast or full lungs). Then, the discrete symptoms are hypothesized to be combined in the higher CNS centers at the subconceptual level as labored breathing, hyperventilation, lung hyperinflation and lung congestion. Next, this perceptual information along with other clusters of symptoms are suggested to be further integrated higher in the CNS at the conceptual level as fatigue, breathing discomfort, and mood. Finally, we hypothesize that our minds are organized such that we can refer to our overall perceptions about a breathing disorder as a global, superconceptual symptom (i.e., undifferentiated breathlessness).

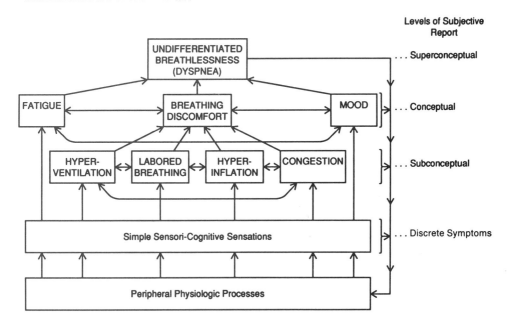

FIGURE 26-1 Pyramidal schema describing the levels of subjective report of dyspnea during bicycle ergometer work. (Adapted from Kinsman RA, Weiser PC. Subjective symptomatology during work and fatigue. In: Simonson E, Weiser PC, eds. Psychological aspects and physiological correlates of work and fatigue. Springfield, IL: Charles C Thomas, 1976:388)

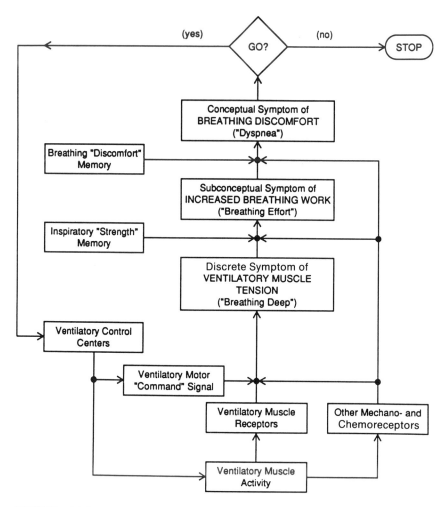

FIGURE 26-2 Schematic feedback diagram of the mechanism for dyspnea showing the interrelations among ventilatory muscle activity, pulmonary mechanics, ventilatory breathing effort, and breathing discomfort.

A simplistic model for the dynamic changes in dyspnea during exertion is shown in Figure 26–2. First, we must constantly decide whether to continue to exercise. If the answer is "yes," then we send a "go" signal to the ventilatory centers. In turn, the medullary ventilatory centers could potentially send one signal to activate ventilatory muscle activity and another to act as a ventilatory motor command reference signal.[7] Information about ventilatory activity is fed back to the medullary ventilatory centers from changes in muscle receptors, chemoreceptors, and mechanoreceptors. The subjective reports of tension as well as breathing depth and breathing rate constitute the most simple and discrete set of breathing sensations. Second, the next higher level of symptom report is referenced to a maximal inspiratory muscle strength memory.[8] The resulting biofeedback signal can become a conscious report of breathing effort. Killian and associates have suggested that the sensation of tension can be distinguished from the more closely correlated sensations of effort and breathlessness.[9] Third, at the conceptual level of ventilatory signal processing, the symptom of breathing discomfort seems to be related to a breathing discomfort memory. Cronan and colleagues compared the hyperventilation from CO_2 rebreathing to exercise hyperpnea and have shown that the symptom of breathlessness can be differentiated from breathing effort.[10]

Currently, our knowledge of the mechanisms underlying dyspnea is still incomplete. Consequently, the perceptual effects of aging, habitual physical activity, anxiety, as well as cardiopulmonary disease may be due to changes that take place at any or all of the levels of our breathing self-biofeedback system.

However, one approach to the treatment of dyspnea consists of assisting patients to use their own ability to regulate their breathing. An effective method for patients to self-regulate their breathing is for them to concentrate on the symptoms of breathing effort and breathing discomfort (i.e., their ratings of dyspnea). In the next section, we will discuss the use of rating scales in assessing and managing dyspnea.

USE OF RATING SCALES FOR DYSPNEA

When to Use Rating Scales for Dyspnea

All of us use evaluation tools such as rating scales. Think of the times when you have asked a client, "How are you doing today?" or "How is your breathing today?" We are constantly monitoring the progress of the patients who are participating in rehabilitation programs.

Detailed discussions of the psychophysical basis of rating scales and their applications are available.[11-13] Briefly, a quantitative relation can be found between a sensory stimulus and the sensation evoked by it. In addition, perception extends sensation, since our perceptual responses can be seen as the interpretation of sensory impressions that are relative to past experiences and, if strong enough, will enter into consciousness and can be subjectively reported. However, to be understood by others, these subjective symptoms need to be rated as a quantitative report (i.e., the experience must be scaled). The type of rating scales available (category, ratio, interval, or combinations) will be discussed later in the How to Use Rating Scales section.

If sensations and symptoms are important components of self-biofeedback and self-regulation, then the subjective evaluation of dyspnea is an integral part of rehabilitation. Furthermore, dyspnea measurements can help with four tasks:

1. Classifying the severity of dyspnea impairment
2. Individualizing rehabilitation programs
3. Monitoring progress
4. Desensitizing those patients who report disproportionately severe dyspnea.

Dyspnea Classification

Dyspnea assessment can be used to classify the severity of the patient's complaint because the symptom of breathlessness is the principal characteristic of pulmonary impairment.

Several schemes for classification are available for chronic obstructive pulmonary disease (COPD). Most investigators believe that the British Medical Research Council (MRC) scale[14] is outdated and not particularly appropriate for general classification or grading of breathlessness severity. Instead of using the MRC scale, unidimensional and multidimensional scales are available and have been used. Selection of the appropriate measuring instrument or tool depends on the question asked and whether short- or long-term intervals are used to assess changes in dyspnea (see the following sections for information on these scales).

Individualization of Dyspnea

Individualization of pulmonary rehabilitation programs can be aided by continually evaluating dyspnea. Ratings of perceived effort have been used to individualize the cardiac rehabilitation components for prescribing exercise therapy and modifying activities of daily living.[15] Likewise, ratings of perceived dyspnea can be employed in individualizing rehabilitation programs for patients with pulmonary disease.[16,17]

Monitoring Dyspnea During Exercise Training

Dyspnea evaluation is being used more frequently for monitoring progress throughout the pulmonary rehabilitation program. Ratings of perceived effort, dyspnea, and leg fatigue can be recorded each session and used to upgrade exercise intensity or to indicate the extent of "bad days." These scales can be used to check your patient's symptoms on bad days or to titrate the target exercise intensity. Furthermore, such scales can be used for the periodic resetting of exercise prescriptions.

Experience has taught us that it is very important to involve the patient in monitoring his or her progress. At the beginning of and periodically during each session, ask each patient to rate his or her severity of dyspnea. These assessments will give you a more objective clue when someone is having a bad day. By commenting on his or her own state of dyspnea, your clients can take charge of the exercise intensity and practice changing the exercise intensity to stay within normal limits (i.e., the exercise prescription).

Desensitization of High Dyspnea Responders

Finally, the application of dyspnea ratings is crucial in desensitizing patients who respond to exertion with disproportionately high dyspnea ratings. Besides establishing that disproportionately severe dyspnea is present in certain patients, the evaluation procedures can assess the individual level of sensitivity to ventilatory sensations and symptoms.

How to Use Rating Scales for Dyspnea

The following is a procedure for incorporating dyspnea evaluation as an important part of a pulmonary rehabilitation program that emphasizes self-regulation. These steps will serve as the framework for applying breathlessness ratings to your program. First, select the type(s) of appropriate dyspnea measuring scales. Second, write clear, concise instructions for the use of the rating scales, profiles, or inventories that you choose. Third, be aware of the limitations in the use of rating scales. Let us now expand the practice of each of these steps.

Rating Instrument Selection

The first step is to select the types of appropriate dyspnea measuring scales or instruments that will be useful to your program. Different aspects of your program require different tools. Basically, there are three aspects of measuring breathlessness: rating the activity that is a threshold for provoking breathing discomfort, rating the intensity of dyspnea at a particular moment during an activity, and rating the complex, multidimensional changes for the different factors of breathlessness that occur over time.

DYSPNEA THRESHOLD SCALES Twenty years ago, the British Medical Research Council (MRC) scale (Table 26–1) was developed to quantitate the level of exertion that provokes breathlessness.[14] It has been included in a larger respiratory disease questionnaire recommended by the American Thoracic Society in 1978.[18] The MRC scale requires patients to estimate the levels of tasks that first provoke dyspnea and to classify them into one of five categories. Many patients can identify the specific tasks on the MRC scale, but some are frustrated by the limited number of available categories and by the lack of clear distinctions among the choices.

Another threshold instrument is a detailed version of the visual analog scale,[19] named the oxygen-cost diagram (OCD). This scale (Fig. 26–3) is also used to classify patients' degrees of dyspnea.[20] The OCD consists of a 100-mm line, along which are listed everyday activities according to the estimated oxygen requirement for performing them. Patients are instructed to mark the point on the line above which they would experience breathing discomfort. Visual analog scales, like the OCD, provide somewhat greater flexibility in rating the threshold of task-induced dyspnea than does the MRC scale. Because the OCD can include a greater variety

---

TABLE 26-1. Modified British Medical Research Council Dyspnea Scale

1. Do you become breathless only on strenuous exertion such as walking up hills?
   Yes (grade 1)
   No
2. Can you walk as far as you like on level ground and keep up with anyone of your age?
   Yes (grade 2)
   No
3. Can you walk as far as you like on level ground at your own pace without stopping?
   Yes (grade 3)
   No
4. Can you move comfortably about the house without becoming breathless?
   Yes (grade 4)
   No (grade 5)

(Adapted from Warly ARH, et al. Grading of dyspnea and walking speed in cardiac disease and chronic airflow obstruction. Br J Dis Chest 1987;81:349)

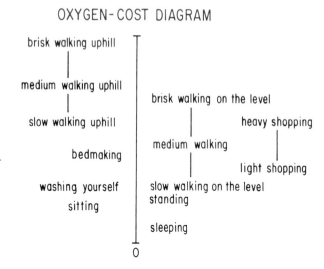

OXYGEN-COST DIAGRAM

FIGURE 26-3 The oxygen–cost diagram. (Adapted from McGavin CR, et al. Dyspnoea, disability, and distance walked: comparison of estimates of exercise performance in respiratory disease. Br Med J 1978;2:241)

of tasks than does the MRC scale, patients have more options in choosing a level of activity that elicits breathlessness. However, some patients require assistance or coaching in marking the vertical line at the appropriate point.

Because the categories are still broad for the MRC scale and OCD, it is difficult to establish how much improvement actually occurred following treatment. In addition, many patients need assistance distinguishing among the choices available. For these reasons, other clinical methods may be selected for measuring the severity of dyspnea.

BREATHLESSNESS INTENSITY SCALES Some practitioners have selected a modification of the Borg category ratio scale[21] to rate perceived dyspnea (RPD). This scale is shown in Figure 26–4 along with similar rating scales for perceived effort and leg fatigue. To use the RPD scale, the patient is instructed to select the number (i.e., category) that corresponds most closely to the level of breathing discomfort. The descriptive phrases used in the RPD refer to degrees of severity of breathing discomfort. One of the advantages of this scale is that it can fit numbers to a positively accelerating exercise physiologic variable such as ventilation.[18] Another advantage is that the patient is instructed to report numbers above 10, if appropriate, so that the maximal value is open-ended to prevent a perceptual ceiling from being obtained. A common error is to use the RPD as a restricted 0 to 10 scale.[21]

Another popular instrument is the visual analog scale (VAS), mentioned earlier, that provides a different perceptual approach to quantifying the severity of dyspnea.[19] A 100-mm line represents the range of severity for the symptom, with the bottom of the scale defined as no breathlessness, whereas the top corresponds to greatest breathlessness (Fig. 26–5). The rating can be made for various activities of daily living or during performance of a specific task, such as walking for a given time or distance. The patient is asked to mark the line at a point that corresponds to his or her severity of breathlessness. The distance from the end labeled "no breathlessness" to the marked point provides the rating of dyspnea. The breathless-

Effort	Breathlessness	Tired Legs
6	0 Not at all	0 Not at all
7 Very, very easy	0.5 Just noticeable	0.5 Just noticeable
8	1 Very slight	1 Very slight
9 Very easy	2 Slight	2 Slight
10	3 Moderate	3 Moderate
11 Easy	4 Somewhat severe	4 Somewhat severe
12	5 Severe	5 Severe
13 Somewhat hard	6	6
14	7 Very severe	7 Very severe
15 Hard	8	8
16	9	9
17 Very hard	10 Very, very severe	10 Very, very severe
18	*	*
19 Very, very hard	*	*
20	? Unbearable	? Unbearable

FIGURE 26-4 Unidimensional rating scales for the rating of perceived effort, dyspnea, and leg fatigue. (Adapted from Borg G. Psychophysical bases of perceived exertion. Med Sci Sports Exerc 1982;14:377)

ness VAS can be limited by the need for assistance in marking the vertical line. Also the top value of this version of the VAS can change with desensitization to the greatest breathlessness level experienced or imagined by the patient.

A simple quasi-linear category scale such as a four- or five-point self-assessment scale has been used to obtain a rough estimate of a patient's breathlessness and how severe it may become. An example of such a category scale is: 0, normal; 1, mild; 2, moderate; 3, severe; 4, very severe.[22] Broad ratings such as this may be helpful in estimating the severity of a patient's pulmonary impairment for a given activity.

VISUAL ANALOG SCALE

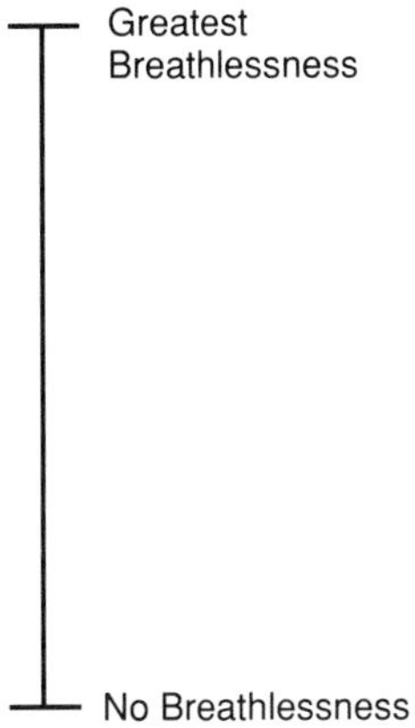

Greatest
Breathlessness

FIGURE 26-5 The visual analog scale. (Adapted from Aitken RCB. Measurement of feelings using visual analogue scales. Proc R Soc Med 1969;62:989)

No Breathlessness

However, this type of instrument cannot be used for precise measurements during exercise testing for grading changes in the severity of dyspnea after an intervention.

These simple scales are limited to the single-dimensional level of the perception of breathlessness. The advantages of these scales are that they are simple and quick to use. However, the perception of breathing discomfort is dependent on not only the intensity, duration, and type of physical activity, but also on other psychophysiologic dimensions.

MULTIDIMENSIONAL SCALES Multi-item inventories or questionnaires have been developed to offer a more comprehensive description of breathlessness and other symptoms that are highly related. Specific dyspnea scales are the Baseline and Transition Dyspnea Indexes[23] and the dyspnea components of the Chronic Respiratory Disease Questionnaire,[24] the Asthma Symptom Checklist,[5] and the Bronchitis and Emphysema Symptom Checklist.[6]

One specific multidimensional approach for quantifying breathing discomfort is the Baseline (BDI) and Transition Dyspnea Indexes (TDI).[23] Ratings are made during a interview by an observer. The BDI requires patients to estimate not only the magnitude of task that provokes breathlessness, but also both the functional impairment (the degree to which activities of daily living are impaired) and magnitude of effort (Table 26–2A). An overall BDI score is obtained by adding the three grades for each component. The TDI is used to measure changes in dyspnea relative to the previous value for the BDI (see Table 26–2B). These indexes are easy to use, reliable, and require less than 5 minutes to administer. Furthermore, the BDI provides a focal score (range, 0 to 12) that summarizes ratings of dyspnea based on one of five grades for each of three test components, and the TDI estimates changes in a patient's breathlessness according to specific criteria by assigning grades to the three components with the sum ranging from -9 (major deterioration) to $+9$ (major improvement).

The Chronic Respiratory Disease Questionnaire (CRQ) has been developed by Guyatt and colleagues[24] to measure quality of life in patients with chronic airflow limitation.[24] Its 20 items measure two dimensions, physical function (which includes shortness of breath and fatigue) and emotional function (including depression, anxiety, frustration, and the extent to which the patient feels in control of, or able to cope with, the illness). Each item is scored during a structured interview by an observer who presents seven response options, a score of 7 indicating the best possible function and a score of 1 the worst possible function. The CRQ was derived from patients' statements about how their lives were adversely affected by their lung disease. It has been extensively tested and found to be reproducible, valid, and responsive to clinically important changes in quality of life which have occurred. However, some patients reported that the effort required to volunteer a list of dyspnea-producing activities of daily living was frustrating and time-consuming, and interviewers were required to receive several hours of instruction and coaching before reliable scores were obtained.

Kinsman and coworkers have combined a series of five-point items in developing the Asthma Symptom Checklist (ASC)[5] and the Bronchitis and Emphysema Symptom Checklist (BESC).[6] They found that the items for dyspnea were associated with the items of the fatigue category. Several colleagues and I have

TABLE 26-2. Dyspnea in COPD: Measurement of Symptoms: The Benchmark of Treatment

A. Baseline Dyspnea Index*

Grade	*Functional Impairment*
4	**No impairment** Patient able to carry out usual activities and occupation without shortness of breath.
3	**Slight impairment** Distinct impairment in at least one activity but no activities completely abandoned. Reduction in work or other activities that seems slight or not clearly caused by shortness of breath.
2	**Moderate impairment** Patient has changed jobs and/or has abandoned at least one usual activity‡ because of shortness of breath.
1	**Severe impairment** Patient unable to work or has given up most or all usual activities because of shortness of breath.
0	**Very severe impairment** Patient unable to work and has given up most or all usual activities because of shortness of breath.
W	**Amount uncertain** Patient is impaired because of shortness of breath, but amount cannot be specified. Details are not sufficient to allow impairment to be categorized.
X	**Unknown** Information unavailable concerning impairment.
Y	**Impaired for other reasons** For example, musculoskeletal problems or chest pain.

Magnitude of Task

4	**Extraordinary** Becomes short of breath only with extraordinary activities, such as carrying very heavy loads on the level, lighter loads uphill, or running. No shortness of breath with ordinary tasks.
3	**Major** Becomes short of breath only with major activities, such as walking up a steep hill, climbing more than three flights of stairs, or carrying a moderate load on the level.
2	**Moderate** Becomes short of breath with moderate or average tasks, such as walking up a gradual hill, climbing fewer than three flights of stairs, or carrying a light load on the level.
1	**Light** Becomes short of breath with light activities, such as walking on the level, washing, or standing.
0	**No task** Becomes short of breath at rest, while sitting, or while lying down.
W	**Amount uncertain** Patient's ability to perform tasks is impaired because of shortness of breath, but amount cannot be specified. Details are not sufficient to allow impairment to be categorized.
X	**Unknown** Information unavailable concerning limitation.
Y	**Impaired for other reasons** For example, musculoskeletal problems or chest pain.

Magnitude of Effort

4	**Extraordinary** Becomes short of breath only with the greatest imaginable effort. No shortness of breath with ordinary effort.
3	**Major** Becomes short of breath with effort distinctly submaximal, but of major proportion. Tasks performed without pause unless the task requires extraordinary effort that may be performed with pauses.
2	**Moderate** Becomes short of breath with moderate effort. Tasks performed with occasional pauses and require longer to complete than the average person requires.

(Continues on p. 488)

TABLE 26-2. Dyspnea in COPD: Measurement of Symptoms: The Benchmark of Treatment (*continued*)

A. Baseline Dyspnea Index*

Grade	*Functional Impairment*
1	**Light** Becomes short of breath with little effort. Tasks performed with little effort or with frequent pauses require 50% to 100% longer to complete than the average person might require.
0	**No effort** Becomes short of breath at rest, while sitting, or lying down.
W	**Amount uncertain** Patient's exertional ability is impaired because of shortness of breath, but amount cannot be specified. Details are not sufficient to allow impairment to be categorized.
X	**Unknown** Information unavailable concerning limitation.
Y	**Impaired for other reasons** For example, musculoskeletal problems or chest pain.

B. Transitional Dyspnea Index†

Grade	*Change in Functional Impairment*
−3	**Major deterioration** Formerly working and has had to stop working and has completely abandoned some of usual activities because of shortness of breath.
−2	**Moderate deterioration** Formerly working and has had to stop working or has completely abandoned some of usual activities because of shortness of breath.
−1	**Minor deterioration** Has changed to a lighter job or has reduced activities in number or duration because of shortness of breath. Any deterioration less than preceding categories.
0	**No change** No changes in functional status because of shortness of breath.
+1	**Minor improvement** Able to return to work at reduced pace or has resumed some customary activities with more vigor than before.
+2	**Moderate improvement** Able to return to work at nearly usual pace or able to return to most activities with moderate restriction only.
+3	**Major improvement** Able to return to work at former pace and able to return to full activities with only mild restriction because of improvement of shortness of breath.
Z	**Further impairment for reasons other than shortness of breath** Patient has stopped working, reduced work, or has given up or reduced other activities for other reasons. For example, other medical problems or being "laid off" from work.

	Change in Magnitude of Task
−3	**Major deterioration** Has deteriorated two grades or more from baseline status.
−2	**Moderate deterioration** Has deteriorated at least one grade but fewer than two grades from baseline.
−1	**Minor deterioration** Has deteriorated less than one grade from baseline. Patient has shown distinct deterioration within grade, but has not changed grades.
0	**No change** No change from baseline.
+1	**Minor improvement** Has improved less than one grade from baseline. Patient has shown distinct improvement within grade, but has not changed grades.

TABLE 26-2. Dyspnea in COPD: Measurement of Symptoms: The Benchmark of Treatment (*continued*)

B. Transitional Dyspnea Index†

Grade   *Functional Impairment*

+2   **Moderate improvement**   Has improved at least one grade, but fewer than two grades from baseline.

+3   **Major improvement**   Has improved two grades or greater from baseline.

Z   **Further impairment for reasons other than shortness of breath**   Patient has reduced exertional capacity, but not related to shortness of breath. For example, musculoskeletal problems or chest pain.

Change in Magnitude of Effort

−3   **Major deterioration**   Severe decrease in effort from baseline to avoid shortness of breath. Activities now take 50% to 100% longer than at baseline.

−2   **Moderate deterioration**   Some decrease in effort to avoid shortness of breath, but not as great as preceding category. Greater pausing with some activities.

−1   **Minor deterioration**   Does not require more pauses to avoid shortness of breath, but does things with distinctly less effort than previously to avoid breathlessness.

0   **No change**   No change in effort to avoid shortness of breath.

+1   **Minor improvement**   Able to do things with distinctly greater effort or more rapidly without dyspnea.

+2   **Moderate improvement**   Able to do things with fewer pauses and distinctly greater effort without shortness of breath. Improvement is greater than preceding category, but not of major proportion.

+3   **Major improvement**   Able to do things with much greater effort than previously with few, if any, pauses. For example, activities may be performed 50% to 100% more rapidly than at baseline.

Z   **Further impairment for reasons other than shortness of breath**   Patient has reduced exertional capacity, but not related to shortness of breath. For example, musculoskeletal problems or chest pain.

---

* The baseline dyspnea index is graded by an observer who asks the patient open-ended questions and selects the appropriate grade of breathlessness based on specific criteria for the three sections. These grades are then added to obtain a baseline focal score (range, 0 to 12).

† The transition dyspnea index is graded in a manner similar to the baseline dyspnea index. An observer questions the patient and selects a grade for each section. The three grades for changes in breathlessness are combined for a transition focal score (range, −9 to +9).

‡ Usual activities refer to requirements of daily living, including maintenance or upkeep of residence, yard work, gardening, and shopping

(Adapted from Mahler DA, et al. The measurement of dyspnea: contents, interobserved agreement, and physiologic correlates of two new clinical indexes. Chest 1984;85:751)

expanded the dyspnea symptom cluster of the ASC and BESC into a Dyspnea Symptom Inventory (Hill KL, Weiser PC, Bell CW, Kinsman RA, Greenspon L, unpublished observations) that is shown in Table 26–3. The items for labored breathing were found to form a factor separate from fatigue and also from mood, hyperventilation, hyperinflation, and congestion (see Fig. 26–1).

The advantages of using multidimensional scales are that they provide a more comprehensive "snapshot" of the patient as well as providing an individual dys-

TABLE 26-3. Breathlessness Inventory: Frequency

Name   *Patient No.*

1. Rate yourself on each item as it relates to your breathlessness during all periods of breathing discomfort.

2. For each of the following items, circle the number that best describes how frequently you have these feelings during periods of breathing difficulty. Circle whether you have (1) Never, (2) Almost Never, (3) Sometimes, (4) Almost Always, or (5) Always, had this feeling *during all periods of breathing difficulty.*

3. Please answer all the items.

	Never	*Almost Never*	*Sometimes*	*Almost Always*	*Always*
Light headed	1	2	3	4	5
Difficult to breathe	1	2	3	4	5
Panicky	1	2	3	4	5
Urge to breathe	1	2	3	4	5
Scared	1	2	3	4	5
Feel like I need air	1	2	3	4	5
Worn out	1	2	3	4	5
Deep breathing	1	2	3	4	5
Uncomfortable breathing	1	2	3	4	5
Lungs full of air	1	2	3	4	5
Upset	1	2	3	4	5
Breathless	1	2	3	4	5
No energy	1	2	3	4	5
Anxious	1	2	3	4	5
Aware of breathing	1	2	3	4	5
Work to breathe	1	2	3	4	5
"Pins and needles" feeling	1	2	3	4	5
Short of breath	1	2	3	4	5
Tired	1	2	3	4	5
Wheezing	1	2	3	4	5
Frightened	1	2	3	4	5
Breathing hard	1	2	3	4	5
Gasping for breath	1	2	3	4	5
Numbness	1	2	3	4	5
Twitching muscles	1	2	3	4	5
Coughing	1	2	3	4	5
Can't get enough air in	1	2	3	4	5
Mucous congestion	1	2	3	4	5
Weak	1	2	3	4	5
Exhausted	1	2	3	4	5
Cramps	1	2	3	4	5
Hard effort to breathe	1	2	3	4	5
Chest congestion	1	2	3	4	5
Tingling in arms and legs	1	2	3	4	5
Disappointed	1	2	3	4	5

TABLE 26-3.   Breathlessness Inventory: Frequency (*continued*)

	Never	*Almost Never*	*Sometimes*	*Almost Always*	*Always*
Lonely	1	2	3	4	5
Stomach hurts	1	2	3	4	5
Stitch in side	1	2	3	4	5
Helpless	1	2	3	4	5
Out of control	1	2	3	4	5
Itching in chest	1	2	3	4	5
Nauseated	1	2	3	4	5
Congested nose	1	2	3	4	5
Angry	1	2	3	4	5
Ears tingle	1	2	3	4	5
Sad	1	2	3	4	5
Desperate to breathe	1	2	3	4	5
Dizzy	1	2	3	4	5
Vision blurred	1	2	3	4	5
Buzzing in ears	1	2	3	4	5

Remember: Answer each item as it relates to your breathlessness during all periods of breathing discomfort.

pnea profile. But the disadvantages are that the administration of the questionnaires takes time and requires concentration by the patient, who may just answer with a set of responses that give the same ratings.

Write Instructions for Use

In the second step, it is crucial to write clear, concise instructions for the use of the rating scales, profiles, or checklists that you chose. Define the sensation or symptom to be rated. Explain the layout of the rating scale explaining that the adjective phrases are to be used to help select the number to be reported. If necessary, anchor the extremes of the scale(s), being careful of the application (e.g., endurance but not explosive exercise). Remind the person that no answer is "right" or "wrong" and that they should focus on being honest and objective. An example set of instructions for the rating of perceived dyspnea follows:

Hold a copy of the rating scale for perceived dyspnea in front of the patient. Tell the patient, "Here is a scale for rating your breathlessness, whatever your type of breathing discomfort might be. Notice that the rating scale is from zero (0) to ten-plus (10+). Zero indicates that you are not at all breathless; 10 tells us that your are very, very severely breathless. During exercise, you might find that your breathing discomfort rating becomes greater than 10; feel free to give a number that matches your breathlessness, for example, 11, 15, and so forth." [Indicate how the patient is to indicate numbers: point, use number of fingers, call out number, or other.] "Remember, there are no right or wrong numbers. So, give the first number that comes to you. Any questions?"

Limitations

Finally, be aware of the limitations in the use of rating scales. Certainly, some individuals tend to underrate and have a low response bias. By stressing being honest, they will upgrade their ratings into a more appropriate range. Their responses, however, are reliable and perhaps indicate that their denial is a real part of their coping mechanism. Another problem is the choice of inadequate adjective definers that can be improved by revising the phrases after a trial period of use.

In summary, these rating scales have been very useful in the assessment and treatment of dyspnea. The first step in becoming familiar with these scales is to include them in the evaluation of dyspnea.

DYSPNEA ASSESSMENT PROCEDURES AND METHODS

The success of pulmonary rehabilitation programs depends upon how well we understand the characteristics of the patient's dyspnea, what types of activities provoke dyspnea, and the frequency and range of dyspnea intensity evoked by these activities. This section summarizes the specific steps taken during the initial and ongoing assessment of the patient to evaluate these characteristics.[25]

History

One of the first steps to evaluate dyspnea severity and peculiarities is a specific and thorough history. As Comroe noted, "Increased ventilation may be a pleasant sensation in a healthy person during exercise, it may be unpleasant but only annoying ('out of breath,' 'breathless'), or it may be incapacitating ('can't get breath'); more specific descriptions of the sensation experienced in the patient's own words will help in separating the various types of breathlessness."[26]

Any initial visit needs to include interviewing for establishing the overall, undifferentiated severity of dyspnea symptomatology. One can do this by selecting the instrument for the classification of dyspnea severity and incorporating it into your initial history. The results will provide the initial estimate of severity to be checked during the subsequent pulmonary exercise testing and will function as the baseline for monitoring progress during rehabilitation.

Include a symptom checklist or questionnaire in your battery of intake forms so that you can characterize the pattern of a patient's (sub)conceptual dyspnea symptoms. These instruments can assist in determining the extent to which congestion, hyperinflation, and increased work of breathing to overcome airway obstruction are important clinical factors. Consequently, these factors will help in determining which aspects of the individual's rehabilitation are to be emphasized.

Use a checklist in your intake battery to evaluate your client's activities of daily living and quality of life. Look for critical activities or areas of life satisfaction that are of particular concern for your patient.

Finally, ask the patients to tell you in their own words just what "breathing difficulty" means to them. Notice at what subjective level (discrete, subconceptual, conceptual, or superconceptual) the individual focuses. Record which aspects of breathlessness are their main concern. Use these results to check your questionnaire and checklist information as you obtain a snapshot of their pulmonary limitations.

Laboratory Findings

Various laboratory studies can provide diagnostic evalution of the cause of dyspnea. In this discussion, we will separate the information that is generated by the pulmonary function testing and exercise testing laboratories.

Chest Radiograph

Although a recent or current chest radiograph is not diagnostic, it can provide important information about heart size and configuration, lung parenchyma, pulmonary vasculature, pleural space, and position of the diaphragm (e.g., hyperinflation).

Pulmonary Function Testing

Spirometry is essential in the evaluation of dyspnea. Measurement of forced vital capacity (FVC) and flow rates is sufficient to diagnose COPD. Measurement of total lung capacity and diffusing capacity can be added to evaluate the presence of restrictive ventilatory defect, interstitial disease, or pulmonary vascular disease. In addition, the measurement of maximal inspiratory and expiratory mouth pressures at residual volume and total lung capacity, respectively, is important for assessing respiratory muscle strength.

Exercise Testing

The diagnostic value of evaluating patients while they exercise is not fully appreciated. First, the correlation of simple spirometric measures such as the 1-second forced expiratory volume (FEV_1) to measures of physical fitness such as maximum oxygen uptake ($\dot{V}O_{2max}$) is poor and only roughly approximate.[27] Exercise testing establishes the direct relation between pulmonary impairment and functional capacity. Second, the patient may have both pulmonary and cardiac impairments, and it is necessary to determine the relative contributions of each before deciding on the therapeutic modalities.[28] Third, since dyspnea on exertion precedes the clinical complaint of dyspnea at rest, exercise testing can reveal cardiovascular or pulmonary disease at an earlier stage.[29] When the patient is evaluated during exercise, even a moderate decrease in physical fitness capacity can be demonstrated to the patient and can reinforce the need to prevent further deterioration.

As the first procedural step for exercise testing, each laboratory must decide which standard values they are willing to accept as normal cardiovascular–pulmonary responses to graded exercise.[28–31] One standard must be set for the peak $\dot{V}O_2$, and the best measure is peak $\dot{V}O_2$ expressed as a ratio of predicted maximal $\dot{V}O_2$. The next standard to be decided is for peak exercise ventilation, and the best measure is the *exercise breathing index* (EBI), defined as the ratio of the highest exercise ventilation expressed relative to the predicted maximal ventilation such as the maximal voluntary ventilation (MVV). The actual measurement of MVV is preferred, rather than estimation from the FEV_1. Another possible standard concerns the determination and standardization of the ventilatory (or anaerobic) threshold. The best standard is the ventilatory threshold expressed as a percentage of the peak $\dot{V}o_2$. Finally, standards for the normal limits of breathlessness can be chosen to evaluate if dyspnea is appropriate for the required ventilation. An appropriate measure for a normal rating of perceived dyspnea (RPD) is the rating at an EBI of 50% MVV. For a group of 123 men of various ages (Fig. 26–6), the mean RPD at 50% MVV was 3.4 ("moderate") and the standard deviation (SD) was 1.8 units.[32] Thus, if a RPD was reported that is more than 2 SD above the mean [i.e., a rating of 7 (very severe)], then this rating of breathlessness can be regarded as disproportionately severe dyspnea.

The next procedural step is to choose the testing procedures for determining cardiopulmonary limitation(s). Several considerations are required for setting up the dyspnea evaluation. First, the evaluation of dyspnea is performed on either a cycle ergometer or treadmill, depending on which is used for the home exercise program. However, most programs prefer to use a cycle ergometer protocol, since

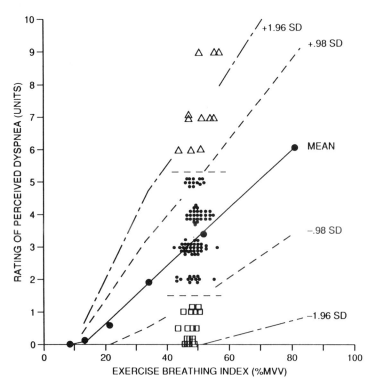

FIGURE 26-6 The rating of perceived dyspnea (RPD) at an exercise breathing index (EBI) of 50% MVV. The data is from a graded cycle ergometer test performed by a group of 123 men of various ages. The *triangles* represent the top 11 dyspnea responders; the *squares* represent the bottom 18 dyspnea responders. The *dashed lines* indicate the 64% and 95% confidence limits above and below the means (*large filled circle*) of the RPD data at selected EBI percentages.

an accurate setting of the work rate on an ergometer that is stationary seems to enable a more effective workup of anxious or elderly patients.

Another consideration involves the determination of the ventilatory threshold, a variable that can be very helpful in the differential diagnosis of dyspnea. During graded exercise testing, the work rate that eventually involves the recruitment of fast twitch motor units also produces an increase of the ventilatory equivalent for oxygen ($\dot{V}i/\dot{V}o_2$) with no change in the ventilatory equivalent for carbon dioxide ($\dot{V}i/\dot{V}co_2$). Under conditions such as poor cardiac output or peripheral blood flow that result in muscle hypoxia, this mechanism is accentuated and occurs at lower work rates. Therefore, it is important to couple both cardiac and pulmonary measurements to determine if hypoxemia is a possible mechanism of dyspnea.

The last concern involves having the individual patient give his or her rating of perceived dyspnea and relating these ratings to exercise physiologic variables such as power output, $\dot{V}o_2$, $\dot{V}co_2$, and ventilation. As a part of exercise testing, try using the rating scales shown in Figure 26–4 to check which symptoms limit the exercise capacity of your patients. Be sure to begin by giving simple, clear instructions for each scale. At the end of each minute or work increment, have the individual verbally or by show of fingers indicate the severity of each symptom.

The final procedural step is to interpret the results of the exercise test to determine the possibility of any cardiopulmonary limitation(s). An excellent analysis of this process is made by Wasserman and coworkers.[28] A summary of their flow chart can be found in Table 26–4.

In summary, seeking the answer to the question, "Is dyspnea due to heart or lung disease?" can be very challenging. Pulmonary function tests need to be an initial part of the workup. Complete exercise testing with arterial blood gas sampling or oxygen saturation monitoring using pulse oximetry often can provide enough information that a reasonable differential diagnosis of the primary organ system can be made. Thus, cardiopulmonary exercise testing can be useful in separating or identifying the various causes or diseases contributing to the symptom of breathlessness.

Psychological Testing

Dyspnea has far-reaching consequences upon psychological functioning. Anxiety and the fear of suffocation result from the perception of dyspnea. Depression may be a closely associated psychological factor. Psychosocial assets (e.g., a vital interest in life, adequate financial resources, good social support, and the ability to manage stress) are important for dealing effectively with the rehabilitation process. Several paper-and-pencil instruments are quick and useful additions to the intake battery.

Assessment Reports

Finally, in the composite summary of the patient's assessment reports, close attention is given to the effect of dyspnea. One important means of evaluating the effectiveness of the treatment plan is to continually assess changes in dyspnea.

Although the intake assessment is the starting point for your rehabilitation patient, the conduct of appropriate management strategies still requires continual

TABLE   26-4.   Overview of Flowchart for Exercise Intolerance

Step 1. Is $\dot{V}O_2$ peak normal?
  If so, is cardiac response normal?
    If so, obese or anxious?
    If not, are ventilatory–perfusion parameters normal?
      If so, check for early cardiovascular limitation
      If not, check for early pulmonary limitation
  If not, go to step 2.
Step 2. Is inspiratory ventilatory threshold determinable?
  If determined, go to step 3.
  If not, go to step 5.
Step 3. Is inspiratory ventilatory threshold normal?
  If so, is peak exercise breathing index near maximal?
    If normal or low, is ECG normal?
    If so, check for poor effort or musculoskeletal limitation.
  If not, check for mild cardiac limitation.
    If high, check for mild pulmonary limitation.
    If low, go to step 4.
Step 4. Is maximal exercise breathing index near maximal?
  If so, is dead space normal?
    If so, check for moderate chronic metabolic acidosis.
  If not, check for pulmonary limitation with poor peripheral oxygenation.
    If not, is $\dot{V}e/\dot{V}CO_2$ at inspiratory ventilatory threshold high?
      If so, check for abnormal pulmonary circulation.
      If not, check for O_2 flow problem from anemia or moderate cardiovascular
        limitation.
Step 5. Are ventilatory–perfusion parameters normal?
  If so, is dead space, normal?
    If so, check for severe cardiovascular limitation or anemia.
    If not, check for malingering, severe peripheral vascular disease or severe chronic
      metabolic acidosis.
      If not, is peak exercise breathing index near maximal?
      If so, check for severe lung limitation.
  If not, is arterial O_2 decreasing?
    If so, is vital capacity low?
      If so, check for severe lung limitation.
      If not, check for severe pulmonary vascular limitation.
    If not, check for severe circulatory limitation.

(Adapted from Wasserman K, et al. *Principles of exercise testing and interpretation.* Philadelphia: Lea
& Febiger, 1987:87)

reassessment of the severity and frequencies of dyspneic episodes. With this requirement in mind, let us turn to considering the strategies available to ameliorate the
discomfort and distress of breathlessness.

MANAGEMENT STRATEGIES FOR
REDUCING DYSPNEA

There are at least seven major approaches for attempting to reduce the sense of
breathlessness in symptomatic patients. Unfortunately, not all of these strategies
have proven scientific efficacy in appropriately designed clinical trials. In fact, re-

sults of different studies may provide conflicting data. In this review we describe the rationale for each of these potential management strategies along with relevant supporting information based on clinical results. Although most of these investigations have examined the problem of dyspnea in patients with COPD, it is possible that these therapeutic options may also be beneficial in patients with other causes of chronic respiratory disease.

Breathing Training

Position

Some relief or improvement in dyspnea can be achieved by body position. Patients frequently discover that the leaning-forward position partially relieves breathing discomfort.[33] Typically, the patient is seated and bends forward at the waist while supporting his or her forearms on the thighs. Sharp and coauthors[34] have suggested that this position enhances the efficiency of the diaphragm because of improved length–tension relationship.[34] If the patient is standing, he or she can lean forward and support his or her arms on a table, shopping cart, or other object. Alternatively, other individual patients may experience relief by lying supine.[34,35] Most patients with chronic lung disease find a best position to alleviate breathlessness by trying different postures when the symptom develops and persists.

Pursed-Lips Breathing

For many patients, pursed-lips breathing (PLB) is a natural response to reduce the severity of dyspnea; for others, PLB must be taught and demonstrated as an important breathing strategy. Directions for PLB are listed in Table 26–5. Pursing the lips provides an external resistance to expiration that actually increases airway pressure and may prevent, at least in part, compression of airways. However, the reduction in dyspnea is more likely related to the accompanying decrease in respiratory frequency and corresponding increase in tidal volume.[36,37] Exhalation should be at least twice as long as inhalation. Tiep and colleagues have reported that PLB can actually increase arterial oxygen saturation.[38] Also, PLB enables patients to gain control over their breathing, rather than passively experience anxiety or panic when breathing becomes distressful.

Paced breathing can be used in conjunction with PLB.[39] Pacing generally refers to inspiring with rest and expiring with an activity (e.g., lifting an object). Pacing incorporates the concept of maintaining a controlled-breathing pattern, especially with increased effort.

TABLE 26-5. Instructions for Pursed-Lips Breathing

1. Breathe in deeply through your nose.
2. Purse your lips together except for the very center as though you are whistling.
3. Breathe out slowly through pursed-lips. This should take at least twice as long as inhaling.
4. The pursed-lips should resist the speed of exhaled air.
5. This sequence can be repeated as needed or several times a day as part of breathing exercises.

Diaphragmatic Breathing

Diaphragmatic breathing refers to active use of the diaphragm during inspiration. Movement of the diaphragm can be detected by having the patient place one hand in the subxiphoid area. When the patient inspires slowly, the hand can feel the abdomen "push out" as the diaphragm contracts (descends). This type of breathing effort can be practiced in seated and supine positions. Exhalation should be slow through pursed-lips.

Relaxation

Anxiety frequently occurs with chronic respiratory disorders. Disproportionately severe dyspnea is one manifestation of anxiety in some patients.[40,41] The usual patient experiences a cluster of symptoms including difficulty in inspiration, rather than expiration, poor exercise tolerance, aggravation of breathing discomfort during social stress, and relief of dyspnea by using alcohol and sedative medications. Cognitive–behavioral treatment programs have recently emphasized breathing retraining for individual COPD patients[42] and also for those who panic.[43,44] One of the authors (PCW) has used breathing retraining for desensitization of the fear of breathlessness in affected individuals. During periods of breathlessness, ratings of dyspnea are used to allow the patient to focus on his or her breathing distress. Accentuated PLB and abdominal contractions during expiration (displayed on a monitor screen) can be used to desensitize a patient from the fear of breathlessness by using biofeedback techniques. Diaphragmatic breathing during inspiration is then added to further assist the patient to gain control of his or her fear and propensity to panic. Finally, the subtle difference between "appropriate" and "inappropriate" dyspnea can be discussed with the patient. Further periods of exercise training both in the laboratory and at home may be useful to decrease the discomfort rating while the patient maintains an objective awareness of breathing mechanics. This type of breathing retraining can become a powerful tool in reducing the magnitude of the breathing distress.

Progressive muscle relaxation can also be an important adjunct to breathing strategies. Generally, this technique incorporates tensing each muscle group for 5 to 10 seconds while inhaling, then relaxing the muscle group while exhaling. This approach associates the release of breath (expiration) with feelings of relaxation.[45] Renfroe demonstrated that progressive muscular relaxation reduced dyspnea, anxiety, and the corresponding respiratory rate in a treatment group compared with a control group over a 4-week period.[46]

Environmental Conditions

Ambient Weather

Patients usually experience an increase in dyspnea with either extreme hot (and humid) or cold (and dry) ambient air conditions. Hot, humid weather may contribute to breathlessness because of higher concentrations of airborne irritants and pollutants; in contrast, cold, dry weather can trigger bronchoconstriction. It appears that the "best" ambient conditions are clear skies with moderate temperature and humidity. Many patients report that staying indoors when extreme conditions occur minimizes breathing discomfort.

Air Movement

Almost all patients who experience severe dyspnea describe symptomatic relief when there is air movement. Typically, the patient will sit by an open window or direct a fan to blow air at his or her face. Schwartzstein and colleagues observed that cold air directed against the cheeks of healthy individuals reduced the sense of breathlessness experienced by hypercapnia and breathing against an inspiratory resistance.[47] Presumably, stimulation of facial receptors in the distribution of the trigeminal nerve can alter perception of breathlessness in these patients.

Exercise Reconditioning

It is generally assumed that regular exercise is beneficial for patients with chronic respiratory diseases, especially COPD. In fact, several controlled studies have demonstrated improvements in exercise endurance and skill performance as part of exercise-reconditioning programs in patients with COPD.[48-52] Although three of these reports describe a subjective reduction in breathlessness after an exercise-training program, valid and reliable methods for measuring dyspnea were not used.[48-50] Strijbos and colleagues randomized 45 patients with symptomatic COPD into a treatment group ($n = 30$) and a control group ($n = 15$).[52] The treatment group participated in a 12-week pulmonary rehabilitation program that included relaxing exercises, breathing retraining, and exercise reconditioning for 2 hours twice a week. The control group received no program. The investigators report that the treatment group showed a significant decrease in Borg ratings of dyspnea at equivalent work loads on the cycle ergometer, whereas the control group showed no change (Fig. 26–7). The results of this clinical trial support overall impressions

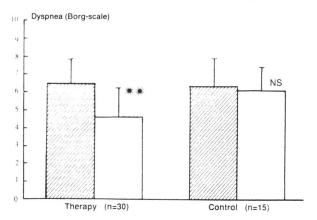

FIGURE 26-7 Borg ratings of breathlessness at equivalent work loads on the cycle ergometer before and after a 12-week pulmonary rehabilitation program (relaxing exercises, breathing retraining, and exercise reconditioning) in a treatment group ($n = 30$) and a control group ($n = 15$). NS, no significant difference; ✳✳, significant difference. (From Strijbos JH, et al. Objective and subjective performance indicators in COPD. Eur Respir J 1989; 2:666, with permission)

and experiences of many health care providers involved in pulmonary rehabilitation programs.

Either physiologic or psychological benefits (or both) may explain any reductions in breathlessness associated with exercise reconditioning. For example, a decrease in exercise ventilation would be expected to diminish the sense of breathlessness.[53] On the other hand, regular exercise training may desensitize the patient to the distress of increased breathing requirements. Despite our limited understanding about the mechanisms of dyspnea, exercise reconditioning has been, and continues to be, a key component of pulmonary rehabilitation programs.

Prescription of exercise should include mode, frequency, intensity, and duration of exercise. Many rehabilitation programs apply the guidelines for developing and maintaining cardiorespiratory fitness established by the American College of Sports Medicine (ACSM) to patients with chronic respiratory diseases.[54] However, there is now no standardized approach for prescribing exercise, especially the intensity component, for pulmonary patients. A target heart rate or target rating of dyspnea obtained from results of a cardiopulmonary exercise test can be used for estimating intensity and providing feedback to the patient (Fig. 26–8).[16] The standard training intensity is 50% of peak exercise capacity.[54] This level of effort is generally tolerable and acceptable for most patients with pulmonary limitation.

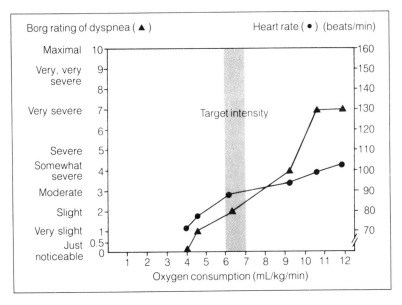

FIGURE 26-8 Method of determining intensity of exercise reconditioning based on results of a cardiopulmonary exercise test. A target heart rate and target rating of dyspnea on the Borg category scale are selected at approximately 50% of peak exercise capacity in this example of a patient with severe COPD. (Faryniarz K, Mahler DA. Writing an exercise prescription for patients with COPD. J Respir Dis 1990; 7:638–644, with permission)

Ries and Archibald have suggested that patients with moderate to severe COPD can exercise at walking speeds on the treadmill that approach peak exercise tolerance.[55] For example, they observed that the average patient could walk for 5 minutes at 3.2 km/hour (2 mph); range 0.96 to 5.0 km/hour (0.6 to 3.5 mph). This intensity was below the anaerobic threshold (AT) which was not detectable in most of their patients.[55] An alternative strategy, recommended by Casaburi and Wasserman, is to have patients train at an intensity above the anaerobic threshold.[56] The rationale for this approach is that exercise ventilation can be reduced in normal subjects only when the exercise training causes a metabolic acidosis (above the AT).[56] However, this intensity of exercise effort may be difficult for pulmonary patients to tolerate, especially when just starting a reconditioning program.

Guidelines for exercise prescription are provided in Table 26–6. Because there is no best method for prescribing exercise intensity, we suggest that the approach be individualized, based on practical considerations as well as trial-and-error attempts at simulating the conditions of training in the laboratory. We believe that long-term compliance and success in reconditioning can best be achieved by starting at a moderate intensity (50% of peak exercise capacity). The corresponding target level of breathlessness could, therefore, range from 2 (slight) to 3 (moderate) or even 4 (somewhat severe) on the Borg category scale. This should minimize patients dropping out and reduce injuries. Over time, the target level of exercise intensity or severity of breathlessness can be gradually increased, depending on the individual patient's response.

Nutritional Manipulations

Nutritional status appears to exert an independent influence on the course of COPD.[57] Both undernutrition and the type of caloric repletion can potentially affect the experience of dyspnea. Approximately one-third of patients with COPD are substantially underweight;[58–60] this is generally associated with reduced maximal respiratory pressures.[61] The corresponding hypothesis is that nutritional repletion

---

**TABLE 26-6. Exercise Prescription Guidelines
for Patients with Pulmonary Disease**

Mode: Activities that involve large-muscle groups and can be maintained continuously, such as walking, treadmill exercise, stationary cycling, rowing, or other.

Frequency: 3–5 days per week; maximum benefits are derived from daily exercise

Intensity: 50% of peak exercise capacity using the corresponding heart rate and/or rating of dyspnea (see Fig. 26–4).

Duration: Goal of 20–30 min of continuous exercise. Initially, the patient may only be able to tolerate 5–10 min; if so, the duration should gradually be increased over several weeks.

Warm-up: A 10–15 min warm-up should precede the exercise period. This can include stretching and flexibility exercises to improve range of motion of major joints.

Cool-down: Gentle stretching and flexibility activities should be part of a cool-down period following the exercise. Focus should be on relaxed breathing.

can enhance respiratory muscle strength and, thereby, diminish the intensity of dyspnea with various activities. Although a number of investigations have been performed evaluating nutritional repletion, the results have been conflicting for the ability to increase body weight or to improve respiratory muscle performance.[62-65] Of note, Efthimiou and associates examined the effect of supplemental oral nutrition in seven poorly nourished patients with COPD in a prospective, randomized study.[65] After 3 months of additional 320 kcal of energy per day, the group increased respiratory muscle strength and showed improvements in breathlessness and general well-being.[65] This is the only investigation that has demonstrated such benefits with nutritional supplementation.

Another concern is that increasing caloric intake in patients with COPD may actually increase carbon dioxide production ($\dot{V}_{CO_2}$). As the level of ventilation is linked closely with $\dot{V}_{CO_2}$, nutritional repletion may augment ventilatory requirements and cause breathlessness. In particular, ingestion of carbohydrates leads to greater $\dot{V}_{CO_2}$ per gram of food than do fats or protein.[66] A low-carbohydrate diet can significantly decrease $\dot{V}_{CO_2}$ and arterial carbon dioxide levels. Therefore, it is possible that a high-fat, low-carbohydrate diet may be beneficial for patients with chronic respiratory disease by decreasing the sense of dyspnea. However, further studies are required before specific recommendations can be made concerning nutritional replacement or supplementation in patients with chronic lung disease, especially for relief of breathlessness.[67]

Psychotropic Therapy

Anxiety or depression (or both) commonly develop in patients with chronic respiratory disease. Either of these conditions can magnify the severity of breathlessness. Benzodiazepines, opiates, and phenothiazines are psychotropic agents that have been considered for relieving the distress of dyspnea. In general, published studies show inconsistent results.

Benzodiazepine drugs could potentially relieve dyspnea by their anxiolytic action or depressive effect on hypoxic ventilatory responsiveness. The results of four studies involving different benzodiazepines are summarized in Table 26–7.[68-71] These overall findings do not support the routine prescription of benzodiazepine medications for treating the symptom of breathlessness. However, in specific situations, a therapeutic trial may be appropriate if anxiety plays a major role in an individual patient's sense of breathlessness and quality of life.

Opiates diminish ventilatory responses and, in large doses, can cause respiratory depression. These agents might ameliorate breathlessness by altering the integration and processing of the dyspnea "signal" in the central nervous system. Woodcock and colleagues reported that a single dose of oral dihydrocodeine (1 mg/kg) decreased breathlessness in patients with COPD.[72] Johnson and associates showed that 15 mg of dihydrocodeine up to three times a day provided less breathlessness (using a daily visual analog scale), compared with placebo, for a 1-week period in patients with chronic airflow obstruction.[73] In contrast, Rice and coworkers found that codeine (30 mg four times a day) did not improve breathlessness in patients with COPD after a 1-month trial, whereas several individuals had

TABLE 26-7. Effects of Benzodiazepine Drugs on Ratings of Dyspnea in COPD

Study	Number of Subjects	Drug	Duration (days)	Change in Dyspnea
Mitchell-Heggs[68]	4	Diazepam	10–32	Improved (not measured)
Woodcock[69]	15	Diazepam	14	None
Eimer[70]	5	Chlorazepate	14	None
Man[71]	24	Alprazolam	7	None

VAS, visual analog scale; OCD, oxygen cost diagram.
(Modified from Mahler DA. Therapeutic strategies. In: Mahler DR, ed. Dyspnea. Mt Kisco, NY. Futura Publishing, 1990).

mild narcotic withdrawal after stopping codeine.[74] In a preliminary report, Eiser and colleagues found that neither single-dose nor extended (2-week) use of oral diamorphine improved dyspnea, compared with placebo therapy, in 14 patients with severe COPD.[75] Finally, Light and associates demonstrated that a single dose of oral morphine (0.8 mg/kg) led to a significant decrease in ratings of dyspnea during cycle ergometry, compared with placebo, in 13 eucapnic patients with COPD.[76] Furthermore, patients improved exercise capacity with morphine, which was related to both decreased ventilation and a reduced perception of dyspnea at a given level of ventilation.[76]

In summary, the efficacy of opiates for relieving dyspnea appears to be highly variable and inconsistent. We agree with the recommendation by Light and colleagues that opiates, including oral morphine, should not now be used *routinely* for treating breathlessness.[76] In addition to the uncertainty of clinical benefit, there are safety concerns about the use of opiates. Potential side effects include respiratory depression, alteration in mental status, drug tolerance, and possible oxygen desaturation during sleep.[74,77] However, opiates are indicated for alleviating the extremely distressful sense of breathing discomfort as part of symptomatic care for patients with terminal respiratory disease. This can provide some comfort for the patient and reassurance for family members.

Phenothiazines are the third type of psychotropic agents that have been used to treat the symptom of dyspnea. Although Woodcock and associates found that promethazine reduced breathlessness during treadmill exercise compared with both placebo and diazepam, an anxiolytic medication,[69] Rice and coworkers did not detect any benefit of promethazine on relieving dyspnea in 14 patients with COPD.[74] Given these conflicting results, there is no clear evidence that phenothiazine drugs should be generally prescribed for relief of dyspnea in symptomatic patients.

Although psychotropic agents are inappropriate for the routine therapy of dyspnea, it is reasonable to consider such therapy in a single-patient clinical trial for a person who experiences persistent breathlessness with functional limitation despite otherwise optimal therapy.[78,79]

Respiratory Muscle Rest

Weakness or fatigue of the respiratory muscle may contribute to the symptom of dyspnea.[80,81] Given the hypothesis that patients with an increased work of breathing owing to respiratory loads (resistive or elastic) develop incipient or chronic respiratory muscle fatigue, resting the muscles of respiration might enhance their function and potentially relieve breathlessness. Initial observational reports by Rochester and coauthors[82] and Braun and Marino[83] suggested that assisted ventilation improved respiratory muscle strength and provided relief of dyspnea in some patients with COPD.

Subsequent studies of external negative-pressure ventilation included a control group for comparison with the study group.[84–88] Although investigators reported symptomatic improvement or reduction in breathlessness, based on comments by individual patients, the symptom of dyspnea was not directly measured in these clinical trials.[84–87] In a preliminary report Martin summarized the results of a randomized trial of external negative-pressure ventilation using a body wrap compared with sham therapy in 184 patients with COPD.[88] Ventilatory support for 8 hours/day failed to improve respiratory muscle strength, exercise performance, arterial blood gas values, dyspnea as measured by the oxygen cost diagram, or quality of life.

It is possible that selected patients with COPD may benefit from respiratory muscle rest using external ventilatory support. However, patient acceptance and tolerance of negative-pressure ventilation are major considerations. From the collective results of randomized, controlled studies,[84–88] external negative-pressure ventilation should not be routinely prescribed for relieving dyspnea in symptomatic patients. However, the application of positive-pressure ventilation by nasal mask may provide an alternative noninvasive approach for resting the respiratory muscles. Clinical trials are needed to evaluate the efficacy of this form of ventilatory support.

Respiratory Muscle Training

At least 18 different studies have evaluated respiratory muscle training in patients with COPD.[89–106] The overall results are conflicting regarding the physiologic and symptomatic benefits. One major limitation of many of these clinical trials is the failure to provide or establish a target for training intensity with feedback to the patient. This feature is critical to provide an effective stimulus load to ensure a training response.

Various investigators have demonstrated that patients with COPD can increase respiratory muscle strength or endurance when training guidelines for frequency, intensity, and duration are met.[94, 97, 101–106] In addition, several reports have suggested that the symptom of dyspnea can be improved as a result of respiratory muscle training.[89, 94, 95, 98, 106] However, only Falk and coworkers[98] and Harver and associates[105] included a control group for comparison with the treatment group. Falk and colleagues[98] reported that the group doing respiratory muscle training had a marked decrease in dyspnea, as measured with a four-question scoring scale. Harver and associates[105] randomized subjects to an 8-week trial of either increasing levels of inspiratory resistance (5 to 35 cmH_2O $L^{-1}sec^{-1}$) or a constant, nominal level of resistance (5 cmH_2O $L^{-1}sec^{-1}$). The inspiratory resistance device provided visual feedback of breath-to-breath changes of inspiratory mouth pressure. The training group showed a significant improvement ($p = 0.003$) in the composite of grades for magnitude of task, magnitude of effort, and functional impairment that contributed to the symptom (Fig. 26–9).[105] The increase in peak inspiratory mouth pressure (PI_{max}) was significantly correlated with two of the categories (task and effort) affecting breathlessness.[105]

A trial of respiratory muscle training may be considered if the patient complains of persistent dyspnea, despite optimal bronchodilator therapy and a regular exercise program; and the measured PI_{max} is decreased without severe hyperinflation.[107] Guidelines for respiratory muscle training include frequency, at least 4 to 5 days/week; intensity, 25 to 35% of PI_{max} measured at functional residual capacity; and duration, two 15-minute sessions or one 30-minute session per day (if this can not be achieved, the intensity can be reduced). Certainly, it is important to quantify the training stimulus (load) and to consider the breathing frequency (12 to 14/minute) and pattern during training. A minimal period of 6 to 8 weeks may be required to demonstrate a training response or symptomatic improvement.

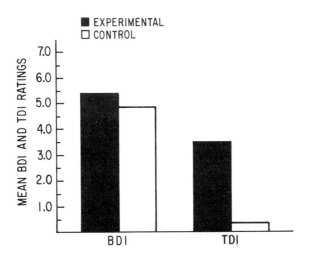

FIGURE   26-9 Scores for baseline (*BDI*) and transition dyspnea indexes (*TDI*) before and after an 8-week program of targeted inspiratory muscle training in experimental (*n* = 10) and control (*n* = 9) groups. There was a significant improvement in dyspnea in the experimental group compared with the control group (*p* = 0.003). (Data from Harver A, et al. Targeted inspiratory muscle training improves respiratory muscle function and reduces dyspnea in patients with chronic obstructive pulmonary disease. Ann Intern Med 1989; 111:117)

FUTURE TRENDS IN
DYSPNEA ASSESSMENT AND MANAGEMENT

Over the last 20 to 30 years, increasing attention has been drawn to investigating the assessment and treatment of the common complaint of breathlessness. Today we find that clinical testing and monitoring of dyspnea during exertion is becoming more common in the pulmonary rehabilitation programs offered by local hospitals and physician groups.

In the near future, the measurement instruments for dyspnea will need further development. Standardized instructions must be devised that ensure clarity, ease of administration, and honest reporting when rating scales are used. Novel approaches to evaluating the perception of dyspnea are conceivable. Refinement of the multidimensional questionnaires requires further development. Overall, the development of a standardized battery of assessment tools and procedures will be most helpful for the processing of multicenter rehabilitation results needed for the documentation of treatment cost-effectiveness.

The management of dyspnea is obviously at an early stage of development. Numerous additional studies are required to evaluate the listed as well as alternative treatment strategies. These studies will examine appropriate patient populations undergoing various strategies, using standardized measurement tools, over sufficient time periods, to generate clinically relevant data. Certainly, one can pick any particular treatment strategy and develop it accordingly. Furthermore, a step approach may be appropriate such that a physician uses step 1; if this is not totally successful, step 2 is used, and then additional steps are incorporated depending on the particular individual characteristics of the patient and his or her specific medical problem.

The assessment and management of dyspnea has been and continues to be a challenge. The mechanism(s) contributing to dyspnea remain an important consideration as well as the demonstration that new methods for evaluating dyspnea and its treatment can actually improve the patient's quality of life. Means said that when ". . . the respiratory organs do meet with embarrassment in the performance of their task, then not only do their movements enter the field of consciousness, but they enter it unpleasantly and produce discomfort, that is to say, dyspnoea."[108] However, Comroe warns us that ". . . all of us, I am sure, will describe the symptom faithfully in the subject's or patient's own words—rather than calling every respiratory complaint 'exertional dyspnoea', a term never used by any patient unless he is a physician!"[109]

REFERENCES

1. Richards DW Jr. The nature of cardiac and of pulmonary dyspnea. Circulation 1953;7:15.

2. Comroe JH. Some theories of the mechanism of dyspnea. In: Howell JBL, Campbell EJM, eds. Breathlessness. Oxford: Blackwell Publishing, 1966.

3. Livingston RB. Sensory processing, perception, and behavior. New York: Raven Press, 1978:19.

4. Kinsman RA, Weiser PC. Subjective symptomatology during work and fatigue. In:

Simonson E, Weiser PC, eds. Psychological aspects and physiological correlates of work and fatigue. Springfield: Charles C Thomas, 1976:388.

5. Kinsman RA, Luparello TJ, O'Banion K, Spector SL. Multidimensional analysis of the subjective symptomatology of asthma. Psychosom Med 1973;35:250.

6. Kinsman RA, Yaroush RA, Fernandez E, Dirks JF, Schocket M, Fukuhara J. Symptoms and experiences in chronic bronchitis and emphysema. Chest 1983;83:755.

7. Gandevia SC. Neural mechanisms underlying the sensation of breathlessness: kinesthetic parallels between respiration and limb muscles. Aust NZ J Med 1988;18:83.

8. Cherniack NS, Altose MD. Mechanisms of dyspnea. Clin Chest Med 1987;8:207.

9. Killian KJ, Gandevia SC, Summers E, Campbell EJM. Effect of increased lung volume on perception of breathlessness, effort, and volume. J Appl Physiol 1984;57:686.

10. Cronan T, Mulholland MB, Leitner J, Altose MD, Cherniack NS. Sensation of dyspnea during hypercapnia, exercise, and voluntary hyperventilation. J Appl Physiol 1990;68:2100.

11. Killian KJ. The objective measurement of dyspnea. Chest 1985;88:84S.

12. Altose MD. Psychophysics—an approach to the study of respiratory sensation and the assessment of dyspnea. Am Rev Respir Dis 1987;135:1227.

13. Mahler DA, Harver A. Clinical measurement of dyspnea. In: Mahler, DA, ed. Dyspnea. Mt Kisco, NY: Futura Publishing, 1990:75.

14. Medical Research Council committee on the aetiology of chronic bronchitis. Definition and classification of chronic bronchitis for clinical and epidemiological purposes. Lancet 1965;1:775.

15. Pollock ML, Wilmore JH, Fox SM III. Exercise in health and disease. Evaluation and prescription for prevention and rehabilitation. Philadelphia: WB Saunders, 1984:255.

16. Faryniarz K, Mahler DA. Writing an exercise prescription for patients with COPD. J Respir Dis 1990;11:638.

17. Weiser PC. Use of perceived dyspnea for exercise training [abstr.] Med Sci Sports Exerc 1990;21:S5.

18. American Thoracic Society epidemiology standardization project. II. Recommended respiratory disease questionnaires for use with adults and children in epidemiological research. Am Rev Respir Dis 1978;118(suppl):7.

19. Aitken RCB. Measurement of feelings using visual analogue scales. Proc R Soc Med 1969;62:989.

20. McGavin CR, Artvinli M, Naoe H, McHardy GJR. Dyspnoea, disability, and distance walked: comparison of estimates of exercise performance in respiratory disease. Br Med J 1978;2:241.

21. Borg G. Psychophysical bases of perceived exertion. Med Sci Sports Exerc 1982;14:377.

22. Pratter MR, Curley FJ, Dubois J, Irwin RS. Cause and evaluation of chronic dyspnea in a pulmonary disease clinic. Arch Intern Med 1989;149:2227.

23. Mahler DA, Weinberg DH, Wells CK, Feinstein AR. The measurement of dyspnea. Contents, interobserver agreement, and physiologic correlates of two new clinical indexes. Chest 1984;85:751.

24. Guyatt GH, Berman LB, Townsend M, et al. A measure of quality of life for clinical trials in chronic lung disease. Thorax 1987;42:773.

25. Mahler DA. Dyspnea: diagnosis and management. Clin Chest Med 1987;8:215.

26. Comroe JH Jr. Dyspnea. Mod Concepts Cardiovas Dis 1956;25:347.

27. Pineda H, Haas F, Axen K, Haas A. Accuracy of pulmonary function tests in predicting exercise tolerance in chronic obstructive pulmonary disease. Chest 1984;86:564.

28. Wasserman K, Hansen JE, Sue DY, Whipp BJ. Principles of exercise testing and interpretation. Philadelphia: Lea & Febiger, 1987.

29. Jones NA. Clinical exercise testing. Philadelphia: WB Saunders, 1988.

30. Hansen JE. Respiratory abnormalities: exercise evaluation of the dyspneic patient. In: Leff AR, ed. Cardiopulmonary exercise testing. Orlando, FL: Grune & Stratton, 1986:69.

31. Weber KT, Janicki JS. Cardiopulmonary exercise testing: physiologic principles and clinical applications. Philadelphia: WB Saunders, 1986:290.

32. Weiser PC, Greenspon LW. Normal values for dyspnea in young and old men during graded cycle exercise [abstr.] Am Rev Resp Dis 1988;137:S335.

33. Barach AL. Chronic obstructive lung disease: postural relief of dyspnea. Arch Phys Med Rehabil 1974;55:494–504.

34. Sharp JT, Drutz WS, Moisan T, Foster J, Machnach W. Postural relief of dyspnea in severe chronic obstructive pulmonary disease. Am Rev Respir Dis 1980;122:201.

35. Barach AL, Beck GJ. Ventilatory effects of head-down position in pulmonary emphysema. Am J Med 1954;16:55.

36. Thoman RL, Stoker GL, Ross JC. The efficiency of pursed-lips breathing in patients with chronic obstructive pulmonary disease. Am Rev Respir Dis 1966;93:100.

37. Mueller RE, Petty TL, Filley GF. Ventilation and arterial blood gas changes induced by pursed lips breathing. J Appl Physiol 1970;28:784.

38. Tiep BL, Burns M, Kao D, Madison R, Herrera J. Pursed lips breathing training using ear oximetry. Chest 1986;90:218.

39. Kohlman-Carrieri V, Janson-Bjerklie S. Coping and self-care strategies. In: Mahler DA, ed. Dyspnea. Mt Kisco, NY: Futura Publishing, 1990.

40. Burns BH, Howell JBL. Disproportionately severe breathlessness in chronic bronchitis. Q J Med 1969;38:277.

41. Rosser R, Guz A. Psychological approaches to breathlessness and its treatment. J Psychosom Res 1981;25:439.

42. Atkins CJ, Kaplan RM, Timms RM, Reinsch S, Lofback K. Behavioral exercise programs in the management of chronic obstructive pulmonary disease. J Consult Clin Psychol 1984;52, 591.

43. Clark DM. A cognitive approach to panic. Behav Res Ther 1986;24, 461.

44. Shear MK, Ball G, Josephson S. An empirically developed cognitive-behavioral treatment of panic. J Integr Eclect Psychother 1987;6:421.

45. Bernstein DA, Borkovec TD. Progressive relaxation training: a manual for the helping professions. Champaign, IL: Research Press, 1973.

46. Renfroe KL. Effect of progressive relaxation on dyspnea and state anxiety in patients with chronic obstructive pulmonary disease. Heart Lung 1988;17:408.

47. Schwartzstein RM, Lahive K, Pope A, Weinberger SE, Weiss JW. Cold facial stimulation reduces breathlessness in normal subjects. Am Rev Respir Dis 1987;136:58.

48. Cockcroft AE, Sanders MT, Berry G. Randomized controlled trial of rehabilitation in chronic respiratory disability. Thorax 1981;36:200.

49. McGavin CR, Gupta SP, Lloyd EL, McHardy GJR. Physical rehabilitation of chronic bronchitis: results of a controlled trial of exercise in the home. Thorax 1977;32:307.

50. Sinclair DJM, Ingram CG. Controlled trial of supervised exercise training in chronic bronchitis. Br Med J 1980;280:519.

51. Chester EH, Belman MJ, Bahler RC, Baum GL, Schey G, Buch P. Multidisciplinary treatment of chronic pulmonary insufficiency. 3. The effect of physical training on cardiopulmonary performance in patients with chronic obstructive pulmonary disease. Chest 1977;72:695.

52. Strijbos JH, Sluiter HJ, Postma DS, Gimeno F, Koeter GH. Objective and subjective performance indicators in COPD. Eur Respir J 1989;2:666.

53. Casaburi R, Wasserman K. Exercise training in pulmonary rehabilitation [editorial]. N Engl J Med 1986;314:1509.

54. American College of Sports Medicine. Position stand on the recommended quantity and quality of exercise for developing and maintaining cardiorespiratory and muscular fitness in healthy adults. Med Sci Sports Exerc 1990;22:265.

55. Ries AL, Archibald CJ. Endurance exercise training at maximal targets in patients with COPD. J Cardiopulm Rehabil 1987;7:594.

56. Casaburi R, Wasserman K, Patessio A, Loli F, Zanoboni S, Donner CF. A new perspective in pulmonary rehabilitation: anaerobic threshold as a discriminant in training. Eur Respir J 1989;2(suppl):618s.

57. Wilson DO, Rogers RM, Wright EC, Anthonisen NR. Body weight in chronic obstructive pulmonary disease. Am Rev Respir Dis 1989;139:1435.

58. Openbrier R, Irwin MM, Rogers RM, et al. Nutritional status and lung function in patients with emphysema and chronic bronchitis. Chest 1983;83:17.

59. Hunter AM, Curey MA, Larsh MW. The nutritional status of patients with chronic obstructive pulmonary disease. Am Rev Respir Dis 1985;124:376.

60. Rochester DF. Body weight and respiratory muscle function in chronic obstructive pulmonary disease [editorial]. Am Rev Respir Dis 1986;134:646.

61. Arora NS, Rochester DF. Respiratory muscle strength and maximal voluntary ventilation in undernourished patients. Am Rev Respir Dis 1982;126:5.

62. Wilson DO, Rogers RM, Sanders MH, Pennock BE, Reilly JJ. Nutritional intervention in malnourished patients with emphysema. Am Rev Respir Dis 1986;134:672.

63. Lewis MI, Belman MJ, Dorr-Vyemura L. Nutritional supplementation in ambulatory patients with chronic obstructive pulmonary disease. Am Rev Respir Dis 1987;135:1062.

64. Knowles JB, Fairbarn MS, Wiggs BJ, Chan-Yan C, Pardy RL. Dietary supplementation and respiratory muscle performance in patients with COPD. Chest 1988;93:977.

65. Efthimiou J, Fleming J, Gomes C, Spiro SG. The effect of supplementary oral nutrition in poorly nourished patients with chronic obstructive pulmonary disease. Am Rev Respir Dis 1988;137:1075.

66. Saltzman HA, Salzano JV. Effects of carbohydrate metabolism upon respiratory gas exchange in normal men. J Appl Physiol 1971;30:228.

67. Wilson DO, Rogers RM, Hoffman RM. Nutrition and chronic lung disease. Am Rev Respir Dis 1985;132:1347.

68. Mitchell-Heggs P, Murphy K, Minty K, et al. Diazepam in the treatment of dyspnea in the "pink puffer" syndrome. Q J Med 1980;49:9.

69. Woodcock AA, Gross ER, Geddes DM. Drug treatment of breathlessness: contrasting effects of diazepam and promethazine in pink puffers. Br Med J 1981;283:343.

70. Eimer M, Cable T, Gal P, Rothenberger LA, McCue JE. Effects of chlorazepate on breathlessness and exercise tolerance in patients with chronic airflow obstruction. J Fam Pract 1985;21:359.

71. Man GCW, Hsu K, Sproule BJ. Effect of alprazolam on exercise and dyspnea in patients with chronic obstructive pulmonary disease. Chest 1986;90:832.

72. Woodcock AA, Gross ER, Gellert A, Shah S, Johnson M, Geddes DM. Effects of dihydrocodeine, alcohol, and caffeine on breathlessness and exercise tolerance in patients with chronic obstructive lung disease and normal blood gases. N Engl J Med 1981;305:1611.

73. Johnson MA, Woodcock AA, Geddes DM. Dihydrocodeine for breathlessness in "pink puffers." Br Med J 1983;286:675.

74. Rice KL, Kronenberg RS, Hedemark LL, Niewoehner DE. Effects of chronic administration of codeine and promethazine on breathlessness and exercise tolerance in patients with chronic airflow obstruction. Br J Dis Chest 1987;81:287.

75. Eiser N, Luce P, Denman W, West C. Effect of oral diamorphine on dyspnea in chronic obstructive pulmonary disease (COPD) [abstr]. Am Rev Respir Dis 1990;141 (suppl):A323.

76. Light RW, Muro JR, Sato RI, Stansbury DW, Fischer CE, Brown SE. Effects of oral morphine on breathlessness and exercise tolerance in patients with chronic obstructive pulmonary disease (COPD). Am Rev Respir Dis 1989;139:126.

77. Woodcock AA, Johnson MA, Geddes DM. Breathlessness, alcohol, and opiates [letter to the editor]. N Engl J Med 1982;306:1363.

78. Guyatt G, Sackett D, Taylor W, Chong J, Roberts R, Pugsley S. Determining optimal therapy: randomized trials in individual patients. N Engl J Med 1986;314:889.

79. Robin ED, Burke CM. Single-patient randomized clinical trial: opiates for intractable dyspnea. Chest 1986;90:888.

80. Black LF, Hyatt RE. Maximal static respiratory pressures in generalized neuromuscular disease. Am Rev Respir Dis 1971;103:641.

81. O'Connell JM, Campbell AH. Respiratory mechanics in airways obstruction associated with inspiratory dyspnoea. Thorax 1976;31:669.

82. Rochester DF, Braun NMT, Lane S. Diaphragmatic energy expenditure in chronic respiratory failure: the effect of assisted ventilation with body respirators. Am J Med 1977;63:223.

83. Braun NMT, Marino WD. Effect of daily intermittent rest of respiratory muscles in patients with severe chronic airflow limitation (CAL). [abstr]. Chest 1984;85(suppl):59s.

84. Gutierrez M, Beroiza T, Contreras G, et al. Weekly curiass ventilation improves blood gases and inspiratory muscle strength in patients with chronic airflow limitation and hypercapnia. Am Rev Respir Dis 1988;138:617.

85. Cropp A, Dimarco AF. Effects of intermittent negative pressure ventilation on respiratory muscle function in patients with severe chronic obstructive pulmonary disease. Am Rev Respir Dis 1987;135:1056.

86. Zibrak JD, Hill NS, Federman EC, Kwa SL, O'Donnell C. Evaluation of intermittent long-term negative-pressure ventilation in patients with severe chronic obstructive pulmonary disease. Am Rev Respir Dis 1988;138:1515.

87. Celli B, Lee H, Criner G, Bermudez M, et al. Controlled trial of external negative pressure ventilation in patients with severe chronic airflow obstruction. Am Rev Respir Dis 1989;140:1251.

88. Martin JG. Clinical intervention in chronic respiratory failure. Chest 1990;97 (suppl):105s.

89. Andersen JB, Dragsted L, Kann T, et al. Resistive breathing training in severe chronic obstructive pulmonary disease: a pilot study. Scand J Respir Dis 1979;60:151.

90. Pardy RL, Rivington RN, Despas PJ, Macklem PT. Inspiratory muscle training compared with physiotherapy in patients with chronic airflow limitation. Am Rev Respir Dis 1981;123:421.

91. Pardy RL, Rivington RN, Despas PJ, Macklem PT. The effects of inspiratory muscle training on exercise performance in chronic airflow limitation. Am Rev Respir Dis 1981;123:426.

92. Bjerre-Jepsen K, Secher NH, Kok-Jensen A. Inspiratory resistance training in severe chronic pulmonary disease. Eur J Respir Dis 1981;62:405.

93. Sonne LJ, Davis JA. Increased exercise performance in patients with severe COPD following inspiratory resistive training. Chest 1982;81:436.

94. Moreno R, Moreno R, Guigliano C, Lisboa C. Entrenamiento muscular inspiratorio en pacientes con limitacion chronica del flujo aereo. Rev Med Chile 1983;111:647.

95. Andersen JB, Falk P. Clinical experience with inspiratory resistive breathing training. Int Rehabil Med 1984;6:183.

96. Ambrosino N, Paggiaro PL, Roselli MG, Contini V. Failure of resistive breathing training to improve pulmonary function tests in patients with chronic obstructive pulmonary disease. Respiration 1984;45:455.

97. Chen HI, Dukes R, Martin BJ. Inspiratory muscle training in patients with chronic obstructive pulmonary disease. Am Rev Respir Dis 1985;131:251.

98. Falk P, Eriksen AM, Kolliker K, Andersen JB. Relieving dyspnea with an inexpensive and simple method in patients with severe chronic airflow limitation. Eur J Respir Dis 1985;66:181.

99. Madsen F, Secher NH, Kay L, Kok-Jensen A, Rube N. Inspiratory resistance versus general physical training in patients with chronic obstructive pulmonary disease. Eur J Respir Dis 1985;67:167.

100. McKeon JL, Turner J, Kelly C, Dent A, Zimmerman PV. The effect of inspiratory resistive training on exercise capacity in optimally treated patients with severe chronic airflow limitation. Aust NZ J Med 1986;16:648.

101. Belman MJ, Thomas SG, Lewis MI. Resistive breathing training in patients with chronic obstructive pulmonary disease. Chest 1986;90:662.

102. Levine S, Weiser P, Gillen J. Evaluation of a ventilatory muscle training program in the rehabilitation of patients with chronic obstructive pulmonary disease. Am Rev Respir Dis 1986;133:400.

103. Larson JL, Kim MJ, Sharp JT, Larson DA. Inspiratory muscle training with a pressure threshold breathing device in patients with chronic obstructive pulmonary disease. Am Rev Respir Dis 1988;138:689.

104. Belman MJ, Shadmehr R. Targeted resistive ventilatory muscle training in chronic obstructive pulmonary disease. J Appl Physiol 1988;65:2726.

105. Harver A, Mahler DA, Daubenspeck JA. Targeted inspiratory muscle training improves respiratory muscle function and reduces dyspnea in patients with chronic obstructive pulmonary disease. Ann Intern Med 1989;111:117.

106. Goldstein R, DeRosie J, Long S, Dolmage T, Avendano MA. Applicability of a threshold loading device for inspiratory muscle testing and training in patients with COPD. Chest 1989;96:564.

107. Mahler DA. Therapeutic strategies: In: Mahler DA, ed. Dyspnea. Mt Kisco, NY: Futura Publishing, 1990.

108. Means JH. Dyspnoea. Medicine 1924;3:309.

109. Comroe JH. Summing up. In: Howell JBL, Campbell EJM, eds. Breathlessness. Oxford: Blackwell Publishing, 1966;223.

DAVID M. ORENSTEIN

Rehabilitation for the Pediatric Patient with Pulmonary Disease

Rehabilitation is an idea and a process long applied to pediatric patients with various pulmonary disorders, yet one that has not been explicitly acknowledged until quite recently. It has been said that ". . . rehabilitation is a therapeutic program designed to minimize the consequences of a permanent or protracted disability," and that rehabilitative efforts differ from standard medical care in that standard medical care attempts to reverse the primary disease process, whereas rehabilitation ". . . concentrates on restoring function."[1] Yet, unfortunately, in the world of pediatric pulmonary disorders, it has been true that the "primary disease processes" often have not been amenable to reversal, and so the thrust of therapy has not been cure, but *restoring*—and very importantly—*preserving* function.

In this chapter, I will discuss the most common pediatric pulmonary disorders, in each one beginning with a definition or description of the problem and its clinical course before turning to a review of traditional therapy and a consideration of physical rehabilitation for the disorder. The discussion of physical rehabilitation will include the acute responses to exercise and the role of exercise testing, and then the responses to repeated bouts of exercise (exercise programs) and the role of exercise prescription.

Obstructive pulmonary disorders are considerably more common in childhood than restrictive defects. Therefore, I will begin the chapter with considerations of asthma, the most common chronic childhood condition of any type, and then cystic fibrosis, the most common inherited life-shortening disease. After these conditions, there will be a section on restrictive defects, principally scoliosis and neuromuscular weakness.

ASTHMA

Asthma is the most common chronic disorder in childhood, accounting for more school days lost and more hospital days than any other single condition.[2] Various epidemiologic studies have placed the incidence of asthma between 1% and 20% of all children. The age of onset is most often between 6 months and 3 years.[3] Asthma is characterized by episodes of airways obstruction, produced by bronchospasm, bronchial and bronchiolar inflammation and edema, and mucous hypersecretion. For the child experiencing these events, there is cough, wheezing, shortness of breath, or a combination thereof. In the susceptible airway, different triggers may be responsible for initiating these episodes. The most common triggers are infection, exercise, cold air, inhaled irritants (e.g., cigarette smoke), and allergies.[3]

Exercise-induced asthma occurs to a greater or lesser degree in nearly everyone with asthma and, in some persons, it is the only obvious manifestation of underlying reactive airways. The factors that lead to exercise-induced asthma include those that lead to cooling and drying the airways. These factors, therefore, include large minute ventilation and cold, dry inspired air.[4] Even before the roles of large minute ventilation and airway cooling and drying were recognized, it was known that some forms of exercise were more likely than others to provoke asthma: running, especially in cold weather, being the most probable, followed by bicycling and swimming.[4] Gold medals have been won by asthmatic athletes in swimming in each of the past six Olympic games.

Asthma can be diagnosed by the typical pulmonary function test findings of obstruction in both large and small airways that reverses after the inhalation of a β-agonist bronchodilator. In situations in which pulmonary function testing is impossible (as in a child younger than 7 years or so) or impractical, the history is often strongly suggestive; for example, few other conditions are characterized by the fairly abrupt onset of cough, shortness of breath, or wheezing immediately after exercise, and the spontaneous resolution of the problem after 20 to 60 minutes. Even when the history is less clear, as with the child who coughs with exercise, has a nocturnal cough, or has prolonged cough with upper respiratory infections, but never wheezes, a therapeutic trial of a bronchodilator may confirm the diagnosis.

The course of asthma is variable, ranging from infrequent mild episodes to chronic disabling obstruction.

Traditional Treatment

Although airway obstruction can be reversed, treatment is most appropriately directed at prevention of obstructive episodes. The avoidance of triggers may be useful when the triggers are things such as cigarette smoke, dog dander, or other avoidable inhaled irritants or allergens. Avoidance will not be effective if the trigger is viral upper respiratory infections, although this has not kept families from trying to isolate their children. The result of such attempts is often detrimental psychologically and is never successful virologically. Avoidance of exertion is often employed for the child who has exercise-induced asthma (EIA). This avoidance can be successful in preventing EIA, but since other methods of blocking EIA are available, and restricted activity is detrimental to children's growth and self-esteem, it should be discouraged.

Pharmacologic means are extremely effective in reversing airway obstruction and in preventing that obstruction. Inhaled β_2-adrenergic stimulants, such as albuterol (Ventolin, Proventil), delivered by metered-dose inhaler (MDI) or by air compressor and nebulizer, are probably the first-line treatment and prevention of choice in 1992. The timing of the inhalations will vary depending on the child's pattern of obstruction: for the child who has asthma only after exercise, the inhalations should precede exercise. For the child who wheezes only with upper respiratory infections, inhalations should be given three times a day, starting with the first sneeze or sniffling heralding such an infection. The child whose problems are more chronic or less predictable should probably use his or her inhalers on a regular three-times-a-day basis. Exercise-induced asthma can be blocked in a fairly large proportion of patients by preexercise inhalation of cromolyn sodium.

Corticosteroids can be extremely helpful for the child with severe asthma unresponsive or incompletely responsive to inhaled or oral β-agonists. For treatment of acute episodes, the corticosteroids are usually administered as oral prednisone, given twice daily for less than a week. Alternate-day prednisone is helpful for many children whose asthma is not controlled by β-agonists and cromolyn. Inhaled nonabsorbed steroids, such as beclomethasone or triamcinolone, have recently emerged as an important adjunct in adults with chronic asthma, and they will almost certainly see increased use in children.[5]

The role of theophylline preparations is undergoing reevaluation. These compounds were formerly considered the first-line drugs for treatment and prevention of airway obstruction, at least in the United States. In recent years, however, there is nearly universal agreement that their relatively narrow therapeutic window, compared with other preparations, has made them at best a third- or fourth-line drug in the outpatient management of patients with asthma.

Physical Rehabilitation

General

If rehabilitation is the attempt to restore function, the first goal in the treatment of children with asthma should be to prevent the loss of function in the first place. Although a cure is not possible, prevention of most of the complications, including loss of function, is realistic. To avoid the general loss of fitness seen in many children with asthma,[6] attention should be paid to avoiding episodes of airway obstruction. This can usually be accomplished by careful attention to the child's history of asthmatic episodes and conscientious administration of bronchodilators (β-agonists) and anti-inflammatory agents (cromolyn, inhaled steroids). Patients, families, and school and sports authorities should be educated about the safety of exercise following bronchodilator inhalation, and about the disadvantages of exercise avoidance.

Exercise Testing

Exercise testing can help to confirm the diagnosis of exercise-induced asthma. The typical response will be demonstrable by pulmonary function testing before and at 3-minute intervals after vigorous running (heart rate = 170 beats per minute or more) for 6 to 8 minutes. Expiratory flow rates will fall by 15% to 20% by 10 to 15 minutes postexercise in a positive test, and will usually revert to baseline after 30 to 60 minutes, or much more quickly after inhalation of albuterol.[4] The EIA response is accentuated by the inhalation of cold, dry air and is ablated if the inspired air is warm and saturated with water vapor.[4] In most children, the exercise test is not needed. A child with known asthma who develops cough or dyspnea with exercise can be assumed to have EIA. Only if standard anti-EIA treatment is not successful should it be necessary to seek laboratory confirmation of the diagnosis.

Exercise Program

Many studies have appeared in the literature over the past few decades suggesting the safety and effectiveness of exercise programs for young patients with asthma. Unfortunately, most of these studies have been subjective and have not quantified exercise stimulus or response, either in terms of airways obstruction, physical working capacity, or physiologic measures of cardiopulmonary fitness. More recent studies, however, have corrected this weakness and, indeed, have confirmed the benefits of aerobic exercise programs for youngsters with asthma. Nickerson and colleagues reported on 15 young asthmatic patients who ran 3.2 km 4 days a week for 6 weeks.[7] These patients took their regular asthma medications, but were not pretreated before their running sessions. Despite developing EIA with these runs, the children increased their exercise tolerance (improved performance on a 12-minute run test) and did not change their daily asthma symptoms, peak flowmeter readings, or their likelihood of developing EIA in the laboratory. We reported a similar 4-month study, except our children were pretreated with albuterol before their thrice-weekly running sessions to prevent EIA during the sessions.[6] We also measured peak oxygen consumption on progressive exercise tests to exhaustion and were able to demonstrate improved cardiopulmonary fitness in the exercising patients with asthma. A control group of comparable children with asthma did not increase their peak oxygen consumption when retested after the same 4 months. Most studies show improved exercise tolerance and no worsening of daily asthma symptoms. However, most studies have either failed to demonstrate a beneficial effect of exercise conditioning on the severity of the underlying airway reactivity, or they have employed faulty methods for examining airway reactivity. Several studies have found patients less likely to develop EIA in response to a standard exercise challenge after they have completed an exercise program than they were on entry into the program. In using the same exercise challenge after the patients have become more fit, however, they have inadvertently given the airways a lighter challenge in terms of minute ventilation. Future studies will have to ensure the same pre- and postconditioning minute ventilation, rather than absolute work load employed, to compare exercise challenges before and after any intervention. Haas and colleagues have controlled for this factor, and their data, alone among studies with this control, suggest that conditioning may, in fact, decrease underlying bronchial reactivity to exercise challenge.[8] Until their results are confirmed, it is impossible to draw firm conclusions about the effect of conditioning on airway reactivity, except to say that it is not harmful.

Tales of successful athletes with asthma now grace magazine and television advertisements, giving evidence that the diagnosis does not preclude exercise, even at an elite level. The 597 athletes who made up the United States Olympic team in 1984 included 67 athletes with asthma. They brought home 15 gold, 21 silver, and 5 bronze medals.

Exercise Prescription

The goal for the average child or adolescent will not be Olympic medals, but should be adopting a normal, active life-style. This can and should include vigorous activity, including competitive athletics if the youngster wants this. The physician's job should not have to be to prescribe a specific exercise program, but rather, to help provide guidance for how the child or adolescent can exercise without encountering asthma. *Any* aerobic, anaerobic, or combination program should be attainable by most children with asthma.

Nonpharmacologic means to this end include recommending tactics for warming and humidifying inspired air, such as wearing a scarf wrapped around the mouth and nose during running or skiing in cold, dry climates. Probably because the air around a swimming pool is considerably warmer and more humid than that around a track or skating rink, swimming is known to be less asthmagenic than running; accordingly, for the youngster who has not yet decided on his or her sport, gentle direction toward swimming or away from track or hockey might be helpful. However, if a young athlete has decided on a particularly asthmagenic sport, he or she need not be discouraged, as evidenced by the performances of Bill Koch, an asthmatic athlete who is the first United States cross-country skier to win an Olympic medal, and Evelyn Ashford, a superb track athlete with asthma. One other nonpharmacologic approach is warmup exercise before the main bout of exercise. Various warmup protocols have been shown to block EIA if exercise is repeated within the ensuing hour.[4]

Pharmacologic means offer the most important approach to allowing patients with asthma to enjoy the active life. Inhalation of albuterol 10 to 20 minutes before exercise will be sufficient to prevent EIA for the large proportion of youngsters. Inhaled cromolyn sodium just before exercise also blocks EIA in most asthmatic subjects. For children in whom these tactics do not suffice to block bronchospasm with exercise, the problem is likely to be worse baseline obstruction or reactivity and will often respond to regular (three-times-a-day) albuterol or cromolyn inhalations or both. Some patients will require long-term steroids, either inhaled or—in the unusually recalcitrant case—oral in addition to the pre-exercise β-agonists and cromolyn.

CYSTIC FIBROSIS

Cystic fibrosis (CF) is the most common inherited life-shortening disease among white populations, with an incidence of 1 in every 2500 live births.[9] Since it is inherited as an autosomal recessive disorder, the gene carrier frequency is as high as 1 : 20. The gene has recently been isolated and cloned and is found on the seventh chromosome. The abnormal protein product of the mutant gene appears to be one of the proteins responsible for ion transport across epithelial surfaces.[10] This abnormality would be consistent with the clinical picture, since patients with CF have abnormal exocrine secretions, with abnormal movement of ions and water across epithelia, making the sweat much saltier than normal, blocking pancreatic ductules, and blocking bronchioles and bronchi leading to a vicious circle of bronchial obstruction, infection, and worsened obstruction. The pancreatic blockage produces pancreatic insufficiency, with malabsorption of fat and proteins, and leads to poor nutrition and growth, often despite a voracious appetite. It is the pulmonary problem that has the most profound influence on morbidity and mortality, with the bronchial obstruction and infection progressing to destruction of the bronchial wall (bronchiectasis) and progressive replacement of pulmonary tissue by fibrosis. The prognosis for patients with CF has improved dramatically in just a few decades. In 1938, when the disease was first recognized by Dr. Dorothy Anderson, life expectancy was a dismal 2 years or less. In 1990, the median age at death was 28 years.[11] This improved outlook can be attributed to several factors, including wider recognition and earlier diagnosis, but especially comprehensive treatment programs.

Traditional Treatment

Comprehensive treatment programs have grown around the 120 Cystic Fibrosis Foundation-approved CF centers around the country. These programs have three main thrusts: pulmonary, pancreatic and nutritional, and psychological.

Pulmonary

The goals of the pulmonary treatment are to treat, or preferably to prevent, the bronchiolar and bronchial obstruction and infection. Methods to minimize obstruction are based on the assumption that obstruction is caused by abnormal secretions that interfere with normal mucociliary clearance mechanisms, infection, bronchospasm, or inflammation and mucosal edema. The abnormally viscous mucus is dealt with by "the ketchup bottle method," namely, chest physical therapy and postural drainage, through which techniques the patient is positioned with the bronchus draining a pulmonary segment pointing downward as the chest is manually clapped above that segment. The idea is to shake the mucus loose with the aid of gravity, so that it can fall into the large central airways, where cough can take over to expel the mucus. The technique, crude though it may be, works.[12,13] Two Canadian studies have shown convincing evidence that patients who perform chest physical therapy do better, both over a 3-week period[12] and a 3-year span.[13]

The role of exercise in promoting mucus clearance is controversial, and will be discussed later.

Infection is treated aggressively with antibiotics, ideally based on recent cultures of respiratory tract secretions. Antibiotics can be given by mouth, by vein, or by inhalation. Some centers employ constant antibiotics, whereas others choose to treat only when there is evidence of increased infection ("pulmonary exacerbations"). It is not yet clear which approach is better.

Bronchospasm is treated with inhaled bronchodilators. Evidence for bronchospasm is clear in some patients, but unclear or absent in others. Furthermore, bronchodilators cause worsened expiratory airflows in a few CF patients, probably because increased bronchomotor tone is required to maintain airway patency in these damaged bronchi, and relaxation of the bronchial smooth muscle takes away that needed support.[14] Nonetheless, some centers prescribe inhaled β-agonists for all their patients, whereas others seldom use these drugs. Even in the absence of clear benefit from bronchial smooth-muscle relaxation, these agents may be helpful by increasing mucociliary transport rates[15] or improving ventilatory muscle contractility.[16]

Inflammation is treated with corticosteroids, especially alternate-day prednisone, in many patients. This treatment has become more common since a 4-year double-blind study from Boston suggested a beneficial role for alternate-day prednisone in terms of improved pulmonary function and growth, and fewer hospitalizations, compared with placebo.[17] Multicenter studies are currently underway to attempt to confirm and refine those results, and to examine the effects of nonsteroidal anti-inflammatory agents.

Nutritional

Nutritional treatment is essential in most patients with CF. Fortunately, this is moderately straightforward, with effective pancreatic enzyme supplements available. In general, several capsules of these enzyme supplements taken with each meal come close enough to correcting digestion and absorption that patients can grow normally. Many patients with CF have not grown well in the past, in part because of their pancreatic insufficiency and, in part, because of what was probably misguided advice to take a low-fat diet. Low fat means low calories, and patients have suffered the consequences, including poor growth and self-esteem, with probably weaker ventilatory muscles and impaired immune mechanisms. Unfortunately, some patients still suffer from undernutrition, despite proper dietary advice and enzyme supplementation. These patients simply cannot take in the increased number of calories dictated by their greater caloric expenditure from ventilatory work, cough, chronic infection, and perhaps a higher cellular metabolic rate.[18] In these few patients, aggressive nutritional rehabilitation is being employed, with nighttime feeding through a gastrostomy, nasogastric, or jejunostomy tube, with good results.[19]

Psychologic aspects of having an inherited, life-shortening disease that may limit exercise tolerance and employability cannot be overlooked. Treating children normally as they grow, including allowing a full active schedule, probably helps the child grow up with good self-esteem. It actually is very impressive how low the rate of depression is in groups of children with CF who were followed in a major CF center.[20] Psychologic support services should be available at most CF centers.

Physical Rehabilitation and Exercise

General

As with asthma, a cure is not yet possible for someone with CF, yet many steps are effective in preventing or delaying the loss of function. For patients with CF, scrupulous attention to pulmonary toilet, with regular postural drainage and aggressive treatment of episodes of increased pulmonary infection and inflammation are essential, and are largely successful in preserving pulmonary function for long periods. Even more than with asthma, preventive care is crucial, since each inadequately treated pulmonary exacerbation probably leads to the formation of just a bit more fibrous tissue. Once scar tissue has formed, it is irreversible. Optimal nutritional treatment with pancreatic enzymes, dietary supplements, and even nocturnal tube feeding where indicated will help the pulmonary treatment succeed.

Exercise Testing

Exercise testing can give useful information in patients with cystic fibrosis. In general, CF patients have reduced exercise tolerance (both in terms of work load achievable on a maximal test and in terms of maximal oxygen consumption), the reduction being proportional to their impairment in pulmonary function (Fig. 27–1). Despite this general correlation between pulmonary function and exercise tolerance, resting pulmonary function tests are not particularly useful for predicting exercise tolerance in the individual patient, since there is such scatter (Fig. 27–2). Although the pulmonary function test at a single time point cannot predict exercise tolerance in an individual patient, changes in an individual's pulmonary status will influence his or

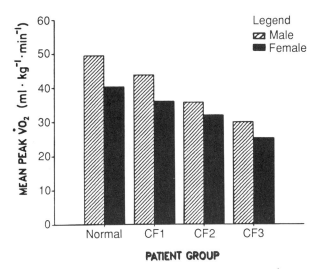

FIGURE 27-1 Mean peak oxygen uptake (ml kg^{-1} min^{-1}) for 56 male and 51 female healthy control subjects, and for 57 male and 52 female CF patients categorized into three groups by degree of pulmonary obstruction: *CF1,* mild obstruction (FEV$_1$ ≥ 70% FVC); *CF2,* moderate obstruction (FEV$_1$ = 50 to 69% FVC); and *CF3,* severe obstruction (FEV$_1$ < 50% FVC). (Orenstein DM, Nixon PA. Patients with cystic fibrosis. In: Franklin BA, Gordon S, Timmis GC, eds. Exercise in modern medicine. Baltimore: Williams & Wilkins, 1988, with permission)

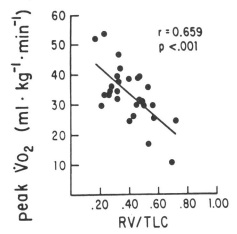

FIGURE 27-2 Peak oxygen uptake ($\dot{V}O_2$) in ml kg^{-1} min^{-1} plotted against residual volume (*RV*)/total lung capacity (*TLC*) for 28 patients. (Orenstein DM, Nixon PA. Patients with cystic fibrosis. In: Franklin BA, Gordon S, Timmis MD, eds. Exercise in modern medicine. Baltimore: Williams & Wilkins, 1988, with permission)

her response to exercise: Cerny and colleagues clearly showed that patients hospitalized for intensive treatment of a pulmonary exacerbation improved their exercise tolerance as they improved lung function.[21]

Most patients with CF, regardless of baseline pulmonary function, maintain gas exchange at their baseline levels during even very vigorous exercise.[22] Exercise desaturation is very unusual if the resting 1-second forced expiratory volume (FEV_1) is above 50% of forced vital capacity (FVC). Of those with FEV_1/FVC less than 50%, most will also maintain their oxygenation, but some will desaturate, and the exercise test is the only tool that can identify which of these severely affected patients will have worsened oxygenation during exertion.[22] Most authorities now recommend exercise testing with oxyhemoglobin saturation monitoring of those patients with resting FEV_1/FVC ratio less than 50% before these patients undertake regular exercise.

Exercise Program

Numerous reports have appeared over the past decade concerning the results of exercise programs for patients with cystic fibrosis. It seems clear that a regular aerobic exercise program, such as jogging[23] or swimming[24] can increase exercise tolerance in patients with CF. The effects of such programs on mucus clearance and resting pulmonary function are less clear. Zach and his Austrian colleagues have reported increased volumes of expectorated mucus with a vigorous 17-day exercise program compared with traditional chest physical therapy[25] and similar results with a 7-week swimming program.[26] In both of these studies, there was also improvement in expiratory airflows during the exercise programs. In contrast, the previously cited studies showed no change in resting pulmonary function. No studies have suggested any worsening in pulmonary function, but the final answer is not yet in on whether exercise programs can increase mucus clearance and improve—or delay the expected deterioration in—pulmonary function, and improve survival in CF.

Exercise Prescription

As with asthma, the most important thing the physician can do vis-a-vis exercise prescription is to remove the *proscription* that has sometimes greeted exercise programs for CF patients. Patients, of all disease severities, should probably be encouraged to adopt a normal active life-style. The best kind of exercise for patients with CF has not yet been determined and is likely not to be identified for some time to come. Despite the burgeoning numbers of studies related to CF exercise programs, few programs have extended beyond 3 or 4 months, and none have compared various programs. Is 30 minutes of jogging three times a week better than more minutes of less intense exercise? For the patient who desaturates during exercise, what is the role of oxygen supplementation? One study has demonstrated that supplemental oxygen will prevent desaturation,[27] yet it is not clear what the long-term effects of oxygen-assisted exercise will be.

Despite these uncertainties, there are some things that can be said about exercise prescriptions for CF patients. Exercise in the heat represents a greater challenge for patients with CF than their healthy peers because of the sweat defect. During 90 minutes of heat chamber exposure and exercise, CF patients lost significantly more sodium and chloride than non-CF controls, a loss that resulted in significant decreases in serum concentrations of these ions in the CF patients.[28] Therefore, patients must be warned to be careful to replace fluids assiduously.

Salt replacement is probably not required during exercise sessions lasting up to 90 minutes in the heat, since patients who ate and drank ad lib were able to replenish electrolytes by 22 hours after exercise and heat stress.[29] It is worth noting that this study was conducted during cool weather, and, after the 90 minutes in the heat chamber, the subjects were not exposed to high ambient temperatures until the next day. There have been no published studies of CF patients' response to repeated bouts of exercise and heat stress in a hot environment.

Further guidance would include the admonition to gym teachers, coaches, and such, not to restrict CF patients because of coughing and not to be alarmed by the hard coughing spells that often accompany vigorous exercise in CF patients. Not only are these coughing spells not dangerous (although they certainly can be tiring and stressful), they are probably helpful in mobilizing mucus.

It is currently the policy at our center to urge youngsters with CF to perform their usual chest physical therapy and postural drainage in addition to their exercise, but we recognize that patients and families often substitute sports participation for the less enjoyable traditional treatments, and we generally do not insist on absolute adherence to our official policy if the child is doing well.

In summary, although the best form of exercise for patients with CF is as yet unknown, aerobic exercise programs can clearly increase cardiopulmonary fitness and exercise tolerance in these patients, while either improving or not affecting pulmonary function. The effect on survival is unknown. Patients with CF when exercising in the heat will lose more sodium and chloride than healthy peers.

RESTRICTIVE PULMONARY DISORDERS

Scoliosis

Scoliosis, which is a lateral curvature of the spine, can be caused by many underlying disorders, including neuromuscular weakness, connective tissue disorders, and various pleuropulmonary processes (including pneumonectomy and empyema). Many cases are congenital and are associated with bone deformities such as hemivertebrae, but the largest numbers of cases are idiopathic. Mild scoliosis has very little cardiopulmonary effect. However, advanced scoliosis can have a profound effect, causing severe pulmonary restriction, with low vital capacity and total lung capacity, resulting in dyspnea on exertion and eventual respiratory failure and death.[30]

Traditional Treatment

In most cases of mild scoliosis, no treatment is needed. In more advanced cases, casting or bracing may be employed and will probably help prevent the progression of idiopathic scoliosis. However, external support, especially casts, may restrict chest wall excursion further, and temporarily add to the ventilatory defect. Severe cases, especially those associated with neuromuscular weakness, may require surgery for internal fixation with Harrington or Luque rods.[30]

Physical Rehabilitation

EXERCISE Exercise intolerance is generally found in patients with moderate to severe scoliosis, in proportion to the ventilatory defect.[30] The intolerance to exercise often is accentuated by underactivity and detraining.[31] Patients also have a relatively high oxygen consumption during submaximal walking,[32] likely an effect of mechanical inefficiency as well as increased oxygen cost of breathing itself.[31] Changes in exercise tolerance with bracing or spinal fusion have been minimal.[31]

EXERCISE PRESCRIPTION There have not been many studies of the effects of exercise programs for patients with idiopathic scoliosis, but there is some suggestion that exercise programs may be beneficial, both in strengthening the trunk muscles, thereby slowing the progression of the scoliosis itself, and in improving maximal aerobic power.[31]

Neuromuscular Disease

Duchenne muscular dystrophy (DMD) is the most common of the severe neurologic or muscular disorders causing a restrictive pulmonary defect in children. It is an X-linked genetic problem, affecting only boys. It results in a progressive weakness of skeletal muscles, beginning with proximal limb muscles. It is first noted sometime before the age of 5, with the youngster having difficulty getting up from the floor. He usually has to "cheat," by using his hands and "walking" them up his thighs until he has pushed himself upright (the Gower maneuver). The weakness progresses, and nearly always renders DMD patients unable to walk by age 10 or 12 years. The ventilatory muscles are almost always affected, with the interesting exception of the diaphragm, which is often spared until very late in the course of the disease. Because the peripheral muscles fail before the ventilatory muscles, dyspnea on exertion is rare,[30,p164] since the child cannot perform enough exercise to outstrip his ventilatory capacity. Respiratory failure usually occurs during the teenage years. Death is caused directly or indirectly by the weakness of the ventilatory muscles in most cases, with ventilatory failure or progressive infection or atelectasis related to ineffective cough. Since the dystrophy may involve the myocardium, some patients die of cardiac failure before their ventilatory muscles fail.

Traditional Treatment

Unfortunately, there is no effective treatment for the progressive muscular weakness. In recent years, more and more patients have been given mechanical ventilatory support, with negative-pressure (usually nighttime) ventilation, as with an iron lung or cuirass ventilator, or with a tracheostomy and intermittent positive-pressure ventilation. Mechanical ventilation may permit survival for years after the onset of ventilatory failure. The ethical and emotional considerations in deciding for or against such support are daunting.

Physical Rehabilitation

EXERCISE Exercise tolerance is very low in patients with DMD, from age 5 or so onward. Exercise testing is not easily accomplished because of the profound weakness. By the time most boys with muscular dystrophy are old enough to understand and cooperate with testing procedures, they are too weak to walk on a treadmill or even support themselves on a cycle ergometer. Even supine exercise is difficult, because the hip internal rotators are so weak that the knees tend to fall outward, making pedaling impossible.[33] Eventually, most patients are unable to perform *any* voluntary muscular activity, even to turn their head to one side for greater comfort. Scratching an itchy nose cannot be done without help.

EXERCISE PRESCRIPTION For years the role of activity in the progression of muscular weakness has been controversial in DMD. Some clinicians felt that exercise hastened the decline, whereas others pointed to the rapid progression in weakness that invariably occurs after the boys become wheelchair-bound as evidence that inactivity led to worse weakness. Few studies have been conducted, but there is some evidence that exercise programs may be able to improve the endurance of ventilatory muscles[30,p289] or of some skeletal muscle (in one study, the muscles of mastication).[34] It seems at this time that there is no reason to prohibit exercise. Further work will need to be done before the role of exercise programs can be defined.

REFERENCES

1. Perry J. Rehabilitation: a definition. In: Nickel VL, ed. Orthopedic rehabilitation. New York: Churchill-Livingstone, 1982:xi.

2. U.S. Department of Health, Education, and Welfare. Illness among children. Children's Bureau Publication no. 405, quoted in Dees SC. Asthma. In: Kendig EL Jr, Chernick V, eds. Disorders of the respiratory tract in children, 3rd ed. Philadelphia: WB Saunders, 1977:623.

3. Phelan PD, Landau LI, Olinsky A. Respiratory illness in children. Oxford: Blackwell Scientific 1982:132.

4. Lemanske RF Jr, Henke KG. Exercise-induced asthma. In: Gisolfi CV, Lamb DR, eds. Perspectives in exercise science and sports medicine, vol 2, Youth, exercise, and sport. Indianapolis: Benchmark Press, 1989.

5. Barnes PJ. A new approach to the treatment of asthma. N Engl J Med 1989;321:1517.

6. Orenstein DM, Reed ME, Grogan FT, Crawford LV. Exercise conditioning in children with asthma. J Pediatr 1985;106:556.

7. Nickerson BG, Bautista DB, Namey MA, et al. Distance running improves fitness in asthmatic children without pulmonary complications or changes in exercise-induced bronchospasm. Pediatrics 1983;71:147.

8. Haas F, Pasierski S, Levine N, et al. Effect of aerobic training on forced expiratory airflow in exercising asthmatic humans. J Appl Physiol 1987;63:1230.

9. Boat TF, Welsh MJ, Beaudet AL, Sly WS, Valle D, eds. The metabolic basis of inherited disease. New York: McGraw-Hill, 1989.

10. Riordan JR, Rommens JM, Kerem B-S, et al. Identification of the cystic fibrosis gene: cloning and characterization of complementary DNA. Science 1989;245:1066.

11. FitzSimmons SC. Patient Registry 1990 Annual Data Report. Cystic Fibrosis Foundation 1992. 6931 Arlington Road, Bethesda, MD 20814.

12. Desmond KJ, Schwenk WF, Thomas E, Beaudry PH, Coates AL. Immediate and long-term effects of chest physiotherapy in patients with cystic fibrosis. J Pediatr 1983;103:538.

13. Reisman JJ, Rivington-Law B, Corey M, et al. Role of conventional physiotherapy in cystic fibrosis. J Pediatr 1988;113:632.

14. Landau LI, Phelan PD. The variable effect of a bronchodilating agent on pulmonary function in cystic fibrosis. J Pediatr 1973:82:863.

15. Wood RE, Wanner A, Hirsch J, Farrell PM. Tracheal mucociliary transport in patients with cystic fibrosis and its stimulation by terbutaline. Am Rev Respir Dis 1975;111:733.

16. Howell S, Roussos C. Isoproterenol and aminophylline improve contractility of fatigued canine diaphragm. Am Rev Respir Dis 1984;129:118.

17. Auerbach HS, Kirkpatrick, Williams M, Colten HR. Alternate-day prednisone reduces morbidity and improves pulmonary function in cystic fibrosis. Lancet 1985;2:686.

18. Shepherd RW, Vasques-Velasquez L, Prentice A, Holt TL, Coward WA, Lucas A. Increased energy expenditure in young children with cystic fibrosis. Lancet 1988;2:1300.

19. Shepherd RW, Holt TL, Thomas BJ, et al. Nutritional rehabilitation in cystic fibrosis: controlled studies of effects on nutritional growth retardation, body protein turnover, and course of pulmonary disease. J Pediatr 1986;109:788.

20. Burke P, Meyer V, Kocoshis S, et al. Depression and anxiety in pediatric inflammatory bowel disease and cystic fibrosis. J Am Acad Child Adolesc Psychiatry 1989;28:948.

21. Cerny FJ, Cropp GJA, Bye MR. Hospital therapy improves exercise tolerance and lung function in cystic fibrosis. Am J Dis Child 1984;138:261.

22. Henke KG, Orenstein DM. Oxygen saturation during exercise in cystic fibrosis. Am Rev Respir Dis 1984;129:708.

23. Orenstein DM, Franklin BA, Doershuk CF, et al. Exercise conditioning and cardiopulmonary fitness in cystic fibrosis: the effects of a three-month supervised running program. Chest 1981;80:392.

24. Edlund LD, French RW, Herbst JJ, et al. Effects of a swimming program on children with cystic fibrosis. Am J Dis Child 1986;140:80.

25. Zach M, Oberwaldner B, Hausler F. Cystic fibrosis: physical exercise versus chest physiotherapy. Arch Dis Child 1982;57:587.

26. Zach MS, Purrer B, Oberwaldner B. Effect of swimming on forced expiration and sputum clearance in cystic fibrosis. Lancet 1981;2:1201.

27. Nixon PA, Orenstein DM, Ross EA, Curtis S. Oxygen supplementation during exercise in cystic fibrosis. Am Rev Respir Dis 1990;142:807.

28. Orenstein DM, Henke KG, Costill DL, Doershuk CF, Lemon PJ, Stern RC. Exercise and heat stress in cystic fibrosis patients. Pediatr Res 1983;17:267.

29. Orenstein DM, Henke KG, Green CG. Heat acclimation in cystic fibrosis. J Appl Physiol 1984;57:408.

30. Shneerson J. Disorders of ventilation. Oxford: Blackwell Scientific, 1988:202.

31. Bar-Or O. Pediatric sports medicine for the practitioner. New York: Springer-Verlag. 1983:243.

32. Lindh M. Energy expenditure during walking in patients with scoliosis. The effect of surgical correction. Spine 1978;3:122.

33. Nixon PA, Orenstein DM. Exercise testing in children. Pediatr Pulmonol 1988;5:107.

34. Kawazoe Y, Kobayashi M, Tasaka T, Tamamoto M. Effects of therapeutic exercise on masticatory function in patients with progressive muscular dystrophy. J Neurol Neurosurg Psychiatr 1982;45:343.

GERILYNN L. CONNORS

SHARON SHNELL-HOBBS

WILLIAM A. SYVERTSEN

Marketing the Pulmonary Rehabilitation Program

Consider the following case study. A Pulmonary Rehabilitation Program (PRP) was developed 8 years ago in an urban 250-bed medical center that had strong physician and community support. Within the last 9 months, a significant decline in patient admissions to the program was noted. The PRP medical director and program coordinator cited factors that could be affecting program admissions, such as a turnover in the medical staff at the facility—resulting in caregivers not being aware of the existence of a PRP or how it could benefit their patients; the spiraling cost of health care, with patients shopping around for the best deal; the opening of a rehabilitation hospital offering inpatient pulmonary rehabilitation; and a new outpatient pulmonary rehabilitation program started in a Comprehensive Outpatient Rehabilitation Facility (CORF), both within a 15-mile radius from their facility. This PRP is facing a classic marketing problem of maintaining a balance between the supply and demand for their services.

Developing PRP awareness through a strategic marketing process is crucial for program success. Physicians, allied health professionals, prospective patients, third-party payers, and the public need to be educated about the mission, goals, objectives, and benefits of a PRP. This chapter will provide the pulmonary rehabilitation expert with the basic concepts needed to employ marketing to its fullest potential for program success. In addition, it will also address several marketing misconceptions.

THE ROLE AND ETHICS OF MARKETING IN HEALTH CARE

The business world has employed the concepts of marketing since the mid-1950s to ensure success.[1,2] Nonprofit organizations first started using marketing between 1969 and 1973.[3] Hospitals initially started using marketing to lure and influence doctors by running advertisements and promotion campaigns to build and promote the image of the hospital.[3] However, it was not until the mid-1980s that hospitals finally understood the true essence of marketing, which came as a result of Diagnosis-Related Groups (DRGs), declining revenues, and greater competition for the same patient. Marketing was no longer viewed as just advertising or a peripheral activity carried out by a specific department in a Health Care Facility (HCF). Marketing became an organized effort directed at attaining the mission of the HCF to effectively serve various areas of human need.

The negative stigma of marketing in the health care arena was strong in the early days. The critics saw marketing as undesirable, unnecessary, a waste of public money, intrusive, manipulative, demeaning, and unethical.[3] This is not surprising since the critics compared marketing with television commercials, "junk mail," newspaper advertisements, pushy sales calls, and mass retailing. These views were misguided, but believed by a variety of people with their own opinions and beliefs. Today, the ethical concerns of health care marketing include inappropriate competition in an area that allows for little or no price shopping; creation of an artificial stimulation of demand targeting only specific markets, therefore, denying the same services to other needy groups; and adding the cost of marketing to the already spiraling cost of health care.[4]

Most of the "unethical" concerns about marketing really focus solely on advertising and promotion, which is only one element of marketing.[4] There are established guidelines for ethics in advertising. The Federal Trade Commission (FTC) prohibits unfair or deceptive advertising, but most HCF advertising is not on a national scale to warrant FTC investigation. In the past, licensed professionals were often prohibited from advertising for clients based upon their code of ethics. However, in the late 1970s, the Supreme Court struck down this ban against advertising stating that bans reduced competition. The American Hospital Association (AHA) published guidelines for hospital advertising in 1977, emphasizing that "the contents of hospital advertising must be measured primarily by the criteria of truth and accuracy."[4]

The American Marketing Association also has a code of ethics for advertising, but as codes go, they are only guides and not enforceable. However, the American Medical Association (AMA) and the Public Relations Society of America (PRSA) have codes of ethics that provide for discipline of individual members if ethics are breached. The AMA may enforce the AMA code by suspending or revoking a violator's membership, and the PRSA bylaws include a detailed mechanism for sanctions against violators. However, the codes apply only to individuals and do not apply to the employer organization. Notably, many physicians and marketing professionals are not members of their respective organizations.

The ultimate goal of a PRP is patient satisfaction. Marketing can help one attain this goal. Advertising, public relations, promotional literature, communications, and academia in and by themselves do not constitute marketing. Marketing is a process of combining business functions with business objectives and is the result of all these factors.[5] Understanding the marketing process allows the employment of marketing to its fullest extent.[6] Marketing strategy, if used and applied properly, can benefit patients and enable a pulmonary rehabilitation program to prosper. This prosperity will, in large part, be due to the development of competitive goals in the areas of patient–consumer needs, efficiency of patient care, education, and cost-effectiveness.[7]

A survey of 3000 consumers from six metropolitan areas in Tennessee confirmed that marketing and, in fact, the advertising component do have a well-defined place in the health care arena.[8] Nonprofit marketing has attained maturity and respect in its "life cycle," as evidenced by the vast array of textbooks and journals addressing the subject.[3] But the basis of all marketing is "truth telling" which is found in the mission statement of the HCF.[4]

MARKETING AND ITS BASIC CONCEPTS

Patients are the consumers in the health care community, actively making choices about their health care and treatment. One must listen to their perceived needs and wants. It is crucial to tailor the program to patients' needs.[9-11] To accomplish this, one must understand the basic concepts of marketing.

Philip Kotler, a leading author in nonprofit marketing, developed a comprehensive definition of *marketing* as follows:[1,2]

> Marketing is the analysis, planning, implementation, and control of carefully formulated exchanges of values with target markets for the purpose of achieving organizational objectives. It relies heavily on designing the organizational's offering in terms of the target markets' needs and desires, and on using effective pricing, communication, and distribution to inform, motivate, and service markets.

The American Marketing Association approved a new definition of marketing in 1985 as follows:[12]

> Marketing is the process of planning and executing the conception, pricing, promotion, and distribution of ideas, goods, and services to create exchanges that satisfy the individual and organizational objectives.

The planning of health services often begins within a health care facility and reaches out to the consumer. The marketing objective is to begin with the consumer to plan health care.[10,13]

Basic marketing concepts must be understood in relation to their application in the pulmonary rehabilitation program setting. Patients, physicians, and third-party payers are consumers in the health care industry, therefore being the potential users of pulmonary rehabilitation. Patients and third-party payers are also the buyers of this health care, being essential components of the marketing picture. Although patients are the main consumers of pulmonary rehabilitation, they most likely will not enter a program without the support of their private physicians or approval (prior authorization) from their insurance. Health care professionals are then, in marketing terms, considered the sellers, deliverers, and providers of health care. Figure 28–1 outlines the marketing terms of pulmonary rehabilitation. The emphasis of marketing is on the user's needs and desires, not on the seller's wants and desires. Health care must be oriented toward the users.[13]

Understanding consumer behavior is vital in identifying the benefits that patient, physician, and third-party payer can expect from a PRP.[9,14] This concept follows that of the supply-and-demand curve of economics. If the patient, physician, and third-party payer demands are increased, then supply must increase to meet the needs of those markets. The patient often equates needs with basic medical care requirements. It is at this elementary stage of health care that the ideals of the patient–consumer and those of the health professional–provider become divided. The health provider is

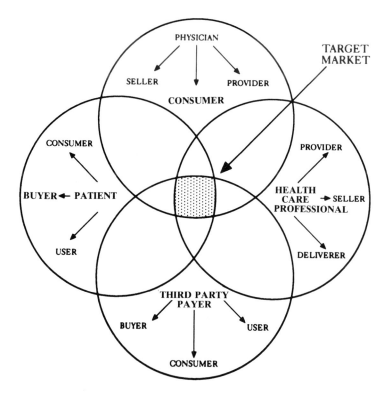

FIGURE 28-1   There are specific marketing terms PRPs must become familiar with. Understanding the basic concepts of marketing and how it relates to the patient, physician, health care professional, and third-party payer will allow the pulmonary rehabilitation team to effectively target the appropriate markets and meet the user's needs and desires.

often technically oriented, whereas the consumer's emphasis is on nontechnical components such as the environment. This nontechnical emphasis then represents benefits to the consumer. In an age when consumers are shopping around for the best health care at the best price, marketing is an essential management component.[13]

DEVELOPING AN EFFECTIVE, STRATEGIC MARKETING PLAN

The initial step in developing an effective pulmonary rehabilitation marketing plan is determining the program's mission, goals, and objectives.[15] The mission statement does not redefine pulmonary rehabilitation, but should explain the overall direction of the PRP and what it is trying to accomplish. Mission statements explain the emphasis or orientation of the PRP, rather than delineating the desired outcomes. Writing a program mission statement will guide the prioritization of activities.

Once the mission statement is written, program goals are determined. The goals are broad statements of intent that the PRP will emphasize, such as market share, profitability, and reputation. These goals must be directly related to the mission of the program. The PRP will generally have a broad goal (see the American Thoracic Society statement defining Pulmonary Rehabilitation in Chapter 1). Specific short- and long-term goals may also be defined by the rehabilitation team members. Listing goals will allow one to note accomplishments, define problems, and direct program planning. Goals should be realistic and attainable, taking into account environmental opportunities and constraints. Involving the entire team in developing the goals aids in acquiring a commitment from each team member to reach the goals developed.

The program goals must then be restated in the form of objectives. Objectives are measurable, allowing for the planning, implementation, and evaluation of the program. These objectives may be stated in terms of the customer–patient, the program, and outcomes. The team needs to consistently evaluate their success or failure in reaching the stated goals and objectives. Marketing must be carried out by everyone on the team, not just by the program director.

An analysis of both the internal components (a program's strengths and weaknesses) and the external components (opportunities and threats) is necessary in managing a program. The SWOT analysis focuses on the Strengths, Weaknesses, Opportunities, and Threats as it relates to a situational analysis in a pulmonary rehabilitation program.[15] A program must analyze the threats and opportunities it is exposed to in the external environment.

This external environment is constantly changing and consists of four components: the public environment, the competitive environment, the macroenvironment, and the market environment. A description of each environment follows.

The Public Environment

A pulmonary rehabilitation program has ongoing relations with many individuals who are considered "publics."[1,9,16] Kotler defines a *public* as a ". . . distinct group of people or organizations or both whose actual or potential needs must in some sense be served."[3] It is important to understand the exchanges of ideas between the program and each of these public groups, the motivation and strategy underlying these transactions, and the types of satisfactions received by these publics. One must examine these publics to understand their perceptions, needs, and function. Figure 28–2 shows the essential publics with whom a pulmonary rehabilitation program must deal to be successful.

A classification of the publics of pulmonary rehabilitation can be achieved by evaluating the functions and levels of involvement each public has relative to the rehabilitation program.[1] There are internal publics, consisting of the pulmonary rehabilitation team depicted in Figure 28–3, and input publics such as suppliers, donors, and regulatory agencies who may have a direct effect on the internal publics. The seller (distributor) of the program may be intermediary publics consisting of merchants, agents, facilitators, and marketing firms, or the internal publics may act directly with the consuming public–client to advertise the pulmonary rehabilitation program. This consuming public can further be divided into client, general publics, local publics, activist publics, and media publics. Figure 28–4 outlines the classification of the many publics of pulmonary rehabilitation.

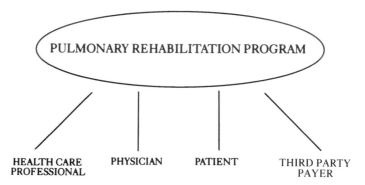

FIGURE   28-2   The essential publics of a PRP are the patient, physician, health care professional, and third-party payer. The success of a pulmonary rehabilitation program depends on the program's relation with and understanding of its essential publics' perception, needs, and functions.

The functions and relations of each public to the PRP may vary. Not every public described may be active or important to the program, but a determination of all publics' relations must be made. Figure 28–5 diagrams the many publics of pulmonary rehabilitation. Those publics whose relations are determined to be important are markets and must be cultivated further. Each public is interrelated. The task of the rehabilitation team is to identify those valued publics, and these publics then become target markets toward which market planning, communication, and implementation

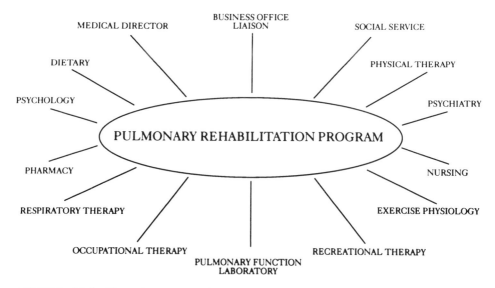

FIGURE   28-3   The pulmonary rehabilitation team makes up the internal publics of pulmonary rehabilitation. An understanding of these internal publics, their function and level of involvement with the program is essential.

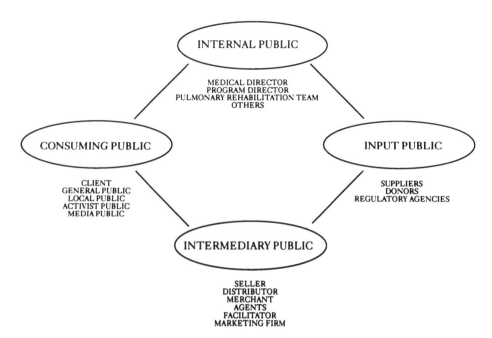

FIGURE   28-4   The classification of the many publics of pulmonary rehabilitation fall into the following categories: internal, input, intermediary, and consuming publics. The many publics of a pulmonary rehabilitation program have varying degrees of function and level of involvement with the program. Not every public may be important, but a determination of which public is important and valued is needed to determine the program's target markets.

are directed. Kotler defines a *market* as the ". . . set of all people who have an actual or potential interest in an exchange and the ability to complete it."[3] The marketing concept is based on the theory of exchanges, which requires two parties to be present, with each party having something valued by the other.[1,2] The PRP exchanges services with the rehabilitation candidates and significant publics. Each target market has needs, desires, perceptions, and satisfactions that the marketer needs to understand.[14] One must evaluate the current and future needs of these customers. Understanding the values of the PRP's markets so that an exchange can occur is what marketing is all about.

The Competitive Environment

The existence of a PRP at a nearby hospital, a competitor, is an important environmental factor to consider. If there are established rehabilitation programs in the community, one must give considerable thought and research toward the need for another program. By evaluating potential competitors during the development of a PRP, one may save the program from disaster and help ensure the likelihood of its success.

Know your competitors. Before you can write an effective marketing plan, you

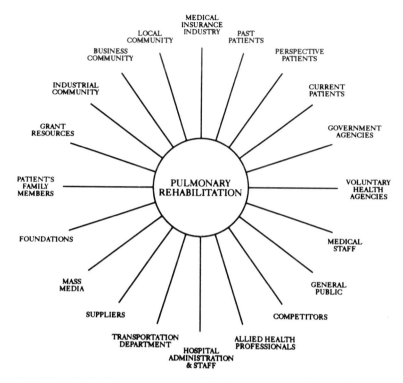

FIGURE   28-5   There are many publics that can have a direct influence on the pulmonary rehabilitation program. It is the responsibility of the program to determine its valued publics. The valued publics then become the target markets to which an exchange of services occurs.

must know who you are up against: the competitor's name, services provided, strengths and weaknesses of the program, the HCF, and past history of the competitor. Remember, you may not always know every competitor, but anyone who can provide the same program benefits to *your* customer is the competition.

For PRP success, three basic questions need to be asked:

1. What business or program are you really in?
2. What is the value of the service the program provides?
3. How different are you from your competition?

This competitive environment can be divided into desire competitors, generic competitors, service form competitors, and enterprise competitors.

In fact, a PRP may face any or all of these major types of competitors in trying to serve their target market. The desire competitors are the patient–target markets' "other" immediate desires. The generic competitors are "other" basic ways in which the patient–target markets may satisfy a specific desire. The service form competitors are other service forms that may satisfy the patient–target market's specific desire. The enterprise competitors are other enterprises offering the same program that can

TABLE 28-1. Example of the Types of Competitors Facing a PRP

Desire Competitors	Generic Competitors	Form Competitors	Enterprise Competitors
Patient asks:			
What desire do I want to satisfy?	How do I want to get a comprehensive program for my lungs?	What form of PRP do I want to go to?	Which outpatient program do I want?
Thorough medical evaluation only	From reading Watching videos	Doctor office Outpatient hospital program	St. John's Hospital Good Sam's Medical Center
Vacation/cruise	Attending BB Club of ALA	CORF	
Comprehensive program for lungs	Go to PRP	Inpatient program Live-in outpatient program	

(Adapted from Kotler P, Andreasen RN. Marketing for health care organizations. Englewood Cliffs, NJ: Prentice-Hall, 1987)

satisfy the patient–target market's specific desire. Table 28–1 is an example of the types of competitors facing a PRP.

By evaluating the different forms of competition, the program team can determine if the program is an effective competitor, and whether the program's strategy must be modified to make it an effective competitor.

The Macroenvironment

The *macroenvironment* looks at the forces creating the environment in which a PRP must operate. This term is defined by Kotler as ". . . the major forces and institutions surrounding and affecting the organization, its markets, and competitors."[1,2] Five main forces of the macroenvironment have been identified: demography, economy, technology, political–legal, and social–cultural. Evaluating the demographic factor includes an assessment of the age and size of the population to be served by the PRP. If the program is located near a retirement center, the emphasis would be directed toward adults, rather than toward children. Trends in birth and death rates also need to be assessed. The cost of the PRP, how much the patient has to pay, and the cost to third-party payers are important environmental factors to consider. What effect will changing medical technology have on the program? Are there governmental agencies or pending legislation that could have a significant bearing on pulmonary rehabilitation programs? And last, cultural developments—values, life-styles, beliefs, and behavioral patterns—need to be assessed to get a total picture of the macroenvironmental factors that affect the market. The macroenvironmental forces are detailed in many publications that look at future trends. Sociology and epidemiology can also help clarify these areas. The main point is to know that macroenvironmental changes will affect the future of a PRP by creating opportunities or by posing threats. These forces represent "uncontrollables" in the program to which it *must adapt.*

The Market Environment

The final external environment to analyze is the *market environment.* This consists of ". . . the groups and other organizations that the focal organization directly works with to accomplish its mission. The main groups in the market environment are the clients, marketing intermediaries, suppliers, and supporters."[3] A PRP should monitor the trends and changes of these key groups to determine their needs, perceptions, preferences, and dissatisfactions.

Once the data is collected, and the mission, goals, and objectives are outlined and set, the information must then be integrated with the long-term strategy of the PRP. One approach for-profit marketers use to integrate the data is the *portfolio planning method,* which ". . . assumes an organization, including non-profits, offer multiple products or services in multiple markets and are constantly facing questions of how to treat simultaneously these sets of existing and potential products or services."[3] From a PRP perspective, consider the following: the program options to which resources will be added (*build*); the program options to be maintained (*hold*); the program options that drain resources owing to poor performance, statistics, or census (*harvest*); the program options to delete because the future is not promising (*divest*); and the program options to add (*new*) for developing the strategic plan of the department. This portfolio is similar to a stock investment for which one has to decide to buy, sell, hold, switch, withdraw, or add to the stocks. The portfolio must be constantly evaluated relative to changing market conditions and performance results of the individual units in the portfolio.

A PRP must develop core marketing strategies that consist of: target markets, a competitive position, and an effective marketing mix.

Target Market Strategy

As discussed earlier, there are many publics with which a PRP may serve or interrelate, but it is to the target market that all the energies of marketing are directed. It may be difficult for a PRP to serve effectively all the markets identified. It is often better to concentrate on specific segments of these markets. A market can be segmented by geographics, behavior, demographics (i.e., age, sex, income), or psychographics.[17] It is important to consider the specific characteristics as well as the current and projected populations of these markets.

Target marketing may focus on five areas:[2] program–market concentration, program specialization, market specialization, selective specialization, or full coverage. The *program–market concentration* looks at a facility concentrating on only one program and only one market segment. The *program specialization* is a facility choosing to offer only one program for all its markets. The *market specialization* consists of the facility choosing to serve only one market segment with all its programs. *Selective specialization* allows a facility to work in several program markets, having no relation to each other, except that each represents an opportunity. *Full coverage* consists of a facility providing a full range of products and programs to serve all market segments.

Once the foregoing target market options are evaluated for a PRP, a determination of the most appropriate market emphasis must be decided.

Competitive Positioning Strategy

Once the target market for the PRP has been chosen, the competitive positioning strategy against the "other" PRPs serving the same target market–patient group must be developed. How can meaningful differences between your program and its competitors be communicated? The method(s) potential patients use to evaluate and choose among programs must be understood. Is the deciding factor location, the hospital landscaping, or program quality? Once you understand the competition, you can develop a successful strategy.

The Market Mix

The market mix consists of product (refers to both products and services), price, place, and promotion.[1,18,19] Each will be discussed in detail. These variables have a direct influence on the level of patient response and are important to the development of a successful relationship with patients.[16]

Product

The major products of a PRP are health care for respiratory patients, education, training, preventative health care, wellness programs, and research.[20–22] The rehabilitation team must continually consider the needs of its consumers. As the consumers' needs change, the pulmonary rehabilitation team must modify its products to meet these changing needs. Reviewing the services provided will help strengthen weak areas, eliminate nonused products, and develop new products to meet the consumers' needs. The program and its products must be designed and implemented to attract consumers. Program options would be another consideration of the products offered by a PRP. Table 28–2 lists various program options a PRP may consider, based upon target market and consumer needs.

Price

The price (cost) of a PRP is dependent on many variables; for example, inpatient versus outpatient programs, physician fees, medical laboratory charges, educational and training material costs, pulmonary function costs, service fees (occupational therapy, physical therapy, and respiratory therapy), and indirect facility expenses (overhead). There are standard costs for a PRP that cannot be avoided, but it is essential to assess what is really necessary for each patient. Potential rehabilitation candidates may be turned away by the total cost of the program, regardless of the benefits they might gain.

The patient is often concerned with the "out-of-pocket" cost as well as the "other" cost. The out-of-pocket cost refers to medical insurance deductibles or charges incurred during a PRP not covered by medical insurance, for which the patient is responsible. Other cost refers to the psychologic, social, or spiritual effects that the program will have on the patient. The patient often feels like a number, a

TABLE 28-2.   PRP Options

Chest Clinic
COPD program
Adult asthma program
Children's asthma program
Cystic fibrosis program
Smoking cessation program
Intensive pulmonary evaluation
Restrictive lung disease program
Pre- and post-lung transplant program

case, or a disease, instead of a person. Wearing everyday clothing, rather than a backless, shapeless gown, helps the rehabilitation inpatient feel more like a person. Other costs are side effects of procedures performed on the patient during the PRP; for example, the discomfort of obtaining arterial blood gas samples (ABGs), the bruising from venous puncture, or the inconvenience of pulmonary function tests.

Place
The positive and negative aspects of the physical location of a PRP must be looked at from the perspective of patients and publics. The time and days a rehabilitation program is offered must be matched to patients' lives and work schedules. Most medical services are offered Monday through Friday, 8:00 AM to 5:00 PM. Many prospective pulmonary rehabilitation candidates cannot afford the loss of a day's wage to enter a program. Identifying times that are most convenient for prospective patients will enhance the likelihood of success. Compromises may be required by both the consumer and provider relative to location and time.

A patient's ability to travel to the site of the program should be evaluated. For example, is the most frequently used patient mode of transportation by automobile, bus, or subway? It is difficult to alter the location of a hospital-based PRP, but the renting of space or a mobile clinic are possible options.

The availability of parking must be considered. Most hospital parking lots are crowded. If rehabilitation patients have to park several blocks from the hospital, forcing them to arrive at the office short of breath, it may result in low attendance at the program's classes.

What are the eligibility criteria for the PRP? How is a candidate admitted to the program, and what is the reception process? One must communicate clearly and regularly with the potential client concerning the pulmonary rehabilitation program's eligibility criteria. The length of time it takes for the patient to get an appointment to be seen by the various rehabilitation team members is important. Patient convenience is crucial. Remember, the team is there to satisfy the patient's needs.

Promotion
The last area of the marketing mix to be discussed is promotion.[18,23] Once the team has developed objectives and identified its publics and target markets, the next important step is to promote the program.

MacStravic has stated that the primary purpose of promotion is ". . . to motivate sufficient numbers of patients to seek appropriate types of services at desired levels."[24] This can be accomplished through information and persuasion, by moving the consumer through a "hierarchy of effects from unawareness to:

- understanding/familiarity
- interest
- decision
- utilization
- satisfaction
- repeated or regular use
- recommendation."[24]

Promotion should begin with the education of the medical and allied health staff of the institution and community where the program is based by developing inservices on pulmonary rehabilitation.[25-32] All team members should be involved in this education process under the leadership of the PRP medical director. The first group toward whom to direct education are those staff physicians who deal with pulmonary patients at the facility where the program is located (e.g., pulmonary internists, thoracic surgeons, allergists). Let these physicians know what services can be offered to their patients. Education also needs to be directed toward emergency room physicians, family practice specialists, and internists in the hospital and in the community. This can be accomplished through inservices or seminars held for these specific groups, offering continuing education credit. The emergency room physicians come in contact with patients with chronic obstructive pulmonary disease (COPD) frequently. These physicians can also initiate a referral system to the pulmonary section for possible rehabilitation candidates.

It is also helpful to direct inservices toward allied health professionals, community organizations such as the American Lung Association, and church groups. Since the potential rehabilitation candidate is often referred to the program, one must develop a network of referrals. It is important to emphasize to the referring physician population that their patients will be discharged back to their care. Only by identifying the educational needs of these specific groups of people will a continuing medical education program on pulmonary rehabilitation succeed.[33]

Holding an open house for the PRP can be beneficial. Reporters from local papers and television and radio stations can be notified of the open house. This is an ideal way of allowing the public and future rehabilitation candidates to see and hear about the rehabilitation program. Such information helps patients make an educated decision about their health care.

The public relations department of the health care facility can aid in publicizing the program by presenting articles in various facility publications, such as the employee, medical, and patient newsletters. This department can also send news releases and stories to the local newspapers covering the program.

During National Pulmonary Rehabilitation (PR) Week, health fairs, or smokeout campaigns, the rehabilitation staff can share its expertise with the public through health screening and education. Table 28–3 shows a sample proclamation for National PR Week, the first week of spring. The staff can provide pulmonary function

TABLE   28-3.   Proclamation for National Pulmonary Rehabilitation Week*

Whereas, lung disease constitutes a critical, social, and economic health problem in the United States; and

Whereas, pulmonary rehabilitation is a vital component of comprehensive quality care of the lung patient, both the public and medical communities are generally unaware of its physical, emotional, and economic benefits; and

Whereas, the incidence of lung disease can be reduced through earlier detection, treatment, prevention, and rehabilitation; and

Whereas, the establishment of a special week each year to promote lung disease awareness, its prevention, and rehabilitation will greatly assist in decreasing its incidence;

Now, therefore, I, _____ , do hereby proclaim the first week of Spring as Pulmonary Rehabilitation Week in our community, and urge all citizens to generously support this worthy effort.

* The first week in spring

testing, blood pressure checks, and literature on lung disease and its prevention at these community programs. The local lung, heart, and cancer societies provide important community educational programs during which team members may also speak. Medical chest conferences are an optimal setting for the presentation of a case study of a pulmonary rehabilitation patient.[34] Each team member can present his or her evaluation of the rehabilitation candidate and recommended treatment at such a conference. This is a way of exposing students, practicing physicians, and allied health professionals to the concepts of pulmonary rehabilitation.

Reaching out to nursing homes, public health agencies, registries, and other home health care programs will help not only in educating these personnel about the pulmonary patient, but will also help in developing referrals from these agencies. Respiratory therapy equipment supply companies and home visiting nurse associations can also benefit from the educational programs. Once valued markets such as these have been identified, the team must make contact with each group.

As mentioned earlier in this chapter, advertising does not equal marketing, but it is an important element of it. In 1977, advertising was accepted as a legitimate and ethical promotional activity by the American Hospital Association and the Federation of American Hospitals.[35,36] Advertising needs to be informative, clearly detailing the PRP's services, and avoiding false or misleading statements. One should not make claims for the quality of the service or care the program provides, because of the possible legal consumer issues that could result. The program's telephone number and mailing address should be incorporated into the advertisement to invite readers or listeners to contact the program office for further information. Any advertisement released must be professional and dignified.[37]

Table 28–4 lists the variety of methods used in advertising, and Table 28–5 lists the "do's and don'ts" of brochure development.

The various sources of health care information for the consumer is often from the primary care physician, the media consisting of direct mailing, newspaper advertisements or television commercials, and by "word of mouth."[38] In fact, direct mail in

TABLE 28-4. **Variety of Advertising Methods**

Brochures
Billboards
Radio
Direct mail
Television
Magazine/newspaper advertisements
Yellow pages/directories

TABLE 28-5. **The "Do's and Don'ts" of Brochure Development**

For patients
- Write in a step-by-step style what is happening, in sequence from the beginning to the end of the program.
- Avoid technical language; if a technical term must be used, define it.
- Illustrate, making diagrams clear and simple; use illustrations to explain complex procedures.
- Avoid negative connotations through words or illustrations.
- Print the brochure on sturdy weight paper (70–80 lb).
- Use photographs that will not become outdated, and that represent your patient population; avoid photographs of patients in bed or immobile.
- Break brochure down into topics if a great deal of explaining must be done; consider a series of brochures, because patients cannot handle too much material in one brochure.
- Include past patients in photographs, along with their comments, testimonials (Be sure to obtain signed photograph releases from patients photographed.).
- Offer reassurance and the positive side of the patient's disease problems in the brochure.
- Choose color appropriately (red can be irritating if used too much, and may signal danger for patients).
- Use bold black type for easy reading, and color for headline or key words.
- Include address, telephone number, and names of contact for the pulmonary rehabilitation program. Cost may also be included if applicable.
- Know your printing budget before you begin developing the brochure.

For Medical Personnel
- Compliment the intelligence of the audience; do not under- or overexplain.
- Include illustrations to avoid reader boredom, such as charts, graphs, or other.
- Include address, telephone numbers, names for contact, and referral information.
- Most of the patient's do's and don'ts apply here as well.
- Avoid including information that may become outdated, requiring frequent brochure revision (e.g., program dates).

one survey showed it was the principal and preferred source of health care information. Radio is often less expensive than television.[37] The yellow pages' directory advertisements usually get people when they are ready to buy or act.[40] In newspaper advertising, be aware of the frequency that the advertisement is run, the variety of space and formats available, whether the newspaper is a daily or weekly, or has zoned editions that allow the advertisements to reach only a specific area. Table 28–6 lists some of the advantages and disadvantages of newspaper and magazine advertising.

Regardless of the types of promotion used in a PRP, a log of the inquiries to the program is helpful to track the source of referral. At the end of the promotion campaign, the program can then assess the types of responses. Table 28–7 shows a sample advertising log that a PRP may use.

With advertising budgets shrinking, the newest idea to hit the market is cooperative image advertisements.[41–43] These advertisements develop meaningful linkages with vendors, often using the advertising theme "partners in quality." The vendor often pays for the advertisement in exchange for being featured or connected with a well-known facility. This type of joint marketing program with a vendor is new and growing, but not without risks. Will the vendor expect the medical facility to purchase more of their products? Will the vendor tarnish the facility's image if the facility chooses not to use their products, or if too many other vendors are chosen?

Cooperative deals can be structured to avoid problems; always involve the HCF purchasing department in such planning. Cooperative promotional programs

TABLE 28-6.   Newspaper/Magazine Advertising Options

Option	Advantages	Disadvantages
Local/regional newspaper	May offer weekday and weekend editions to reach increased readership May offer inserts to target specific audience (e.g., health care insert), *TV Guide* May offer local editions to target specific communities	May be more expensive than advertising in other publications. Beware of oversaturation of readership. Advertisements run intermittently
Small newspaper syndicate	May be less expensive than advertising in other publications Readership may include segment of community likely to utilize PRP services	Circulation may be smaller than local/regional newspaper
Magazine	May offer inserts to target specific audience May offer local editions to target specific communities	May be more expensive than advertising in other publications

TABLE 28-7. Sample Advertising Log

Publication:
Date Advertisement Appeared:

Date Call Received	Name	Address	Phone	Info Sent	Enrolled

may be made between a HCF and local business such as retail outlets and banks.[44,45] This joint sponsorship is growing and can be seen with television stations in their struggle to meet the current, frantic demand for accurate medical information.

MARKET IMPLEMENTATION

The final steps in the strategic marketing plan process are to develop the organizational structure, tactics, and benchmarks, then to implement and assess the market strategy chosen. Implementing the market strategy is now done. Kotler has referred to marketing as the ". . . philosophical alternative to force."[1,2] The purpose of marketing is not to force an idea, product, or service on a group of people, but to design a product–program tailored to meet the needs of the consumer. There is no specific style of marketing for a PRP. Choose a style that meets the program's goals and objectives within the restraints of the institution represented. The program must constantly reevaluate patients' and publics' needs. One way of accomplishing this is to give patients and referring physicians program evaluation forms and questionnaires to obtain feedback on the program. This information can then be used to strengthen or change weak areas within the program.

There are two major benefits a PRP can achieve from market implementation. The first is to increase the satisfaction of its target markets (e.g., patients, publics, physicians, third-party payers, and other health professionals), thereby increasing patient referral. The second benefit is the development of an efficient marketing strategy.

"These benefits of bringing marketing thought into an organization are not without some cost."[1,2] Orienting a pulmonary rehabilitation team to marketing involves attitude awareness with possible change. A marketing orientation includes helping the team members understand that they are there to satisfy and meet the consumer–patient needs, however difficult. Accumulation of technical knowledge, which may mean hiring a marketing specialist, is the other potential cost involved in the marketing orientation.

Once an understanding of the basic concepts of marketing has been achieved by a pulmonary rehabilitation team proceeding with a market audit, the implementation of the data must then be carried out.[1,14,16,18,46] The audit may not answer all the questions raised, but it will allow a program to develop a plan for implementation. The plan must include short- and long-range goals being reviewed regularly.

MARKETING OF THE FUTURE

What will be the future of government regulations, the national economy, local geographic occurrences, or third-party reimbursement changes on the PRP? You may not always have control over these issues, but their effect will be felt by the program.

Marketing into the 21st century will see quality, health outcome measures and smarter markets; advances in treatment and therapy approaches; rising costs, yet frozen prices and market segmentation; and consumer market information as *key* challenges for the next decade.[47]

Marketing fails for lack of a vision or mission and lack of understanding what the customer means to the program. Nurture positive relationship with the four Ps: physicians, patients, payers, and publics.[48]

Marketing is a philosophy involving the management and specific concepts relating to consumer needs, wants, and desires. Marketing and management go hand in hand. Each involves a planning process and implementation. They must harmonize or else failure occurs.[49] In health care marketing[50]

Physicians want quality.
Patients want convenience.
Payers want low cost.

SUMMARY

Marketing is a term becoming more familiar in the health care industry, and if its strategy is applied to the development of a PRP, it will likely succeed. The basic concepts of marketing that must be understood by the pulmonary rehabilitation team members include knowing who are your consumers, providers, referrers, sellers, payers, and deliverers. Once this is understood and outlined, target markets and publics can be identified.

To ensure effectiveness of marketing, a strategic plan must be developed. The market audit does just this, consisting of an examination of the external market environment, the internal market system, and the market mix (product, price, place, and promotion). Too often the words *marketing* and *promotion/advertising* are thought to be synonymous, but advertising is just one element of marketing.

The last phase of the marketing process is to implement your findings for a successful PRP. This is done through short- and long-range goals. The marketing process will develop program awareness for the benefit of both the patient and the program, but it must be continually reviewed and updated. *Remember, marketing is an ongoing process.*

Pulmonary Rehabilitation Program Sample Marketing Plan

I. Determine the PRP mission, goals, and objectives.

PRP Mission Statement: Offer a comprehensive rehabilitation program to the members of our community.

PRP Goal: Increase patient enrollment in the PRP.

PRP Objective: Increase patient enrollment in the PRP by 20% within the next fiscal year.

II. Analyze the PRP external environment:

A. *Public Environment* (from Fig. 28–5)

1. Medical staff—turnover—Physicians not aware of PRP existence and benefits.
2. Competitors—Inpatient PRP in rehabilitation hospital, outpatient PRP in CORF.
3. Business community/government agencies (third-party payers)—Increased cost of health care—decreased patient health care benefits—patients' comparison shopping for least expensive health care services.

B. *Competitive Environment* (from Table 28–1)

1. Desire competitors—Patient has choice of going on a cruise or entering a comprehensive pulmonary rehabilitation program.
2. Generic competitors—Read books on lung problems, watch videos from the American Lung Association on lung disease, or attend a PRP.
3. Service form competitors—Inpatient PRP in rehabilitation hospital offering a golf clinic for PRP participants, outpatient PRP in CORF offering a cruise vacation for PRP participants, and a 6-week outpatient PRP from outpatient hospital setting.
4. Enterprise competitors—St. John's Rehabilitation Hospital, our program, or the CORF.

C. *Macroenvironment*

1. Demography—High percentage of community residents (within 15-mile radius), are over age 55, according to our hospital's community affairs department statistics.
2. Economy—High percentage of community residents have Medicare insurance only (no secondary health care insurance), and are on a fixed income, according to our hospital's community affairs department statistics.
3. Technology—Our hospital is implementing computerization of medical records within the next fiscal year. Each hospital department is to share the burden of computerization of records costs, which may increase the cost of PRP (to be determined in the future).
4. Political—Recent legislation has mandated an increase in the Medicare deductible, resulting in increased out-of-pocket expenses for PRP participants with Medicare insurance (who have no secondary insurance carrier).
5. Social/cultural—High percentage of community residents are Hispanic. Hospital statistics demonstrate that this population segment does not use the hospital's services proportional to the percentage of Hispanic people in the community.

D. *Market Environment*

1. Clients—PRP program survey showed prospective PRP participants (sampled from the Better Breathers Club and private physician practices) desired an

(continued)

ongoing exercise program for pulmonary rehabilitation patients. This service is not being offered currently by inpatient PRP in rehabilitation hospital or outpatient PRP in CORF.

2. Marketing intermediaries—Hospital community relations department recently cut personnel and nonpersonnel expense budget. PRP coordinator notified that PRP staff would have to bear increased responsibility for cost and time to market the PRP.

3. Suppliers—PRP interdisciplinary team members have the opportunity to market the PRP to physicians and prospective patients when working in their respective departments (during non-PRP work hours).

4. Supporters—Survey of medical staff who have referred patients to PRP revealed the physicians desired the establishment of an ongoing exercise program for post-PRP participants, as their patients fail to continue exercising after completing the PRP, and lose the physical improvement they have gained during the PRP.

III. Assess the PRP Strengths, Weaknesses, Opportunities and Threats (SWOT)

   A. *Strengths*

      1. Eight-year history of PRP program statistics have demonstrated the efficacy of the PRP in the following areas: improved patient stamina, decreased hospitalization rate, decreased physician office visit rate, decreased patient depression and anxiety scores.

      2. Historically strong physician and community support of the hospital center services due to excellent professional reputation of the hospital providers in the community.

   Inpatient PRP in the rehabilitation hospital and outpatient PRP in the CORF are new programs. Quantity is still unknown and there is no proved track record.

   B. *Weaknesses*

      1. Cost of PRP higher than outpatient PRP at CORF.

      2. Decrease in marketing budget of community affairs department—decreased availability of personnel and supply resources to market PRP.

   C. *Opportunities*

      1. Our PRP able to expand to offer an ongoing exercise program for pulmonary rehabilitation patient graduates.

      2. Neither rehabilitation hospital nor CORF PRP offers ongoing exercise program.

   D. *Threats*

      1. No threats exist for an ongoing exercise program post PRP at this time.

      2. Be aware that the rehabilitation hospital and CORF PRP may start an ongoing exercise program but at this time neither program has a facility to hold the ongoing exercise program.

IV. Long-term strategy of the PRP

   A. Program option(s) to *build*—PRP extracurricular activity, such as pilot day trip by bus to local botanical garden.

   B. Program option(s) to *hold*—Cosponsorship of local pulmonary education program with nonprofit organization (ALA). Feeds enrollment of participants in PRP.

   C. Program option(s) to *harvest*—Asthma rehabilitation program for children (low enrollment in program, and high percentage of community residents are 55 years or older) and draining resources.

   D. Program option(s) to *divest*—Preventative pulmonary health class. Insurance does

not cover cost of the class for participants and statistics show that the class does not feed enrollment of participants in PRP.
  E. Program option(s) *new*—Ongoing exercise program for PRP participants.
V. Develop core marketing strategies
  A. *Target market*—Market specialization, emphasize development of new ongoing exercise program and improve marketing of existing PRP program to population segment of residents over 55 years.
  B. *Competitive positioning strategy*—Emphasize long-standing history of PRP success, excellent professional reputation of providers and medical center in community, trust of community residents in hospital staff and services (known quality).
  C. *Market mix*
    1. Product
      a. Cosponsorship of pulmonary education program with nonprofit organization (ALA).
      b. Outpatient PRP (6-week program at medical center).
      c. Ongoing exercise program for PRP participants (at local senior center).
    2. Price
      a. More expensive than outpatient PRP at CORF, but assistance available to eliminate patient's out-of-pocket expense through grant money.
    3. Place
      a. Advantages of a pulmonary education program (ALA cosponsor) and ongoing exercise program held at local senior center:
        • Convenient, ample parking on flat terrain
        • Wheelchair access (parking and building facilities)
        • Convenient bus access (stops in front of senior center)
        • Midafternoon schedule of programs in response to survey of patients demonstrating preferred time
      b. Advantages of outpatient PRP held at hospital
        • Parking for PRP participants reserved outside classroom
        • Wheelchair access (parking and building facilities)
        • Convenient bus access (stops outside hospital)
        • Morning and afternoon program schedules to accommodate patient preferences
    4. Promotion
      a. Physicians—PRP presentations at medical staff meetings to educate new medical staff concerning PRP existence and benefits.
        • Thank you notes to physicians referring patients to PRP
        • Ensure rapid turnaround of patient progress reports in PRP to referring physician
      b. Prospective patients—Participation of PRP staff in community health fairs
        • PRP presentations to community organizations (e.g., senior centers, church groups)
        • Participation of PRP staff in employee health fairs (e.g., pulmonary function screenings)
VI. Implement marketing strategies
  A. Ongoing assessment of marketing effectiveness
  B. Remember, marketing is an ongoing process

REFERENCES

1. Kotler P. Marketing for nonprofit organizations. Englewood Cliffs, NJ: Prentice-Hall, 1975.

2. Kotler P, Clarke RN. Marketing for health care organizations. Englewood Cliffs, NJ: Prentice-Hall, 1987.

3. Kotler P, Andreasen AR. In: Strategic marketing for non-profit organizations, 3rd ed. Englewood Cliffs, NJ: Prentice-Hall, 1987.

4. Critelli-Schick I, Schick T. In the market for ethics: marketing begins with values. Health Prog 1989;Oct:72.

5. Kaplan MD. What it is, what it isn't. Marketing Hosp 1979;Sept:176.

6. Clarke R, Shyavitz L. Marketing information and market research—valuable tools for managers. Health Care Manage 1981;Winter:73.

7. Friedman E. Does market competition belong in health care. Hospitals 1980;Jul:47.

8. Johns HE, Moser HR. An empirical analysis of consumers' attitudes toward hospital advertising. Health Care Superv 1987;7(4):11.

9. Garton T. Marketing health care: its untapped potential. Hosp Prog 1978;Feb:46.

10. McMillan NH. Marketing: a tool that serves hospital's survival instincts. Hospitals 1981;Nov:89.

11. MacStravic RE. Health care marketing needs rational, ethical approach. Hosp Prog 1980;May:60.

12. AMA Board approves new marketing definition. Marketing News 1985;Mar:1.

13. Flexner W, Berkowitz E. Marketing research in health planning: a model. Publ Health Rep 1979;94:503.

14. MacStravic RE. Marketing: changing prospective patients' behavior. Hosp Prog 1979;Jun:47.

15. Higgins JM. The planning process and organizational purpose. In: The management challenge. An introduction to management. New York: Macmillan Publishing, 1991:145.

16. Walter CM. Academic medical center applies marketing audit to specific service. Hospitals 1981;Sept:90.

17. Sapienza AM. Psychographic profiles: aid to health care marketing. HCM Rev 1980;Fall:53.

18. MacStravic RE. Marketing by objectives for hospitals. Rockville, MD: Aspen Systems, 1980:5.

19. Shapiro B. Marketing for nonprofit organizations. In: Montana P, ed. Marketing in nonprofit organizations. New York: AMACOM, 1978:16.

20. Longe M, Ardell D. Wellness programs attract new markets for hospitals. Hospitals 1981;Nov:115.

21. Galvagni W. Hospitals diversity to thrive in a competitive environment. Hospitals 1981;Apr:131.

22. Kuntz EF: Businesses may be steady buyers of hospitals' wellness programs. Mod Health Care 1981;Aug:104.

23. Bates D. Special demands on nonprofit PR. In: Montana P. ed. Marketing in nonprofit organizations. New York: AMACOM, 1978:55.

24. MacStravic RE. Marketing health care. Germantown: Aspen Systems, 1977.

25. Wang V, Terry P, Flynn B, Williamson J, Green L, Faden R. Evaluation of continuing medical education for chronic obstructive pulmonary diseases. J Med Educ 1979;54:803.

26. Linn B. Continuing medical education impact on emergency room burn care. JAMA 1980;244:565.

27. Manning P, Lee P, Denson T, Gilman N. Determining educational needs in the physician's office. JAMA 1980;244:1112.

28. Ad Hoc Committee on CME of AAMC. Continuing education of physicians: conclusions and recommendations. J Med Educ 1980;55:149.

29. Stein LS. The effectiveness of continuing medical education: eight research reports. J Med Educ 1981;56:103.

30. Newborn VB. Whose reality: ramifications for marketing in adult education. J Continuing Educ Nurs 1981;12(5):17.

31. Hauf BJ. Nurse response to continuing education: relevant factors in marketing success. J Continuing Educ Nurs 1981;12(5):10.

32. Grubb AW. Role, relevance, cost of hospital education and training debated. Hospitals 1981;Apr:75.

33. Yoder Wise PS. Needs assessment as a marketing strategy. J Continuing Educ Nurs 1981;12(5):5.

34. Cooper SS. Methods of teaching—revisited case method. J Continuing Educ Nurs 1981;12(5):32.

35. Flexner W, Berkowitz E. Media and message strategies: consumer input for hospital advertising. Health Care Manage Rev 1981;Winter:35.

36. Cooper P, Robinson L. Health care marketing management, a case approach. Rockville, MD: Aspen Systems, 1980:88.

37. Lee JM. Marketing ensures success of maternity care program. Hospitals 1980;Dec:91.

38. Jensen J. Direct mail the primary, preferred source of healthcare information for consumers. Mod Healthcare 1989;Sept 15:94.

39. Radio spots triple calls for mental health. Profiles Healthcare Marketing 1989:Oct:42.

40. Eisenhart T. What's right, what's wrong with each medium. Business Marketing 1990;Apr:40.

41. Harms J. Developing an effective occupational health marketing plan. J Ambulatory Care Marketing 1989;3(1):11.

42. Perry L. Link-up with vendor can stretch ad budget. Mod Healthcare 1990;Apr 9:52.

43. Television reaches a broad community. Profiles Healthcare Marketing 1989;Oct:32.

44. Exter TG: The baby boomers turn 40. Healthcare Forum J 1989;Jan/Feb:19.

45. Perry L. Hospitals trying ventures with various businesses. Mod Healthcare 1990;Apr 16:60.

46. Walter CM. Academic medical center features image analysis in marketing audit. Hospitals 1981;Aug:91.

47. Bezold C, Peck JC, Kurent H. The "smarter markets" of the 1990s. Healthcare Forum J 1989;Jan/Feb:32.

48. Stier, R. Creating an effective marketing team. Healthcare Executive, 1989;May/June:36.

49. Morley AP, Brown SW. Marketing isn't always the cure. Physician's Manage 1989;Feb:127.

50. OR Manager, monthly newsletter for OR decision makers 1990;Jan:6(1):1.

JUDITH L. RADOVICH

JOHN E. HODGKIN

GEORGE G. BURTON

ALAN R. YEE

Cost Effectiveness of Pulmonary Rehabilitation Programs

The containment of health care costs is one of the highest priorities in the United States today. Many economists, business leaders, and politicians have spoken out on the rising cost of health care. Health care costs in 1988 were estimated to be about 12% of the nation's economy.[1] In 1987 national health care expenditures totaled more than 500 billion dollars in the United States. In 1988 the overall inflation rate was 4.1%, but the rate of increase of the medical care component of the Consumer Price Index was 6.5%.[2] The cost of health care in 1991 was estimated to be 740 billion dollars, representing 13.1% of the gross national product.

In analyzing the cost benefits of pulmonary rehabilitation one needs to take into account several questions:

1. Do pulmonary rehabilitation programs (PRPs) reduce the cost of health care to third-party payers such as Medicare?
2. Do these programs affect the Social Security system favorably by delaying the need for people to take early retirement or to go on permanent disability?
3. Do PRPs decrease the number of sick days taken by working patients with COPD?
4. Do they help return patients to the work force?
5. Do hospitals benefit from a reduction of inpatient days (this would be helpful in the era of DRGs)?
6. With many health maintenance organizations capitating hospitals and physicians, can PRPs reduce physician office or emergency room visits?
7. Not to be forgotten, are PRPs affordable for the patients?

Designing PRPs to meet all these needs definitely presents a challenge and a need for some answers to these questions.

ECONOMIC IMPACT OF CHRONIC
OBSTRUCTIVE PULMONARY DISEASE

Recent statistics have reported the effect of chronic obstructive pulmonary disease (COPD) on the national economy. Since 1987, COPD has been ranked fifth in the leading causes of death of individuals 65 years of age or older. The death rate per 100,000 population for COPD has increased from 1970 (13.2 : 100,000) to 1990 (35.5:100,000). Statistics show an increase in the number of people who have COPD and die of it. Also, the proportion of the population that is 65 years of age and older is increasing rapidly. Life expectancy at age 65 in 1978 was 16.3 years past 65. In 1987, this increased to 16.9 years more. Older persons want to lead more healthy, active, and enjoyable lives and want to reduce the influence of chronic problems, such as respiratory diseases, on their lives.[2]

Another way of measuring the effect of health care on the economy is to look at restricted activity days and bed disability days. In 1977, people 65 years and older had 36.5 days/person when they were unable to engage in usual activities; in 1987, this rate decreased to 30.3. In 1977, the same group of people had 14.5 days/year per person of bed disability and, in 1987, this figure decreased to 14.0 days. Obviously, any factor that would decrease these restricted activity days and bed disability days would help the economy.[2]

Chronic obstructive pulmonary disease also affects people younger than 65 years old. The U.S. Health and Prevention Profile notes that, in 1980, 115,000 years of potential life were lost because of COPD, and this figure increased to 132,000 years in 1987. If one considers years of potential life lost per 1000 population because of COPD, the figure is 0.6 years.[2]

Thus, COPD has a tremendous influence on the national economy, Medicare, and other third-party payers. Can pulmonary rehabilitation be cost-effective for the national economy and third-party payers?

COST-EFFECTIVENESS STUDIES

Cost-effectiveness studies of pulmonary rehabilitation have been reported in the literature for quite some time. In 1970 to 1977, Loma Linda University Medical Center's pulmonary rehabilitation program[3] studied 80 patients with COPD. The patient's average age was 62, and the mean 1-second forced expiratory volume (FEV_1) at entry was 1.33 L. Data was collected on the number of hospital days per patient 1 year before beginning the PRP and then up to 5 years after the program. Each patient studied had completed a comprehensive PRP including education, exercise modalities, and home visits. During the year preceding the program, each patient averaged 17.41 hospital days. At 1 year after the program the average number of hospital days per patient had dropped significantly to 7.78 days, and after year 2 to 4.91 days. Continued drops were seen from year 3 to 2.74 days and year 4 to 2.22 days. After the fifth year, the average number of hospital days per patient had increased slightly to 3.26 days (Figure 29–1). A total of 27 patients died during the 5-year follow-up period, but the tabulations were adjusted to account for this population change. Figure 29–2 shows the average hospital days each year per patient for only the 53 surviving patients.

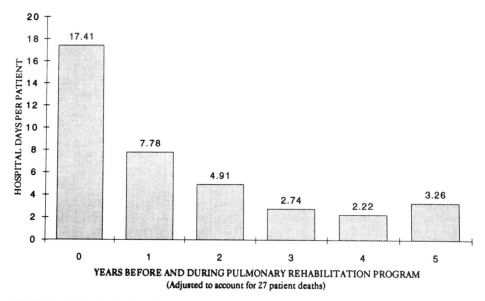

FIGURE   29-1   Analysis of hospital days before and during a pulmonary rehabilitation program at Loma Linda University Medical Center, a 5-year study conducted on 80 patients. Data were collected from 1970 to 1977. (Dunham JL, et al. Cost effectiveness of pulmonary rehabilitation programs. In: Hodgkin JE, Zorn EG, Connors GL, eds. Pulmonary rehabilitation: guidelines to success. Boston: Butterworths, 1984, with permission)

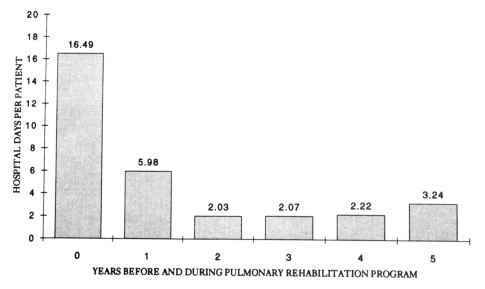

FIGURE   29-2   Analysis of hospital days before and during a pulmonary rehabilitation program at Loma Linda University Medical Center for the 53 patients alive 5 years after the program. (Dunham JL, et al. Cost effectiveness of pulmonary rehabilitation programs. In: Hodgkin JE, Zorn EG, Connors GL, eds. Pulmonary rehabilitation: guidelines to success. Boston: Butterworths, 1984, with permission)

In 1978, the average cost per hospital day at LLUMC was 400.00 dollars. With the data from only the 53 survivors, hospitalization for the year before the program cost approximately 349,600 dollars (Fig. 29–3). Cost of hospitalization for the first year after the program was approximately 126,800 dollars, for the second year 43,000 dollars, for the third year 43,900 dollars, for the fourth year 47,100 dollars, and for the fifth year 68,700 dollars. Total hospital costs for all 53 survivors for the total 5-year postprogram period equalled 329,500 dollars. This 5-year total was less than the cost of hospitalization for the year before the start of the program.

It was estimated that LLUMC's PRP, in 1982 cost 452.00 dollars/year per patient to provide a pulmonary rehabilitation program, including extensive follow-up by home visits. The average cost for pulmonary rehabilitation (PR) for the 53 survivors was approximately 24,000 dollars/year. The first-year hospital cost of 126,800 dollars plus the rehabilitation cost of 24,000 dollars totaled 150,800 dollars. This total reflected a savings of 198,800 dollars for the first year postprogram alone. And these savings reflected 1978 costs, not 1990 costs.

In 1976 Hudson and associates also reported a similar reduction in hospital days following a PRP.[4] They studied 70 patients, but reported on 44 of the patients who were still living 4 years postprogram. The 44 survivors average entry-level FEV_1 was 1.07 L. The PRP included education, exercises, and home visits. Figure 29–4 shows the number of hospital days pre- and postprogram. Again, at 1990 costs, this represents a significant savings.

Hudson and coworkers then analyzed the data again, adding back in the 20 patients who had died before the end of the study, on whom complete data were

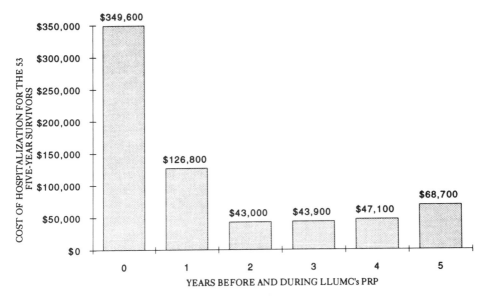

FIGURE   29-3   Years before and during LLUMC's pulmonary rehabilitation program. (Dunham JL, et al. Cost effectiveness of pulmonary rehabilitation programs. In: Hodgkin JE, Zorn EG, Connors GL, eds. Pulmonary rehabilitation: guidelines to success. Boston: Butterworths, 1984, with permission)

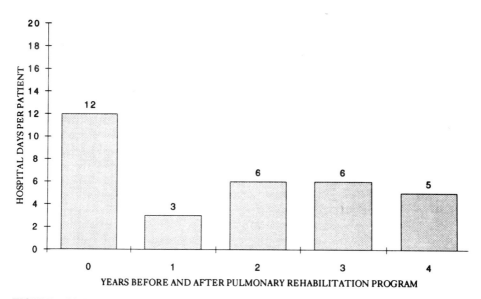

FIGURE 29-4 Summary of number of hospital days before and following a respiratory rehabilitation program for 44 survivors in the study reported by Hudson and associates. (Hudson LD, et al. Hospitalization needs during an outpatient rehabilitation program for severe CAO. Chest 1976;70:606, with permission)

available. They found that there were 10 hospital days per patient during the year before the PRP. Hospital days dropped to 5 days per patient after year 1 and continued at 5 hospital days per patient after year 2.

The PRP group at Barlow Hospital studied 96 COPD patients, with 74 surviving for approximately 1 year after they completed the program.[5] The average patient age was 65 and the mean entry level FEV_1 was 0.87 L. Each patient received a complete PRP including education and exercise components as inpatients. Their workers reported 38 hospital days per patient preprogram and a significant reduction to only 12 days per patient postprogram in the 74 survivors group. When they looked at the total 96 patients, they reported 42.5 hospital days per patient pre-PRP followed by 18.9 hospital days 1 year postprogram.

These three studies share several similarities. They all offered similar modalities in their PRPs and looked at the number of hospital days for at least 1 year before the program and at least 1 year postprogram. The mean FEV_1 for these groups ranged from 1.33 to 0.87 L. Barlow's and Hudson's groups were "sicker" than LLUMC's, at least by entry level FEV_1 data. It was interesting to note that the patients with lower FEV_1s had more hospital days postprogram, but still showed a decrease in hospital days when compared with the year preceding the PRP.

In 1983, a group at St. Joseph's Hospital in Stockton, California reported benefits from their PRP.[6] All patients had symptomatic COPD, but an average FEV_1 was not reported. All patients completed a 10-week outpatient PRP, including education and exercise. Postprogram they found a significant decrease in oxygen consumption, minute ventilation, and heart rate at comparable exercise levels on a treadmill. They also reported the number of hospital days pre-PRP and the number of hospital days 1 year postprogram for 57 patients. This patient group averaged 8.72 hospital days per patient preprogram and only 0.60 hospital days 1 year postprogram. Of the 57 patients, 16 accounted for all the hospital days preprogram and only 4 patients were hospitalized during the first year postprogram.

The average cost of a hospital day during June 1980 to November 1981 at St. Joseph's was approximately 1470 dollars. The decrease in the number of hospital days from a total of 497 to 34 represented a savings of 217,610 dollars in inpatient charges. St. Joseph's listed their program cost at approximately 1000 dollars.

Baystate Medical Center studied 55 patients with a mean FEV_1 of 1.17 L.[7] Thirty patients (group 0) received pulmonary rehabilitation in individual sessions, and 25 patients (group 1) were seen for 6 weeks in a group session. Data was collected for the 12 months before the program and up to 6 months postprogram. They reported a mean decrease in hospital days postprogram of 5.43 per patient for group 0 and 4.52 days for group 1. They did note a significant increase in phone calls to the PRP postprogram, but did not see a significant increase in emergency room or physician office visits.

In 1988, the PRP group at Eisenhower Medical Center reported data collected over 11 years.[8] They looked at the number of inpatient hospital days before and after PRP and discussed program costs. They also reported morbidity and mortality data. For their cost analysis they randomly selected 150 patients who had been initially evaluated for the PRP. The mean age of these patients was 68 years for men and 61 years for women. The mean entry level FEV_1 was 1.19 L. They divided these 150 patients into three groups, based on the portions of the PRP they had completed. Group 1 had been interviewed only, group 2 received only education, and group 3 received the complete PRP with exercise.

Group 1 was hospitalized a total of 1069 days or 4.28 days/patient per year (Table 29–1) for the 5 years before the program, and their total hospital days increased to 1570 or 6.28 days/patient per year for the 5 years postprogram. Group 2 (who received education only) also showed an increase in the total number of hospital days, from 586 or 2.73 days/patient per year, to 946 or 3.78 days/patient per year. Only group 3 (who completed a full PRP) showed a decrease in hospital days. Their total hospital days for the 5 years before the PRP were 801, or 3.2 days/patient per year, and decreased to 417, or 1.67 days/patient per year. The Eisenhower investigators estimated that an average cost per hospital day in 1987

TABLE 29-1. Average Number of Hospital Days per Patient per Year for the 5 Years Before and After the PRP at Eisenhower Medical Center[8]

	Group 1*	*Group 2†*	*Group 3‡*
For the 5 yr pre-PRP	4.24	2.34	3.2
For the 5 yr post-PRP	6.28	3.78	1.67

* Group 1: Interview only; did not participate in the PRP.
† Group 2: Received education only.
‡ Group 3: Received the complete PRP, including exercise.

was 1193 dollars. Group 1 increased the cost of hospitalization from 1,275,317 dollars for the 5 years before the PRP to 1,873,010 dollars for the 5 years following the program. Group 2 increased the cost of hospitalization from 699,098 dollars to 1,128,578 dollars. Only group 3 showed a savings in the cost of hospitalization. The prior 5 years cost 955,593 dollars, but the 5 years postprogram decreased to 497,481 dollars, or a total 5-year savings of 458,112 dollars. The Eisenhower Medical Center group estimated that their pulmonary rehabilitation program cost an average of about 1900 dollars/patient, or 95,000 dollars for 50 patients. For the 50 patients in group 3, the savings after the program costs were subtracted equaled 363,112 dollars, or 7262 dollars/patient for the 5 years postprogram.

Clearly, these studies show that pulmonary rehabilitation is cost-effective in at least decreasing the number of hospital days after a pulmonary rehabilitation program. This type of data has been successfully used to justify the benefit of pulmonary rehabilitation to third-party payers, such as Medicare. Most of the components of outpatient pulmonary rehabilitation programs have been recognized as reimbursable services through Medicare since at least 1980.[9]

A group from the Center for Behavioral Medicine at San Diego University in San Diego, California, showed cost benefits from pulmonary rehabilitation using an exercise program.[10] They reported on the number of well years of life produced by a PRP and were able to show that the program was cost-effective. They used the Health Policy Model to evaluate the number of well years produced. The Health Policy Model is a flexible tool in that it can compare different types of health care programs objectively. For example, it can compare inpatient versus outpatient programs, dialysis versus pulmonary rehabilitation programs, and so on, and establish the number of well years that these programs produce. Kaplan and Bush[10] published rough criteria indicating what they considered the cost of a cost-effective well year. Their mathematical formula to assess cost-effectiveness was

$$C/E = \frac{C_{rx} + C_{morb}}{E},$$

where C_{rx} represented the costs of an exercise program and C_{morb} stood for treatment cost savings from reduced morbidity; E represented the number of well life years. Any well year that cost less than 20,000 dollars was considered cost-effective. Well years at the 20,000 to 100,000 dollar range could be considered controversial, but still justifiable, but well years costing more than 100,000 dollars were questionable when compared with other health care expenditures. The San Diego group showed improved health status in their group and produced a total of 4.41 well years. The cost of those well years was 24,256 dollars. By Kaplan's guidelines this behavioral exercise program falls into the justifiable category and consequently was considered cost-effective. For further comparison, a typical renal dialysis program (which is considered effective medical treatment) costs more than 50,000 dollars to produce a well year, and a hypertension screening program costs about 10,000 dollars to produce a well year.

The San Diego State University study looked at the number of well years produced, because of the incredible effect of COPD on the economy. Statistics reviewed in the article show that costs for COPD in 1972 were 4.55 billion dollars; 803

million dollars of that figure were for hospital costs, physician services, and prescription medications; 3.05 billion dollars were spent for disability payments. Also mentioned was that COPD was more costly as a cause of disability than as a cause of death because many patients lived 20 to 30 years or longer with COPD. Patients with COPD have approximately 34 days of restricted activity per 100 persons per year. These statistics point to the value of increasing the number of well years for COPD patients.

EFFECTS ON OCCUPATIONAL DISABILITY

Another way to measure cost-effectiveness of PRPs is to determine if program graduates can be returned to the work force or can achieve a delay in the onset of disability. In 1983 and 1984, it was estimated that more than 16,000 individuals per year received Social Security disability benefits for the first time owing to COPD. These individuals do not start reporting significant limitations in activity until their mid-50s to 60s. Consequently, it is the older worker, limited by a progressive respiratory disease, who is seeking out PRPs. These individuals are generally not good candidates for vocational rehabilitation training.[11]

Studies over the years have reported the effectiveness of PRPs in returning patients to gainful employment. In 1970 Petty's group reported on 182 patients with COPD who had participated in a PRP for 2 years.[12] Of these patients, 60 were working at least part-time but the remainder (122) were not gainfully employed. The working patient's average age was 58 years, but the nonworkers was 62. The working group also had better FEV_1s (1.02 L) compared with 0.91 L for the nonworkers. The working group also had significantly greater exercise tolerance at the end of the program.

In 1969, Haas and Cardon reported data on 252 COPD patients whom they had studied for 5 years.[13] They divided these patients into three groups. Group 1 received a complete PRP as outpatients, group 2 received PR as inpatients and group 3 consisted of outpatients from another hospital who received standard care for COPD, but did not participate in a PRP. The average age for all three groups was approximately 57 years. Haas and Cardon reported that 25% of groups 1 and 2 were able to assume full-time employment, but only 3% of group 3 were working full time (Table 29–2). This table also shows that Group 1 and 2 were more independent in self-care and had fewer participants placed in extended care facilities.

In 1988, Holle and coauthors reported on 52 patients who had completed a PRP.[14] The average age was 58, and the average FEV_1 was 33% of predicted. The number of participants employed is unknown, but the study did find that those patients who worked were more productive and reported less time off work. All patients reported a significant improvement in their ability to do household and work-related activities. They commented that a real estate agent was able to double his income because he could now show more homes and that a longshoreman was able to return to work. The final treadmill evaluation showed that subjects were able to generate 73% more peak power (peak METs) and 250% more work completion (MET-min), whereas there was no significant change in $\dot{V}e_{max}$, HR_{max}, FEV_1, or oxygen saturation.

TABLE   29-2.   Five-Year Follow-up of 252 Male Patients*

	Group 1	Group 2	Group 3
Average age (yr)	56½	56½	57
% Full-time employed	25%	25%	3%
% Independent in self-care	19%	19%	5%
% Placed in extended care facilities	8%	8%	17%
% Dead	22%	22%	42%

* Comparison of Patients receiving respiratory rehabilitation and standard medical care (group 1, outpatients; group 2, inpatients) with a control group (group 3) of patients who received only standard care.
(Data from Haas A, Cardon H. Rehabilitation in chronic obstructive pulmonary disease. Med Clin North Am 1969;53:593)

These three studies[12–14] reported an average age of 57 years or older. Because of age alone these people generally would not be considered good candidates for a formal vocational rehabilitation program. The amount of time and cost to train them versus the benefit of years of continued employment is generally not thought to justify the time and cost of training. However, more benefit might be obtained from returning these patients to their previous jobs or helping them adapt their skills to less-demanding work within their own work environment. Further evaluation of patients' work ability may help determine who can return to their jobs.

The official American Thoracic Society statement, adopted in 1981, lists vocational evaluation as an additional service for PRPs.[15] Disability and the need for vocational rehabilitation are further discussed in Chapter 18.

Dr. Donald Dudley, a psychiatrist who has devoted many years to the study of COPD patients, comments on vocational rehabilitation potential for the older COPD patient.[16] He points out that productive work often leads to physical discomfort, such as disabling shortness of breath. Also, good motivation is needed for successful vocational rehabilitation. Often COPD patients lack this motivation (for one reason or other). Returning to work or learning a new job involves a great deal of "life change," and most people find this an uncomfortable process. He found that only 10% of patients complied with a vocational rehabilitation PRP component, whereas 90% cooperated with the other PR modalities. He feels that vocational rehabilitation or learning of new job skills is seldom possible for COPD patients. He felt that those patients most likely to benefit from a vocational rehabilitation program would have to be younger, have a better prognosis, and have skills and aptitudes that would help them with their new jobs. Patients with asthma would fall in this category. Also, with earlier detection of COPD by office spirometry, the long-term effects of the disease may be altered favorably.

Kass and coworkers have made a significant contribution in establishing criteria to determine individuals disabled by COPD.[17] They studied the vocational rehabilitation potential in a group of 147 COPD patients and concluded that patients with an FEV_1 of less than 50% of predicted and an MVV of less than 40% of predicted were unlikely to benefit from vocational rehabilitation training. They did note that patients who were still working were better candidates for vocational rehabilitation training.

Petty and his group found that many COPD patients have a difficult time learning new skills, because COPD and its associated hypoxemia can affect immediate memory as well as cause visual and perceptual dysfunctions.[18] Patients with COPD are often anxious, depressed, and concerned about physical illness.

In summary, if COPD patients are to be good candidates for vocational rehabilitation, they need to be younger, have their disease detected earlier, and have less severe disease.

The PRPs can help patients return to work and help them be more productive with less absenteeism. Pulmonary rehabilitation may even have an influence on some COPD patients to help them delay accepting disability or early retirement.

HEALTH-RELATED BENEFITS

Cost-effectiveness studies have already shown that pulmonary rehabilitation is helpful for patients unable to return to work by helping to decrease the need for hospitalization. It may also decrease the need for other health care services, such as home health agencies, emergency room visits, and visits to doctors' offices. Fewer patients may need placement in extended care facilities, as indicated by Haas and Cardon's 1969 study.[13]

Stillerman and colleagues[19] looked at the number of emergency department visits and visits to doctors' offices following PR and found no increase in the number of these visits.

Cost-effective PRPs must demonstrate that program expenses should be in line with health-related benefits. The COPD literature (many examples found in this volume) supports the notion that pulmonary rehabilitation has significant health-related benefits. This chapter attempts to demonstrate that PRPs have helped COPD patients decrease the need for hospitalization and other health care services and returned people to work or delayed disability or early retirement when possible. Certainly these savings have made a substantial contribution to national health care costs.

DEVELOPMENT OF A COST-EFFECTIVE PROGRAM

Pulmonary rehabilitation programs have operated on an inpatient as well as outpatient basis. Most are hospital-based, but some are located in other outpatient facilities such as physicians' offices or American Lung Association offices. However, when Medicare started reimbursing hospitals for inpatient care through the diagnostic-related groups (DRG) system, it became more advantageous to emphasize outpatient PRPs so that hospital stays could be decreased.[20] Also Medicare does not pay for hospital stays of relatively stable patients unless patients are in a certified rehabilitation unit.[21,22]

Braun and coauthors described a cost-effective pulmonary rehabilitation program in the rural areas of Wisconsin.[23] Wisconsin has COPD patients in rural areas that could benefit from PR but who cannot afford an expensive inpatient stay in a hospital in a large urban area. However, the long travel distances made outpatient programs unfeasible. Wisconsin has many rural hospitals with fewer than 100 beds, but these hospitals lack trained personnel to develop and run a PRP. The University of Wisconsin Center for Health Services (UWCHS) developed a PRP. Health professionals from the outlying rural areas who wanted to establish PRPs were then trained by UWCHS and a member of the UWCHS team was available to go out to the rural hospital to help establish the program. The UWCHS then continued involvement with each rural PRP with regular visits and provided a yearly 1-day seminar to update material. They were also available by telephone for specific patient problems if needed. UWCHS paid for all the training costs.

After 1 year, this decentralized program was felt to be successful. At the rural patients' first follow-up visits they demonstrated increased exercise tolerance and were continuing to use the techniques taught to them. This program showed that pulmonary rehabilitation could be done in a small rural hospital successfully and at a reasonable cost to the patient.

Callahan reported on a 12-hour group program at the offices of the American Lung Association in New Mexico. In 1985 her program charge to the patient was 56.25 dollars/patient per year. She did not comment on how this program was reimbursed. She found good patient compliance and an attrition rate below 5%.[24]

Little Company of Mary Hospital has had a PRP for more than 10 years and they report good success with fewer than three full-time employees.[25] They mention that one can have a multidisciplinary team by using specialized team members only when needed for a few hours a week. They use volunteers and receive contributions from community organizations, such as durable medical equipment companies, to support social activities for their program participants and graduates.[25]

Bickford and Hodgkin reported on the results of a national survey of PRPs that was conducted in 1987.[21] Most programs were in the outpatient setting, largely owing to reimbursement issues. Twenty-eight percent offered instruction on a one-to-one basis, 30% used a group format, and the remainder used a mixed group–individual format. Eighty-five percent of the programs used a multidisciplinary team consisting of at least two different disciplines. Team members included physicians, dietitians, respiratory therapists, nurses, social workers, physical and occupational therapists. Of the programs, 95% offered educational lectures, and 84% had exercise training sessions. The average program charge was 1232 dollars. Major differences in reimbursement were reported across the nation and the consensus was that programs should have measurable objectives to show the effectiveness of program components and to only bill for services that Medicare considers reimbursable.

Now that we know what type of patients to see, what type of program to offer, what allied health professionals are needed, and how to obtain maximum reimbursement, how does one develop a cost effective program?

Nicol and associates outlined three major components that are necessary to consider when planning a cost-effective PRP: strategic planning, budgetary process, and program promotion.

Strategic Planning

Strategic planning studies both the internal and external environment to establish a need for pulmonary rehabilitation. External environment issues would focus on establishing a need for a program based on the estimated number of patients in the community with COPD, would take into account the number of established PRPs in the community, and would explore the potential for adequate reimbursement. The internal environment study would consider program space needs, the availability of trained personnel to operate the program, if the program has good administrative support, and if it fits into the facility's goals and mission statement. Is there a physician with specialized training in the treatment of COPD that is available to be a medical director and supports the PRP? Only when the need is established for a PRP and the host facility agrees to support program development is one ready to move to the budgetary process.

Budgetary Process

The budgetary process outlines how to achieve a cost-effective program. It addresses the issues of program costs and expected revenue. Most facilities already have budgetary processes in place so it will be up to the individuals developing a program to make sure that the program costs versus benefits are in line. Program costs to be addressed include personnel, space for the service, and necessary equipment and supplies. Revenue sources need to be detailed.

Many questions need to be asked. For example, how many patients or patient visits per year must a program have to cover personnel, equipment, and office space costs? Will a "break-even" program meet the hospital's goals? How long will it take for the program to become self-sufficient and pay back startup costs?

Program Promotion

Careful planning should result in a cost-effective program, but initial and ongoing promotion cannot be overlooked if a program is going to continue to be cost-effective. The community may have enough patients with COPD for several programs, but if patients and their physicians are not aware of the benefit of PRPs, they will not use them. Appropriate promotional efforts will help provide programs with a steady supply of needy COPD patients.

PATIENT AFFORDABILITY

A cost-effective program should also be affordable to the participants. Probably the most important consideration to the patient is that his or her health insurance will help cover the program's cost. The PRPs have been shown to reduce the number of emergency department visits, doctor's office visits, and reliance on other health care providers.[7,10,13,19] All these effects help to decrease the cost of health care to the program participants.

An interesting note on attrition rates was reported by Shenkman.[20] She studied 40 patients of whom 29 failed to complete a PRP. Of the 29 patients who failed to complete the program, 18 had an income level of 10,000 to 15,000 dollars; however, the income level for the 11 patients completing the program was higher than 15,000 dollars/year. Many PRP participants are retired and on fixed incomes. If their health insurance does not pay all or most of the program cost, it is unlikely that they will be able to participate in a PRP. It would be worthwhile to explore tax-deductible charitable donations to hospitals to help especially needy patients. Most patients will report that a PRP is cost-effective (to them) if they have been able to decrease their symptoms and improve their quality of life, at an acceptable net cost to themselves.

SUMMARY

Pulmonary rehabilitation is cost-effective to the national economy, to third-party payers such as Medicare, and most important, to pulmonary patients. The savings from the reduction in hospital days alone is significant. It is worthwhile to evaluate program participants' vocational rehabilitation potential and help them return to their jobs or perhaps delay the onset of disability or retirement. The PRPs may help such patients lose less time from work because of illness.

Cost-effective programs can be developed. Probably the most important issues to consider are how to get more COPD patients referred to PRPs, and how to improve the level of reimbursement.

In our experience, it appears that the most successful programs share the major asset of dedicated and caring personnel, who not only devote their work hours to helping COPD patients, but also volunteer time outside of their jobs to help these people have better lives. These employees feel rewarded by the successes that their patients experience, another example of program effectiveness!

REFERENCES

1. Farnham A. No more health care on the house. Fortune 1989;Feb 27:71.
2. Center for Disease Control. United States health and prevention profile. U.S. Department of Health & Human Services. DHHS Publication No. (PHS) 90-1232. Hyattsville, MD: National Center for Health Statistics, 1990;Mar: 23, 24, 210.
3. Dunham JL, Hodgkin JE, Nicol J, Burton GG. Cost effectiveness of pulmonary rehabilitation programs. In: Hodgkin JE, Zorn EG, Connors GL, eds. Pulmonary rehabilitation: guidelines to success. Boston: Butterworth Publishers, 1984:389.
4. Hudson LD, Tyler ML, Petty TL. Hospitalization needs during an outpatient rehabilitation program for severe CAO. Chest 1976;70:606.
5. Johnson NR, Tanzi F, Balchum OJ, Gunderson MA, DeFlorio G, Hoyt A. Inpatient comprehensive pulmonary rehabilitation in severe COD: Barlow Hospital study. Respir Ther 1980;May/Jun:17.
6. Wright RW, Larsen DF, Monie RG, Aldred RA. Benefits of a community-hospital pulmonary rehabilitation program. Respir Care 1983;28:1474.
7. Bria W, Stillerman R, Lemoine M, Niles D, Soldega A. Effect of pulmonary rehabilitation on health care utilization. Chest 1987;92:153s.
8. Sneider R, O'Malley JA, Kahn M. Trends in pulmonary rehabilitation at Eisenhower Medical Center: an 11-years' experience (1976–1987). J Cardiopulm Rehabil 1988;11:453.
9. Porte P. Legislation and respiratory rehabilitation. Respir Care 1983;28:1498.
10. Toevs CD, Kaplan RM, Atkins CJ. The costs and effects of behavioral programs in chronic obstructive pulmonary disease. Med Care 1984;22:1088.

11. Kanner R. Impairment and disability evaluation and vocational rehabilitation. In: Hodgkin JE, Petty TL, eds. Chronic obstructive pulmonary disease: current concepts. Philadelphia: WB Saunders, 1987:172.

12. Petty TL, MacIlroy ER, Swigert MA, Brink GA. Chronic airway obstruction, respiratory insufficiency, and gainful employment. Arch Environ Health 1970;21:71.

13. Haas A, Cardon H. Rehabilitation in chronic obstructive pulmonary disease. Med Clin North Am 1969;53:593.

14. Holle RH, Williams DV, Vandree JL, Starks GL, Schoene RB. Increased muscle efficiency and sustained benefits in an outpatient community hospital-based pulmonary rehabilitation program. Chest 1988;94:1161.

15. Pulmonary rehabilitation: official American Thoracic Society position statement. Am Rev Respir Dis 1981;124:663.

16. Dudley DL, Martin CJ, Masuda M, et al. The psycho-physiology of respiration in health and disease. New York: Appleton-Century-Crofts, 1969:313.

17. Kass I, Dyksterhuis JE, Rubin H, Patil KD. Correlation of psychophysiologic variables with vocational rehabilitation outcome in patients with COPD. Chest 1975;67:433.

18. Petty TL, Branscomb BV, Farrington JF, Kettek LJ, Lindesmith LA. Community resources for rehabilitation of patients with COPD and cor pulmonale. Inter-society commission. Circulation 1974;49:A-4.

19. Stillerman R, Bria W, Lemoine M, Niles D, Soldega A. Effect of pulmonary rehabilitation program format on health care utilization. Chest 1987;92:153s.

20. Shenkman B. Factors contributing to attrition rates in a pulmonary rehabilitation program. Heart Lung 1985;14:57.

21. Bickford LS, Hodgkin JE. National pulmonary rehabilitation survey. Respir Care 1988;33:1033.

22. Hodgkin JE, Asmus RM, Connors GA. Pulmonary rehabilitation: designing a program that works. J Respir Dis 1987;8(12):55.

23. Braun SR, Driscoll S, Anderegg A, Barb J, Smith FR, Reddan WG. A decentralized rehabilitation program for chronic airway obstruction disease patient in small urban and rural areas of Wisconsin: a preliminary report. Public Health Rep 1981;96:315.

24. Callahan M. A prudent pulmonary rehabilitation program. Am J Nurs 1985:1368.

25. Nelson M. Putting some PEP into pulmonary rehabilitation. Respir Manage 1988;Jul/Aug:30.

26. Nicol J, Hodgkin JE, Connors G, et al. Strategies for developing a cost-effective pulmonary rehabilitation program. Respir Care 1983;28:1451.

GERILYNN L. CONNORS

LANA HILLING

SHARON GRINDAL

WILLIAM K. WILKISON

30

Reimbursement: A Determinant of Program Survival

Why do I need to know all the business office jargon of reimbursement? My job is to provide the highest quality of care possible to patients with lung disorders. The pulmonary rehabilitation program director's background is clinical with management involvement. Directors have chosen pulmonary rehabilitation because of the desire to work with patients with lung disease and to increase their quality of life. Program directors are experts in the pulmonary rehabilitation field, but must now also become experts in the reimbursement arena. With the diagnosis-related groups (DRGs), hospital cutbacks, and the volatile, ever-changing reimbursement practices, pulmonary rehabilitation directors have been forced to restructure their programs. Program survival is synonymous with reimbursement.

The intent of this chapter is to provide the pulmonary rehabilitation director and staff with the working knowledge of reimbursement from past to present. Understanding health care policy, third-party liability, the role of the business office in pulmonary rehabilitation reimbursement, and insurance terminology is just a start to avoiding unnecessary communication barriers. Reimbursement is a dynamic entity always changing and, at this critical period in the history of pulmonary rehabilitation, the director must become an expert in reimbursement. To know is to survive, to ignore will result in program suicide.

HISTORICAL PERSPECTIVE

Before the advent of Medicare and Medicaid programs, health care was covered under private insurances or paid privately. The first insurance program was established by the federal government in 1778 to provide merchant seamen with hospital care.[1] At that time, marine insurance was designed to protect the owners of vessels in world trade, which was later followed by fire insurance, life insurance, worker's compensation, and health and hospital insurance plans.[2] As early as 1900, a few states became involved with worker's compensation laws and by 1920, these laws were accepted by 42 states. Cash payments for a worker's time lost from the job because of injury or illness was the first benefit, later followed by coverage for health care and rehabilitation services.

The Medicare and Medicaid programs evolved over a 53-year period, starting with Theodore Roosevelt's Bull Moose party platform in 1912. The Bull Moose party platform first promoted the idea of having national health insurance.[1,2] Then in 1935 when the Social Security Act was passed, Congress submitted bills that called for equal access to health care, since the major source of health care financing was provided by not-for-profit, prepayment, or commercial insurance plans. During the Truman administration in 1949, a bill was introduced calling for comprehensive and universal health care coverage. This domestic legislation was stalled in Congress for years because of political squabbles debating whether it was politically feasible and if it should be narrowed in scope. Congress feared that this general medical insurance plan would be a "giveaway" program independent of need, would help the "well-off" American, cause a glut of demand for services beyond the supply capacity, and create excessive federal control of physicians, leading to socialism in America. Truman's advisors narrowed the eligibility of the plan to persons aged 65 years who had contributed to a Social Security program during their past employment. Intense debate occurred over some form of national health insurance from 1949 to 1965, when at last the Medicare and Medicaid laws were finally passed under the guidance of the Kennedy and Johnson administrations. The laws were amendments to the Social Security Act, which incorporated proposals from three sources: the Johnson administration to limit coverage of hospital and nursing home care financed through Social Security; the American Medical Association plan for "elder care" providing comprehensive benefits, but with limited eligibility; and the Republican Byrne proposal which was not compulsory and covered physician services and drugs. The Byrne proposal was also financed by general federal revenues instead of Social Security.[3] The complexity between governmental process and social policy is great, as seen in the health insurance arena. This legislation represents a singular approach to health care financing, since it establishes age-based entitlements and health care regardless of need.

OTHER WORLD INSURANCES

National health insurance programs that include people of all ages and income levels can be found throughout the major industrialized nations, except South Africa and the United States.[3,4] In 1883, Germany saw its first national health insurance. Britain passed national health service legislation in 1946. And the reform of the Italian health care system to national insurance occurred in 1978.

A brief description of the German socialized health care system follows. Each working person pays a monthly premium (depending on income) toward health care coverage. Unemployed persons can make an elective contribution. Most physicians are part of the national health care system and are thoroughly investigated when placed on a health care list. Patients may also choose a private physician who is not listed and self-pay. If they choose to do this, they may also pay an additional premium for private pay insurance. Patients purchase a *Krankenschein* or "sick permit" for a very small amount of money (approximately 25 cents). The Krankenschein is good for 3 months. When medical care is needed, the Krankenschein is presented to the physician. Medical bills are prepared in multiple copies: one bill goes to the Krankenkasse (cashier) and the other goes to the patient. The patient ensures the bill is correct and authorizes payment. This can be difficult with older persons who do not open their mail or do not understand the bill. It often has to be submitted many times. Respiratory care modalities in the home setting are very rare; for example, if the patient is ill enough to be receiving oxygen, they are considered ill enough to be hospitalized.

In Eastern European countries, a common custom for affluent patients is to bring gifts to the physicians to receive special care.[5] Regardless of the country, custom, or national health insurance program, the issues are the same—providing health care for the people.

SOURCES OF REIMBURSEMENT

Payment of medical care is by third-party payers or by the patient. A *third-party payer* is an organization that pays or insures medical/health expenses on behalf of its beneficiaries, members, or clients. Therefore, the patient receiving the medical service is considered the *first party*, the provider of the medical service is considered the *second party*, and the organization paying for the medical service is the third party (Fig. 30–1). A further explanation of the different sources for reimbursement can be seen in Table 30–1, which will be expanded on in the text.[6] Not all of these

TABLE   30-1.   Sources of Reimbursement

Nongovernmental health insurance programs
  Private, single, or group health insurance plans
  Health maintenance organizations (HMO)
  Preferred provider organizations (PPO)
  Medicare supplement

Federal and state health insurance programs
  Medicare
  Medicaid
  Uncompensated services (Hill–Burton)
  Comprehensive outpatient rehabilitation facility (CORF)
  Veterans administrative benefits
  Civilian health and medical programs of the uniformed services (CHAMPUS)
  Federal workers insurance

Auxiliary liability and casualty insurance programs
  Automobile insurance, related to auto accidents
  Worker's compensation, related to accidents on the job
  Business insurance coverage, related to injuries sustained on business premises
  Homeowners insurance, related to injuries sustained on the owner's premises
  Malpractice insurance on providers of health care
  Product and service liability insurance related to product or service-caused injuries

Other options of reimbursement
  Senior care
  Rehabilitation hospitals
  Grants

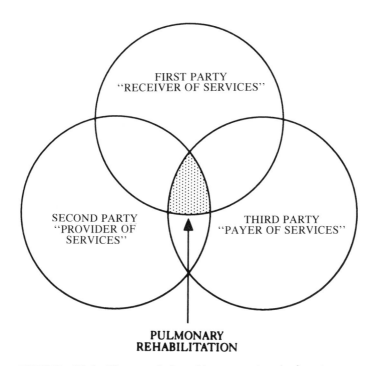

FIRST PARTY
"RECEIVER OF SERVICES"

SECOND PARTY
"PROVIDER OF
SERVICES"

THIRD PARTY
"PAYER OF SERVICES"

**PULMONARY
REHABILITATION**

FIGURE   30-1   The correlation of insurance terminology to
pulmonary rehabilitation is necessary for effective communication
with the insurance industry and for program reimbursement.
Pulmonary rehabilitation involves first-, second-, and third-party
involvement, with each party having a specific function as it
relates to pulmonary rehabilitation. Understanding the party
function is essential to ensure reimbursement for the program.

third-party payers have a direct relation to pulmonary rehabilitation. The major
sources for reimbursement (third-party payers) include the federal and state government programs, Blue Cross and Blue Shield plans, and commercial health insurance
companies.[1] A description of the major sources for reimbursement is presented in the
following section.

NONGOVERNMENTAL HEALTH
INSURANCE PROGRAMS

Private Health Insurance Programs

Nongovernmental private health insurance programs transfer individual risk to the
insured through a premium and are regulated by the state insurance commission.
Insurance was developed to protect people from economic losses. The first private
insurance was established at Baylor University Hospital in 1929 and was called
prepayment. It consisted of a group of school teachers who paid 50 cents per month
for a guarantee of up to 21 days of hospital care at no additional cost.[1] When the
depression occurred in the 1930s, the hospitals liked the Baylor group idea as a way to
keep solvent. Next came the Blue Cross plan which became the first organization to

develop financial protection to its subscribers against economic loss by hospitalization. At this time, payment for services was negotiated between the hospital and the plans. Then in 1939, the California State Medical Society organized the first Blue Shield plan, covering comprehensive medical and surgical services during a hospitalization for a premium of 1.70 dollars.[1] Blue Cross and Blue Shield plans were multiplying rapidly as well as were the number of plan subscribers. In 1948, the Supreme Court ruled that unions could negotiate health insurance benefits for their members. The Internal Revenue Service stepped into the scene ruling health insurance premiums paid by employers were considered a business expense and premiums paid by employees were not considered taxable income. These changes caused such an explosion in subscribers over the years that by 1978, approximately 83 million people had Blue Cross coverage and about 70 million people had Blue Shield coverage. Commercial insurances that were either mutual (owned by policy holders) or stock (outside ownership) also entered the health insurance market offering insurance for a number of personal risks. Over 700 commercial insurance companies wrote most of the health insurance policies in 1978.[7]

Health Maintenance Organizations

Prepaid Group Practice (PGP) was the original term used for Health Maintenance Organizations (HMO), and the first such group was Kaiser-Permanente. The Kaiser-Permanente Medical Care Program was developed in the 1930s by Henry J. Kaiser to keep his workers healthy and on the job. Kaiser was building pipelines and dams in remote locations quite a distance from physicians and hospitals. When Kaiser began building ships in World War II, the greatest problem he faced in meeting the war production quota was absenteeism caused by illness. So the Kaiser Health Clinic was started at numerous job sites to keep the workers healthy and productive.[8]

The HMOs use prospective payment, retrospective, cost-based remuneration that ensures the "get what you pay for and pay for only what you get" philosophy.[1,4] Primary care services are provided through the organization's physicians or through special contracts with private physicians. Hospital care is also covered under the plan. In 1973, the HMO act was passed which allowed the HMOs to qualify as Medicare providers. Each state legislation approves an HMO before it is allowed to operate in the state.

Preferred Provider Organizations

Preferred Provider Organizations (PPOs) represent another managed health care system on the rise. Health care purchasers want to control the cost of the health care provided yet offer flexibility to its beneficiaries.[9] The PPO is set up as a limited group of health care providers who agree to "discount" their fees to attract customers. The PPO may contract with an employer, insurance company, or other health care purchaser (i.e., HMOs, other PPOs). The negotiated fees for services provided by the PPO are normally below the usual market costs. The purchaser, in return, guarantees a patient–customer volume to the PPO with a quick response time for payment of services rendered. Even though the patient–customer is not locked into a specific PPO, the purchaser may offer incentives to the patient–customer to use the PPO by decreasing deductibles and coinsurance payments. The PPOs originally started out in the physician and hospital arena, but nonphysician groups (i.e., dentists, chiropractors, physical therapists) are now also developing PPOs.

Medicare Supplement

The last type of private health insurance is the Medicare supplement that developed after 1965 for Medicare beneficiaries who wanted an increase in coverage that was not provided by the Medicare program. Today, there are many options available in all areas of private health insurance, and it can become confusing to the subscriber as well as to the program director. The state's department of insurance has consumer guides on health insurance and is an excellent resource for consumer information and complaints.[10]

FEDERAL AND STATE HEALTH INSURANCE PROGRAMS

Medicare

When Medicare and Medicaid laws passed in 1965, the federal government became the largest third-party payer for health care services, and this continues to grow by leaps and bounds with the "graying of America." Medicare became an extension of Social Security, but it is not a national health insurance, since it applies only to the elderly and disabled, not to the entire population. Medicare is a program of contributory social insurance for beneficiaries and not a welfare program, since Part A (hospital care) is financed by Social Security contributions and Part B (physician and medical services) is voluntary and financed by contributions and general revenues.[1,11] When Medicare began, it was an entitlement program protected from annual appropriations and budgetary fluctuations.[4]

Medicare's initial administrative responsibilities were three-fold, to:[4]

1. Take care of the elderly
2. Develop reimbursement and regulatory procedures to keep providers happy
3. Satisfy the political hierarchy that Medicare expenditures were legal according to law

The Social Security Administration (SSA) had only dealt with beneficiaries, but when Medicare came under the SSA, it was faced with dealing with providers as well. The terms and rates for provider reimbursement under Medicare was described in the statutes, but in very *vague* language. This left the burden of decisions to the Medicare administrators and fiscal intermediaries. Third-party payers responsible for Medicare Part A are called *fiscal intermediaries,* and third-party payers responsible for Medicare Part B are called *carriers.* A description of the coverage under Medicare Part A and B is seen in Table 30–2. In fact, in the early years of Medicare, the delegation of administrative duties was left to the intermediaries and carriers, along with their own interpretation of responsibilities and control of claim payments. Regulatory powers were not used by Medicare to promote uniformity, consistency, or coordination of

TABLE 30-2. Explanation of Medicare Coverage

Part A: *INTERMEDIARIES* **Hospital Insurance**	Part B: *CARRIERS* **Medical Insurance**
Hospital care	Physician services
Skilled nursing facility	Outpatient hospital services*
Home health care	Durable medical equipment
Hospice care	"Other" medical services/supplies not covered by hospital insurance CORF

* All hospital outpatient services are covered by intermediaries, not carriers.

the administrative forces that implemented it, but allowed the providers and private intermediaries and carriers the responsibility to determine cost and quality.[4,12] Medicare expenditures varied with the demand for services, and the cost varied with supply, demand, and technology. In fact, technology was a prime reason for the spiraling cost of Medicare.[12,13] Before 1969, the Social Security Administration made little effort to control reimbursement or even to define "reasonable costs."[4] Review and control of Medicare was not dealt with in Washington, but in hundreds of state and local entities, both public and private. The Professional Standards Review Organization (PSRO) is one such entity for which physician peers evaluate medical decisions, formulate standards, and review Medicare use.[12] Over 200 PSROs do utilization review. The Certificate of Need (CON) was a state-enacted review of capital expenditures. With the development of utilization review, prospective rate setting, capital expenditure review, and health maintenance organizations (HMOs discussed earlier), the control of health providers was in the "central" hands of state-based, public organizations, or local organizations in the private sector.[4]

In 1977, Medicare underwent its biggest administrative reorganization since its inception in 1966, by leaving the Social Security Administration and going under the Health Care Financing Administration (HCFA). The HCFA is a department under the Health, Education and Welfare (HEW) secretary and this newly created department combined the administration of both the Medicare and Medicaid programs. The HCFA became a policy administrator to address Medicare. Also in 1977, to assist in the administration of Medicare, Congress passed the Medicare/Medicaid antifraud and abuse amendments. The purpose of this amendment was to enhance uniformity and quality of reporting, which led HCFA to develop a new System for Uniform Hospital Reporting (SUHR) in 1978. This new system would eliminate the hospital's ability to maximize reimbursement. The HEW administrators wanted to develop a common language and standard procedures for hospitals.

When Medicare started in 1965, there was no definable art and science known as Respiratory Therapy (RT). Therefore, there is no mention of respiratory therapy anywhere in the Medicare or Medicaid statutes. Iron lungs and oxygen tents can be found in the original statutes, but nothing on respiratory therapy. This exclusion continues to "haunt" the respiratory care profession today, causing us to fight for coverage for the patient population we work with.[14,15] In fact, in 1972, Medicare started to cover rehabilitation benefits for the disabled under SSA, and for individuals with end-stage renal disease.[2] During this period, amendments to Medicare allowed HMOs to be included in Medicare in a new "Part C" HMO option. The political caution allowing HMOs to be included was seen in the stringent writing of the provisions allowing this to happen.[4]

An old axiom HCFA has adhered to states, "If the service is reimbursable, it will be performed. If it is not, it won't."[14] As advances in treatment and technology continue, Medicare provision changes will continue. These changes will be more difficult, since the overall cost of medical care is spiraling higher and higher daily. In 1991, over 34 million elderly and disabled persons were enrolled in Medicare, with the overall cost reaching 104 billion dollars.

In 1977, Washington was concerned that the former approaches to controlling the cost of health care were not working.[4] A leaner, more efficient health care system was needed. Payment for Medicare coverage started out as retrospective, cost-based reimbursement. But on October 1, 1983, HCFA started to phase in payment rates for hospital admissions based on 467 Diagnosis-Related Groups (DRGs).[16–19] This changed Medicare from reimbursing by cost to reimbursing as priced per procedure, giving the Medicare administrators a powerful set of directive tools for the first time. The old system had abstract vocabulary relating to actual and reasonable cost. Medicare gathered, reviewed, and reimbursed the actual cost incurred by the providers in the old system, but lacked authority and consistency. The development of DRGs gave clearer terminology for the classification of hospital admissions, making it a prospective payment system, putting the government into a *proactive* role, and allowing the development of agendas for change. The DRGs changed Medicare from a cost system to a pricing system, resulting in the following:

1. The first time (1983) since the establishment of Medicare (1965) that the program bureaucracy, HCFA, had a role in initiating changes in the Medicare program.
2. The Medicare administrators now have a strong set of directive tools.
3. The DRGs have moved the public health insurance system of the United States (at least Medicare) toward a continental style of corporalized negotiators.
4. Medicare has changed from a claims-processing system to a rate-setting system.

In 1988, the Medicare Catastrophic Coverage Act expanded the Medicare benefits even more since Medicare began in 1965.[20] The goal was to ease the financial burden of the elderly and disabled by providing expanded Medicare coverage, but because of the nation's budget deficit, this act was repealed.

The future atmosphere of Medicare reimbursement will continue toward rate setting, as seen now in the physician services section.[21] Ambulatory Patient Groups (APGs) are being considered by Medicare as an approach to controlling outpatient costs.[22] They are being developed for HCFA by Health Systems International. Reimbursement would be based on the procedure or test and not on diagnosis.[23,24] This type of prospective payment system would likely be adopted eventually by non-Medicare third-party payers.[25] There is also talk that Medicare will begin to weigh cost as a factor in deciding if payment for new procedures, devices, and drugs is warranted. Cost will determine the future of expansion, continuation, or termination of services. Some have said this is the start of rationing medical technology. Table 30–3 gives the reader a chronologic development of health insurance in the United States from past to present. Now if we only knew what the future held for health care reimbursement.

Medicare Intermediaries

Each facility has an insurance intermediary acting as a liaison between the health care provider and Medicare. The intermediary is usually assigned to a hospital and, generally speaking, is a function of geographics. Intermediaries have evolved into state-oriented agencies. For example, an intermediary may service the entire country; yet may establish regions with designated personnel to handle all claims within that region. *Program directors should know who their intermediary is.* The intermediary must follow policies established by HCFA; however, HCFA has given intermediaries latitude to *interpret* general policy statements broadly or specifically. Most state intermediaries do not have specific pulmonary rehabilitation guidelines or policy established for Medicare reimbursement.[26,27] Without this specific reimbursement policy statement, the intermediary may search for a document on a broader level and use it as a rationale for their decision to reimburse or deny payment or, in fact, may simply create its own policy. Realistically, Medicare is not in the business of quality patient care, but aims to fulfill its obligation under the law for the least possible cost.

If there is no specific policy for an intermediary justifying reimbursement, the absence of policy may be the reason for denial. Yet another intermediary, given the same scenario, may provide reimbursement because reimbursement is not specifically prohibited, or it seems reasonable. As a result, different intermediaries, all reading from the same manual, have derived totally different policies dealing with reimbursement for pulmonary rehabilitation programs throughout the United States.

Some intermediaries send out policy or bulletin statements to the hospital and expect the department receiving the statements to provide copies to the departments or programs affected.[26,28] Other intermediaries send policy statements to specific individuals within the hospital. Some intermediaries are very organized and can provide current policy quickly and accurately. Other intermediaries consider it the hospital's responsibility to be knowledgeable of the multitude of amendment changes. An expanded discussion of intermediary policy for reimbursement may be found in the documentation section of this chapter.

Intermediaries may develop forms to simplify their request for needed data to determine reimbursement.[28,29] The HCFA documents, such as the UB82 (HCFA 1450) or HCFA 1500, are vehicles by which Medicare intermediaries can control the consistency and quality of information they receive. These forms also guide the provider.[30] The UB82 is the "bill" sent to the payer for the services rendered. The UB82 must be completed correctly for the bill to be processed. Errors on the UB82 may cause delays in payment or even an audit. Sample revenue codes that may be used

TABLE   30-3.   A Chronologic Development of Health Insurance in the United States

1778	Federal government establishes hospital care for merchant seamen
1912	First mention of national health insurance by Theodore Roosevelt's Bull Moose party platform
1920	42 states enact worker's compensation laws
1929	First private insurance established at Baylor University Hospital
1930s	Blue Cross plan first organized financial protection to its subscribers
1930s	Kaiser developed health clinics at job sites, the first HMO
1935	Social Security Act passed calling for equal access to health care
1939	California State Medical Society organized first Blue Shield plan
1948	Unions negotiate health insurance benefits for members and IRS rules on premiums as business expense for employers and nontaxable income for employees
1949	Truman administration introduces bill for comprehensive and universal health care coverage, but caused great debate in the legislature for the next 16 years
1965	Medicare and Medicaid legislation passes as amendments to the Social Security Act
1965	Medicare supplement insurances develop
1969	State and local PSROs and CON developed to review and control Medicare reimbursements
1972	Rehabilitation benefits for the disabled and individuals with end-stage renal disease get coverage under Medicare
1973	HMO Act passed to qualify HMOs as Medicare providers, "Part C," HMO option
1977	Medicare leaves SSA to be administered by HCFA, a department under HEW Secretary
1977	Medicare/Medicaid antifraud and abuse amendments pass to assist in the administration of Medicare/Medicaid
1978	HCFA develops a new system for uniform hospital reporting to enhance uniformity and quality
1982	CORF regulations established
1983	DRGs phased in for hospital admissions based on 467 DRGs, a prospective payment-rate setting system
1984	Tax Reform Act (the Deficit Reduction Act) makes changes in many domestic spending programs to reduce federal expenditures, especially laboratory testing
1986	Congress requires HCFA to establish PPS for outpatient services by October 1, 1991, ambulatory patient groups
1986	Omnibus Reconciliation Act gives states the option to expand Medicaid coverage as it pertains to respiratory care services for home ventilator-dependent individuals
1988	Medicare Catastrophic Coverage Act expands Medicare benefits, but because of the nation's budget deficit, it is repealed
1991	Over 34 million elderly and disabled people enrolled in Medicare, costing over 104 billion dollars

TABLE   30-4.   Sample Billing Codes

Services Billed	Revenue Code*
Respiratory therapy	410
Other respiratory services	419
Physical therapy	420
Occupational therapy	430
Pulmonary function laboratory	460
Other therapeutic services	949

* Medicare intermediaries and third-party payers may differ for the revenue codes required to bill for pulmonary rehabilitation services. Check with the insurance company for questions on billing PR and the revenue codes used.

on the UB82 when billing for pulmonary rehabilitation services are listed in Table 30–4. Each Medicare intermediary and third-party payer may stipulate the revenue codes to be used for billing pulmonary rehabilitation services.

As stated earlier, the hospital's Medicare intermediary is determined by geographics, so why would a hospital or corporation want to change their Medicare intermediary? This is not a choice that the hospital makes just because it wants to. A request must be submitted with legitimate business reasons to HCFA. If HCFA determines the facility has sufficient grounds for change, the request may be granted. When a facility proposes an intermediary change, it is generally a one-time, one-way event. One particular reason HCFA may allow a change is when many hospitals composing a corporation have to deal with different intermediaries which, in turn, make the hospital audits and cost reports a nightmare for the corporation. The corporation evaluates the available intermediaries, decides which is doing the best job and, in turn, asks to be affiliated with that one intermediary. Instead of numerous intermediaries, the corporation then has one intermediary for all hospitals in the corporation *independent of geographics.*

Whether it is a new pulmonary rehabilitation program or an already established program with an intermediary change, the program director should have a written program protocol to offer the hospital intermediary if one is available.[27] This helps provide the intermediary with a document and assists them with the decision to reimburse services provided in pulmonary rehabilitation.

Medicaid

The original purpose of Medicaid in the 1965 Social Security Act Amendments was to provide aid for dependent children and poor families. It is considered a "poor" peoples' program which aids welfare recipients and is funded jointly by federal and state agencies. Medicaid now covers less than half the poor in the United States, because nearly half of its dollars go to nursing home care of the indigent elderly.

The eligibility and benefit limits for Medicaid are set by federal law, but the state can take these rules and develop their own criteria. The state Medicaid program is administered through either a state organization, private insurance companies, or a combination of both.

The 1986 Omnibus Budget Reconciliation Act gave states the option of extending the Medicaid program to include reimbursement for home respiratory care services for ventilator-dependent individuals. States that choose not to provide this option under the Medicaid program make it necessary to legislate the option into law. Then the law dictates what the state does.[20]

A legislative bill passed in late 1989 in California amends the state's Welfare and Institutional Code to include respiratory care practitioner services (including pulmonary rehabilitation) as a benefit in the California Medicaid program called Medi-Cal.[31] The California Society of Respiratory Care is currently meeting with Medi-Cal administrators and policy makers to determine how the respiratory care services under Medi-Cal can be implemented by writing regulations and developing fee schedules.

Uncompensated Services

Health services provided at no charge or at reduced charges for people unable to pay are called uncompensated services under Titles VI (Hill-Burton) and Titles XVI of the Public Health Service Act.[32] A hospital that receives grants or loans (including construction, modernization, or equipment loans) is mandated under law to provide uncompensated services.

If a pulmonary rehabilitation candidate has no insurance (third-party payer or governmental program coverage) and the annual family income is not more than double the national poverty income level, the potential patient may be eligible for coverage of the program through uncompensated services. Check with your hospital business office for this specific determination.

Comprehensive Outpatient Rehabilitation Facility

A *comprehensive outpatient rehabilitation facility* (CORF) is a Medicare-certified health care facility that is defined as

> . . . a nonresidential facility that is established and operated exclusively for the purpose of providing diagnostic, therapeutic, and restorative services to outpatients for the rehabilitation of injured, disabled, or sick persons, at a single fixed location, by and under the supervision of a physician.
> (Code of Federal Regulations, 42: Section 485.51)[14,33,34]

Included in CORF services are: physicians' services, physical therapy, occupational therapy, speech–language pathology, respiratory therapy, prosthetic device services, orthotic device services, psychologic services, nursing care services, drugs, biologicals, supplies, appliances, equipment, and evaluation of the home environment. The regulations state in Section 410.100 (3e) that respiratory therapy services are

. . . services for the assessment, diagnostic evaluation, treatment, management, and monitoring of patients with deficiencies or abnormalities of cardiopulmonary function. These services include:

1. Application of techniques for support of oxygenation and ventilation of the patient and for pulmonary rehabilitation.
2. Therapeutic use and monitoring of gases, mists, and aerosols and related equipment.
3. Bronchial hygiene therapy.
4. Pulmonary rehabilitation techniques, such as exercise conditioning, breathing retraining and patient education in the management of respiratory problems.
5. Diagnostic tests to be evaluated by a physician, such as pulmonary function tests, spirometry and blood gas analysis.
6. Periodic assessment of chronically ill patients and their need for respiratory therapy.

There are several requirements in Section 410.105 that must be met for respiratory therapy services to be covered as CORF services. First, a physician must refer the individual to the facility and must also certify that the individual needs skilled rehabilitation services. Furthermore, the physician must provide the CORF with the individual's significant medical history, current medical findings, diagnosis(es), contraindications to any treatment modality, and rehabilitation goals. Second, all services must be furnished while the individual is under a physician's care, and they must be furnished on site at the CORF, except for the home evaluation visit. Finally, a written treatment plan prescribing the type, amount, frequency, and duration of services to be furnished, along with the diagnosis and rehabilitation goals, must be established and signed by a physician before treatment is begun. This treatment plan must be reviewed and updated at least every 60 days by the treatment team, and the physician must certify or recertify that the plan is being followed, that the patient is making progress, and that the treatment is having no harmful effects on the patient.

Included in the regulations are numerous requirements that facilities must meet to be certified by Medicare as a CORF. These include rules and regulations concerning personnel qualifications, clinical records, physical environment, and utilization review. An initial certification is granted to CORFs by Medicare upon successful inspection of the facility, its programs, policies, and procedures. Medicare then reinspects and recertifies all CORFs on a yearly basis.

There are several advantages for pulmonary rehabilitation programs to be provided in a CORF setting. First, the services are readily reimbursed by Medicare Part B-CORF, using a single procedure code (90020 for the initial visit, and 90060 for subsequent interim visits). These codes are specifically from the Health Care Procedure Code System for Medicare and do not always apply to other insurance companies. When billing Medicare for services provided to a patient in a CORF, it is necessary to send some materials from the patient's chart along with the bill. These include, at the very least, a copy of the current pulmonary rehabilitation orders and a signed treatment plan. Various Medicare intermediaries across the country require additional items, such as test interpretations and progress notes. In any event, it is important to document progress toward the patient's rehabilitation goals as necessary so that the therapy program does not appear to be one of maintenance. Second, the goal-directed, multidisciplinary environment of a CORF is very conducive to an effective, goal-oriented team approach. And third, the outpatient rehabilitation setting allows the patient to feel more at home than they might in a more institutionalized hospital setting.

Veteran Administration Benefits

The Veterans Administration (VA) provides care for service-connected veterans in the outpatient or inpatient setting, usually through one of their VA hospitals, clinics, or through a contract with an outside facility.[6] The VA patient does not pay out-of-pocket for services provided if the services are offered at the VA facility. Services contracted undergo a very complex process, and the regional political environment determines the funding for each VA facility within its region.

The VA hospitals are inconsistent when it comes to offering pulmonary rehabilitation services. There are no written policies or guidelines concerning referral to or reimbursement of pulmonary rehabilitation for VA patients. If a VA facility decides to provide pulmonary rehabilitation as one of their programs, they can do so. The problem comes with trying to find staffing, space, and supplies for such a program. The federally funded VA programs will depend on what is geographically available and appropriate for that particular facility. The VA patients interested in pulmonary rehabilitation should contact their closest VA hospital for information.

Civilian Health and Medical Programs of the Uniformed Services

The Civilian Health and Medical Programs of the Uniformed Services (CHAMPUS) is a government health care program covering *dependents* of military personnel (alive or deceased) and *retired* military personnel under aged 65 and their dependents.[6] Military personnel separating from the military (not retiring) are no longer eligible for CHAMPUS. Also, retired military personnel 65 years of age or older receive Medicare benefits. The CHAMPUS insurance coverage is often through private insurance companies, such as Blue Cross/Blue Shield. CHAMPUS has specific requirements for documentation of services rendered for reimbursement to occur, and knowledge of these requirements is important.[30]

Federal Workers Insurance

Government employees, such as postal service and civil service employees, have health benefit plans available to them. Health care coverage depends on the specific health care plan chosen by the employee.[35] Employees and their spouses and family should contact their health benefits department to determine applicable coverage for pulmonary rehabilitation, since insurance policy benefits for federal workers change frequently.

AUXILIARY LIABILITY AND CASUALTY INSURANCE

There are numerous insurance programs listed in Table 30–1, under auxiliary, liability, and casualty insurances, for people who sustain an injury from an automobile accident, an occupational accident, or from negligence of a liable party. This section will expand only on the Worker's Compensation program.[6]

Worker's Compensation Program

Each state has worker's compensation laws to represent a person's losses sustained from a work-related injury or disease.[6] The law covers compensation for medical expenses and lost wages. Each state determines the coverage limits available to this patient group. The Occupational Safety and Health Administration (OSHA) now requires screening spirometry of workers at work sites with potential occupational respiratory hazards, to avoid a disastrous health outcome and liability. It is possible for a patient, because of a work-related injury (i.e., federal black lung benefits), to have Medicare as a secondary payer to Workman's Compensation. Worker's compensation is an area of reimbursement for pulmonary rehabilitation directors to investigate further.

OTHER OPTIONS OF REIMBURSEMENT

Senior Membership Program

Specific financial programs for seniors have been developed in various hospitals in the United States. The financial program may be constructed differently with varying eligibility requirements. The hospital business office will have the specifics of the senior membership program if offered at your institution.

Rehabilitation Hospital

In a national survey, 97% of pulmonary rehabilitation programs reported that they accept outpatients, and 49% will work with inpatients as well.[36] Only 3% work only with inpatients.[36] With the rehabilitation hospital now exempt from DRGs, expansion to this type of facility is the current trend. However, the changes seen in outpatient reimbursement to a prospective rate-setting DRG arena is likely to affect rehabilitation hospitals in the future as well.

Grants

Grants may provide some financial support for some programs. Sources of grants include foundations, charitable organizations, universities, medical schools, and the federal government.[37]

As of 1985, there were 22,000 private grant-making foundations of various sizes with total resources of 50 billion dollars and annual grants of about 4 billion dollars.[38,39] The foundation's resources are maneuverable by their choice of selection, thereby shaping and altering the course of events. Getting money from a foundation is not impossible *if* the following requirements are met:

- The foundation the grant application is sent to must be interested in the project.
- Proposal submission and deadlines must be met.
- The proposal can prove that the organization submitting the request is capable of providing the service proposed.
- A strong case is built in support of the request, showing why the applicant deserves it.
- The dollar amount requested is consistent with the support levels of the foundation.
- The applicant should be willing to maintain a relation with the foundation, reporting regularly on the progress of the grant.
- The applicant does the necessary "homework" covering the specific goals, budget, time constraints, staffing needs, and such, in detail.

The process of seeking foundation support is a specialized, detailed, systematic process involving extensive research with detailed communication. The grant proposal must be tailored to the specific foundation, since over 1 million grant proposals are submitted yearly and only 7% are funded.[40,41] There are five basic types of foundations in the United States:

1. General purpose foundations
2. Special-sponsored foundations
3. Company-sponsored foundations
4. Family foundations
5. Community foundations

The Foundation Center Libraries (national and local) carry tremendous files of information on foundations and grant writing, and can be an invaluable resource.[13,43] Most state libraries also keep files on Internal Revenue Service (IRS) tax returns (990AR) for specific foundations, which represent the annual reports of the foundation's money distribution. These tax returns include a list of all the grants made during the year, with the name and address of each recipient, the amount, and the purpose of the grant. This can prove to be very valuable information to a grant writer. The *Foundation Directory* and the *Annual Register of Grant Support* are reference books containing information on thousands of private, company-sponsored, and community foundations. A source for federal grants is the *Catalog of Federal Domestic Assistance* and the *Federal Register, Commerce Business Daily*.[41]

Federal grants (i.e., National Institutes of Health) are usually given to universities. The small community hospital may be able to "get a piece of the pie" from a university grant if a close-working relation can be developed so the community hospital is seen as a "satellite" facility, necessary for the research project to attain the number of patients needed.

Preparing a grant proposal is the cornerstone for success in grant writing. There are five distinct types of grant proposals:[41]

1. Program proposals
2. Research proposals

3. Planning proposals
4. Training proposals
5. Technical assistance proposals

Once a determination has been made for the type of grant needed, the writing begins. A proposal should include a cover letter, proposal abstract, introduction, problem–needs assessment, program objectives, procedures–methods, personnel evaluation, budget, future funding, and the necessary attachments to be included.[40] Many books are written specifically on grant writing, and reference should be made to them to avoid unnecessary errors in writing and submitting a grant.

Some foundations and federal agencies have specific application forms to be filled out for a grant to be awarded. Once the grant is submitted, it is not uncommon for 6 to 9 months to pass before a response is heard. Grant writing is *not* an easy process and involves time and energy, but the rewards are worth the effort.

DOCUMENTATION FOR REIMBURSEMENT

Pulmonary rehabilitation is a young discipline in the health care arena, trying to grow up in a time when regulatory changes occur rapidly. Consequently, directors of pulmonary rehabilitation programs must be familiar with the facility's business office responsibilities concerning third-party payer reimbursement for the program. Pulmonary rehabilitation programs are based on a team approach, and a person from the business office should be considered a vital team member. Together, a rapport may be developed to address reimbursement issues that occur in the program. This liaison with the business office should be the program director's first step in understanding reimbursement.

When a reimbursement problem arises with a patient's claim, the first step is to determine why. Technical problems are often the cause, but these errors can stem from various departments such as the pulmonary rehabilitation department, the medical records department, or the billing department. Table 30–5 details where and why errors may arise for patient claim denial with third-party payers. It is important for the program director to establish the reason for claim denials so correction of the problem can occur, resulting in payment of the services rendered.

There are no "golden rules" for documentation, but specific do's and don'ts apply.[44,45] Third-party payers may develop specific policy statements for the reimbursement of pulmonary rehabilitation services. The Medicare intermediary, Blue Cross of California, has published a bulletin for providers under their jurisdiction that outlines the intermediary's interpretation for pulmonary rehabilitation reimbursement.[26]

The HCFA, in response to a 1990 inquiry from the American Association of Respiratory Care (AARC) to establish greater uniformity in handling of pulmonary rehabilitation claims under Medicare, has advised their Medicare Part-B carriers about the potential usefulness of the *Blue Cross of California Pulmonary Rehabilitation Guidelines* to assist in processing pulmonary rehabilitation claims.[26,46] The HCFA suggested the *California Medicare Blue Cross Pulmonary Rehabilitation Guidelines* might help minimize problems in the processing of pulmonary rehabilitation claims.[46]

TABLE 30-5. Where and Why Errors Occur Resulting in Denial of Claims

Department	Type of Errors	The Reasons*
Pulmonary rehabilitation	Technical documentation	Charting date not the same as billing date; charting incomplete; medical necessity not established from submitted documentation; noncovered service
Medical records	Technical	Incomplete records sent for audit; audit deadline date not met
Billing office	Technical billing	UB82 errors, start of care date same as onset date; billing codes incorrect; improper diagnosis used

* Tables 30-7 and 30-9 expand on the reasons for denial of patient claims.

So the second step to take in understanding pulmonary rehabilitation reimbursement is to determine your facility's Medicare intermediary and find out if a policy exists for pulmonary rehabilitation reimbursement. If a policy is nonexistent, take this opportunity to extend your expertise to the third-party payer in developing such a document or sharing the California Medicare Blue Cross Bulletin on Pulmonary Rehabilitation with them.[7,26] Reviewing current third-party payer guidelines for reimbursement for outpatient respiratory therapy, physical therapy, occupational therapy, or speech therapy services, is also helpful in understanding the trends for reimbursement of the third-party payer.[7]

Pulmonary rehabilitation documentation for reimbursable services should reflect the need for professional supervision of the treatment or constant professional judgment. The medical necessity of the pulmonary rehabilitation treatment is the foundation stone for documentation. Table 30–6 highlights the documentation needs of a pulmonary rehabilitation program for optimizing reimbursement. Periodic review of the patient's progress by the pulmonary rehabilitation team physi-

TABLE 30-6. Pulmonary Rehabilitation Treatment Documentation Needs for Reimbursement

- Individualized to patient needs
- Reasonable and necessary for diagnosis
- Individualized toward patient goals and accomplished in a predictable time frame
- An insurance policy (i.e., Medicare, Blue Cross, or other) benefit
- Objective, measurable and functional
- Matched to itemized ledger on bill according to date of service and duration of treatment

cian or other team members is important to determine the patient's achievement of goals and objectives established in the treatment program. Is the treatment restorative and rehabilitative, as opposed to preventative? Changes in the patient's treatment plan are based upon the patient's progress, and documentation must show the changes that occur.

Preventative care and maintenance is never a Medicare benefit and almost never a benefit under third-party payer thinking.[1,7] Education is not a Medicare benefit, but the AMA National Commission on the Cost of Medical Care stated that educational programs were important in providing the patient–consumer with the knowledge and assistance to make cost-effective utilization decisions.[1,2] Table 30–7 summarizes *noncovered* Medicare services and Table 30–8 summarizes *covered* Medicare services. It is always necessary to be aware of the types of covered services when charting on a patient. If progress is not shown owing to an exacerbation of the patient, documentation of this is critical so the claim will not be denied. Each treatment session should be documented carefully in a systematic format. During the initial evaluation, the following information should be documented in the patient's record:

- Diagnosis
- Subjective findings
- Estimate of rehabilitation potential

TABLE 30-7. Medicare Noncovered Services

Preventative services
Health promotion
Education to increase knowledge
Research
Maintenance care
Support group
Team conference
Documentation time
Discharge summary
Nutritional counseling
Social services
Biofeedback for relaxation training
Poor rehabilitation potential exists with patient
Prepackaged programs
Routine exercise
Unreasonable and unnecessary care
Duplication of service with OT, PT, RN, RT
Routine screening evaluations
Films/videos
Routine psychologic evaluation and treatment
Treatment not medically necessary

TABLE   30-8.   **Services Covered by Medicare**

Treatment reasonable and necessary
Services individualized
Services provided are of a skilled level of care
Patient demonstrates rehabilitation potential
Medically necessary
Skilled intervention needed
Specific problems identified to necessitate treatment
Education or training related to self-management treatment

- Objective findings
- Frequency and duration of treatment
- Treatment goals
- Intervention or plan of action
- Precautions, if applicable

The format for documenting progress of each treatment session may be accomplished in a variety of styles, from the Subjective, Objective, Assessment, and Plan (SOAP) format, to narrative, notes, grids, or flowsheets. Regardless of the charting style, it must be organized and easily followed by the team members who review the notes, or by third-party payers who may perform an audit.[45]

The team conference, changes in the treatment plan, and the discharge summary are other areas of pulmonary rehabilitation documentation. When completing the discharge summary, the following areas should be covered:

- Attainment of goals
- Functional status of patient at discharge compared with that at program admission (i.e., specific improved ADLs, exercise tolerance)
- Training sessions given to the patient
- Home program plan
- Follow-up care

All documentation should be signed, dated, legible, and completed in black ink. Thorough documentation is vital.[45] Remember, the medical records used to determine medical necessity when being audited is the documentation.

Programs that experience Medicare reimbursement difficulties should query the intermediary. Whether being audited or denied, the program director should find out what steps to take in adjudicating claims denied and the reasons for the denial. The billing office receives the claim correction notices that provide the reasons for denial. With this information, the pulmonary rehabilitation program can develop a plan to correct errors, deficiencies, and inconsistencies. Quality assurance in the charting arena is critical.

Different systems can be used to govern reimbursement. Current Procedural Terminology (CPT-4) is a coding system at the service level (what was done for the patient). Whereas International Classification of Diseases (ICD)-9-CM is a coding at the diagnostic level (what is wrong with the patient). Both systems can be used jointly to govern reimbursement. As CPT coding becomes more refined, there will be more and more items available and more services on an outpatient basis will have CPT codes assigned to them. As of July 1, 1987, hospitals were instructed to change from ICD-9-CM coding to CPT-4 coding for outpatient procedures.[47,48]

Close supervision to address the issue of digital accuracy of inputting the claim by the billing office (such as dates, policy numbers, start of care, diagnosis, and plan of care/assessment form) to the third-party payer is important.[28–30] There are a lot of opportunities for claims to be delayed or denied because of a technical flaw at this step. Flaws such as these may prevent the claim from ever getting to the point at which the intermediary can look at what pulmonary rehabilitation service was being submitted for the patient. Table 30–9 expands the list of PRP technical errors that can result in full or partial claim denial.

When it comes to patients understanding their pulmonary rehabilitation charges on the bill, the following suggestions may alleviate problems and confusion. The patient, before entering the pulmonary rehabilitation program, should have a complete understanding of what his or her responsibility is concerning the financial aspects of the program (the program fee). Completeness of admission registration is critical to allow prompt filing of the claim to third-party payers. It is helpful to keep a copy of the patient's outpatient registration form in your pulmonary rehabilitation chart. If components of the program are not covered by third-party payers, the patient should understand and agree in writing to be responsible for those components. Development of a fee-structured payment plan for non-covered components may still allow patients to participate in the pulmonary rehabilitation program and should be agreed to and signed by the patient before starting the program. Billing can be frustrating both to the program and the patient. There-

TABLE 30-9. Potential Technical Errors from the Pulmonary Rehabilitation Department

Incomplete physician orders

Nonspecific orders

Frequency and duration of treatment not specific (i.e., 1–3 times/wk for 2–4 wk)

Blanket order for pulmonary rehabilitation

PRN care order

Orders do not match specific services provided

Unsigned and dated orders, and certifications

Use of physician signature stamp

No cosignature for PT/OT aide or exercise physiologist on daily notes

Billing for services not documented

Itemized services billed on financial ledger do not match daily documentation

Services rendered not a Medicare benefit

Lack of need documented in initial assessment

Lack of patient progress toward goals

fore, every effort must be made to assure that the billing process is completed as efficiently and accurately as possible at the conclusion of the program.

Staff or patients who have comments or concerns about the issues of reimbursement for pulmonary rehabilitation should not hesitate to contact their congressional representatives or insurance company. It is only when concerns are communicated that the initial steps can be taken to resolve difficulties in reimbursement.[7,27,49]

Awareness leads to control. By working together, programs can continue to grow, mature, and demonstrate expertise in handling insurance difficulties. The pulmonary rehabilitation program staff needs to be involved in the cost containment of the program. Table 30–10 lists ways for the team to achieve this. Reimbursement is crucial for program survival, but cost containment is also necessary and a key element in program management.

SUMMARY

The 1988, National Pulmonary Rehabilitation Survey,[36] responses to program reimbursement showed program costs were covered by a combination of private insurance and Medicare for 51% of the patients, by Medicare for only 45%, and by an HMO for 9%. Six percent of the patients had no insurance. The diversity of program reimbursement is seen in the survey, but untapped reimbursement avenues do exist for pulmonary rehabilitation program directors who look beyond the routine third-party payers.[32,50,51]

As pulmonary rehabilitation experts, we must not become isolated in a world of constant change.[25] Many pulmonary rehabilitation programs direct their attention to the end-stage lung disease patient instead of focusing on the need for earlier detection, treatment, and prevention of lung disease. The average age of the pulmonary rehabilitation candidate is older than 65, so treating patients earlier in the disease process means reaching a younger population that would benefit from pulmonary rehabilitation and help reduce medical costs. The insurance industry has a commitment to make insurance affordable, and the medical profession must also assist in making medical care affordable.[2] As pulmonary rehabilitation experts, we need to show the cost saving of pulmonary rehabilitation programs to third-party payers. Pulmonary rehabilitation for the lung-impaired patient is today's challenge

TABLE 30-10. Cost Containment Strategies for Pulmonary Rehabilitation

- Determine patient eligibility for program admission
- Individualize program for patient
- Develop patient goals and objectives to achieve success
- Discharge patient if progress not shown
- Show cost-effectiveness of the program through outcomes
- Determine specific goals and objectives for the program
- Document the patient's improved ability to make personal and societal health care decisions postprogram
- Rehabilitating patients earlier in the disease process will help reduce medical costs

and tomorrow's option. In 1988, Hodgkin stated that an effective pulmonary rehabilitation program is no longer a luxury but a necessity for lung patients.[52] This is even more true today. Let us continue to strive for pulmonary rehabilitation program recognition in the third-party payer industry. Remember, program survival is up to us.

REFERENCES

1. LeBrun P, Miller JM, Raichel TM. Financing for health education services in the United States. Prepared by Blue Cross and Blue Shield Association per HHS Contract 200-79-0916, 1980.

2. Mittelmann M. Rehabilitation issues from an insurer's viewpoint: past, present, future. Arch Phys Med Rehabil 1980;61:587.

3. Guccione AA. Needs of the elderly and the politics of health care. Phys Ther 1988;68:1386.

4. Brown LD. Technocratic corporatism and administrative reform in medicine. J Health Politics Policy Law 1985;10:579.

5. Bunch D. Hungary: a dynamic country in the midst of change. AARC Times 1990;14(1):30.

6. Health Care Financing Administration. Guide to third party liability. US Dept of Health and Human Services. US Government Printing Office 1980;311-168:421.

7. Simmock P, Bauer DW. Reimbursement issues in diabetes. Diabetes Care 1984;7:291.

8. Nielsen WA. The golden donors, a new anatomy of the great foundations. New York: Truman Talley Books, 1985:3.

9. Horting M. Preferred provider arrangements: selecting the plan that's right for your practice. Clin Manage 1987;7(2):34.

10. State of California Department of Insurance. Buyer's guide to insurance information. Consumer Service Bureau, Dec 1986.

11. U.S. Department of Health and Human Services, Healthcare Financing Administration. Medicare 1991 handbook. Rockville MD: 1991, Publ HCFA 10050, 1991.

12. Ruby G, Banta HD, Burns AK. Medicare coverage, medicare costs and medical technology. J Health Politics Policy Law 1985;10:141.

13. Purtilo RB. Saying "no" to patients for cost-related reasons, alternatives for the physical therapist. Phys Ther 1988;68:1243.

14. Porte P. Legislation and respiratory rehabilitation. Respir Care 1983;28:1498.

15. Dobson A, Langenbrumer JC, Pelovitz SA, Willis JB. The future of Medicare policy reform: priorities for research and demonstrations. Health Care Financing Rev 1986;Annu Suppl:1.

16. Ellis RP, McGuire TG. Insurance principles and the design of prospective payment systems. J Health Econ 1988;7:215.

17. Fetter RB, Freeman JL, Mullin RL. DRGs: how they evolved and are changing the way hospitals are managed. Pathologist 1985;Jun:17.

18. Russell LB, Manning CL. The effect of prospective payment on medicare expenditures. N Engl J Med 1989;320:439.

19. Dore D. Effect of the Medicare prospective payment system on the utilization of physical therapy. Phys Ther 1987;67:964.

20. Momii KR, Wilson CN. The Medicare Catastrophic Coverage Act of 1988: implications for respiratory care. Respir Care 1989;34:201.

21. Ortbals DW. Effect of Medicare/Medicaid reimbursement policies on diagnostic methodology in the physician's office. Diagn Microbiol Infect Dis 1986;4:1435.

22. Alternate care. Trouble ahead: PPS outpatient radiology limits. Hospitals 1988;Apr:72.

23. Grimaldi PL. Inching toward prospective payment for outpatient hospital care. Nurs Manage 1987;18:26.

24. Lutz S. Ambulatory patient groups: the new DRG challenge. Mod Healthcare 1989;Dec:20.

25. Korcok M. Will DRG payments creep into all U.S. health insurance plans? Can Med Assoc J 1984;130:912.

26. Provider Services Department, Blue Cross of California. Pulmonary rehabilitation guidelines. Medicare Bull 224. Blue Cross of California 1987:1.

27. American Diabetes Association task force on financing quality health care for persons with diabetes. Third–party reimbursement for diabetes outpatient education. 1986.

28. Mutual of Omaha Insurance Company, Supply Department. Medicare Division, Nebraska. HCFA Form 700/701/702, 1989.

29. Provider Services Department, Blue Cross of California. Therapy information update form. Medicare Bull 1989; 256 (Spec Iss), April.

30. CHAMPUS/CHAMPVA News. Wisconsin, 1988; Sept.

31. Lopez B. Alternate-site RC reimbursement: one AARC affiliates' success story. AARC Times 1991;15:58.

32. Providers guide to uncompensated services regulations. 1988;Feb:1.

33. Comprehensive outpatient rehabilitation facility. Fed Reg Nov 14, 1986;51(220):41332.

34. Comprehensive outpatient rehabilitation facility. Rules and regulations. Fed Reg Dec 15, 1982;47(241):56282.

35. United States Office of Personnel Management, retirement and insurance group. 1990 enrollment information guide and plan comparison chart; for US Postal Service Employees. Washington, DC. 1989:RI70-2.

36. Bickford LS, Hodgkin JE. National pulmonary rehabilitation survey. In: Hodgkin JE, ed. Pulmonary rehabilitation symposium. J Cardiopulm Rehabil 1988;8(11):473.

37. Bunch D. Getting reimbursed for your pulmonary rehabilitation program. AARC Times 1988;12(3):52.

38. Shellow JR. A guide to national grantmakers. In: Shellow JR, ed. Grant seekers guide. New York: Moyer Bell, 1985:91.

39. Shellow JR. A guide to regional and local grantmakers. In: Shellow JR, ed. Grant seekers guide. New York: Moyer Bell, 1985:269.

40. Shellow, JR. Approaching the grantmaker and preparing a proposal. In: Shellow JR, ed. Grant seekers guide. New York: Moyer Bell, 1985:31.

41. Grasty WK, Sheinkopf KG. Successful fundraising. A handbook of proven strategies and techniques. New York: Charles Scribner's Sons, 1982:262.

42. Shellow JR. Appendix IV. The foundation center. In: Shellow JR, ed. Grant seekers guide. New York: Moyer Bell, 1985:467.

43. Shellow JR. Appendix V. State grantmaking directories. In: Shellow JR, ed. Grant seekers guide. New York: Moyer Bell, 1985:481.

44. Bernstein F, Eguchi K, Messer S, et al. Documentation for outpatient physical therapy. Clin Manage 1987;7:28.

45. Elkousy NM, Komorowski D, Foto M, Welch MA, Doyle P. Outpatient pulmonary rehabilitation: a Medicare fiscal intermediary's viewpoint. In: Hodgkin JE, ed. Pulmonary rehabilitation symposium. J Cardiopulm Rehabil 1988;11:492.

46. Brown C. AARC waits for word on CLIA '88. AARC Times 1990;14(9):11.

47. Carter K. New reimbursement rules for outpatient services will mean more work, higher costs for hospitals. Mod Healthcare 1987;Aug:78.

48. Horting M. Filing insurance claims. Clin Manage 1987;7(2):24.

49. American Diabetes Association. Position statement. Third-party reimbursement for outpatient diabetes education and counseling. Diabetes Care 1990;13:36.

50. Horting M. Marketing strategies: how to enhance reimbursement for PT services. Clin Manage 1987;7(2):36.

51. Seltzer MS. Appendix II. The funding search renewed. In: Shellow JR, ed. Grant seekers guide. New York: Moyer Bell, 1985:459.

52. Bunch D. Pulmonary rehabilitation: the next ten years. AARC Times 1988;12(3):54.

JOHN E. HODGKIN

Benefits and the Future
of Pulmonary Rehabilitation

As emphasized in the preceding chapters, pulmonary rehabilitation requires the use of many individually tailored treatment modalities and a management system that can be used to help the patient achieve and maintain the highest functional capacity possible. Table 31–1 outlines the components of a pulmonary rehabilitation program. Many benefits have been reported by pulmonary rehabilitation programs using these components of care;[1-3] however, information is still accumulating concerning the specific benefits of each individual component.[4,5] The overall benefits reported for pulmonary rehabilitation programs, the demonstrated benefits for each individual component of care, and the future of pulmonary rehabilitation will be discussed in this chapter.

OVERALL BENEFITS
OF PULMONARY REHABILITATION

A summary of benefits reported through the use of the pulmonary rehabilitation modalities described in this book are listed in Table 31–2. Many patients achieve a reduction in respiratory symptoms as well as a reversal of anxiety and depression and an improvement in ego strength.[6-8] For most patients all programs have reported an enhanced ability to carry out activities of daily living (ADL),[9-20] improved exercise ability,[21-45] and better quality of life.[9-20,46,47] Some patients are able to continue or return to gainful employment.[9,12,48-51]

A reduction in the number of days of hospitalization required by patients with chronic obstructive pulmonary disease (COPD) following pulmonary rehabilitation has been reported by several groups.[4,7,14,19,52-58] Patients at Loma Linda University Medical Center had a reduction from approximately 19 days of hospitalization in the year before the pulmonary rehabilitation program down to slightly over 6 days of hospitalization per year in the year after completion of the program.[52] This trend has continued for the 8 years for which follow-up data are available.[4] Some might suggest that this reduction in days of hospitalization simply reflects the deaths of the sickest patients during the initial years of follow-up, leaving healthier patients toward the end. However, the curve for hospital days required over the 8-year period for only

TABLE 31-1. Components of Pulmonary Rehabilitation

General

Patient and family education
Proper nutrition including weight control
Avoidance of smoking and other inhaled irritants
Avoidance of infection (immunization, other)
Proper environment
Adequate hydration

Medications

Bronchodilators
Expectorants
Antimicrobials
Corticosteroids
Cromolyn sodium
Digitalis
Diuretics
Psychopharmacologic agents

Respiratory therapy techniques

Aerosol therapy
Oxygen therapy
Home use of ventilators

Physical therapy modalities

Relaxation training
Breathing retraining
Chest percussion and postural drainage
Deliberate coughing and expectoration

Exercise conditioning

Occupational therapy

Evaluate activities of daily living
Outline energy-conserving maneuvers

Psychosocial rehabilitation

Vocational rehabilitation

TABLE 31-2. Demonstrated Benefits of Pulmonary Rehabilitation

Reduction in respiratory symptoms

Reversal of anxiety and depression and improved ego strength

Enhanced ability to carry out activities of daily living

Increased exercise ability

Better quality of life

Reduction in hospital days required

Prolongation of life in selected patients (i.e., use of continuous oxygen in patients with severe hypoxemia)

those patients still surviving at the end of 8 years is very similar to the curve reflecting data for all of the patients (Fig. 31–1). This decrease in hospital days obviously can result in a substantial reduction in cost by helping the patient function more adequately in an outpatient setting (see Chapter 29).

Although the decrement in 1-second forced expiratory volume (FEV_1) for a normal population is estimated to be 20 to 30 mL/year,[59,60] the reported decrement for patients with COPD ranges from 40 to 80 mL/year.[61–68] No study yet reported has shown a significant alteration in the mean rate of decrease in the FEV_1 in COPD patients with significant respiratory impairment.

It has commonly been stated that there is no evidence that good comprehensive care (i.e., pulmonary rehabilitation) for patients with COPD improves survival. Whereas, it is clear that oxygen therapy significantly improves survival in COPD patients who are seriously hypoxemic,[69,70] many believe that the other aspects of care commonly used in these persons do not significantly prolong life. There have been some reports in recent years suggesting that pulmonary rehabilitation can lead to improved survival.

In a study comparing 252 rehabilitated COPD patients with 50 control subjects selected from an outpatient clinic, Haas and Cardon reported 5-year mortality rates from respiratory failure of 22% in the rehabilitated patients compared with 42% in the control subjects.[12]

In a study by Petty and associates,[61] 182 COPD patients (mean FEV_1 0.94 L)

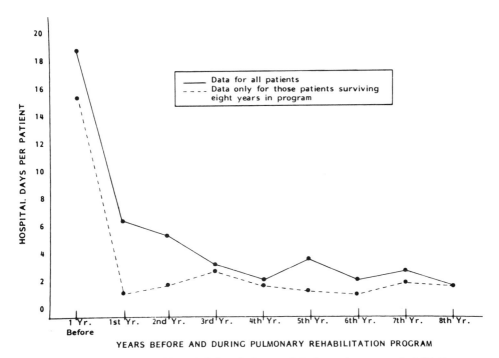

FIGURE   31–1   Analysis of hospital days before and during pulmonary rehabilitation program, Loma Linda University Medical Center.

were accepted for pulmonary rehabilitation between 1966 and 1968. Survival at 5 years was 41% and at 10 years 17%. The patients who participated in this program in Denver did have a significantly improved survival at 2.5 years when compared with the only other study of COPD patients residing at a similar high altitude [i.e., the Veterans Administration (VA) cooperative study by Renzetti and coworkers].[67] Survival at 2.5 years in the Petty study was 67% compared with 50% in the VA cooperative study. Petty has also reported a slightly better survival in patients participating in his pulmonary rehabilitation program compared with matched control patients who received ordinary care in the same community.[71]

In a report by Hodgkin and associates,[72,73] patients (mean FEV_1 1.53 L) participating in a university hospital pulmonary rehabilitation program showed significantly better long-term survival than in most previous reports (i.e., 5-year survival was 86% and 10-year survival was 64%). Patients in this study had chronic bronchitis or emphysema, or both (patients with asthma were excluded). Of particular note is that pulmonary function was less impaired in these patients than in patients studied by Burrows,[74] Postma,[66,75] and Petty.[61] In an attempt to compare patients from this pulmonary rehabilitation program with those of like severity getting "ordinary care," but not participating in a formal pulmonary rehabilitation program, patients with an FEV_1 above 1.24 L from this study were compared with patients with a similar level of pulmonary impairment from the Burrows Chicago study.[62] Patients from the pulmonary rehabilitation program of Hodgkin and associates with an FEV_1 above 1.24 L had a significantly better survival rate at 2 to 7 years of follow-up than patients with similar impairment in the Burrows study. The authors point out that the improved survival rate in the group, as a whole, was probably because the patients entering this study had milder disease. However, they also suggested that the good comprehensive respiratory care, including careful follow-up, they received through the pulmonary rehabilitation program might also be responsible for some of the improved survival compared with that in earlier studies.

Sneider and colleagues reported more recently on the experience of patients participating in their pulmonary rehabilitation program between 1976 and 1987.[58] During this time, 1592 patients were evaluated; however, only 212 patients (mean FEV_1 1.19 L) completed the entire pulmonary rehabilitation program. Patients with a reactive airway disease component were not specifically excluded from this study population. Survival at 5 and 10 years was 86% and 66%, respectively. Of particular interest was the comparison performed by Sneider and associates of their 212 patients completing the pulmonary rehabilitation program with the 921 patients with similar impairment who did not complete the rehabilitation program and with a group of 100 randomly selected patients with similar pulmonary impairment who died of COPD at the same hospital over a 10-year period.[58] Five-and 10-year survival was significantly better in those completing the full pulmonary rehabilitation program than in the other two groups from the same community and cared for at the same hospital.

Burns and coauthors reported on the results of patients (mean FEV_1 0.97 L) completing a pulmonary rehabilitation program between 1977 and 1987.[76] Subjects in this study had emphysema or chronic bronchitis. Survival figures from this study were better than in the Burrows Chicago study.[74] Survival in the Burrows Chicago study (200 COPD patients with a mean FEV_1 1.04 L) was 52% at 5 years and 23% at 10 years, compared with 58% at 5 years and 32% at 10 years in the Burns and associates study.

One of the largest studies to suggest that good comprehensive care may improve survival in patients with COPD is the National Institutes of Health intermittent positive-pressure breathing (NIH/IPPB) trial.[77,78] In this study, a definite effort was made to exclude asthmatics and include only those patients with typical COPD (985 patients with a mean FEV_1 1.03 L). The age and level of pulmonary impairment was similar to those of subjects in the Burrows Chicago study.[74] A comparison of patients from the NIH/IPPB study was made with those from the Burrows Chicago group. Survival was similar in patients with the least obstruction (postbronchodilator FEV_1 above 42.5% of predicted) but, as shown in Figure 31–2, in more obstructed patients, survival was greater in the NIH/IPPB patients than in the Burrows Chicago group. The most obvious potential explanation for this would seem to be that the Burrows group did not exclude hypoxemic patients, as was done in the NIH/IPPB study. The first 3 years of the Burrows study preceded the widespread use of home oxygen therapy, which was given to patients in the NIH/IPPB study who became significantly hypoxemic during the study. This is a reasonable explanation for survival differences among patients with the most severe obstruction (FEV_1 below 30.5% of predicted); 22% of the NIH/IPPB patients in this category eventually received home oxygen therapy. However, only 12% of the less-obstructed patients (FEV_1 of 30.5% to 42.5% of predicted) in the NIH/IPPB study received home

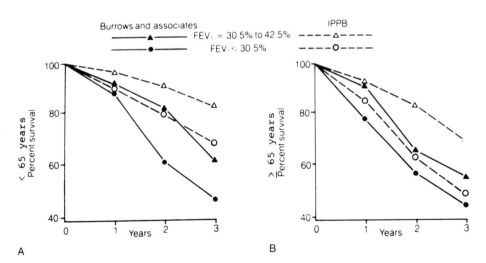

FIGURE 31–2 Comparison of survival in the NIH IPPB trial (*open symbols*) with that of patients in the Burrows Chicago study (*closed symbols*). (**A**) patients <65 years of age at the start of the studies; (**B**) patients ≥65 years of age. *Circles* are patients with baseline postbronchodilator FEV_1 <30.5% predicted; *triangles* are patients with baseline postbronchodilator FEV_1 30.5–42.5% predicted. (*From* Anthonisen NR, et al: Prognosis in chronic obstructive pulmonary disease. Am Rev Respir Dis 1986; 133: 14–20, with permission. Courtesy of the American Lung Association.)

oxygen, so this is not likely to account for mortality differences between these two groups. It is certainly possible that survival was better in the NIH/IPPB patients because of the careful assessment, education, and intense follow-up (i.e., good comprehensive respiratory care) they received as being part of a clinical trial.

The factors that affect survival in patients with COPD have recently been reviewed.[79] The patient's postbronchodilator FEV_1 and age have been reported to be the best predictors of survival.[71,78,79] It seems logical that if one is to achieve a significant reduction in the rate of respiratory function deterioration and definite prolongation of life, the principles of pulmonary rehabilitation discussed in this book must be applied earlier in the course of the disease, rather than waiting until severe, irreversible impairment of function is present.

BENEFITS OF INDIVIDUAL COMPONENTS OF CARE

General Care

Although there is little published data relating to the value of education for respiratory patients, teaching patients about their disease process and its treatment is an integral part of pulmonary rehabilitation (see Chapter 5).[3,80,81] A pulmonary rehabilitation knowledge test has been developed and validated.[82] Education of COPD patients can indeed improve their knowledge of the disease.[81,83]

A careful initial and ongoing evaluation of nutritional factors and diet patterns can be of major help to patients with COPD. In obese patients, a weight-reduction program can lessen the work of breathing, resulting in reduced dyspnea. A high-protein diet, with multiple small feedings, can help prevent or reverse weight loss. Adequate protein in the diet may help reverse the diminished respiratory muscle strength observed in poorly nourished individuals.[84] Proper nutrition may help patients resist respiratory infections,[85] and may help restore the ventilatory response to hypoxemia[86] and hypercapnia[87] in severely malnourished individuals.

A reduced body weight has been reported to be a predictor of survival, independent of the FEV_1.[88] Currently, data is insufficient to determine whether adequate nutrition support in undernourished patients with COPD can significantly alter their survival. There are, however, a couple of short-term studies that suggest that further clinical research to help answer this question is justifiable (see Chapter 17).[89,90]

Cessation of smoking is fundamental to achieving both subjective and objective improvement. Stopping smoking generally results in an improved appetite, decreased dyspnea, a reduction in cough and sputum, and improved pulmonary function.[91,92] Smoking has been shown to increase the risk of getting an influenza infection.[93]

One of the most impressive studies to show that stopping smoking can improve survival in COPD patients was that reported by Postma and associates (Fig. 31–3).[75] (For a comprehensive discussion of smoking cessation, see Chapter 8.)

Influenza vaccinations on a yearly basis and a one-time pneumococcal vaccine help reduce the risk from these specific infections. Since dehydration can thicken sputum, promote atelectasis, and drop cardiac output, adequate hydration should be promoted.

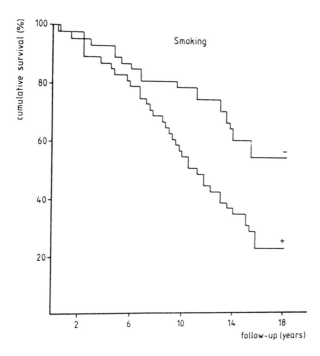

FIGURE 31–3 Cumulative survival curves of continuing smokers ($+$) and ex-smokers ($-$). (Postma DS, Sluiter HJ. Prognosis of chronic obstructive pulmonary disease: the Dutch experience. Am Rev Respir Dis 1989; 140:S100, with permission. Courtesy of the American Lung Association.)

Medications

Almost all patients benefit from a consistent program of medications, as described in Chapter 9. On the other hand, all these agents have significant side effects and, when not used appropriately, can lead to a worsening of the patients' conditions. Bronchodilators not only help relieve bronchospasm, but also can enhance mucociliary clearance. Antimicrobial agents limit the airway irritation and inflammation that result from bacterial respiratory infections. Corticosteroids lessen airway inflammation and the adverse effects of allergy; in addition, they facilitate bronchodilator action. Cromolyn sodium can reduce the need for corticosteriods and hospitalizations in many patients with bronchial asthma. Digitalis is useful for patients with left ventricular failure, and diuretics are beneficial for the fluid retention of both left ventricular decompensation and cor pulmonale. A proper use of psychopharmacologic agents can significantly improve some COPD patients' ability to function effectively.[94]

Respiratory Therapy Techniques

Aerosol Therapy

Various devices have been used to aerosolize bronchodilators, corticosteroids, mucolytic agents, bland mist, and antimicrobials. Although there is little support for aerosolization of the latter three agents, clearly inhalation of bronchodilators and corticosteroids are of tremendous benefit. Inhalation of a sympathomimetic medication accomplishes much faster bronchodilation, with less systemic side effects, than oral ingestion or parenteral administration of the same agent. Inhalation of beclomethasone, triamcinolone, or flunisolide accomplishes much of the corticosteroid benefit, while avoiding significant systemic side effects. (See Chapter 10 for a discussion of aerosol therapy.)

Oxygen Therapy

Supplemental oxygen has clearly been shown to lessen the adverse effects of significant hypoxemia, such as pulmonary hypertension, polycythemia, and neuro-psychologic dysfunction, in COPD patients. Specifically, patients with an arterial PO_2 of 55 mm Hg or less on room air (O_2 saturation $\leq$ 88%) or a PaO_2 less than 60 mm Hg (O_2 saturation < 90%) and evidence of polycythemia or right heart dysfunction, when stable, have achieved a significant prolongation of life with continuous oxygen when compared with nocturnal oxygen only.[69,70] Patients who develop significant hypoxemia during exercise testing can improve their exercise tolerance by using supplemental oxygen during exercise training.[21,95–99] Nocturnal oxygen is beneficial for patients with sleep apnea or arrhythmias resulting from nocturnal hypoxemia.[100–102] The use of supplemental oxygen in patients with severe hypoxemia can result in a survival rate similar to that of those patients with similar levels of impairment (i.e., FEV_1, but without severe hypoxemia) (Fig. 31–4).[78]

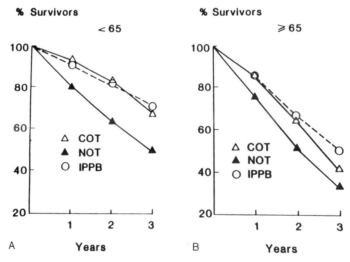

FIGURE 31–4 Comparison of survival in the NIH IPPB and NOTT trials. All patients had baseline FEV_1 <30% predicted. (**A**) Data from patients <65 years of age at the beginning of the studies; (**B**) patients ≥65 years of age. Circles are patients in the IPPB trial; open triangles are hypoxemic patients receiving continuous oxygen therapy; closed triangles are hypoxemic patients receiving 12 hours of nocturnal oxygen therapy. (From Anthonisen NR, et al. Prognosis in chronic obstructive pulmonary disease. Am Rev Respir Dis 1986; 133:14, with permission. Courtesy of the American Lung Association.)

Intermittent Positive-Pressure Breathing

Although IPPB therapy has been used for many years in patients with pulmonary disorders, there is no evidence that in outpatients with chronic disease such therapy has any advantage over less expensive and simpler methods of aerosol therapy, such as cartridge inhalers or compressor nebulizers. The National Heart, Lung and Blood Institute-sponsored study comparing IPPB devices with compressor nebulizers in outpatients with COPD showed no difference in morbidity or mortality between subjects in the two groups.[77] This evaluation in approximately 1000 patients did not demonstrate any role for periodic IPPB treatments in outpatients with COPD. The continuous use of IPPB (continuous mechanical ventilation) is important for the rehabilitation of individuals requiring ventilator assistance (see Chapter 20).

Physical Therapy Modalities

Relaxation Training

Relaxation techniques, such as biofeedback or listening to soothing music, can help anxious patients reduce fear and tension and are recommended especially for persons of the high-fear–high-anxiety personality type.[103] Some relaxation exercises, such as contracting and then relaxing skeletal muscle groups, can help reduce dyspnea and anxiety in patients with COPD.[104] Other demonstrated benefits include a slowing of the respiratory rate and heart rate, as well as lowering oxygen consumption.[105,106]

Breathing Retraining

Training patients with COPD to slow their respiratory rate, with a prolonged exhalation (with or without the use of pursed-lips), helps control dyspnea, and results in improved ventilation, increased tidal volume, decreased respiratory rate, and a reduced alveolar–arterial oxygen difference.[107–112] Such a breathing pattern not only helps relieve dyspnea, but can improve the ability to exercise and carry out activities of daily living. The benefits of pursed-lips breathing are often discovered by patients before instruction from health care providers.

An improvement in respiratory muscle strength and endurance can be accomplished through voluntary normocapnic hyperpnea[113–117] and inspiratory resistive loading.[118] Although ventilatory muscle endurance training can result in improved exercise capacity in some COPD patients,[116–119] the role of such training as part of a pulmonary rehabilitation program is yet to be determined. There is as yet no evidence that respiratory muscle training adds to the improved quality of life or enhanced activity level that can be achieved through exercise training using the lower or upper extremities.

Deliberate Cough, Chest Percussion, and Postural Drainage

Teaching patients how to cough properly can result in more effective expectoration. The forced expiration technique for coughing has been recommended for expectorating sputum.[120,121] Postural drainage, when accompanied by chest percussion or vibration, has also been recommended to help clear secretions from obstructed airways. A comprehensive review of chest physical therapy was recently published.[122] In the outpatient setting, postural drainage should be reserved for those patients with large amounts of sputum (i.e., > 30 mL/day).[123] There is no evidence that postural drainage is beneficial in COPD patients with smaller amounts of sputum during acute exacerbations of COPD[124] or in those with uncomplicated pneumonia.[125] (See Chapter 12 for a review of chest physical therapy.)

Exercise Conditioning

Exercise training should be an essential component of any pulmonary rehabilitation program. Many studies have reported an enhanced exercise level following such general conditioning exercises as walking, bicycle riding, and swimming.[21-45,126] One of the greatest benefits of exercise conditioning is to allow patients to do more work for any given oxygen consumption. In effect, patients become more efficient, while increased muscular strength and endurance enable them to accomplish more. As a result, the patients can better tolerate daily activities. Although exercise training has little effect on pulmonary function, it has been shown to improve sleep, appetite, and tolerance of dyspnea. Recent studies demonstrate that COPD patients can exercise at a considerably higher percentage of their maximal exercise capacity than has been used in the past.[127-129] Exercise training above the anaerobic threshold has been reported to achieve more benefit than training at a lower intensity level in those COPD patients who can exercise to a high enough intensity to reach an anaerobic threshold.[130-132] Adding upper extremity exercise training to traditional lower extremity training has been recommended for COPD patients.[133-135] (See Chapter 14 for a comprehensive discussion concerning a proper approach to exercise training in patients with respiratory disease.)

Occupational Therapy

An occupational therapy evaluation will help identify short- and long-term reasonable goals for the patient, will disclose tasks important for the patient that are precluded by functional limitations, and will reveal patterns of daily activities in which energy can be conserved for other productive and worthwhile activities. A home visit will often disclose unexpected architectural barriers and often leads to significant improvement in the patient's ability to function in his or her real world (see Chapter 13).

Psychosocial Rehabilitation

Patients disabled from COPD usually exhibit emotional reactions, such as depression, fear, anxiety, hostility, and denial, all of which impair functional capacity.[6] Psychotherapy, sometimes requiring a psychologist or psychiatrist, and the appropriate use of psychopharmacologic agents can help such patients better cope with their disease process (see Chapter 15). Sexual dysfunction is often a crucial obstacle to overall rehabilitation[136] and should be addressed positively (see Chapter 16). The attitudes transmitted by the entire rehabilitation team and the interactions among the patients themselves contribute significantly to the psychologic rehabilitation of the patients.

Vocational Rehabilitation

Although some individuals will be able to continue working in their current occupations, many others will need to either quit their jobs or to alter the type of work performed. A proper evaluation and categorization of the patient's capacities are important for successful rehabilitation. The goals of vocational and functional rehabilitation may vary after a careful evaluation of the patient. Possible goals would include

- Returning the patient to the job he or she is holding
- Returning the patient to the same occupational field or plant, but in a different job or location
- Changing the occupational field to a totally different one in which the patient can use previous training or existing skills
- Job retraining and reemployment
- Entering the patient in a sheltered workshop program
- Retraining the individual in daily self-care with an eye to conservation of effort and efficiency of motion[137]

When a patient is employed in an unhealthy environment, or if further progression of disease is anticipated and continued employment therefore unlikely, it may be desirable to train the patient for a sedentary occupation in anticipation of the future course of the disease (see Chapter 18).

FUTURE CHALLENGES OF PULMONARY REHABILITATION

While no slowing of the rate of pulmonary function deterioration has been shown, reports of improvement in survival through pulmonary rehabilitation were reviewed earlier in this chapter. Clearly, instituting a comprehensive respiratory care program earlier in the course of a patient's disease will provide more potential for favorably altering the course of the disease.

Unfortunately, only 20% to 35% of participants in most smoking cessation programs quit permanently. An enhanced effort needs to be directed toward the prevention of respiratory diseases, rather than waiting until significant respiratory impairment has occurred to begin instituting therapy.

Although some modalities—including bland mist inhalation, aerosolization of mucolytic agents, aggressive oral hydration, some phases of breathing retraining, postural drainage, and some psychologic support programs—lack scientific validation, these techniques have been integral in programs with documented overall success. Even though these methods have much anecdotal support and are employed by persons with a great deal of experience in pulmonary rehabilitation, their inclusion in any rehabilitation program should be combined with an open mind toward redefinition of their indications and value.

Visiting nurse associations and such socially oriented service programs as Meals on Wheels and Homemakers exist in many locations; however, the establishment of such services in every community would substantially enhance the ability for pulmonary rehabilitation programs to provide adequate support.

Each member of the pulmonary rehabilitation team needs to be aware of the factors that can lead to failure of rehabilitation so that the potential for success can be optimized. Reasons for failure include lack of competent and dedicated medical supervision, inclusion of inappropriate patients, lack of individualization so that the very sick and the nearly well get the same treatment, poor communication with referring physicians, lack of objective documentation, excessive commercialization, poor organization of the program, lack of personal access between the patients and the program on an ongoing basis, failure to establish realistic goals, and lack of flexibility in the therapeutic offerings.

One of the major limitations continues to be the failure of many primary care physicians to refer their pulmonary patients for rehabilitation. Teams must redouble their efforts to familiarize these physicians with the benefits of rehabilitation.

The problem faced by some patients and programs to have pulmonary rehabilitation paid for needs to be resolved. Third-party payers must be educated about the cost savings (e.g., reduction in hospital days) that can be achieved through pulmonary rehabilitation.

Steps should be taken to ensure that the special needs and problems of respiratory patients are incorporated into the curricula of allied health schools, including nursing, respiratory therapy, physical therapy, occupational therapy, and dietetics. Psychologists, psychiatrists, chaplains, social workers, and others involved in counseling patients and their families need to be knowledgeable about the special needs of respiratory patients to fully meet their needs.

The routine use of spirometry in the office can assist in identifying respiratory disease before clinical signs and symptoms appear. Decreasing the number of persons who smoke remains the key to a major reduction in disability from respiratory disease.

REFERENCES

1. Hodgkin JE, ed. Chronic obstructive pulmonary disease: current concepts in diagnosis and comprehensive care. Park Ridge, IL: American College of Chest Physicians, 1979.

2. Make BJ. Pulmonary rehabilitation: myth or reality? Clinics in Chest Med 1986; 7(4):519.

3. Hodgkin JE, Farrell MJ, Gibson SR, et al. Pulmonary rehabilitation: official ATS statement. Am Rev Respir Dis 1981;124:663.

4. Hodgkin JE. Pulmonary rehabilitation: structure, components, and benefits. In Hodgkin JE, ed. Pulmonary rehabilitation symposium. J Cardiopulm Rehabil 1988;8:423.

5. Ries AL. Position paper of the American Association of Cardiovascular and Pulmonary Rehabilitation. Scientific basis of pulmonary rehabilitation. J Cardiopulm Rehabil 1990;10:418.

6. Dudley DL, Glaser EM, Jorgenson BN, Logan DL. Psychosocial concomitants to rehabilitation in chronic obstructive pulmonary disease. Chest 1980;77:413, 544, 677.

7. Agle DP, Baum GL, Chester EH, Wendt M. Multidiscipline treatment of chronic pulmonary insufficiency: 1. Psychologic aspects of rehabilitation. Psychosom Med 1973; 35:41.

8. Fishman DB, Petty TL. Physical, symptomatic, and psychological improvement in patients receiving comprehensive care for chronic airway obstruction. J Chronic Dis 1971;24:775.

9. Kass I, Dyksterhuis JE. The Nebraska COPD rehabilitation project: a program to

identify the factors involved in the rehabilitation of patients with chronic obstructive pulmonary disease: a multidisciplinary study of 140 patients. Final Report, Social and Rehabilitation Service, DHEW Project RD-2517-m. Omaha: University of Nebraska, Dec 1971.

10. Daughton DM, Fix AJ, Kass I, Patil KD, Bell CW. Physiological–intellectual components of rehabilitation success in patients with chronic obstructive pulmonary disease (COPD). J Chronic Dis 1979;32:405.

11. Miller WF, Taylor HF, Pierce AK. Rehabilitation of the disabled patient with chronic bronchitis and pulmonary emphysema. Am J Public Health 1963;53(suppl):18.

12. Haas A, Cardon H. Rehabilitation in chronic obstructive pulmonary disease: a five-year study of 252 male patients. Med Clin North Am 1969;53:593.

13. Cherniack RM, Handford RG, Svanhill E. Home care of chronic respiratory disease. JAMA 1969;208:821.

14. Petty TL, Nett LM, Finigan MM, Brink GA, Corsello PR. A comprehensive care program for chronic airway obstruction: methods and preliminary evaluation of symptomatic and functional improvement. Ann Intern Med 1969;70:1109.

15. Kimbel P, Kaplan AS, Alkalay I, Lester D. An in-hospital program for rehabilitation of patients with chronic obstructive pulmonary disease. Chest 1971;60(suppl):6S.

16. Shapiro BA, Vostinak-Foley E, Hamilton BB, Buehler JH. Rehabilitation in chronic obstructive pulmonary disease: a two-year prospective study. Respir Care 1977;22:1045.

17. White B, Andrews JL Jr, Mogan JJ, Downes-Vogel P. Pulmonary rehabilitation in an ambulatory group practice setting. Med Clin North Am 1979;63:379.

18. Krumholz RA. Pulmonary outpatient rehabilitation: a four-year follow-up. Ohio State Med J 1973;69:680.

19. Moser RM. Rehabilitation of the COPD patient. Lesson 40 in weekly update: pulmonary medicine. Princeton, NJ: Biomedia, 1979.

20. Balchum OJ. Rehabilitation in chronic obstructive pulmonary disease. Arch Environ Health 1968;16:614.

21. Pierce AK, Paez PN, Miller WF. Exercise therapy with the aid of a portable oxygen supply in patients with emphysema. Am Rev Respir Dis 1965;91:653–659.

22. Miller WF. Rehabilitation of patients with chronic obstructive lung disease. Med Clin North Am 1967;51:349.

23. Woolf CR, Suero JT. Alterations in lung mechanics and gas exchange following training in chronic obstructive lung disease. Dis Chest 1969;55:37.

24. Bass H, Whitcomb JF, Forman R. Exercise training: therapy for patients with chronic obstructive pulmonary disease. Chest 1970;57:116.

25. Woolf CR. A rehabilitation program for improving exercise tolerance of patients with chronic lung disease. Can Med Assoc J 1972;106:1289.

26. Rusk HA. Pulmonary problems. In: Rehabilitation medicine, 3rd ed. St Louis: CV Mosby, 1971.

27. Schrijen F, Jezek V. Haemodynamic variables during repeated exercise in chronic lung disease. Clin Sci Mol Med 1978;55:485.

28. Nicholas JJ, Gilbert R, Gabe R, Auchincloss JH Jr. Evaluation of an exercise therapy program for patients with chronic obstructive pulmonary disease. Am Rev Respir Dis 1970;102:1.

29. Unger KM, Moser KM, Hansen P. Selection of an exercise program for patients with chronic obstructive pulmonary disease. Heart Lung 1980;9:68.

30. Brundin A. Physical training in severe chronic obstructive lung disease. Scand J Respir Dis 1974;55:25.

31. Wasserman K, Whipp BJ. Exercise physiology in health and disease. Am Rev Respir Dis 1973;112:219.

32. Degre S, Sergysels R, Messin R, et al. Hemodynamic responses to physical training in patients with chronic lung disease. Am Rev Respir Dis 1974;110:395.

33. Alpert JS, Bass H, Szucs MM, Banas JS, Dalen JE, Dexter L. Effects of physical training on hemodynamics and pulmonary function at rest and during exercise in patients with chronic obstructive pulmonary disease. Chest 1974;66:647.

34. Shephard RJ. Exercise and chronic obstructive lung disease. Exerc Sport Sci Rev 1976;4:263.

35. Hughes RL, Davison R. Limitations of exercise reconditioning in COLD. Chest 1983;83:241.

36. Mall RW, Medeiros M. Objective evaluation of results of a pulmonary rehabilitation program in a community hospital. Chest 1988;94:1156.

37. Cockcroft AE, Saunders MT, Berry G. Randomized controlled trial of rehabilitation in chronic respiratory disability. Thorax 1981;36:200.

38. McGavin CR, Gupta SP, Lloyd EL, McHardy JR. Physical rehabilitation of chronic bronchitis: results of a controlled trial of exercises in the home. Thorax 1977;32:307.

39. Sinclair DJM, Ingram CG. Controlled trial of supervised exercise training in chronic bronchitis. Br Med J 1980;280:519.

40. Busch AJ, McClements JD. Effects of a supervised home exercise program on patients with severe chronic obstructive pulmonary disease. Phys Ther 1988;68:469.

41. Strijbos JH, Koeter GH, Meinesz AF. Home care rehabilitation and perception of dyspnea in chronic obstructive pulmonary disease (COPD) patients. Chest 1990;97:109S.

42. Chester EH, Belman MJ, Bahler RC, et al. Multidisciplinary treatment of chronic pulmonary insufficiency: 3. The effect of physical training on cardiopulmonary performance in patients with chronic obstructive pulmonary disease. Chest 1977;72:695.

43. Carter R, Nicotra B, Clark L, et al. Exercise conditioning in the rehabilitation of patients with chronic obstructive pulmonary disease. Arch Phys Med Rehabil 1988;69:118.

44. Holle RHO, Williams DV, Vandree JC, Starks GL, Schoene RB. Increased muscle efficiency and sustained benefits in an outpatient community hospital-based pulmonary rehabilitation program. Chest 1988;94:1161.

45. Tydeman DE, Chandler AR, Graveling BM, Culot A, Harrison BDW. An investigation into the effects of exercise tolerance training on patients with chronic airways obstruction. Physiotherapy 1984;70:261.

46. Atkins CJ, Kaplan RM, Timms RM, Reinsch S, Lofback K. Behavioral exercise programs in the management of chronic obstructive pulmonary disease. J Consult Clin Psychol 1984;52:591.

47. Guyatt GH, German LB, Townsend M. Longterm outcome after respiratory rehabilitation. Can Med Assoc J 1987;137:1089.

48. Petty TL, MacIlroy ER, Swigert MA, Brink GA. Chronic airway obstruction, respiratory insufficiency, and gainful employment. Arch Environ Health 1970;21:71.

49. Lustig FM, Haas A, Castillo R. Clinical and rehabilitation regime in patients with chronic obstructive pulmonary disease. Arch Phys Med Rehabil 1971;53:315.

50. Kass I, Dyksterhuis JE, Rubin H, Patil KD. Correlation of psychophysiological variables with vocational rehabilitation outcome in patients with chronic obstructive pulmonary disease. Chest 1975;67:433.

51. Fix AJ, Daughton D, Kass I, et al. Personality traits affecting vocational rehabilitation success in patients with chronic obstructive pulmonary disease. Psychol Rep 1978;43:939.

52. Burton GG, Gee G, Hodgkin JE, Dunham JL. Respiratory care warrants studies for cost-effectiveness. Hospitals 1975;49:61.

53. Hudson LD, Tyler ML, Petty TL. Hospitalization needs during an outpatient rehabilitation program for severe chronic airway obstruction. Chest 1976;70:606.

54. Lertzman MM, Cherniack RM. Rehabilitation of patients with chronic obstructive pulmonary disease. Am Rev Respir Dis 1976;114:1145.

55. Jensen PS. Risk, protective factors, and supportive interventions in chronic airway obstruction. Arch Gen Psychiatry 1983;40:1203.

56. Johnson HR, Tanzi F, Balcham OJ, et al. Inpatient comprehensive pulmonary rehabilitation in severe COPD. Respir Ther 1980;May/Jun:15.

57. Nichol J, Hodgkin JE, Connors G, et al. Strategies for developing a cost-effective pulmonary rehabilitation program. Respir Care 1983;28:1451.

58. Sneider R, O'Malley JA, Kahn M. Trends in pulmonary rehabilitation at Eisenhower Medical Center: an 11-years' experience (1976–1987). In: Hodgkin JE, ed. Pulmonary rehabilitation symposium. J Cardiopulm Rehabil 1988;11:453.

59. Ferris BG Jr, Anderson DO, Zickmantel R. Prediction values for screening tests of pulmonary function. Am Rev Respir Dis 1965;91:252.

60. Kory RC, Callahan R, Boren HG, Syner JC. Veterans Administration–Army cooperative study of pulmonary function. I. Clinical spirometry in normal men. Am J Med 1961;30:243.

61. Sahn SA, Nett LM, Petty TL. Ten-year follow-up of a comprehensive rehabilitation program for severe COPD. Chest 1980;77(suppl):311.

62. Burrows B, Earle RH. Course and prognosis of chronic obstructive lung disease. N Engl J Med 1969;280:397.

63. Boushy SF, Thompson HK, North LB, Beale AR, Snow TR. Prognosis in chronic obstructive pulmonary disease. Am Rev Respir Dis 1973;108:1373.

64. Diener CF, Burrows B. Further observations on the course and prognosis of chronic obstructive lung disease. Am Rev Respir Dis 1975;111:719.

65. Emergil C, Sobol BJ. Longterm course of chronic obstructive pulmonary disease: a new view of the mode of functional deterioration. Am J Med 1971;51:504.

66. Postma DS, Burema J, Gimeno F, et al. Prognosis in severe chronic obstructive pulmonary disease. Am Rev Respir Dis 1979;119:357.

67. Renzetti AD Jr, McClement JH, Litt BD. The Veterans Administration cooperative study of pulmonary function. III. Mortality in relation to respiratory function in chronic obstructive pulmonary disease. Am J Med 1966;41:115.

68. Davis AL, McClement JH. The course and prognosis of chronic obstructive pulmonary disease. In: Current research in chronic respiratory disease. Proceedings of the 11th Aspen emphysema conference. Arlington, VA: DHEW, 1968:219.

69. Medical Research Council working party. Longterm domiciliary oxygen therapy in chronic hypoxic cor pulmonale complicating chronic bronchitis and emphysema. Lancet 1981;1:681.

70. Nocturnal oxygen therapy trial group. Continuous or nocturnal oxygen therapy in hypoxemic chronic obstructive pulmonary disease: a clinical trial. Ann Intern Med 1980;93:391.

71. Petty TL. Pulmonary rehabilitation. Am Rev Respir Dis 1979;122(suppl):159.

72. Bebout DE, Hodgkin JE, Zorn EG, Yee AR, Sammer EA. Clinical and physiological outcomes of a university-hospital pulmonary rehabilitation program. Respir Care 1983;28:1468.

73. Hodgkin JE, Branscomb BV, Anholm JD, Gray LS. Benefits, limitations and the future of pulmonary rehabilitation. In: Hodgkin JE, Zorn EG, Connors GL, eds. Pulmonary rehabilitation: guidelines to success. Boston: Butterworth, 1984.

74. Traver GA, Cline MG, Burrows B. Predictors of mortality in chronic obstructive pulmonary disease. Am Rev Respir Dis 1979;119:895.

75. Postma DS, Sluiter HJ. Prognosis of chronic obstructive pulmonary disease: the Dutch experience. Am Rev Respir Dis 1989;140(suppl):S100.

76. Burns MR, Sherman B, Madison R, et al. Pulmonary rehabilitation outcome. J Respir Care Pract 1989;2:25.

77. Intermittent positive pressure breathing trial group. Intermittent positive pressure breathing therapy of chronic obstructive pulmonary disease. Ann Intern Med 1983;99:612.

78. Anthonisen NR, Wright EC, Hodgkin JE, et al. Prognosis in chronic obstructive pulmonary disease. Am Rev Respir Dis 1986;133:14.

79. Hodgkin JE. Prognosis in chronic obstructive pulmonary disease. In: Hodgkin JE, ed. Chronic obstructive pulmonary disease. Clin Chest Med 1990;11(3):555.

80. Gilmartin ME. Patient and family education. Clin Chest Med 1986;7:619.

81. Neish CM, Hopp JW. The role of education in pulmonary rehabilitation. In: Hodgkin JE, ed. Pulmonary rehabilitation symposium. J Cardiopulm Rehabil 1988;11:439.

82. Hopp JW, Lee JW, Hills R. Development and validation of a pulmonary rehabilitation knowledge test. J Cardiopulm Rehabil 1989;7:273.

83. Ashikaga T, Vacek PM, Lewis SO. Evaluation of a community-based education program for individuals with chronic obstructive pulmonary disease. J Rehabil Res Dev 1980;46:23.

84. Arora NS, Rochester DF. Respiratory muscle strength and maximal voluntary ventilation in undernourished patients. Am Rev Respir Dis 1981;126:5.

85. Wilson DO, Rogers RM, Hoffman RM. Nutrition and chronic lung disease: state of the art. Am Rev Respir Dis 1985;132:1347.

86. Doekel RC Jr, Zwillich CW, Scoggin CH, Kryger M, Weil JV. Clinical semistarvation: depression of hypoxic ventilatory response. N Engl J Med 1976;295:358.

87. Askanazi J, Weissman C, La Sala PA, Milic-Emili J, Kinney JM. Effect of protein intake on ventilatory drive. Anesthesiology 1984;60:106.

88. Wilson DO, Rogers RM, Wright EC, Anthonisen NR. Body weight in chronic obstructive pulmonary disease. The National Institutes of Health intermittent positive pressure breathing trial. Am Rev Respir Dis 1989;139:1435.

89. Wilson DO, Rogers RM, Pennock BE, Keilly J. Nutritional intervention in malnourished emphysema patients. Am Rev Respir Dis 1985;131(part 2):61.

90. Efthimiou J, Fleming J, Gomes C, Spiro SG. The effect of supplementary oral nutrition in poorly nourished patients with chronic obstructive pulmonary disease. Am Rev Respir Dis 1988;137:1075.

91. Buist AS, Nagy JM, Sexton GJ. Effect of smoking cessation on pulmonary function: a 30-month follow-up to two smoking cessation clinics. Am Rev Respir Dis 1979;120:953.

92. Camilli AE, Burrows B, Knudson RJ, et al. Longitudinal changes in forced expiratory volume in one second in adults. Am Rev Respir Dis 1987;135:794.

93. Kark JD, Legiush M, Rannon L. Cigarette smoking as a risk factor for epidemic A (HI,NI) influenza in young men. N Engl J Med 1982;307:1042.

94. Glaser EM, Dudley DL. Psychosocial rehabilitation and psychopharmacology. In: Hodgkin JE, Petty TL, eds. Chronic obstructive pulmonary disease: current concepts. Philadelphia: WB Saunders, 1987.

95. Barach AL. Ambulatory oxygen therapy: oxygen inhalation at home and out-of-doors. Dis Chest 1959;35:229.

96. Bradley BL, Garner AE, Billiu D, et al. Oxygen-assisted exercise in chronic obstructive lung disease: the effect on exercise capacity and arterial blood gas tensions. Am Rev Respir Dis 1978;118:239.

97. Cotes JE, Gilson JC. Effect of oxygen on exercise ability in chronic respiratory insufficiency. Lancet 1956;1:872.

98. Leggett RJE, Flenley DC. Portable oxygen and exercise tolerance in patients with chronic hypoxic cor pulmonale. Br Med J 1977;2:84.

99. Stein DA, Bradley BL, Miller WC. Mechanisms of oxygen effects on exercise in patients with chronic obstructive pulmonary disease. Chest 1982;81:6.

100. Kearley R, Wynne JW, Block AJ, Boysen PG, Lindsey S, Martin C. The effect of low flow oxygen on sleep disordered breathing and oxygen saturation. Chest 1980;78:682.

101. Tirlapur VG, Mir MA. Nocturnal hypoxemia and associated electrocardiographic changes in patients with chronic obstructive airways disease. N Engl J Med 1982;306: 125.

102. Tiep BL. Longterm home oxygen therapy. In: Hodgkin JE, ed. Chronic obstructive pulmonary disease. Clin Chest Med 1990;11:505.

103. Sexton DL. Relaxation techniques and biofeedback. In: Hodgkin JE, Petty TL, eds. Chronic obstructive pulmonary disease: current concepts. Philadelphia: WB Saunders, 1987:99.

104. Renfroe KL. Effect of progressive relaxation on dyspnea and anxiety in patients with chronic obstructive pulmonary disease. Heart Lung 1988;17:408.

105. Benson H. The relaxation response. New York: Morrow, 1975.

106. Benson H, Kotch JB, Crassweller KD. The relaxation response: a bridge between psychiatry and medicine. Med Clin North Am 1977;61:929.

107. Mueller RE, Petty TL, Filley GF. Ventilation and arterial blood gas changes induced by pursed lip breathing. J Appl Physiol 1970;28:784.

108. Motley HL. The effects of slow deep breathing on the blood gas exchange in emphysema. Am Rev Respir Dis 1963;88:484.

109. Paul G, Eldridge F, Mitchell J, Fiene T. Some effects of slowing respiration rate in chronic emphysema and bronchitis. J Appl Physiol 1966;21:877.

110. Sergysels R, Willeput R, Lenders D, et al. Low frequency breathing at rest and during exercise in severe chronic obstructive bronchitis. Thorax 1979;34:536.

111. Thoman RL, Stoker GL, Ross JC. The efficacy of pursed-lips breathing in patients with chronic obstructive pulmonary disease. Am Rev Respir Dis 1966;93:100.

112. Tiep BL, Burns M, Kao D, Madison R, Herrera J. Pursed lips breathing training using ear oximetry. Chest 1986;90:218.

113. Leith DE, Bradley ME. Ventilatory muscle strength and endurance training. J Appl Physiol 1976;41:508.

114. Peress L, McClean P, Woolf C, Zamel N. Respiratory muscle training in severe chronic obstructive pulmonary disease. Am Rev Respir Dis 1979;119(4, part 2):157.

115. Celli BR. Respiratory muscle function. Clin Chest Med 1986;7:567.

116. Pardy RL, Reid WD, Belman MJ. Respiratory muscle training. Clin Chest Med 1988;9(2):287.

117. Belman MJ, Mittman D, Weir R. Ventilatory muscle training improves exercise capacity in chronic obstructive pulmonary disease patients. Am Rev Respir Dis 1980; 121:273.

118. Pardy RL, Rivington RN, Despas PJ, Macklem PT. The effects of inspiratory muscle training on exercise performance in chronic airflow limitation. Am Rev Respir Dis 1981;123:426.

119. Larson JL, Kim MJ, Sharp JT, Larson DA. Inspiratory muscle training with a pressure threshold breathing device in patients with chronic obstructive pulmonary disease. Am Rev Respir Dis 1988;138:689.

120. Pryor JA, Webber BA, Hodson ME, Batten JC. Evaluation of the forced expiration technique as an adjunct to postural drainage in treatment of cystic fibrosis. Br Med J 1979;2:417.

121. Sutton PP, Parker RA, Webber BA, et al. Assessment of the forced expiration technique, postural drainage and directed coughing in chest physiotherapy. Eur J Respir Dis 1983;64:62.

122. Faling LJ. Chest physical therapy. In: Burton GG, Hodgkin JE, Ward JJ, eds. Respiratory care: a guide to clinical practice, 3rd ed. Philadelphia: JB Lippincott, 1991:625.

123. Murray JF. The ketch-up bottle method. N Engl J Med 1979;300:1155.

124. Anthonisen P, Riis P, Sogaard-Andersen T. The value of lung physiotherapy in the treatment of acute exacerbations in chronic bronchitis. Acta Med Scand 1964;175:715.

125. Graham WGB, Bradley GA. Efficacy of chest physiotherapy and intermittent positive-pressure breathing in the resolution of pneumonia. New Engl J Med 1978;299:624.

126. Barach AL, Gickerman HA, Beck GJ. Advances in treatment of nontuberculous pulmonary disease. Bull NY Acad Med 1952;28:353.

127. Hodgkin JE, Litzau KL. Exercise training target heart rates in chronic obstructive pulmonary disease. Chest 1988;94:30S.

128. Ries AL, Archibald CJ. Endurance exercise training at maximal targets in patients with chronic obstructive pulmonary disease. J Cardiopulm Rehabil 1987;7:594.

129. Carter R, Nicotra B, Clark L, et al. Exercise conditioning in the rehabilitation of patients with chronic obstructive pulmonary disease. Arch Phys Med Rehabil 1988;69:118.

130. Wasserman K, Sue DY, Casaburi R, Moricca RB. Selection criteria for exercise training in pulmonary rehabilitation. Eur Respir J 1989;2(suppl 7):604S.

131. Casaburi R, Wasserman K, Patessio A, et al. A new perspective in pulmonary rehabilitation: anaerobic threshold as a discriminant in training. Eur Respir J 1989;2(suppl 7):618S.

132. Casaburi R, Patessio A, Ioli F, et al. Reductions in lactic acidosis and ventilation as a result of exercise training in patients with obstructive lung disease. Am Rev Respir Dis 1991;143:9.

133. Celli BR, Rassulo J, Make BJ. Dyssynchronous breathing during arm but not leg exercise in patients with chronic airflow obstruction. N Engl J Med 1986;314:1485.

134. Ries AL, Ellis B, Hawkins RW. Upper extremity exercise training in chronic obstructive pulmonary disease. Chest 1988;93:688.

135. Ellis B, Ries AL. Upper extremity exercise training in pulmonary rehabilitation. J Cardiopulm Rehabil 1991;11:227.

136. Selecky PA. Sexuality and the COPD patient. In: Hodgkin JE, Petty TL, eds. Chronic obstructive pulmonary disease: current concepts. Philadelphia: WB Saunders, 1987.

137. Matzen RV. Vocational rehabilitation: the culmination of physical reconditioning. Chest 1971;60(suppl):21S.

Index

Page numbers followed by *f* indicate figures; those followed by *t* indicate tabular material.

ISBN 0-397-51065-9

9 780397 510658